Bioinformatics

Bioinformatics

B. G. Curran   **R. J. Walker**
S. C. Bhatia

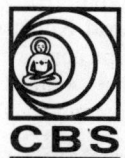

CBS

CBS Publishers & Distributors Pvt. Ltd.

New Delhi • Bengaluru • Chennai • Kochi • Kolkata • Mumbai
Hyderabad • Nagpur • Patna • Pune • Vijayawada

ISBN: 978-81-239-1828-0 (PB)
ISBN: 978-81-239-1825-9 (HB)

First Edition: 2010
Reprint: 2017

Published by **Satish Kumar Jain** and produced by **Varun Jain** for
CBS Publishers & Distributors Pvt. Ltd.,
4819/XI Prahlad Street, 24 Ansari Road, Daryaganj, New Delhi - 110002
delhi@cbspd.com, cbspubs@airtelmail.in • www.cbspd.com
Ph.: 23289259, 23266861, 23266867 • Fax: 011-23243014

Corporate Office: 204 FIE, Industrial Area, Patparganj, Delhi - 110 092
Ph: 49344934 • Fax: 011-49344935
E-mail: publishing@cbspd.com • publicity@cbspd.com

Branches:
- *Bengaluru:* 2975, 17th Cross, K.R. Road, Bansankari 2nd Stage,
  Bengaluru - 70 • Ph: +91-80-26771678/79 • Fax: +91-80-26771680
  E-mail: cbsbng@gmail.com, bangalore@cbspd.com
- *Chennai:* No. 7, Subbaraya Street, Shenoy Nagar, Chennai - 600030
  Ph: +91-44-26681266, 26680620 • Fax: +91-44-42032115
  E-mail: chennai@cbspd.com
- *Kochi:* Ashana House, 39/1904, A.M. Thomas Road, Valanjambalam,
  Ernakulum, Kochi • Ph: +91-484-4059061-65
  Fax: +91-484-4059065 • E-mail: cochin@cbspd.com
- *Kolkata:* 6-B, Ground Floor, Rameshwar Shaw Road, Kolkata - 700014
  Ph: +91-33-22891126/7/8 • E-mail: kolkata@cbspd.com
- *Mumbai:* 83-C, Dr. E. Moses Road, Worli, Mumbai - 400018
  Ph: +91-9833017933, 022-24902340/41 • E-mail: mumbai@cbspd.com

Representatives:

- Hyderabad: 0-9885175004
- Patna: 0-9334159340
- Vijayawada: 0-9000660880
- Nagpur: 0-9021734563
- Pune: 0-9623451994

Printed at:
India Binding House, Noida, UP (India)

Preface

The study of bioinformatics has gained enormous importance with the tremendous pace of growth in computational sciences. In its broadest sense, the term bioinformatics can be considered to mean information technology applied to the management and analysis of biological data. It is the science of using information to understand biology. In bioinformatics, biology, computer science and mathematics merge into a single discipline. Strictly speaking, bioinformatics is a larger subject of the computational biology, the application of quantitative analytical techniques in modeling biological systems. Thus, bioinformatics is the marriage of biology and information technology.

Biological data are being produced at a phenomenal rate as seen in genomic repository of nucleic acid and protein sequences. The three-fold aim of bioinformatics includes organizing and preservation of data, development of tools and resources and analysis of data and interpretation of results using tools. Thus, it is the science of storing, extracting, organizing, analyzing, interpreting and utilizing biological information.

This textbook provides the physical scientist, whether mathematician, computer scientist, statistician or astrophysicist with a biological framework to understand the question a life scientist would pose in the context of the computational issues, for the various computational tools now available, along with introduction to their underlying mathematical foundations. Hence, this book can be used as a bridge towards homologation of these field.

This book on bioinformatics deals with topics such as basic concepts of bioinformatics, biochemistry, cell and molecular biology, molecular genetics and their database and computers and their applications in bioinformatics.

The text is divided into six sections. Section I deals with basic concepts of bioinformatics. Chapter 1 is devoted to bioinformatics technology and its review. Section II focuses on biochemistry, cell and molecular biology. Chapter 2 studies biochemistry and bioinformatics and describes basic cellular structure and biological decoding of the genome. The processes of transcription, RNA and translation constitute the pathway that leads to conversion of genetic information in the linear sequence of base in genomic DNA into linear amino sequences of functional proteins. Considering this, Chapter 3 explains transcription and translation. Section III discusses molecular genetics and their database. Chapter 4 highlights the basic concepts of genomics. Chapter 5 concentrates on molecular genetics which gives the readers an understanding of the long range regulation of genomes, the *in silico* detection of the elements that impact long range control and the molecular genetic basis of disease as a consequence of replication. Chapters 6 and 7 deal with genome mapping and gene identification respectively. Most databases are built from sequences of genes, genomes and proteins. However, little is understood about how Macromolecules (nucleic acid) give structure, function and analysis of multicellular organisms like plants and animals. Keeping this in mind, chapter 8 focuses on proteome analysis.

Section IV concentrates on computers and their applications in bioinformatics. Chapter 9 is devoted to installing bioinformatics software in a server-based computing environment. This chapter discusses the strategies for installing programs for a server-based molecular biology software resource, accessed by a large user base. Chapter 10 deals with management of a server-based bioinformatics resources and describes the strategies for managing server-based molecular biology software resource, accessed by diverse users of community. Chapter 11 offers an insight into databases. Bioinformatics is characterized by an abundance of data stored in very large databases. The practical computer technologies related to very large databases are discussed with an emphasis on object-oriented database methods. Chapter 12 concentrates on statistics and provides an in-depth discussion of statistical techniques applicable to molecular biology, gene prediction and quantifying uncertainty in sequencing results. Chapter 13 focuses on data visualization techniques that apply to bioinformatics, from methods of generating 2d and 3d renderings of protein structures to graphing the results of statistical analysis of protein structures. Chapter 14 discusses sequence and alignment analysis which forms the basis for a number of applications in molecular biology. Chapter 15 studies data mining. The aim of this chapter is to study various data mining techniques, using technologies such as the Perl language, that are uniquely suited to searching through data strings. Chapter 16 focuses on pattern matching and covers a variety of pattern-matching approaches, using molecular biology as a working context. The strengths and weaknesses of various pattern-matching approaches have been also discussed. Gen Bank or any other biological database for that matter serves little purpose unless the database can be easily searched and entries retrieved in a usable format. Considering this, chapter 17 deals with information retrieval from biological databases.

Section V focuses on 'applications of bioinformatics'. Chapter 18 deals with innovations in bioinformatics, such as in nucleic acid sequence database, gen bank, protein sequence database, protein engineering technology, hybrid technologies, DNA chip technology, discovery of drugs plus many other fields.

Section VI concentrates on predictive methods and analysis. Chapter 19 studies predictive methods using nucleotide sequences. Various interpretation methods that rely primarily on detection of functional patterns, rather on comparison with other individual sequences discussed in detail. Chapter 20 highlights predictive methods using protein sequences. Various computational techniques that allow for biological discovery based on the protein sequences are discussed. Chapter 21 deals with phylogenetic analysis. In phylogenetic analysis, one composes the results of evolutionary processes, be it shape and size of specific bones or patterns of DNA or protein sequences in an attempt to determine how different groups or species may have been derived during evolution. Chapter 22 focuses on phylogenetic prediction. The exponentially increasing amount of data accessible in digital form over the internet from gene sequences to published references – to the experimental methods used to determine specific sequences, is only accessible through advanced search engine technologies. Keeping this in mind, search engine technologies related to the major online bioinformatics resources have been dealt with in Chapter 23. Accurate and informative biological annotation of sequence records is critical in every attempt to determine the function of a diseased gene by similarity to a gene that was isolated and sequenced because of its biological function. Keeping this in mind, Chapter 24 discusses submission of DNA sequences to the databases.

Such a wide coverage makes this book a treatise on the subject. Glossary, Appendices, References and Index have been provided as the end for quick reference. Diagrams, figures and tables supplement and text. All the topics have been covered in a cogent and lucid style to help the reader grasp the information quickly and easily. It will not be wrong to hold that this textbook on Bioinformatics is an essential reading for all students and teachers of life sciences, biotechnology, bioinformatics and engineering as well as the researchers in these and allied fields. This textbook has been prepared with meticulous care, aiming at making the book error-free. Constructive suggestions are always welcome from the readers of this book.

Readers should note that names of the websites mentioned in this book are subject to change or removal as all websites undergo regular maintenance and updation of the data in their database

B. G. Curran
R. J. Walker
S. C. Bhatia

Contents at a Glance

Contents

SECTION V

Applications of Bioinformatics in Industry and Research *403-414*

SECTION VI

SECTION I

BASIC CONCEPTS OF BIOINFORMATICS

Chapter 1

Bioinformatics Technology: A Review

INTRODUCTION

In its broadest sense, the term bioinformatics can be considered to mean information technology applied to the management and analysis of biological data. From 1950 onwards, large amount of sequence data related to various living organisms have been collected and stored in databases.

Since it is not very convenient to compare the sequences of several hundred nucleotides and amino acids by hand, several computational techniques were developed. Where data can be amassed faster than they can be analysed and utilised, there is a great need for professionals who can use software to digest this ever-growing mass of information.

Bioinformatics is the combination of biology and information technology. It is the branch of science that deals with the computer-based analysis of large biological data sets. Bioinformatics incorporates the development of databases to store and search data and of statistical tools and algorithms to analyse and determine relationships between biological data sets, such as macro-molecular sequences, structures, expression profiles and biochemical pathways.

The discipline encompasses any computational tools and methods used to manage, analyse and manipulate large sets of biological data. Essentially, bioinformatics has three components:

1. The creation of databases allowing the storage and management of large biological data sets.
2. The development of algorithms and statistics to determine relationships among members of large data sets.
3. The use of these tools for the analysis and interpretation of various types of biological data, including DNA, RNA and protein sequences, protein structures, gene expression profiles and biochemical pathways.

DEFINITION

Bioinformatics is defined in various ways. Some of the definitions are as follows:

1. Bioinformatics is the use of computer in solving information problems in life sciences; mainly it involves the creation of extensive electronic database on genomes and protein sequences. Secondarily it involves techniques such as the three-dimensional modelling of biomolecules and biological systems.
2. Bioinformatics is a computational management of all kinds of biological informations, including genes and their products, whole organisms or even ecological systems.

3

3. Bioinformatics is an integration of mathematical, statistical and computational methods to analyse biological, biochemical and biophysical data. It deals with methods of storing, retrieving and analysing biological data, such as nucleic acid and protein sequences, structures, functions, pathways and genetic interactions.
4. Bioinformatics is the storage, manipulation and analysis of biological information via computer science. Bioinformatics is an essential infrastructure underpinning biological research.

SEQUENCING DEVELOPMENT

Before 1945, there was not even a single quantitative analytical method available for any one protein. However, significant progress with chromatographic and labelling techniques over the next decade eventually led to the elucidation of the first complete sequence, that of the peptide hormone insulin.

The sequence of the first enzyme ribonuclease was completed by 1960. By 1970, around 50 proteins with more than 150 residues had been sequenced and by 1980, the number was estimated to be around 1600. Today more than 3,00,000 sequences are available.

The term bioinformatics first came into use in the 1990s and was originally synonymous with the management and analysis of DNA, RNA and protein sequence data. Computational tools for sequence analysis had been available since the 1960s but this was a minority interest until advances in sequencing technology (Topic B1) led to a rapid expansion in the number of stored sequences in databases such as GenBank (Topic C2). Now the term has expanded to incorporate many other types of biological data, for example protein structures, gene expression profiles and protein interactions. Each of these areas requires its own set of databases, algorithms and statistical methods, some of which are discussed in this book.

Initial Attempts

Initially a majority of protein sequences were obtained by the manual process of sequential Edman degradation–dansylation. A very important step towards the rapid increase in the number of sequenced proteins was the development of automated sequences which, by 1980, offered a 10^4 fold increase in the sensitivity compared to the procedure implemented by Edman and Begg in 1967.

The first complete protein sequence assignment using mass spectrometry was achieved in 1980. This technique played a vital role in the discovery of the amino acid γ-carboxyglutamic acid and its location in the N-terminal region of prothrombin.

During 1960s and 1970s scientists were finding it difficult to develop methods to sequence nucleic acids. When the techniques were available, the first techniques to emerge were applicable only to RNA (ribonucleic acid), especially transfer–RNAs (tRNA). tRNAs were ideal materials for this early work, because they are short (typically 74–95 nucleotides in length) and because it is possible to purify individual molecules.

Advanced Techniques

DNA (deoxyribonucleic acid) consists of thousands of nucleotides and assembling the complete nucleotide sequence of an entire chromosomal DNA molecule is a very big task. With the advent of gene cloning and PCR, it became possible to purify defined fragments of chromosomal DNA. This paved the way for the development of fast and efficient DNA sequencing techniques.

By 1977, two sequencing methods had emerged, using chain termination and chemical degradation approaches. These techniques with some minor modifications laid the foundation for the sequence revolution of the 1980s and 1990s and the subsequent birth of bioinformatics.

The polymerase chain reaction (PCR) due to its sensitivity, specificity and potential for automation, is considered the front-line analytical method for analysing genomic DNA samples and constructing genetic maps. Over the years, incremental improvements in basic PCR technology have enhanced the power and practice of the technique.

Since the introduction of the first-semi-automated sequence in 1987, coupled with the development of PCR in 1990 and fluorescent labelling of DNA fragments generated by the Sanger dideoxy chain termination method, there have been large-scale sequencing efforts which have contributed greatly. Technologies for capturing sequence information have also become advanced over a period of time.

In the early 1980s, researchers could use digitiser pens to manually read DNA sequences from gels. Then came image-capture devices, which were cameras that digitised the information on gels. In 1987 Steven Krawetz, helped to develop the first DNA sequencing software for automated film readers.

In the early 1990s, J. Craig Venter and his colleagues devised a new method to find genes. Rather than taking the single base chromosomal DNA, Venter's group isolated messenger RNA molecules, copied these mRNA molecules into DNA molecules and then sequenced a part of the DNA molecule to create expressed sequence tags or ESTs. These ESTs could be used as handles to isolate the entire gene.

The EST approach also has generated enormous databases of nucleotide sequences and the development of the EST technique is considered to have demonstrated the feasibility of high throughput gene discovery, as well as provided a key impetus for the growth of the genomics industry.

Sequence Deposits

At the start of 1998, more than 3,00,000 protein sequences have been deposited in publicly available nonredundant databases, and the number of partial sequences in public and proprietary expressed sequence tag (EST) databases was expected to run into millions. By contrast, the number of 3D structures in the protein data bank (PDB) is still less than 20000.

The United States department of energy (DoE) initiated a number of projects in 1980s to construct detailed genetic and physical maps of the human genome. Their aim was to determine the complete nucleotide sequence of human genome and to localise the estimated 30000 genes.

Work of such a great dimension required the development of new computational methods for analysing genetic map and DNA sequence data and demanded the design of new techniques and instrumentation for detecting and analysing DNA. To benefit the public most effectively, the projects also necessitated the use of advanced means of information dissemination in order to make the results available as rapidly as possible to scientists and physicians. The international effort arising from this vast initiative became known as the human genome project (HGP).

Role of Computers in Bioinformatics

Bioinformatics is largely although not exclusively a computer-based discipline. Computers are important in bioinformatics for two reasons. First, many bioinformatics problems require the same task to be repeated millions of times. For example, comparing a new sequence to every other sequence stored in a database or comparing a group of sequences systematically to determine evolutionary relationships. In such cases, the ability of computers to process information and test alternative solutions rapidly is indispensable. Second, computers are required for their problem-solving power. Typical problems that might be addressed using bioinformatics could include solving the folding pathway of a protein given its amino acid sequence or deducing a biochemical pathway given a collection of RNA expression profiles.

Computers can help with such problems, but it is important to note that expert input and robust original data are also required.

Internet

Biological information is stored on many different computers around the world. The easiest way to access this information is for the computers to be joined together in a network. A computer network is a group of computers that can communicate, for example over a telephone system, therefore allowing data to be exchanged between remote users. A typical computer network is shown in Fig. 1.1. For transfer, data are first broken into small packets (units of information), which are sent independently and reassembled when they arrive at their destination. If information is sent from computer A to computer C, it can travel via two different routes. In one case computer B acts as a router and in the other case computers D and E both act as routers. The availability of different routes through the network means that communications can be maintained between computers A and C even if part of the network is unavailable, for example if computer B ceases to function.

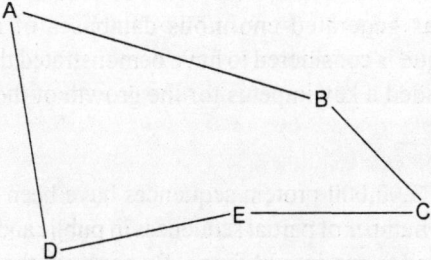

Fig. 1.1. A simple computer network.

The Internet is an international network of computers derived from an earlier system, ARPAnet, developed by the US military. The Internet as we know it began in 1970, when four American universities were connected together for the first time allowing the rapid exchange of scientific data. The number of computers linked to the Internet has grown exponentially over the last 35 years and it is now estimated that over 30 million computers have access, many of them personal computers in people's homes. Information transfer over the Internet is governed by a set of protocols (procedures for handling data packages) called TCP/IP. TCP is the transmission control protocol, which determines how data is broken into packages and reassembled. IP is the internet protocol, which determines how the packets of information are addressed and routed over the network. To access the Internet, a computer must have the correct hardware (generally a network card and/or a modem), the appropriate software and permission for network access. Many institutions have automatic access to the Internet, but private users must subscribe to an internet service provider (ISP).

World Wide Web (www)

The world wide web (www) is a way of exchanging information over the Internet using a program called a browser. A number of browsers are available for working on the www, the most widely used of which are Internet Explorer and Netscape Navigator. Most computers are sold nowadays 'Internet ready' with the appropriate hardware and one or both of these browser programs installed as standard. The www was developed in 1992 and allows the display of information pages containing multimedia objects (e.g. text, images, audio and video) in a special format called hypertext. In a hypertext document, text is displayed normally and can be read and manipulated like any other text document, but some words and objects are highlighted in a different colour and these are known as hypertext links (or simply hyperlinks). Clicking on a hyperlink directs the browser to access another hypertext document, which might be on the same computer or might be on any other computer linked to the Internet. The new document may have its own hyperlinks and thus the process can be repeated allowing the user to move rapidly from computer to computer around the world downloading information as he or she goes (this is commonly known as surfing the web or surfing the net).

The www works on the basis that each hypertext document has a unique address known as a uniform resource locator (URL). URLs take the format http://restofaddress, where http://identifies the protocol for communication over the www (hypertext transfer protocol) and 'restofaddress' provides a location for the hypertext document on the Internet. Every computer on the Internet has an IP address, which is in the form of four integers conventionally separated by dots. Associated with this is a text version of the address, for example http://www.bios.co.uk, which is the publisher's address. The equivalent IP address for the publisher is 195.172.6.15. If a local user tries to contact http://www.bios.co.uk, how does the browser find the correct site? The local computer first contacts Internet computers called Domain Name Servers (DNSs) that try to understand parts of the address starting with the most significant (right hand) part. For example, most text addresses have a country abbreviation, in this case 'uk' for United Kingdom, but American addresses do not since the Internet was an American invention. If the computer one is trying to access is providing a service on the www, it is known as a web server. This means there are numerous files available for browsing, and each can be identified by a unique URL. Such files are specified by extra characters separated from the main Internet address by a solidus (/).

For example, the URL http://www.bios.co.uk/bioinformatics refers to a subdirectory on the publisher's web server that corresponds to the web site accompanying this book. Once the DNS has found the Internet name for the server, it is for the server itself to work out what do about any extensions to the URL such as '/bioinformatics'.

Useful Bioinformatics Sites

For absolute beginners, we have listed nine good starting points for bioinformatics on the www (Table 1.1). Each of these gateway sites is comprehensive, has many useful links and is well maintained and stable. Time spent browsing and using these sites will provide an accurate feeling for the bioinformatics resources available on the Internet.

Searching the Internet

Although the nine web sites listed in Table 1.1 provide some of the best starting points for bioinformatics on the www, there is a great deal of specialist biological data that cannot be accessed directly from these sites. Finding relevant data on the Internet is made simpler by the availability of general-purpose search engines, such as Google, Yahoo, Lycos, AltaVista and Hotbot. These tools search the entire Internet for pages that contain particular keywords or phrases, and they can also be used to search for files of a particular type, such as image files or video files. For example, one might search the Internet using the phrase 'alcohol dehydrogenase' to find pages containing information about that enzyme. Alternatively, one might look for image files of a particular insect or flower or video files of frog development. Relevant sites are displayed as a list of hits, with hyperlinks allowing direct access to the page of interest. The problem with general-purpose search engines is that they have not been developed specifically with molecular biology in mind and the information they provide can be irrelevant or misleading, especially if the search term used has other connotations.

Table 1.1. Nine good starting points for bioinformatics on the www.

Uniform resource locator (URL)	Note
General bioinformatics 'gateways'	
http://www.ncbi.nlm.nih.gov/	National centre for biotechnology information homepage. A resource for public databases, bioinformatics tools and applications. Links to many useful sites and resources for bioinformatics software
http://www.ebi.ac.uk/	The European bioinformatics institute outstation (EMBL). A resource for biological databases and software, much of which has excellent tutorialsupport
http://www.expasy.ch/	The expert protein analysis system (ExPASy) molecular biology server. Maintained by the Swiss institute of bioinformatics (SIB). Provides links, databases and software resources for the analysis of protein sequences, structures and expression
http://www.embl-heidelberg.de/	European molecular biology laboratory homepage
http://www.gmd.de/Welcome.en.html	German national centre for information technology homepage
http://links.bmn.com/	The BioMedNet gateway to thousands of biological websites, includes a search facility and provides descriptions of each of the websites listed
Genome projects	
http://wit.integratedgenomics.com/GOLD/	Genomes on line database, with links to genomic databases and progress reports on genome projects
http://www.genome.ad.jp/kegg/	Kyoto encyclopaedia of genes and genomes. A very comprehensive Japanese site including metabolic maps
Computing notes	
http://foldoc.doc.ic.ac.uk/foldoc/index.html	Free online dictionary of computing (FOLD). A good place to look up meanings of computer jargon

As an alternative to search engines, the home pages of academic institutions or biotechnology companies can also be a good place to start. Many universities for example, maintain comprehensive web sites with pages for staff to describe research projects and display data and such sites often contain hyperlinks to sites of related interest.

NCBI

The national centre for biotechnology information (NCBI) was established in 1988 in USA as a division of the national library of medicine and is located on the campus of the national institute of health in Bethesda, Maryland.

The role of the NCBI is to develop new information technologies in aiding our understanding of the molecular and genetic processes that underlie health and diseases. Its specific aims include the creation of automated systems for storing and analysing biological information, the development of advanced methods of computer-based information processing, the facilitation of user access to databases and software and the coordination of efforts to gather biotechnology information worldwide.

NCBI also maintains GenBank, the NIH DNA sequence database. Groups of annotators create sequence data records from the scientific literature and together with information acquired directly from authors, data are exchanged with the international nucleotide databases, EMBL and DDBJ.

Entrez

Just like SRS for EMBnet, Entrez facility was evolved at NCBI to allow retrieval of molecular biology data and bibliographic citations from NCBI's integrated databases. Entrez permits related articles in different databases to be linked to each other, whether or not they are cross-referenced directly.

Entrez provides access to DNA sequence (from GenBank, EMBL and DDBJ), protein sequence (from SWISS-PROT, PIR, PRF SEQDB, PDB and translated protein sequence from the DNA sequence databases), genome and chromosome mapping data, 3D protein structures from PDB and the PubMed bibliographic database.

Links between various databases are a strong point of NCBI's system. The starting point for retrieval of sequence and structures is called Entrez. Entrez is a www-based data retrieval system. It integrates information held in all NCBI databases. It is the common front-end to all the databases maintained by the NCBI and it is extremely easy to use. In total, Entrez links to 11 databases (Table 1.2). Entrez can be accessed via the NCBI web site at the following URL: http://www.ncbi.nlm.nih.gov/Entrez/.

Table 1.2. The databases covered by Entrez, listed by category.

Category	Databases
Nucleic acid sequences	Entrez nucleotides: Sequences obtained from GenBank, Ref Seq and PDB
Protein sequences	Entrez protein: Sequences obtained from SWISS-PROT, PIR, PRF, PDB and translations from annotated coding regions in GenBank and Ref Seq.
3D structures	Entrez molecular modelling database (MMDB)
Genomes	Complete genome assemblies from many sources
PopSet	From GenBank, set of DNA sequences that have been collected to analyse the evolutionary relatedness of population
OMIM	Online Mendelian Inheritance in Man
Taxonomy	NCBI taxonomy database
Books	Bookshelf
ProbeSet	Gene Expression Omnibus (GEO)
3D domains	Domains from the entrez molecular modelling database (MMDB)
Literature	PubMed

Aims and Tasks of Bioinformatics

The underlying principle of bioinformatics is that, biological polymers such as nucleic acid molecule and proteins, can be transformed into sequences of digital symbols. Besides, only limited numbers of alphabets are required to represent the nucleotide and amino acid monomers.

This flexibility of analysing the biomolecules with the help of limited alphabets resulted in the flourishing of bioinformatics. The growth and performance of bioinformatics rely on the developments in computer hardware and software. The simplest tasks used in bioinformatics concern the creation and maintenance of databases of biological information.

Essentially bioinformatics has three components: (i) the creation of databases allowing the storage and management of large biological data sets; (ii) the development of algorithms and statistics to determine relationships among members of large data sets; and (iii) the use of these tools for the analysis and interpretation of various types of biological data, including DNA, RNA and protein sequences, protein structures, gene expression profiles and biochemical pathways.

Aims

The aims of bioinformatics are as follows:
1. To organise data in a way that allows researchers to access existing information and to submit new entries as they are produced.
2. To develop tools and resources that aid in the analysis and management of data.
3. To use these tools to analyse the data and interpret the results in a biologically meaningful manner.

Tasks

The tasks in bioinformatics involve the analysis of sequence information. This involves the following:
1. Identifying the genes in the DNA sequences from various organisms.
2. Developing methods to study the structure and/or function of newly identified sequences and corresponding structural RNA sequences.
3. Identifying families of related sequences and the development of models.
4. Aligning similar sequences and generating phylogenetic trees to examine evolutionary relationships.

Besides these, one of the important dimensions of bioinformatics is identifying drug targets and pointing out lead compounds.

Areas

Bioinformatics deals with the following areas:
1. Handling and management of biological data including its organisation, control, linkages, analysis and so on.
2. Communication among people, projects and institutions engaged in the biological research and applications. The communication may include e-mail, file transfer, remote login, computer conferencing, electronic bulletin boards or establishment of web-based information resources.
3. Organisation, access, search and retrieval of biological information, documents and literature.
4. Analysis and interpretation of the biological data through the computational approaches including visualisation, mathematical modelling and development of algorithms for highly parallel processing of complex biological structures.

Application of Bioinformatics

Biocomputing has found its application in many areas. Apart from providing the theoretical background and practical tools for scientists to explore proteins and DNA, it also helps in many other ways.

In understanding the meaning of sequences, two distinct analytical themes have emerged: (i) in the first approach, pattern recognition techniques are used to detect similarity between sequences and hence to infer related structures and functions; and (ii) *ab initio* prediction methods are used to deduce 3D structures and ultimately to infer function directly from the linear sequence. The direct prediction of protein three-dimensional structure from the linear amino acid sequence is the objective of bioinformatics.

Sequence homology analysis

One of the driving forces behind bioinformatics is the search for similarities between different biomolecules. Apart from enabling systematic organisation of data, identification of protein homologs has some direct practical uses. Theoretical models of proteins are usually based on experimentally solved structures of close homologs.

Wherever biochemical or structural data are lacking, studies could be carried out in yeast like lower organisms and the results can be applied to homologs in higher organisms such as human. It also simplifies the problem of understanding complex genomes by analysing simple organisms first and then applying the same principles to more complicated ones. This would result in identifying potential drug targets by checking homologs of essential microbial proteins.

Drug design

The adoption of a bioinformatics-based approach to drug discovery provides an important advantage. With bioinformatics, genotypes associated with patho-physiological conditions could be defined, which might lead to the identification of potential molecular targets. Given the nucleotide sequence, the probable amino acid sequence of the encoded protein can be determined using translation software.

Sequence research techniques could then be used to find homologs in model organisms; and based on sequence similarity it is possible to model the structure of the specific protein on experimentally characterised structures. Finally, docking algorithms could design molecules that could bind to the model structure, leading the way for biochemical assays to test their biological activity on the actual protein.

Predictive functions

Through large-scale screening of data, one can address a number of evolutionary, biochemical and biophysical questions. We can identify: (i) specific protein folds associated with certain phylogenetic groups, (ii) commonality between different folds within particular organisms, (iii) the degree of folds shared between related organisms, (iv) the extent of relatedness derived from traditional evolutionary trees, and (v) the diversity of metabolic pathways in different organisms.

One can also integrate data on protein functions, given the fact that particular protein folds are often related to specific biochemical functions. Combining expression information structural and functional classifications of proteins, one can predict the occurrence of a protein fold in a genome, which is indicative of high expression levels. In conjunction with structural data, one can compile a map of all protein-protein interactions in an organism.

Medical areas

Applications in medical sciences have centred on gene expression analysis. This usually involves compiling expression data for cells affected by different diseases and comparing the measurements against normal expression levels. Identification of genes that are expressed differently in affected cells provides a basis for explaining the causes of illness and highlights potential drug targets.

With this information one can design compounds that bind to the expressed protein. Given a lead compound, microarray experiments can be used to evaluate responses to pharmacological intervention; it can also help in providing early tests to detect or predict the toxicity of trial drugs.

If bioinformatics is combined with experimental genomics, a lot of advances could be made to revolutionise the future healthcare program. This involves postnatal genotyping to assess susceptibility or immunity from specific diseases and pathogens; prescription of a unique combination of vaccines; minimising the healthcare costs of unnecessary treatments and anticipating the onslaught of diseases later in life, which could lead to guidance for nutrition intake and early detections of any illness.

In addition, drug-based treatments could be tailored specifically to the patient and disease, thus providing the most effective course of medication with minimal side effects. Human genome project will benefit forensic sciences, pharma industries, discovery of beneficial and harmful genes, contribute to a better understanding of human evolution, diagnosis of disease and disease risks, genetics of response to therapy and customised treatment, identification of drug targets and gene therapy.

Intellectual property rights

Intellectual property rights (IPR) are essential part of today's business. IPRs are the means to protect any intangible asset. Examples of IPR are Patent, Copyright, Trademark, Geographical Indication and Trade Secret. A patent is an exclusive monopoly granted by the Government to an inventor over his invention for limited period of time.

Major areas of bioinformatics which need intellectual property protection are: (i) analytical and information management tools (e.g. modelling techniques, databases, algorithms, software, etc.), (ii) genomics and proteomics, and (iii) drug discovery/design.

Innovations

Majority of bioinformatics innovation involves applications of computer-implemented protocols or software in collecting and/or processing biological data. These inventions fall within the general category of computer related inventions called inventions implemented in a computer and inventions employing computer readable media. These inventions have two aspects: (i) software, and (ii) hardware.

For example, a computer based system for identifying new nucleotide sequence clusters from a given set of nucleotide sequences based on sequence similarity may comprise an input device, a memory and a processor as hardware components of the system and a data set or method of operating instructions stored in the memory and operable by the processor as a software for the system. Patent protections would be invaluable in protecting methods, which use computational power, such as sequence alignments, homology searches and metabolic pathways modelling.

Genomics and proteomics

Genomics involves isolation and characterisation of gene and assigning a function or use to the gene sequence, i.e. either expression of a particular protein or identification of the gene as a marker for a particular disease. This work involves a great deal of laboratory experiments as well as computational techniques. These techniques can also be protected under IPR.

Proteomics involves purification and characterisation of proteins using technologies like 2D electrophoresis, multidimensional chromatography and mass spectroscopy. The application of these techniques, to characterisation and finding relation of the protein, i.e. marker with a particular disease is challenging, time consuming and needs heavy investment.

Drug design by modelling which involves computer and computation can also be protected under IPR. Table 1.3 gives some examples of patents in bioinformatics.

Table 1.3. Some examples of patents in bioinformatics.

Code number	Specific title
US 6,355,423	Methods and devices for measuring differential gene expression
US 6,334,099	Methods for normalisation of experimental data
US 5,579,250	Method of rational drug design based on *ab initio* computer simulation of conformational features of peptides
WO 98/15652	DNA sequencing and RNA sequencing using sequencing enzyme
EPI 108779	Spatial structures of at least one polypeptide
EPO 807 687	Recombinant protease purification and computer program for use in drug design.

Instant Notes Bioinformatics www Site

This book makes reference to many databases and computer software tools that are available on the world wide web as well as various informative web sites. Although the addresses for many of these resources are listed in the book, the Internet is constantly evolving and such addresses are subject to change on a regular basis.

For convenience, links to all the sites discussed in the text can be found on an accompanying www site (http://www.bios.co.uk/inbioinformatics). The www site also contains further information, updates and links that are not found in this book.

SECTION II

BIOCHEMISTRY, CELL AND MOLECULAR BIOLOGY

## Chapter 2

Biochemistry and Bioinformatics

INTRODUCTION

Genomics and bioinformatics have the power to transform all facets of society. From anthropology to agriculture, medicine to manufacturing, virtually all disciplines undeniably will be changed by these promising fields. The goal of genomics is to mine the genomes of all relevant organisms to identify genes and their encoded products that govern the biological reactions that provide fuels, food, fibre and other materials essential for our health. In addition to feeding the burgeoning world population, genomics/bioinformatics-based discovery will lead us to safer and more nutritious foods; self-resistant crops; disease-resistant animals; foods with prolonged shelf life; an understanding of why pathogens are virulent; and novel bio-based 'smart molecules' such as alternative fuels, pharmaceuticals and environmental sensors. Access to the genetic codes of microbes, plants and animals will enable a clearer understanding of how life evolved on our planet. Training in genomics/bioinformatics requires a unique amalgam of skills in statistics, computer science (including algorithm development and database management), engineering, analytical chemistry and of course, genetics and molecular biology. This chapter introduces venerable, fundamental concepts in molecular biology from a contemporary genomics/bioinformatics perspective using a language-based approach.

NUCLEIC ACIDS AND PROTEINS

Definition of Nucleic Acids

Any of several complex compounds occurring in living cells, usually chemically bound to proteins to form nucleoproteins. Nucleic acids are of high molecular weight and are easily changed by many mild chemical reagents. They contains carbon, hydrogen, oxygen, nitrogen (15–16 per cent) and phosphorus (9–10 per cent).

The fundamental units of nucleic acid are nucleotides; nucleic acids are polynucleotides in which the nucleotides are linked by phosphate bridges. Upon extensive heating in the presence of water (hydrolysis), nucleic acids yield a mixture of purines and pyrimidines, D-ribose or D-deoxyribose and phosphoric acid. Nucleic acids are sub-divided into two types: (i) ribonucleic acid (RNA), containing the sugar D-ribose, and (ii) deoxyribonucleic acid (DNA) containing the sugar D-deoxyribose.

Proteins

A complex high polymer containing carbon, hydrogen, oxygen, nitrogen and usually sulphur and comprised of chains of amino acids connected by peptide linkage (—CO.NH—). Proteins occur in the cells of all living organisms and in biological fluids (blood plasma, protoplasm). They are synthesised by plants largely because of the nitrogen-fixing ability of certain soil bacteria. Their molecular weight may be as high as 40 million (tobacco mosaic virus). They have many important functional forms: enzymes, haemoglobin, hormones, viruses, genes, antibodies and nucleic acids. They also comprise the basic component of connective tissue (collagen), hair (keratin), nails, feathers, skin, etc. Some have been synthesised in the laboratory.

The sequence of amino acids in the polypeptide chain is of critical importance of genetics. Proteins can be hydrolysed to their constituent amino acids and can be broken down into simpler forms by proteolytic enzymes. They form colloidal solutions and behave chemically as both acids and bases simultaneously. They are denatured by changes in pH, by heat, ultraviolet radiation and many organic solvents.

Simple proteins contain only amino acids; conjugated proteins contain amino acids plus nucleic acids, carbohydrates, lipids, etc. On the basis of solubility they can be classified as albumins (water-soluble), globulins (insoluble in water but soluble in aqueous salt solutions) and prolamines (soluble in alcohol-water mixtures but not in alcohol or water alone). A number of proteins have been synthesised, notably the hormone insulin. Proteins are an essential component of the diet, occurring chiefly in meat, eggs, milk and fish. Edible proteins suitable for human food as well as cattle feed can be produced from micro-organisms grown in carbonaceous or nitrogenous media to form yeast-like materials. Paraffinic hydrocarbons (methane) and petroleum-derived ethyl alcohol can be used as growth media for protein biosynthesis. Industrial applications of proteins include plastics, adhesives and fibres derived from casein and soyabean protein, but these have been declining in recent years. Special forms in which proteins are commercially available include textured proteins for food products, protein hydrolysate and liquid predigested protein, both for medical use.

Molecular Biology

A sub-division of biology that approaches the subject of life at the molecular level. This applies to phenomena occurring within the cell nucleus, where the chromosomes and genes are located. These structures, which determine heredity, are in turn composed of nucleic acids, which direct the selection and assembly of amino acids in the dividing chromosomes. Much of the essential mechanism of life can be understood by study of specific protein molecules (DNA and RNA) and their determination of the amino acid composition of the genes.

Many different kinds of molecules are components of living cells: carbohydrates, lipids, proteins, nucleic acids. All can be studied at the molecular level, including biosynthesis and assembly, atomic and molecular architecture, physio-chemical properties, cellular targeting, and function. The common denominator among these avenues of investigation is the genes aligned along lengthy DNA strands. Stretched end-to-end, the genome would extend 2 to 3 metres in a normal human cell. Genes encode information for synthesising molecules and their assembly into cellular structures.

Molecular biology focuses on the structure and activity of these genes, which can be defined in two broad, fundamental ways:

1. The flow of information within a cell. One very famous descriptor of this activity is the Central Dogma of Molecular Biology. In its original concept, the Dogma was stated as seen in Scheme 1:

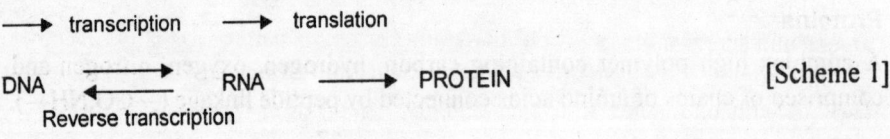

[Scheme 1]

By this scheme, DNA was considered to be self-replicating (→), providing information in the form of a template for the precise duplication of one DNA molecule, the double helix, into two copies; the intracellular flow of information would continue to follow a strict path by transcription of a gene copy in the form of RNA, followed by interpreting the language of nucleic acids (nucleotides) into the language of proteins (amino acids) via translation of the RNA into a polypeptide chain. As seminal advances were made in the 1970s and 1980s, modifications were added to the central dogma that involved reverse transcription of RNA into DNA (typical of many dangerous retroviruses such as HIV-1, the AIDS virus), and self-replication of RNA molecules.

2. Heredity, or the flow of information between cells (as during cell division; binary fission in bacteria and mitosis in higher cells) and through the generations of an organism (typically mediated by eggs and sperm, produced through meiosis). The chromosomal basis of inheritance is founded on the process of DNA replication, and requires an intimate understanding of the functional architecture of the DNA molecule.

Role of molecular biology in contemporary terms, genomics and bioinformatics

The term genome, refers to the complete set of genetic information found within an individual organism. Our understanding of molecular biology has enabled the establishment of a simple organisational hierarchy (Fig. 2.1) that provides a useful scaffold for this discussion. We see that the genome is the all encompassing term for hereditary instructions, whereas the nucleotide is the fundamental chemical building block for the genetic material. Therefore, the genome is composed of the entire collection of nucleotides polymerised into long DNA strands. In the human genome, approx 3×10^9 nucleotides comprise one copy of our genome, condensed into each egg and sperm cell. This hierarchy can be annotated for human by adding additional numerical values (Fig. 2.2) to illustrate the interrelationship between the genome and other molecular units that collectively define our genetic material.

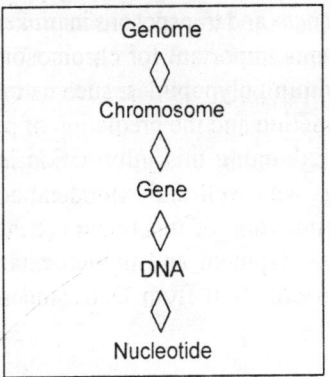

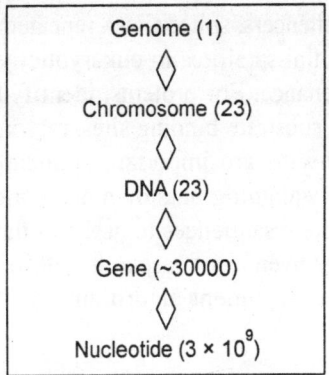

Fig. 2.1. Simple organisational hierarchy of genetic material.

Fig. 2.2. Numerically annotated hierarchy of genetic material.

In Fig. 2.2, we find that each copy of the human genome is subdivided into 23 chromosomes. (When an egg and sperm unite during fertilisation, the newly formed zygote contains 46 chromosomes, or two genome copies; most cells in our body are in this diploid state; eggs and sperm in the offspring remain haploid with one genomic copy). Individual chromosomes contain one DNA double helix, so each haploid genome is composed of 23 individual DNA duplexes. Distributed among these 23 helices are an estimated 30,000 genes (although human gene approximations have ranged from 30,000–1,00,000). Nucleotides are bonded together to create the 23 individual DNA chains. Sizes of the 23 chromosomes range from 50×10^6 to greater than 250×10^6 nucleotides.

This hierarchy now allows us to define a 'completely sequenced genome'. Using high-throughput molecular technology and robotics in concert with sophisticated computer algorithms, it is now possible to assemble the precise order of the four nucleotide building blocks that comprise the single DNA helix within each chromosome. When such sequences are available for all chromosomes in an organism, the genome has been sequenced. Genome sizes range from about 2 million nucleotides for single bacterial chromosomes to $1,00,000 \times 10^6$ for some amphibians and plants. Each report of a completely sequenced genome represents an explosion of data that adds to the rapidly expanding international databases.

Storing of data, accessed, manipulated, managed and analysed

Here, computer science and molecular biology partner into the new and rapidly emergent field of bioinformatics. It is the goal of bioinformatics to make sense of nucleotide sequence data (and for proteins or Proteomics, amino acid sequence data). Assume that as we read this sentence, there are no spaces between words nor punctuation marks delimiting the boundaries of written thought. This same sentence might appear as:

assumethataswereadthissentencetherearenospacesbetweenwordsnorpunctuationmarks delimitingtheboundariesofwrittenthought

If this were a DNA sequence written in the language of the four nucleotide building blocks, or a protein sequence inscribed in the language of the 20 amino acids, informatic methodologies would be employed to extract and make sense of information encrypted in what superficially appears as a nonsense string. Bioinformatics as applied to DNA sequences would be exploited to find individual genes in the form of protein coding sequences (exons), expanses of nucleotides that might interrupt gene regions (introns), domains within the DNA that might control the expression of individual genes (e.g. promoters, enhancers, silencers, splice sites), repeated elements (insertion sequences and transposons in prokaryotes; micro and mini-satellites in eukaryotic genomes) and other elements important for chromosome and gene maintenance. For proteins, identifying important domains within polypeptides, such as catalytic active sites, substrate binding sites, regions of protein-protein interaction and the prediction of protein-folding pathways are important applications of bioinformatics. Exhuming this information is often conducted by aligning unknown nucleotide (or amino acid) strings with well-understood expanses of DNA or protein sequences to assist in the identification and determination of functional architecture. One popular avenue of research within Bioinformatics is the development and implementation of sophisticated alignment algorithms for the purpose of mining information from DNA and protein sequences.

Language of DNA in the genomics era: nucleotides and the primary structure of nucleic acid

This chapter is written in the English language that is composed of a 26-letter alphabet. Users of the language string letters into words, words into sentences, sentences into paragraphs and so forth. The precise order of the letters conveys definition and meaning. Similarly, chains of DNA (and RNA) are polymers of four different chemical letters or nucleotide bases; the precise order of polymerisation is called the primary structure of nucleic acid and embedded within the primary structure is the definition of gene content.

The molecular structure of nucleotides also dictates important chemical properties of DNA. Nucleotides are composed of three chemically distinct precincts that confer functionality (Fig. 2.3). These include a deoxyribose (DNA) or ribose (RNA) sugar, phosphate groups bonded to the 5' carbon in the deoxyribose (or ribose) sugar and one of four nitrogenous bases (B; Fig. 2.3) that are attached to the 1' carbon. For DNA, the bases are: the purines, adenine (A) and guanine (G); the pyrimidines, cytosine (C) and thymine (T). Uracil (U), a pyrimidine that replaces T in RNA. When the complete DNA sequence of a genome is reported, it is actually the primary structure or precise polymerisation order, of the nitrogenous bases that are published as a simple string of As, Gs, Cs and Ts. Sugars and phosphate groups remain invariant in the DNA chain (Fig. 2.4). The phosphate groups and deoxyribose (or ribose) sugars are highly polar and confer upon DNA (and RNA) the property of solubility in aqueous environments such as the interior of cells. At physiological pH, the phosphate group is ionised (deprotonated) conferring a net negative charge onto the nucleic acid polymer (Fig. 2.4). In contrast, the nitrogenous bases are nonpolar entities that are 'driven' into seclusion, away from aqueous environment.

The interior of a DNA double helix provides such an environment; it is these hydrophobic forces, along with the additive Van der Waals interactions (0.1–0.2 kcal/mole) among the bases now stacked in the interior of the helix, that help stabilise the double helical structure. However, it is the unique arrangement of atoms within the nitrogenous bases that provides most of the stability to the double helix. When A is juxtaposed with T and G is adjacent to C, the opportunity now exists for hydrogen bonding between hydrogen atoms of lower electronegativity resulting in a partially positive character and oxygen atoms of high electronegativity with a partially negative character (Fig. 2.5). This pairing behaviour is often referred to as complementarity between bases (A and T, G and C). Hydrogen bonds (1–10 kcal/mole) formed precisely between the two complementary base pairs (A and T; G and C) stabilise the association between the two DNA chains resulting in the double helix.

The specific pairing we have postulated immediately suggests a possible copying mechanism for the genetic material.

What this statement was intended to convey is that each of the two strands in a DNA duplex, by virtue of their complementary, can act as an informational template to specify the primary structure of the second strand in a double helix (Fig. 2.6). It is the principle of complementarity that provides the foundation for the faithful duplication of DNA, requisite to transmitting the genetic material at cell division and across generations. Semi-conservative DNA replication, in which the new daughter helices each contain one parental and one newly synthesised strand (Fig. 2.6) is the initial step in the Central Dogma of Molecular Biology and at the mechanistic level provides the foundation for many procedures involved in genome sequencing. Nucleotides represent the basic chemical building blocks of the DNA or RNA chain. However, chromosomes are extremely long polymers of nucleotides cemented together. The glue between adjacent nucleotides in a nucleic acid chain is the phosphodiester bond (Fig. 2.4). Formation of the phosphodiester bond in nature is catalysed by the enzyme DNA polymerase (Fig. 2.6, oval). Amazingly, the enzyme recognises three substrates in a simultaneous fashion: (i) a free 3'-OH group of the nucleotide representing the growing end of a DNA chain (Fig. 2.4, –OH), (ii) the template DNA (the opposite strand in a double helix) that provides instructions for the next nucleotide to be added in the form of complementary information (Fig. 2.6, DNA strands), and (iii) the appropriate nucleotide to be added to the growing end of the chain. The nucleotide to be added next into the polymer is in the form of a high energy deoxynucleotide triphosphate (dNTP; Fig. 2.3).

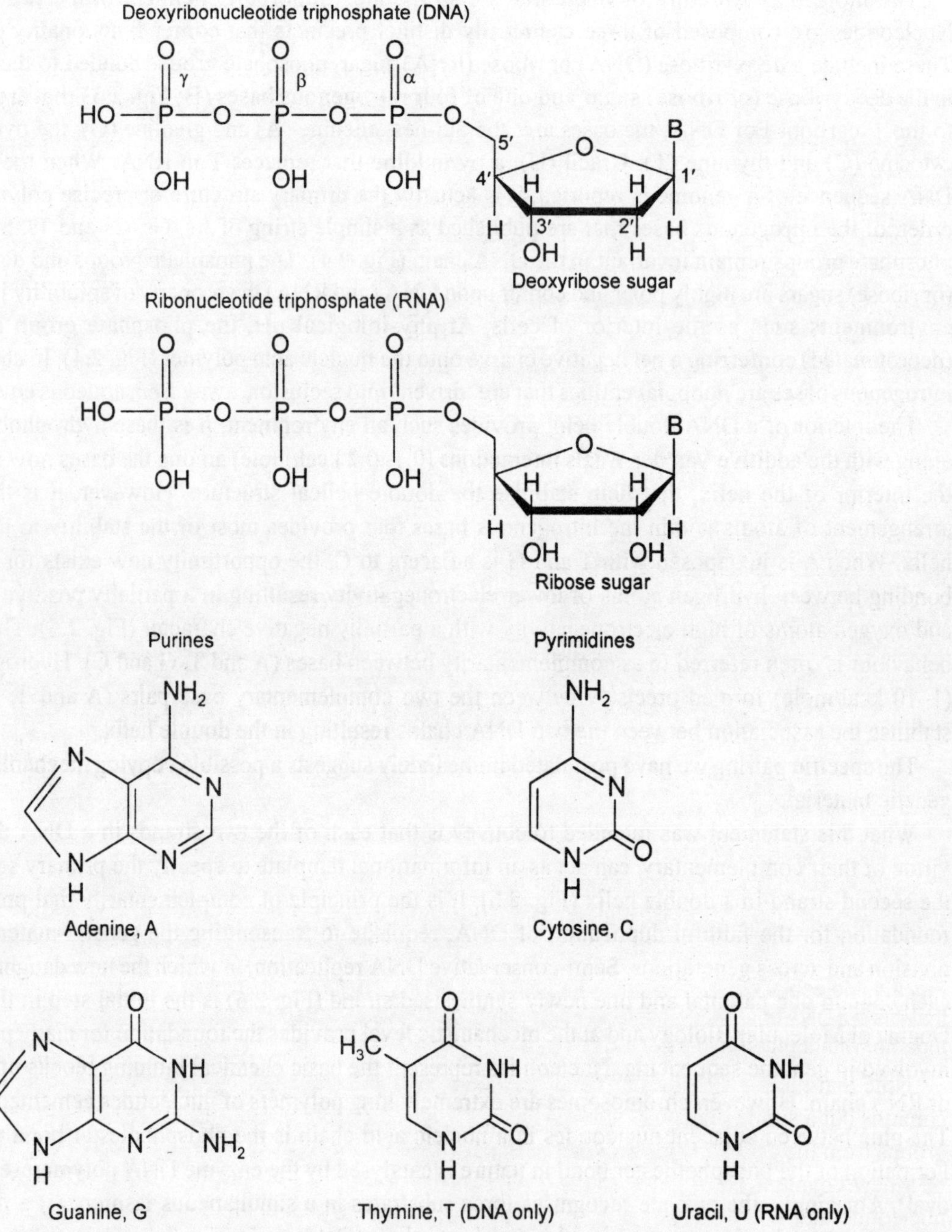

Deoxyribonucleotide triphosphate (DNA)

Ribonucleotide triphosphate (RNA)

Purines

Adenine, A

Guanine, G

Pyrimidines

Cytosine, C

Thymine, T (DNA only)

Uracil, U (RNA only)

Fig. 2.3. Molecular structure of nucleotides, the building blocks of DNA and RNA. The 1' → 5' numbering convention used to designate carbons in the deoxyribose and ribose sugars is annotated only on the deoxyribose sugar. 'B' extending from the 1' carbon of deoxyribose and ribonucleotides represent the purine and pyrimidine nitrogenous bases. Designation of the different phosphate groups (α, β, γ) are depicted on the deoxyribose nucleotide.

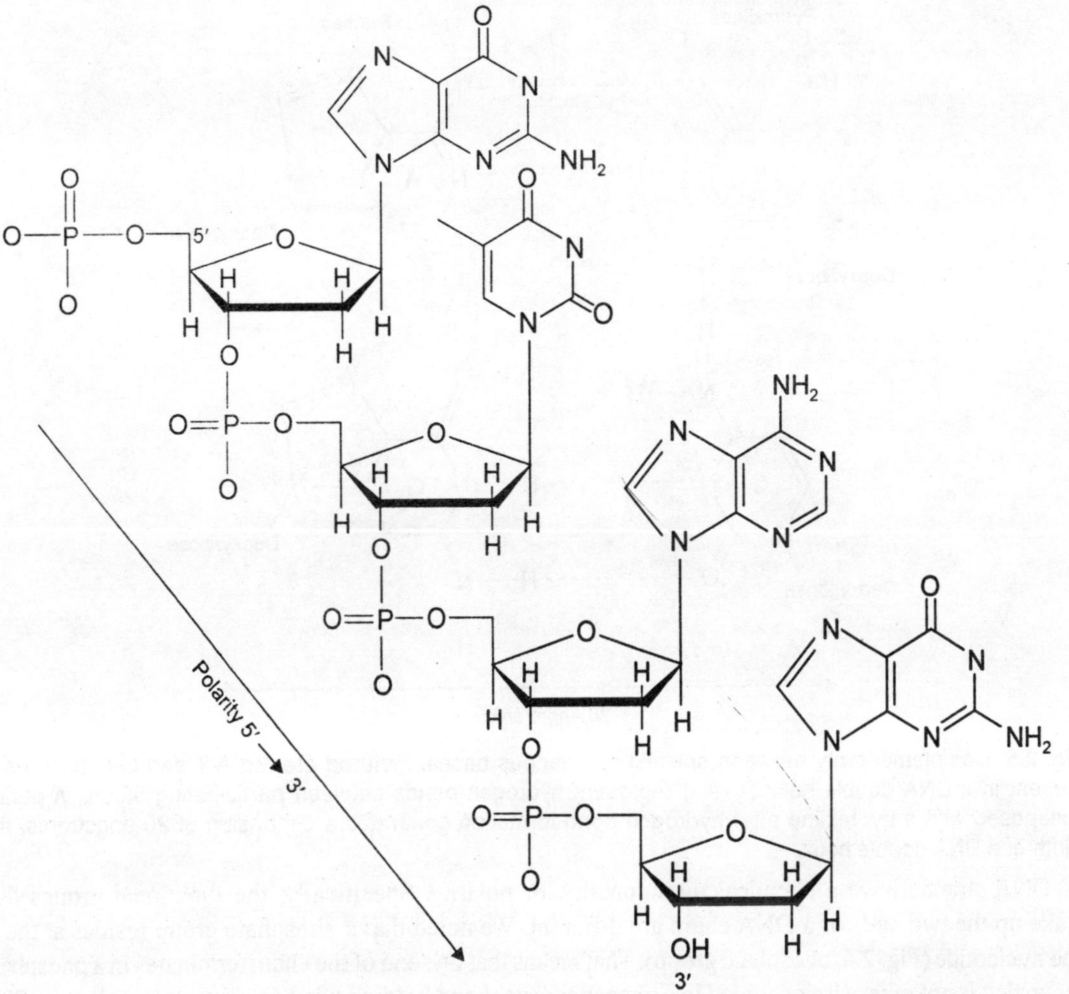

Fig. 2.4. Molecular structure of the tetranucleotide GTAG. The H present at 2' carbon of each sugar indicates that this is a DNA chain composed of deoxynucleotides. Phosphates involved in cementing adjacent nucleotides together with a phosphodiester bond.

Note that the phosphodiester bond cementing two adjacent nucleotides together in the DNA chain contains but a single phosphate group (Fig. 2.4). The energy released by the excision of two phosphate groups from the dNTP during polymerisation is recruited by DNA polymerase to catalyse the formation of a new covalent bond between the 3'-OH of the preceding nucleotide and the α-phosphate of the nucleotide that will be added (Fig. 2.3). The overall chemical reaction for the polymerisation of DNA can be written as shown in Equation 2.1:

$$(dNMP)_n + dNTP \rightarrow (dNMP)_{n+1} + PP_i \qquad \qquad ... (2.1)$$

In Equation 2.1, n represents the number of nucleotides already polymerised in the DNA chain, dNMP represents any nucleotide polymerised into a DNA chain (note only one phosphate, a Monophosphate defines the precise structure of a phosphodiester bond) and PP_i is inorganic phosphate, the two phosphates released from the deoxynucleotide triphosphate during addition of a nucleotide to a growing DNA chain.

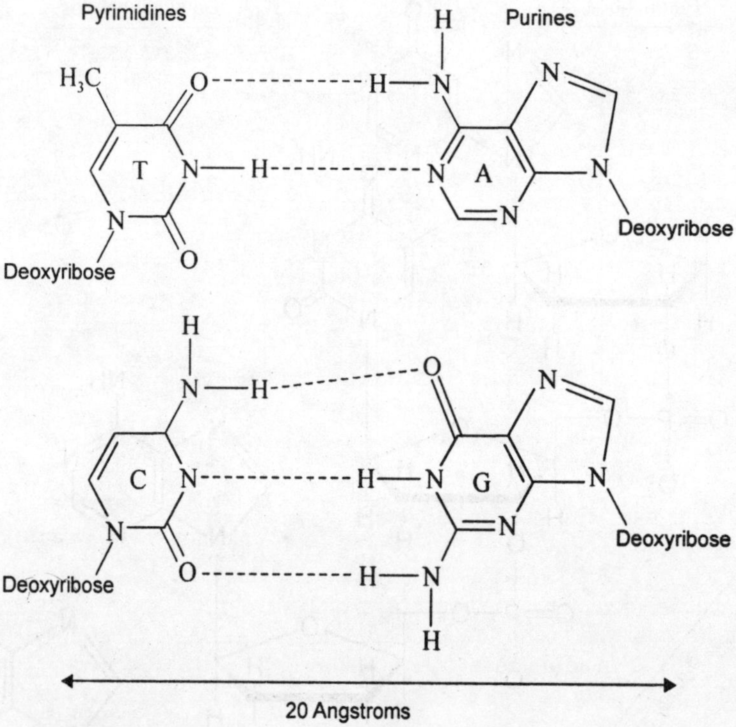

Fig. 2.5. Complementarity between specific nitrogenous bases. Pictured are the A-T and G-C base pairs present in a DNA double helix (- - - -) represent hydrogen bonds between participating atoms. A purine juxtaposed with a pyrimidine after hydrogen bond formation generates a dimension of 20 angstroms, the width of a DNA double helix.

DNA strands have a chemical directionality, or polarity. Specifically, the functional groups that make up the two ends of a DNA chain are different. We noted that a phosphate group resides at the 5' end nucleotide (Fig. 2.4, phosphate group). That means that one end of the chain terminates in a phosphate group that is not otherwise occupied in a phosphodiester bond holding two adjacent nucleotides together. There will also be one 3'-OH group (Fig. 2.4, –OH group) not engaged in cementing two nucleotides together in the polymer.

This unoccupied -OH group will be found at the opposite end of the chain. Thus, the polarity of a DNA chain is arbitrarily defined as 5' → 3' and DNA sequences are recorded and read in this fashion. Hence, the sequence ^{5}P-GTAG–OH^3 (shown in Fig. 2.4) would offer very different informational content than ^{5}P-GATG-OH^3, the simple reversal of the above sequence. Importantly, the two extended chains in a double helix reveal an opposite or antiparallel polarity (Fig. 2.6). If we again take the tetranucleotide sequence: ^{5}P-GTAG-OH^3 and now write this molecule in the form of a double helix, obeying all the rules of base pair complementarity, the correct depiction would be:

$$^5\text{P-GTAG-OH}^3$$
$$|\ |\ |\ |$$
$$^3\text{HO-CATC-P}^5$$

where the vertical lines denote hydrogen bonds between the complementing nucleotide bases in each strand.

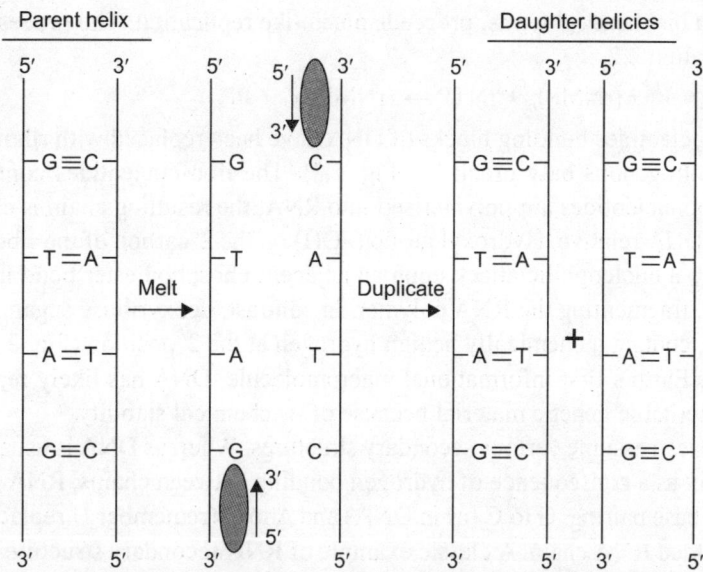

Fig. 2.6. Base pair complementarity is the basis for faithful duplication of the double helix. Chains of a DNA helix are pictured in an antiparallel configuration. Horizontal lines between the complementing bases denote hydrogen bonds (Fig. 2.4). DNA polymerase (oval) polymerises DNA in a 5' to 3' in an antiparallel direction on each strand. Each new daughter helix is composed of an original stand and a newly synthesised chain, indicative of semi-conservative replication.

Complementarity provides an important check for the precision of sequencing in the laboratory. When a nucleotide sequence is determined for one strand of a DNA duplex, the sequence of the opposite strand is easily predicted. Sequencing both strands of a gene region permits an infallible determination of a DNA sequence because of the cross-check provided by base pairing within the double helix. You may see the term 'single pass' in some reports of genomic sequencing efforts, meaning that only one strand of the DNA was sequenced, but a single time. There is some inherent error as the sequence is not experimentally validated by its complement, but single-pass sequencing is useful for rapidly deducing the information content of a genomic region.

Transcription: converting the informatics of DNA into a working RNA copy

Transcription or gene expression is the second step in the Central Dogma. Controlling gene expression at the level of transcriptional regulation is the subject of more papers published in Molecular Biology than any other topic. The process of transcription involves duplicating a gene sequence encoded in the DNA into an RNA copy. RNA, like DNA, is written in the language of nucleotides, although uracil (U) is substituted for thymine (T) in RNA molecules. The structural similarities between T and U (Fig. 2.3) allow for either base to hydrogen bond with A. Chemical languages are not changed for RNA synthesis because both DNA and RNA are polymerised nucleotide chains. Information in DNA is simply copied and this process is referred to as transcription. If the gene encodes a protein, the RNA draft is called messenger or mRNA. The end-products of some genes are simply RNA copies, not protein. Typically, these are genes that encode transfer RNAs (tRNAs) and ribosomal RNAs (rRNAs), both components of the translation apparatus.

Transcription, in biochemical terms, proceeds much like replication. The process can be described by the familiar Equation 2.2.

$$(rNMP)_n + rNTP \rightarrow (rNMP)_{n+1} + PP_i \qquad \qquad ...(2.2)$$

The deoxyribonucleotides building blocks of DNA have been replaced with ribonucleotides, one of which carries the nitrogenous base uracil (U; Fig. 2.3). The ribo-nucleotides contain a ribose sugar (Fig. 2.3). When ribonucleotides are polymerised into RNA, the resulting chain is chemically unstable relative to its close DNA relative. Hydroxyl group (–OH) on the 2' carbon of the ribose sugar (Fig. 2.3) in RNA can undergo a nucleophilic attack upon an adjacent phosphodiester bond in an RNA polymer and break the bond, fragmenting the RNA polymer. In contrast, deoxyribose sugars, the constituent of the DNA backbone, contain a chemically benign hydrogen at the 2' position (Fig. 2.3). Although RNA is thought to be the Earth's first informational macromolecule, DNA has likely replaced RNA as the primary source of heritable genetic material because of its chemical stability.

RNA, like DNA, can assume various secondary structures. Whereas DNA is usually found as a rigid rod-like double helix as a consequence of hydrogen bonding between chains, RNA polymers typically exhibit intra-strand base pairing, G to C (as in DNA) and A to U (remember U replaces T in RNA). The result is a highly folded RNA chain. A classic example of RNA secondary structure is that assumed by tRNA, which folds into the well-recognised cloverleaf conformation (Fig. 2.7). RNA secondary structures provide important architectural features that influence function. Many RNA molecules, for example, are catalytic ribozymes, including the peptidyltransferase activity of the ribosome (which catalyses the formation of peptide bonds). Its precise folding is required for this activity. Secondary structure at the 5' end of an mRNA molecule often influences the ability of the ribosome to engage the initiation of protein synthesis and provides a check point for controlling gene expression at the post-transcriptional level.

Embedded within the primary sequence of DNA are sequences that control the initiation or termination of transcription. In effect, these are the primary regulators of gene expression. These signals are promoters, enhancers, silencers, terminators and other sites along the DNA chains that are targets for DNA binding proteins. For example, promoters may be targets for RNA polymerases and other general transcription factors (TFs); enhancers provide docking sites for the proteins that are also needed to activate transcription, called transcriptional activation factors (TAFs); silencers bind proteins that inhibit or suppress transcription. One goal of genomics and bioinformatics initiatives is to identify these elements within genomic sequences and address questions regarding commonalities, among controlling elements for different genes. These strategies are helpful in providing a means to understand how genes residing at great distances along the DNA chain or on different chromosomes, may be coregulated in response to environmental cues.

Language of protein in the genomics era: amino acids and the functional architecture of proteins

The central goal of genomics and bioinformatics is to understand the complete set of information encoded in a genome. Most of this information will reside in the ensemble of genes that dictates cellular functionality and the 'assembly' of an organism. The end-product of most expressed genes is a protein, and the entire set of proteins elaborated by a specific cell type or by an organism is defined as the proteome.

The language of proteins is composed of an elaborate, 20 amino acid chemical alphabet. As with nucleic acids, the primary structure of a protein (the precise order of its amino acids) helps dictate the structure of a polypeptide. By analogy with nucleotides, we can dissect the chemical anatomy of amino acids to understand their role in directing protein structure.

The typical structure of an amino acid is:

$$\text{R}$$
$$|$$
$$\text{NH}_2\text{–CH–COH}$$

There are two important chemical features characteristic of this simple structure that are important for understanding the conformation of proteins. First, we note a chemical polarity to amino acids, with an N- or amino-terminal end (the NH_2-amino group) and a C- or carboxy-terminal end (the –COOH or carboxylic acid groups). Here we can draw an analogy with the chemical polarity of nucleotides defined by the 5' phosphate and 3'-OH groups. The NH_2-CH-COOH 'backbone' is common among all 20 amino acids. Just as nucleotide bases are distinguished by one of four nitrogenous bases, amino acids differ from each other by the presence of one of 20 side chains or R-groups. These R-groups are the information content of amino acids when polymerised into proteins, just as the nitrogenous bases are the informational component of nucleic acid chains.

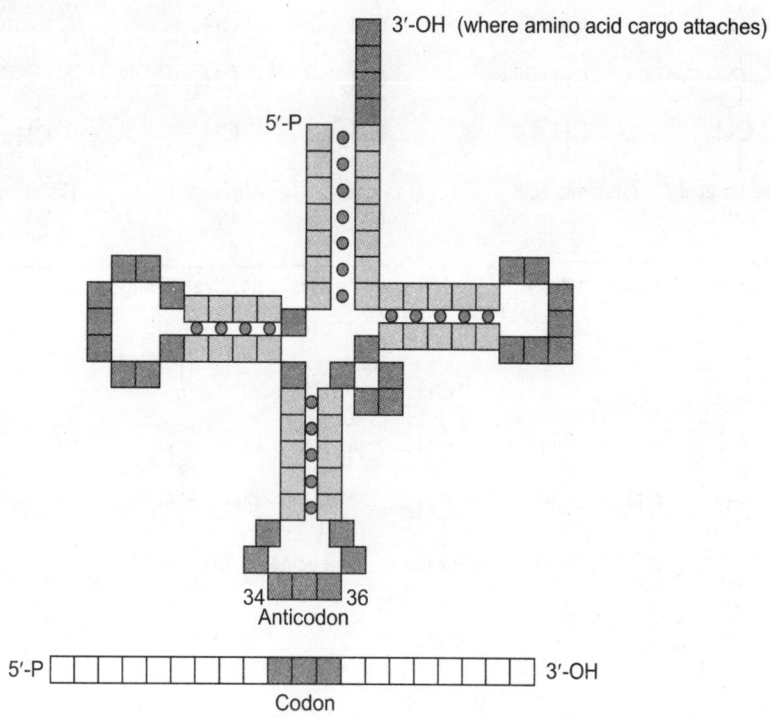

Fig. 2.7. A transfer RNA (tRNA) molecule acting as an interpreter between the language of nucleic acids (DNA and RNA) and the language of amino acids (proteins). A tRNA, pictured as a polymer of 76 individual ribonucleotides (individual squares), is folded into the universal cloverleaf structure by virtue of intra-molecular hydrogen bonding between complementing bases. The black dots denote base-pairing by hydrogen bonds to form stems. Gray squares are unpaired nucleotides, forming loops. The triplet anticodon nucleotides (34–36) are shown recognising and interacting via hydrogen bonding with the appropriate triplet codon within an mRNA molecule.

The 20 side chains can be catalogued into three major groups depending on whether the R-group is nonpolar, polar or charged at physiological pH (+ charge = basic; charge = acidic). Figure 2.8 catalogues all 20 amino acids in these groups.

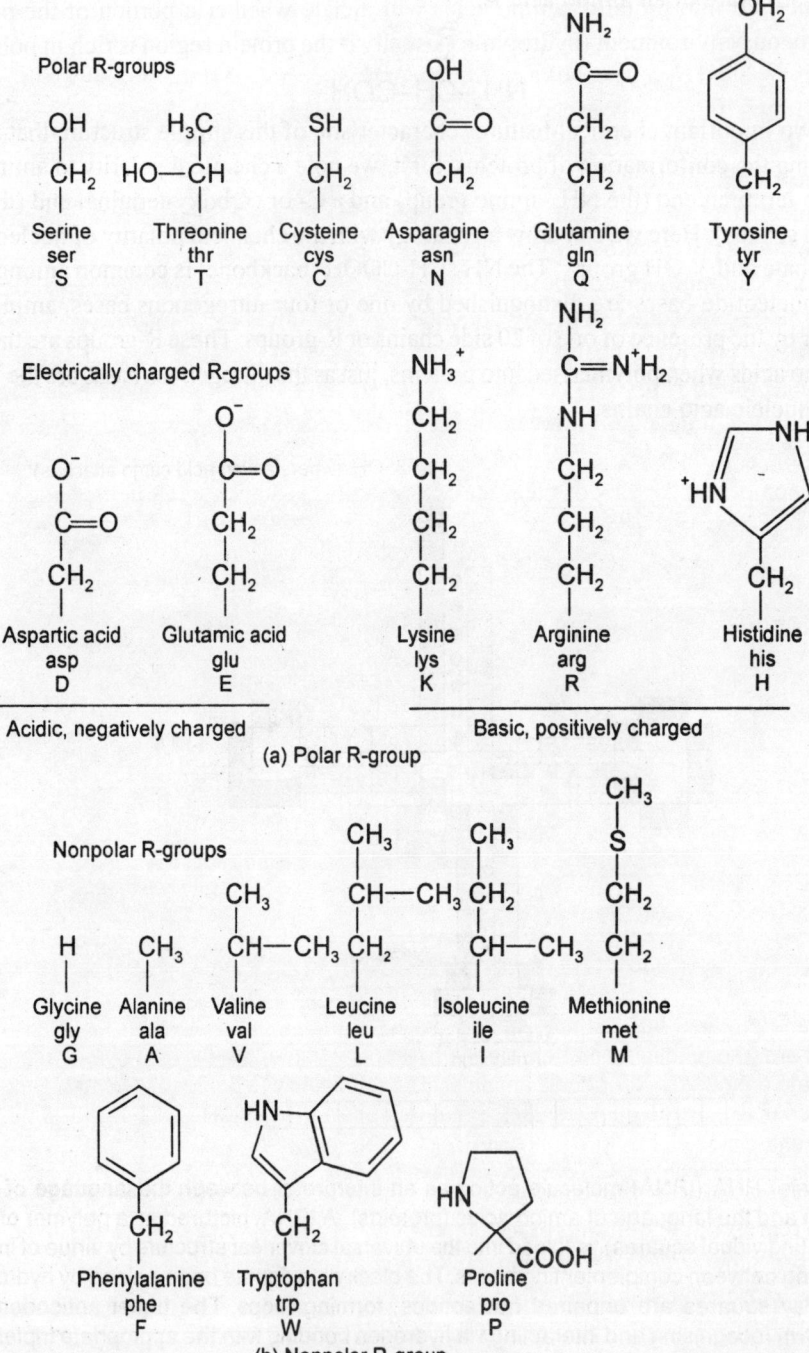

Fig. 2.8. Molecular structure of the 20 amino acid side-chains (R-groups), listed according to chemical character (A, polar or B, charged). Beneath each structure is the name of the R-group, is three-letter designation, and its single letter designation. In an amino acid, the individual side-chain is attached to by a covalent bond to the common backbone NH_2–CH–COOH, where C indicates the position of attachment.

When polymerised into proteins, amino acids will dictate whether a portion of the polypeptide is soluble in an aqueous environment (hydrophilic) usually if the protein region is rich in polar or charged amino acids or is repelled by a water-like environment (hydrophobic) if the protein chain is locally rich in nonpolar R-groups. By sequestering nonpolar amino acids within the interior of a globular protein and exposing polar and charged amino acids to the exterior, proteins in an aqueous environment are forced to assume a three-dimensional or 'tertiary' conformation.

Proteins involved in membrane function provide an excellent example of how the precise distribution of amino acids within a polypeptide polymer govern structure/function relationships within a biological system (Fig. 2.9). Membranes are composed of lipids, nonpolar hydrocarbons that present a hydrophobic environment. Proteins embedded in membranes serve many functions, including communicating with the environment and providing channels for transit of essential metabolites into and out of cells. A typical membrane protein (Fig. 2.9) contains a series of trans-membrane domains composed almost exclusively of nonpolar, uncharged amino acids (small darker dots) that seek a hydrophobic environment within the interior of a membrane, as well as segments that interact with the aqueous interior and exterior of cells comprised by runs of polar and charged amino acids (small lighter dots).

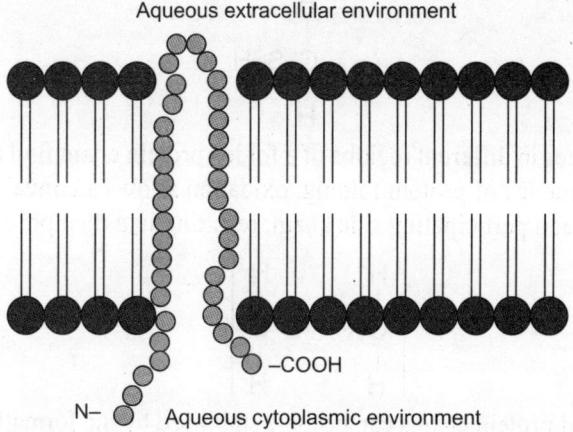

Fig. 2.9. Membrane proteins: An example of how amino acid distribution dictates structure and function. Pictured in black are phospholipids that create the hydrophobic interior of a lipid bilayer membrane. Small darker dots indicate nonpolar, hydrophobic amino acid constituents of a polypeptide chain. Small lighter dots represent polar, charged, amino acid residues that are capable of interacting with the aqueous, hydrophilic environments on either side of the cell membrane. Such trans-membrane protein domains typify proteins that serve as channels and as receptors to perceive external stimuli.

Amino acids represent the building blocks of proteins. Adjacent amino acids are glued together via a peptide bond (see Scheme 2). Two adjacent amino acids would exhibit the following structure shown in Scheme 2. As with the synthesis of DNA, polymerisation of amino acids into proteins involves a condensation/dehydration reaction that results in a peptide bond.

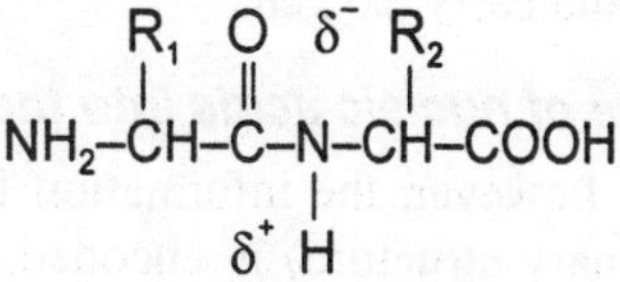

$$\underset{\delta^+ \text{H}}{\text{NH}_2-\text{CH}-\overset{\text{O}}{\overset{\|}{\text{C}}}-\overset{\delta^-}{\text{N}}-\text{CH}-\text{COOH}}$$

[Scheme 2]

R1 and R2 represent two different side chains. Each amino acid with their unique side-chain is typically given a three-letter or a single letter designation (Fig. 2.8). If the dipeptide depicted above is composed of the amino acids glycine and phenylalanine, the peptide would be written NH_2-GLY-PHE-COOH or NH_2-GP-COOH or most often 'GP'. Note that proteins also have a chemical polarity, arbitrarily written from the N-terminal ® C-terminal direction. Thus the dipeptide 'GP' would be a very different from 'PG'. Chemical polarity serves an important role in the informational content of nucleic acids and proteins, as well as in how we annotate the primary structure of both macromolecules.

The oxygen and nitrogen atoms present in the peptide bond are electronegative. As such, the oxygen takes on a partial negative charge (δ^-) and the hydrogen covalently bonded to nitrogen a partial positive charge (δ^+). In a protein with hundreds of peptide bonds, this charge distribution is a recurrent theme, and hydrogen bonding (as in nucleic acids) between the partially charged H and O atoms occurs resulting in important secondary structures known as the α-helix and the β-pleated sheet. The α-helix is a coil, much like the a telephone handset cord; the β-pleated sheet adds a flattened, sheet-like topology to specific domains of the folded protein, much like a tightly routed 'switchback' on a hiking trail.

One additional contributor to protein folding is offered by the chemical composition of the side-chain featured by the amino acid cysteine. The R-group for CYS (or C) is:

$$
\begin{array}{c}
H \\
| \\
-C-S-H \\
| \\
H
\end{array}
$$

When two CYS residues in different regions of a folded protein chain find themselves in the vicinity of each other as a consequence of protein folding, oxidation allows a covalent bond (below) to form between the S atoms in each participating side chain, resulting in a disulphide bridge:

$$
\begin{array}{cc}
H & H \\
| & | \\
-C-S-S-C- \\
| & | \\
H & H
\end{array}
$$

We observe that folded protein chains can become stabilised by the formation of disulphide bridges, contributing to the overall topography of the polypeptide. Unlike DNA, every individual protein assumes a unique three-dimensional, tertiary conformation that is necessary for catalytic activity (in the case for enzymes) or to play structural roles within the cell. Tertiary structure, then, is determined by a combination of factors that include the precise order of amino acids (the primary structure), formation of secondary structures in the form of α-helices or β-pleated sheets and folding due to the generation of disulphide bridges, then driven by hydrophobic and hydrophilic interactions between amino acids and their environment. An even higher level of structure is achieved because many active proteins are not monomers (one properly-folded polypeptide chain), but subunits that must interact with other properly folded proteins to form an active quarternary structure. One popular example is the protein haemoglobin, the oxygen carrier protein in our red blood cells. Active haemoglobin is a tetramer comprised of two α and two β subunits in erythrocytes of adult human. In isolation, these individual protein subunits are inactive, but when they come together they bind and carry oxygen.

Translation: converting the language of nucleic acids into the language of proteins

Proteins are composed of amino acids, however, the information for directing the precise order of amino acids within a peptide (the primary structure) is encoded within DNA and its constituent nucleotides. Conversion between any two languages requires a translator and no less is true in the cell. The molecular interpreter is the ribosome, the cellular site where polymerisation of amino acids into protein occurs. Translation is the final step in the Central Dogma.

The primary sequence of the nucleotides within DNA, and its RNA copies, can be considered a code that requires deciphering. Proteins are composed of 20 different amino acids and the first question regarding the code is 'How many nucleotides are required to specify one amino acid in a protein sequence?' This question led to the concept of the coding ratio: number of nucleotides required to encode one amino acid, or the number of nucleotides/amino acid. There are four nucleotides (A, G, C, T). Thus if one nucleotide encoded one amino acid (coding ratio = 1), the genetic code could only accommodate 4 amino acids. This is not sufficient to encode 20 amino acids. If the coding ratio were two, there are $4^2 = 16$ possible dinucleotide combinations and 16 amino acids could be encoded. The requirement to encode 20 amino acid is not quite achieved with a doublet code. A coding potential of 64 amino acids (4^3) is achieved with a coding ratio of three and hence the triplet codon (three contiguous nucleotides along the DNA or RNA chain) encodes the information for a single amino acid (Table 2.1). The 64 codon carrying capacity of this code far exceeds the necessary requirement to encode 20 amino acids. However, the code is redundant; i.e. the same amino acid is often encoded by several different nucleotide codons that are synonyms. For example, the amino acid leucine (LEU) is encoded by six different triplets (Table 2.1).

Table 2.1. Universal genetic code.

First 5'	Second				Third 3'
	U	C	A	G	
U	Phe	Ser	Tyr	Cys	U
	Phe	Ser	Tyr	Cys	C
	Leu	Ser	Tyr	Stop	A
	Leu	Ser	Tyr	Trp	G
C	Leu	Pro	His	Arg	U
	Leu	Pro	His	Arg	C
	Leu	Pro	Gln	Arg	A
	Leu	Pro	Gln	Arg	G
A	Ile	Thr	Asn	Ser	U
	Ile	Thr	Asn	Ser	C
	Ile	Thr	Lys	Arg	A
	Met	Thr	Lys	Arg	G
G	Val	Ala	Asp	Gly	U
	Val	Ala	Asp	Gly	C
	Val	Ala	Glu	Gly	A
	Val	Ala	Glu	Gly	G

Three codons do not encode any amino acid. They are termination or stop codons that delimit the C-terminal end of the protein, where translation stops. Continuing with our analogy of languages, termination codons serve as the period to end a sentence.

The mRNA copy of the information encoded in DNA is translated into a protein in groups of three nucleotides. Translation typically commences at an AUG (methionine, MET) codon that also signals the initiation of translation. This sets the reading frame, one of three possible ways any mRNA molecule can be read in groups of triplets. To illustrate the concept of a reading frame, let us create an mRNA molecule as a sentence in the English language that consists of words with only three letters: 'The fat cat ate the big rat.' When read as triplets, this rendition makes sense to us. But read in triplets from a different start point, the sentence could also be read '..T hef atc ata tet heb igr at..' or even in a third frame as '..Th efa tca tat eth ebi gra t..'. A triplet code implies there are three possible reading frames within a mRNA molecule. The AUG start codon establishes the correct reading frame, the one that makes sense.

This is defined as an open reading frame that typically begins with a start codon (AUG) and ends with one of three termination codons (UAG, UGA, UAA). Gene discovery within genomic sequences, annotating genes and using sequence information for alignments relies on these features of the nearly universal genetic code (Table 2.1).

Clearly, a molecular adaptor is required to decipher each triplet codon and deliver the correct amino acid into the growing protein chain. This adaptor is a specific tRNA molecule of about 76–80 nucleotides in length (Fig. 2.7). Typically residing at nucleotides 34–36 is a set of three continuous nucleotides, a triplet anticodon with base pair complementarity to a codon along the mRNA chain (Fig. 2.7). At the 3' end of this molecule the corresponding amino acid cargo is carried (Fig. 2.7, Table 2.1). The mRNA and tRNAs congregate at the ribosome, a complex cellular, organelle with multiple functions that include: (i) transiting along the mRNA chain in three nucleotide (codon) intervals, (ii) capturing the tRNA dictated by the appropriate anticodon/tRNA combination, (iii) catalysing the hydrolytic removal of the amino acid from the tRNA adaptor, and (iv) condensing the same amino acid to the growing peptide by formation of a peptide bond. This same series of reactions occurs in a sequential fashion, three nucleotides at a time, for each codon found in the mRNA. Translation is an energetically expensive and complex process; three high energy molecules at ATP or GTP are invested to add each amino acid to a growing protein chain.

A Perspective

Modern genomics and bioinformatics is really a new kind of linguistics. Nature, through dynamic evolutionary forces, inscribes genetic information in the form of long nucleotide chains or genomes. Deciphered by the cell using steps in the Central Dogma, the end-products of sensible nucleotide strings (the genes) are highly versatile proteins whose three-dimensional structure dictates function. The universal genetic code was cracked over four decades ago. Yet, how genomes encode traits that make each organism and species different from each other and each individual within a species unique, remained encrypted information until now. With the advent of DNA and protein methodologies, genomes no longer present themselves as molecular hieroglyphics.

STRUCTURE AND FUNCTION OF CELL ORGANELLES

The myriad biochemical reactions that comprise life processes are too numerous and complex to be carried out entirely by simple diffusion-mediated interactions between enzymes and substrates. Instead, sequences of biochemical reactions must be efficiently organised and integrated with other sets of reactions by the cell. Two fundamental structural elements are used by eukaryotic cells to organise and integrate these reactions: membranes and a cytoskeletal system. An elaborate system of cellular membranes, in the form of the plasma membrane, membrane-bound organelles and the nuclear envelope, has evolved to provide reaction surfaces and to organise and compartmentalise molecules involved in specific metabolic pathways. Other cytosolic biochemical reactions, as well as the organisation of membranous organelles within the cell, are regulated by interactions with the cytoskeletal system. Consequently, enzymes and proteins involved in biochemical reactions can be located in the cytosol, within membranes, on the surfaces of membranes, within the interior of membrane-bound compartments or in association with the cytoskeleton. The elaboration of these structural elements has allowed for the sophisticated level of biochemical integration that exists in living eukaryotic cells.

Over two hundred different types of cells are found in higher animals, including human and the interaction of these diverse cell types is responsible for the formation and functioning of tissues and organs. Different types of cells carry out specialised functions, but all cells face similar sets of challenges to exist. In general, cells must maintain a barrier against and sensing mechanisms to interact with, their external environment; synthesise and recycle their structural and enzymatic components; repair physical or chemical damage; grow and reproduce; and generate energy for all of these activities. These generalised functions, as well as the more, specialised functions of individual cell types, are all performed by cell organelles. Cell organelles perform the basic functions that allow cells to survive and replicate, and are dynamic entities that become modified to help specialised cells carry out specific functions. For example, all cells contain a cytoskeletal filamentous system that functions in maintenance of cell shape and allows for some degree of movement, but muscle cells contain far greater numbers of these filaments to carry out the contractile activity that comprises muscle activity.

Classically, the phrase cell organelle has been used to denote distinct membrane bound structures that are readily visible by light or electron microscopy and possess characteristic morphological features that make them readily identifiable in essentially all eukaryotic cells. Such structures include the plasma membrane, ER, Golgi apparatus, lysosomes, peroxisomes and mitochondria (Fig. 2.10). The structure and function of these organelles, as well as the cytoskeleton and nucleus, are described in this section. Because membrane structure plays fundamental roles in organelle function, the basic features of membrane organisation will be considered first.

Membrane Structure

Cell membranes are composed of lipid and protein, which are assembled into two opposing layers called the lipid bilayer. Four major types of phospholipids and cholesterol comprise most of the lipid portion of the bilayer. The phospholipids include the choline-containing lipids phosphatidylcholine and sphingomyelin and the amine-containing lipids phosphatidylethanolamine and phosphatidylserine. All of these phospholipids possess hydrophilic polar heads and two hydrophobic fatty acid tails. The membrane bilayer represents an energetically favourable conformation of these lipids in that the tails associate with each other to form a hydrophobic environment in the centre of the bilayer, with the polar heads facing outward to interact with the charged aqueous environment of the cytoplasm, organelle lumen or extracellular space. The hydrophobic region resulting from the association of lipid tails creates a barrier to the passage of charged molecules, and only small uncharged molecules, or lipid-soluble molecules, can freely penetrate the lipid bilayer. Cholesterol, which is shorter and stiffer than phospholipids, can comprise up to about 50 per cent of the total membrane lipid. The hydroxyl end of cholesterol interacts with the polar heads of phospholipid molecules, with the rest of the molecule in the same plane as the fatty acid tails of phospholipids. Its presence in membranes is thought to help prevent phase transitions by stiffening membranes at higher temperatures, while also maintaining membrane fluidity at lower temperatures. Although cholesterol is prevalent and equally represented in both bilayers of a membrane, the major phospholipids are asymmetrically distributed, with higher concentrations of choline-containing phospholipids present in the noncytoplasmic layer (i.e. the layer facing organelle lumens and the layer of the plasma membrane facing the extracellular matrix) and higher concentrations of amine-containing phospholipids in the layer facing the cytoplasm.

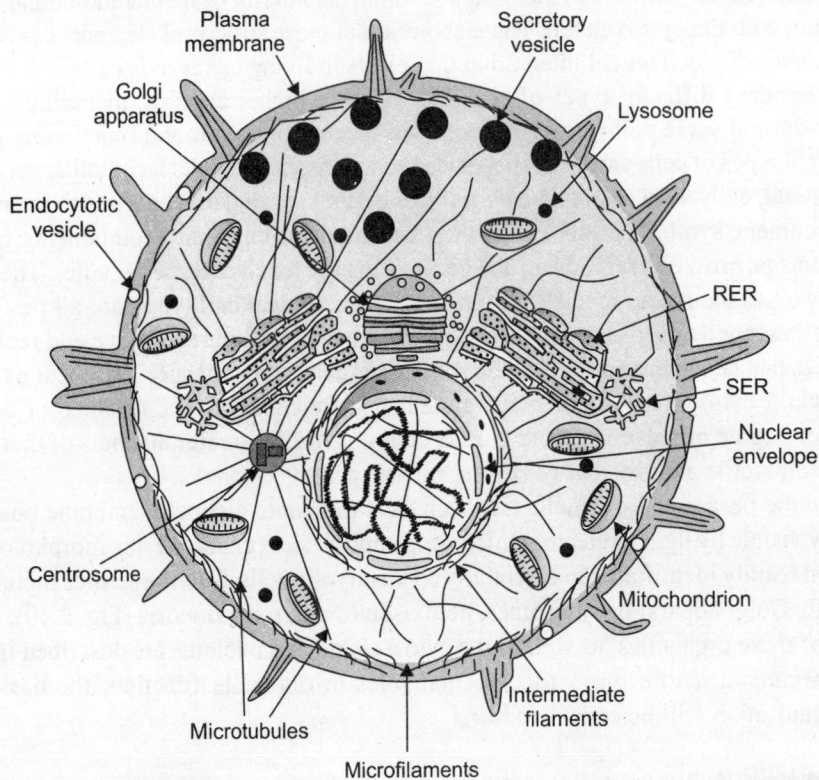

Fig. 2.10. Overview of cell organisation. Diagram of the major cell organelles, including the cytoskeleton and nucleus. This drawing depicts a single idealised cell and so does not include the cell-cell and cell-ECM junctions elaborated by cells in tissues.

In addition to lipid, membranes are also composed of protein. Membrane proteins are either classified as integral membrane proteins if they penetrate or are anchored in the bilayer or as peripheral membrane proteins if they are just associated with the surfaces of the bilayer. Integral membrane proteins are difficult to remove from membranes, usually requiring disruption of the lipid bilayer (e.g. with detergents) to be released. Peripheral proteins are easier to remove from membranes, as they are generally held in place by protein-protein interactions. Integral membrane proteins can penetrate the bilayer completely a single time (single-pass proteins) or multiple times (multi-pass proteins). They can also be anchored in the membrane through covalent attachments to lipid molecules in the bilayer.

A number of membrane lipids and proteins are glycosylated. Glycosylation of membrane components takes place in the ER and Golgi apparatus. Because glycosylation occurs exclusively within the interior (or lumen) of these organelles, the sugar groups of glycoproteins and glycolipids all face toward the lumenal surface of membranes of organelles and the extracellular matrix (ECM) side of the plasma membrane. Glycosylation of membrane lipids and proteins is thought to help protect membranes and in the case of the plasma membrane, to help identify the cell and to assist in the adhesion of cells to the ECM.

Membrane lipids and proteins carry out a number of functions. In addition to serving as the structural framework of the membrane, they mediate the functions of all membranes of the cell. Membrane lipids can form specialised subdomains composed of specific lipid population (lipid rafts) that appear to facilitate localised membrane function, and some membrane lipids are intimately involved in signal transduction events. Membrane proteins carry out a wide variety of functions, including serving as membrane channels, carriers and pumps; transducing cytoplasmic and extracellular signals; targeting membranes to specific locations; and adhering membranes to each other and to the ECM.

Plasma Membrane

The plasma membrane encloses the cytoplasm of a cell and carries out multiple functions. It forms both a barrier to and an interface with, the cellular environment. The plasma membrane is a selectively permeable barrier that, by regulating what enters and exits a cell, is a primary determinant of the composition of the cytoplasm. The plasma membrane is associated with sensing mechanisms that transduce environmental information into a cytoplasmic or nuclear response. The plasma membrane is involved in cell-cell and cell-ECM attachments and also contains cell-specific molecules that help identify cells, thereby helping to establish the appropriate position and arrangement of each cell in the body.

Barrier functions

The hydrophobic nature of the central region of the lipid bilayer serves as a barrier to charged or large hydrophilic molecules; thus, the lipid bilayer is impermeable to small ions (e.g. Na^+, K^+, Cl^-) and proteins. Only small, uncharged molecules (e.g. CO_2, H_2O) or molecules freely soluble in lipid (e.g. steroid hormones, dioxin) are able to pass directly through the lipid bilayer. In this way, the plasma membrane is selectively permeable. However, materials can be transported into and out of the cell by specific transport mechanisms carried out by the plasma membrane. The carbohydrate moieties of glycolipids and glycoproteins also serve as barriers by impeding the access of molecules to the surface of the plasma membrane, which can also serve to protect plasma membranes exposed to harsh environments (e.g. the stomach and intestinal lumen).

Transport functions

Because the lipid bilayer is impermeable to most types of organic molecules, the cell must possess mechanisms to move materials between the cytoplasm and the external environment. Two approaches are used by the cell to move material into and out of the cytoplasm:
1. Transport through the membrane.
2. Transport involving membrane flow.

Transport through the plasma membrane

Transport through membranes is mediated by integral membrane proteins, which help conduct material past the hydrophobic lipid bilayer in a number of ways. Integral membrane proteins can form channels by associating to form pore-like structures in the membrane. Such channels allow for diffusion of molecules small enough to fit through them. This type of transport allows for the flow of molecules down their concentration gradient and an expenditure of energy is not needed if the channel is open. Thus, molecules can move through protein channels by passive diffusion. Examples include ion channels that allow for the passage of ions such as Na^+ and K^+ and the connexons in gap junctions, which allow for the passage of molecules <1000 daltons through the plasma membrane. Whether these channels are open or closed is tightly regulated in order to prevent the constant leakage of small molecules into or out of the cell. Integral membrane proteins can also act as carriers that bind specific molecules and help them traverse the lipid bilayer. Binding of the appropriate molecule to carrier proteins results in a conformational change in carrier protein structure such that the ligand is conveyed across the membrane. This type of transport is also driven by the concentration gradient of the ligand and does not require the expenditure of energy by the cell. An example of transport by this method of facilitated diffusion includes glucose transporters in the basolateral membranes of intestinal epithelial cells.

Cells must also transport molecules against their concentration gradients and this type of transport is carried out by integral membrane proteins that act as pumps and requires the expenditure of energy. This is referred to as active transport and is an essential process in living cells. Examples include a number of different ion pumps, which keep the cytoplasm relatively low in Na^+ and high in K^+. Ion pumps are vital elements of the plasma membrane and it has been estimated that as much as one-third or more of the energy consumed by a living cell is used to actively transport Na^+ out of the cell. The concentration gradient of certain ions established by these membrane pumps can itself serve as a motive force for other transport mechanisms. For example, in addition to moving out of a cell by facilitated diffusion, glucose is actively transported into cells by integral membrane proteins that bind both glucose and Na^+. Because these transporters bind both Na^+ and glucose, the high concentration of Na^+ outside the cell relative to the cytoplasm drives the movement of both Na^+ and glucose into the cell, against the concentration gradient of glucose.

Acquisition of glucose from the small intestine is an elegant example of how active transport can be coupled with facilitated diffusion to move molecules past epithelia. The apical membrane of intestinal epithelial cells contain Na^+-coupled active transporters that move glucose against its concentration gradient to accumulate in the cytoplasm. Consequently, the concentration of glucose is higher in the cytoplasm of these cells than in the extracellular spaces underlying them, and carrier proteins in the basolateral membranes of these cells allow for the facilitated diffusion of glucose out of the cell (down its concentration gradient) and into the circulation. It can be seen from this example that directional transport of molecules past epithelial cells requires that integral membrane transport proteins occupy specific locations within the plasma membrane (i.e. either the apical or basolateral membrane). How transporters are organised within the plasma membrane is determined by specific targeting mechanisms acting in conjunction with cell junctions and the cytoskeleton.

Transport involving membrane flow

In addition to movement of materials through membrane channels, carriers and pumps, the plasma membrane mediates the transport of material into and out of cells by membrane flow. Internalisation of extracellular material can occur by entrapment in membrane-bound vesicles that pinch off from the plasma membrane and are transported into the cytoplasm for processing. This process, called endocytosis, can be subdivided into a number of different categories based on the mechanics of how the formation of vesicles occurs at the plasma membrane and includes the formation of clathrin-coated vesicles from coated pits and the formation of nonclathrin-coated vesicles derived from structures called caveolae.

Clathrin-coated vesicles comprise a major pathway in which specific extracellular molecules are recognised and bound to the plasma membrane prior to internalisation. This process involves membrane receptors, which are integral membrane proteins of the plasma membrane that recognise specific ligands. The best understood example of this process involves how cholesterol is taken up by cells. In the circulation, cholesterol is packaged in low-density lipoprotein (LDL) particles, which are small particles composed of protein and cholesterol esters. Specific LDL receptors are present in the plasma membrane that bind and anchor LDL particles to the surface of the cell. Occupied LDL receptors form clusters in the membrane that recruit adapter proteins and the cytoplasmic protein clathrin. Clathrin molecules assemble beneath receptor clusters to form a basketwork that deforms the plasma membrane into an invagination referred to as a coated pit. Continued assembly of the clathrin coating results in the continued invagination, pinching off and release of a membrane-bound coated vesicle containing LDL receptor and LDL cargo into the cytoplasm. Once the vesicle is formed, the clathrin coating is disassembled and the clathrin recycled to the plasma membrane to assist in the formation of more coated pits. The clathrin-free vesicle then fuses with a membrane-bound compartment called an endosome, which, in addition to receiving vesicles from the plasma membrane, also receives lysosomal vesicles filled with hydrolytic enzymes packaged by the Golgi apparatus. Membrane-bound structures containing a mixture of LDL particles and acid hydrolases then arise from the endosome to form mature lysosomes. During this process, LDL dissociates from the LDL receptor in the acidic endosomal environment and vesicles enriched in LDL receptor pinch off from the endosome to be recycled back to the plasma membrane. Digestion of LDL particles occurs in the lysosome, followed by the release of cholesterol from the lysosome into the cytoplasm of the cell. This process of receptor-mediated endocytosis is used to concentrate and internalise a number of extracellular molecules. Other common features of receptor-mediated endocytosis include the recycling of both clathrin and the receptor; the fusion of internalised vesicles with endosomes; and the formation of lysosomes (digestive organelles) for material internalised by this route.

A second endocytotic pathway exists that does not involve clathrin and may bypass delivery of internalised material to lysosomes. In this pathway, which appears to involve both receptor-mediated endocytosis as well as the nonspecific internalisation of extracellular fluid, vesicles are created from clathrin-free invaginated membrane regions called caveolae. Caveolae are associated with specialised membrane domains with distinct phospholipid contents called lipid rafts. Invagination and formation of vesicles in these areas does not require clathrin, and the vesicles formed may be transported directly to the Golgi apparatus or endoplasmic reticulum instead of the endosomes and lysosomes. Presumably this route is used for material that would be damaged or degraded by exposure to lysosomal enzymes. Many cells display a constitutive formation and internalisation of these vesicles in a process sometimes referred to as pinocytosis or cell drinking.

Signalling functions

The plasma membrane serves as the interface with the cell environment and possesses a number of mechanisms to detect and transduce specific extracellular signals. Integral membrane proteins that serve as signal receptors can be categorised into three broad classes: ion channel-linked receptors, G-protein-linked receptors and enzyme-linked receptors.

Ion channel-linked receptors undergo conformational changes upon ligand binding, opening a membrane channel permeable to small ions. Examples of this type of receptor include some types of neurotransmitter receptors. G-protein-linked receptors are integral membrane proteins that, upon ligand binding, activate small GTP-binding proteins (G-proteins), which in turn activate other effector molecules, including ion channel-linked receptors and various enzymes (e.g. adenylate cyclase). Thus, G-protein-linked receptor activity can lead to ion transients across the plasma membrane or the generation of second messengers such as cAMP. Examples of G-protein-linked receptors include polypeptide hormone receptors. The third class of membrane-associated signalling molecules are enzyme-linked receptors, which upon ligand binding activate an enzyme activity, which is usually a protein kinase or a guanylyl cyclase. Examples of enzyme-linked receptors are growth factor receptors, whose tyrosine kinase activity is an important regulator of the cell cycle.

In addition to membrane receptors involved in signal transduction events, cells possess other types of receptors not associated with the plasma membrane. For example, steroid hormones (e.g. estrogen and testosterone) are lipid soluble and pass directly through the lipid bilayer without the need to bind to proteins exposed on the external face of the plasma membrane. Receptors for these types of signalling molecules are found in the cytoplasm and nucleus.

Cell junctions

Specialisations of the plasma membrane also help cells adhere to each other and to the ECM. They form barriers against the diffusion of material between cells of an epithelium and form channels between adjacent cells. All of these functions are carried out by cell junctions.

Cell-cell barrier junctions

It is important for the body to prevent the passage of material between epithelial cells. For example, a major function of intestinal and bladder epithelia is to prevent the direct passage of the contents of the intestine and bladder into the body cavity. The ability of epithelia to form effective barriers between different compartments is owing to the presence of special cell-cell junctions called occluding, or tight, junctions. Tight junctions are composed of linear arrays of the integral membrane proteins occludin and claudin; forming a barrier between cells as strands of occludin encircling the apical part of adjacent epithelial cells line up and bind to each other. Epithelia that form strong barriers to intercellular leakage contain many tight junction strands, whereas more leaky epithelia generally display fewer strands. Occludin and claudin molecules are associated with other cytoplasmic proteins that appear to furnish some linkages with the cytoskeleton. Extensive cytoskeletal interactions, such as those associated with adhesive-type cell junctions, are not readily apparent in tight junctions.

Cell-cell adhesive junctions

These specialisations of the plasma membrane allow cells in an epithelium to bind tightly to each other and can be subdivided into two categories: adherens junctions and desmosomes. Adherens-type cell-cell junctions form belt-like arrays encircling the apical part of epithelial cells and are associated with a thick band of microfilaments. Zonulae adherens are comprised of integral membrane proteins belonging to the cadherin family of proteins, a number of the linking proteins that interconnect cadherins to microfilaments, including vinculin and catenin and associated microfilaments. Cadherins from adjacent cells bind tightly to each other in the presence of Ca^{2+} and the chelate of Ca^{2+} promotes cell dissociation. Interestingly, β-catenin functions not only as an adherens plaque protein, but also as a transcription factor in the nucleus. Thus, β-catenin may serve as a sensing device that translates changes in cell-cell adhesion into changes in gene activity.

Desmosomes are punctate cell-cell adhesive junctions that are associated with the intermediate filament cytoskeleton. Like adherens junctions, they are also composed of cadherin integral membrane proteins and proteins that interlink cadherins and the associated cytoskeletal filament system. One type of desmosomal cadherin is a protein called desmoglein and the major linking protein of desmosomes is a member of the plakin family of proteins called desmoplakin. Desmosomal intermediate filaments form dense bundles that interconnect desmosomal plaques, thus strengthening cell-cell attachments that contribute to the mechanical integrity the epithelium.

Cell-cell communicating junctions

Two types of cell-cell junctions, gap junctions and synapses, constitute specialisations of the plasma membrane that allow cells to communicate with each other. Gap junctions are punctate structures that electrically couple cells through channels that provide for direct cytoplasmic communication between adjacent cells. Gap junctions are composed of clusters of pore-like structures, called connexons, that span the lipid bilayer and allow passage of molecules smaller than 1000 daltons. Connexons, made up of hexameric arrays of the integral membrane protein connexin, line up between adjacent cells to form continuous, tightly sealed channels from cell to cell. These connections maintain a barrier against leakage of material to, or from the extracellular compartment, but ions and small molecules can diffuse from cell-to-cell to permit electrical coupling.

The electrical coupling of gap junctions perform vital functions in propagating the contraction of cardiac muscle. The conformation of connexons is regulated by Ca^{2+} such that they remain open in low concentrations of Ca^{2+}, but close in the presence of higher concentrations Ca^{2+}.

In addition to the direct coupling of cells at gap junctions, neurons also communicate with each other at synapses. At synapses, cells release neurotransmitters in quantal fashion by the regulated exocytosis of membrane-bound vesicles. Neurotransmitters rapidly diffuse across a narrow extracellular space to bind to specific receptors on the plasma membrane of the adjacent cell. These receptors are either ion channels or in some cases, G-protein-linked receptors. When stimulated by a neurotransmitter, ion channels open, allowing Na^+ to enter the cell by diffusing down its concentration gradient, thereby depolarising the plasma membrane. G-protein-linked receptors that bind neurotransmitter release activated G-proteins that may subsequently activate and open other ion channels. Depolarisation of the plasma membrane is conducted down the body of the stimulated cell, and can trigger the release of the neurotransmitter at synaptic junctions between the stimulated cell and other adjacent cells. In this way, signalling activity is propagated between cells interconnected by synapses.

Cell-ECM adhesive junctions

Cells elaborate two types of cell-ECM junctions that assist in their adherence to the ECM. Hemidesmosomes anchor epithelial cells to underlying connective tissue and are associated with intermediate filament cytoskeletal fibres, whereas focal contacts can be formed by many types of cells and involve microfilament-associated linkages with the extracellular matrix. Hemidesmosomes resemble half-desmosomes where proteins called integrins form the integral membrane component, linked to intermediate filaments by members of the plakin family of proteins. Integrins are also the integral membrane proteins of focal contacts, and are connected to bundles of microfilaments by vinculin, tal in, and other linking proteins. Focal contacts are associated with protein kinases, called focal adhesion kinases (FAKs). FAKs are thought to help transmit the status of cell-ECM linkage at focal contacts to the cytoplasm and nucleus. Normal (noncancerous) cells must usually be in contact with a substrate to divide and FAKs may be involved in relaying contact information to regulatory elements of the cell cycle.

Cell protection and cell identity

Many proteins and lipids of the plasma membrane possess covalently-linked sugar groups. These sugar groups are asymmetrically distributed and are presented exclusively on the ECM side of the membrane. Plasma membrane glycoproteins and glycolipids serve important roles in both protecting the membrane and in identifying specific cell types. Epithelial cells lining the small intestine elaborate a thick glycocalyx that helps to protect them against the harsh digestive conditions of the intestinal lumen. Examples of cell recognition processes involving glycoproteins and glycolipids include the patterns of antigens on red blood cells responsible for blood groupings. Another example involves the initial adhesion of neutrophils to capillary endothelium in areas of inflammation. During inflammation, endothelial cells express the integral membrane protein P-selectin, which contains a lectin domain that recognises a four sugar group (N-acetylglucosamine, galactose, fucose and sialic acid) present on glycoproteins and glycolipids of neutrophils. Neutrophils adhere to endothelial cells expressing P-selectin. This facilitates their subsequent migration past the capillary bed to reach the sites of inflammation.

Endoplasmic Reticulum

The ER is a prominent organelle in most cells, and its total membrane area can constitute more than half of all the membrane of a cell. ER membranes delimit enclosed spaces that vary in shape from flattened sheets, or cisternae, to branching tubules, to distended sacs; the total enclosed lumenal space can occupy 10 per cent or more of the cell volume. A number of distinct functions are carried out by the ER. The ER is the primary site of synthesis of membrane lipids and integral membrane proteins for all membranous organelles (ER, Golgi, lysosomes, endosomes, secretory vesicles and plasma membrane) except mitochondria and peroxisomes. It is also the site of production of secreted proteins and lumenal proteins of ER, Golgi and lysosomes. In addition, the ER functions in lipid synthesis, detoxification reactions and Ca^{2+} regulation.

ER can be categorised as either rough (RER) or smooth (SER). RER is so designated owing to the presence of numerous ribosomes bound to the cytoplasmic surface of the cisternal membranes, whereas SER lacks associated ribosomes. These different forms of ER are specialised for different functions; RER is the site where integral, lumenal and secretory proteins are synthesised, whereas SER is the major site of detoxification and lipid synthesis.

Protein synthesis

Protein synthesis takes place on ribosomes, which are either located free in the cytoplasm or attached to membranes of the ER (forming RER). Cytoplasmic proteins (e.g. cytoskeletal proteins) are synthesised by free ribosomes, whereas proteins associated with membranes (including the plasma membrane) or the lumenal compartments of membrane-bound organelles, as well as proteins destined for secretion, are synthesised by RER. The lipid components of membranes are also made by the ER, and both protein and lipid are delivered to the plasma membrane and most organelles by membrane flow. This involves the transport and fusion of membrane-bound vesicles between ER, the Golgi apparatus, and other target organelles. Exceptions to this pattern of membrane biogenesis and renewal include mitochondria and peroxisomes. Interestingly, most proteins of mitochondria, and all peroxisome proteins, are made by free ribosomes and subsequently delivered to these organelles via transport mechanisms that move individual proteins into or past their membranes. Membrane lipids are delivered to these organelles by transport proteins that extract lipid from ER membranes and insert them in the membranes of mitochondria and peroxisomes.

Whether ribosomes remain free in the cytoplasm or are bound to ER is determined by the amino acid sequence of the polypeptide chain as it emerges from the ribosome. ER-associated proteins possess a signal sequence that functions in docking the polypeptide to the membranes of the ER. The signal sequence is recognised and bound by a signal recognition particle or SRP. The SRP in turn binds to a SRP receptor in the membrane of the ER. A protein translocator apparatus forms a pore in the ER membrane through which growing polypeptide chains can pass. It also associates with the SRP and SRP receptor, and receives the protein as translation proceeds. Thus, proteins with signal sequences are injected directly into the membrane of the ER as they are synthesised. The signal sequence, which is hydrophobic, remains inserted into the lipid bilayer while the rest of the protein spools past as it elongates. The relative orientation of the signal sequence influences whether the N or C-terminus of the polypeptide is threaded into the ER lumen. Soluble lumenal proteins spool all the way through the bilayer and a signal peptidase then clips the protein at the signal sequence, liberating the protein into the lumen. Single and multi-pass membrane proteins are thought to achieve their conformations by internal stop-transfer and start-transfer sequences, which interact with the bilayer to either promote the passage of the growing polypeptide chain through the bilayer (start-transfer sequences) or halt the transmembrane passage (stop-transfer sequences). Multiple start and stop-transfer sequences therefore can result in a polypeptide chain that doubles back and forth to penetrate the bilayer at multiple points, forming loops in both the cytoplasm and ER lumen.

A number of post-translational modifications of proteins occur in the ER, as well as in the Golgi apparatus. Chaperone proteins that help direct the correct folding of newly synthesised protein are present in the ER cisternae; disulphide bonds form and many proteins are glycosylated or may have glycolipid anchors added. Glycosylation is carried out by the initial assembly of sugars into polymeric structures attached to the membrane lipid dolichol. The assembled carbohydrate group is then transferred from dolichol to the protein. The glycoprotein may be processed in the ER by trimming some sugars and addition of others. Further processing of glycoproteins, and the formation of glycolipids, are major functions of the Golgi apparatus.

Lipid synthesis

In addition to synthesis of proteins for membranes, lysosomes and secretory vesicles, the ER is also responsible for the synthesis of most membrane lipid for all organelles (including mitochondria and peroxisomes). Enzymes involved in lipid synthesis are embedded in the membrane of the ER, with their active sites facing the cytoplasm. Fatty acids are added to glycerol phosphate to form phosphatidic acid, which then receives various head groups. Phosphatidylcholine, phosphatidylserine and phosphatidylethanolamine are formed in this way and initially added to the cytoplasmic leaflet of the ER lipid bilayer. Phospholipid translocators (flippases) are present in the membrane that transfer choline-containing phospholipids from the cytoplasmic half to the lumenal half of the bilayer. These translocators keep the total numbers of phospholipid molecules approximately equal between the two layers, but give rise to membrane asymmetry in the distribution of these lipids. Sphingomyelin synthesis is more complex; serine is first attached to fatty acids to form ceramide, which is exported to the Golgi apparatus, where phosphocholine head groups are added. Mitochondria and peroxisomes appear to receive their membrane lipid from the ER through the activity of phospholipid exchange proteins, which transfer phospholipids between membrane systems by extraction and insertion of individual lipid molecules. In addition to membrane lipid synthesis, the ER plays important roles in other aspects of lipid metabolism. For example, steroid hormones are synthesised from cholesterol in the SER.

Detoxification

Harmful substances that are relatively insoluble are difficult to clear from the cell. Such substances can occur as either environmental contaminants or as products of metabolism. SER contain a variety of enzymes that are able to process insoluble toxicants to make them more water-soluble and amenable for excretion. The best studied detoxification enzymes are members of the cytochrome P450 family of enzymes. Liver hepatocytes are among the most active cells involved in detoxification reactions and contain large amounts of SER that house the P450 enzymes. The quantity of SER within a cell can fluctuate in response to different levels of exposure to toxic compounds.

Ca²⁺ Regulation

The ER membrane contains Ca^{2+}-ATPases that actively transport cytoplasmic Ca^{2+} into the ER lumen. This activity keeps cytoplasmic Ca^{2+} levels very low, which is necessary to allow Ca^{2+} to effectively function as a signalling molecule. In electrically excitable cells, depolarisation of the plasma membrane promotes influx of Ca^{2+} from outside the cell; in nonexcitable cells, however, most of the Ca^{2+} released into the cytoplasm comes from the ER. ER membranes contain Ca^{2+} release channels that are activated by inositol triphosphate (IP3), a signalling molecule released by the activation of certain G-protein-linked receptor proteins at the plasma membrane. The contraction of muscle cells is triggered by Ca^{2+} and these cells possess an extensive and specialised SER system, the sarcoplasmic reticulum, that contains a second type of Ca^{2+}-release channel in the SER membrane. After release from the ER, Ca^{2+} concentrations are lowered in the cytoplasm by the activity of plasma membrane and ER pumps.

Golgi Apparatus

The Golgi apparatus functions as the post office of a cell, packaging and directing different types of cargo from the ER to different organelles and the plasma membrane. In addition to packaging and targeting membrane-associated protein and lipid, as well as secreted protein, to their appropriate destinations, the Golgi apparatus modifies certain proteins and lipid received from the ER. Glycolipids are formed in the Golgi by the addition of oligosaccharide chains to ceramide; in addition, further processing of glycoproteins continues in the Golgi.

The Golgi apparatus is made up of a set of flattened, membrane-bound cisternae and associated tubulovesicular elements and membrane-bound vesicles in the process of being transported between ER, Golgi and other locations. The stacks of Golgi cisternae are biochemically distinct and the entire stack is polarised, so that a *cis* or entry face and a *trans* or exit face, exist. The *cis* face lies adjacent to ER and is the site of vesicular traffic back and forth between the ER and Golgi. The *trans* face is the site of formation of a number of types of vesicles that convey material to the plasma membrane, produce secretory vesicles and form lysosomes. Integral membrane proteins, membrane lipids and soluble cisternal protein formed by the ER traverse the Golgi and are targeted to their appropriate destinations by this organelle. Three major routes of export from the Golgi occur: (i) constitutive delivery of membrane-bound vesicles to the plasma membrane, (ii) formation of secretory vesicles whose exocytosis is regulated, and (iii) formation of lysosomes. Specific targeting signals are associated with the formation of lysosomal vesicles and secretory vesicles; however, the path way from the Golgi apparatus to the plasma membrane appears to be largely constitutive and unregulated, forming a default pathway.

Proteins destined to be secreted in a regulated manner (e.g. release of hormones from endocrine cells) are concentrated and packaged in membrane-bound vesicles formed by the *trans* Golgi. These secretory vesicles are stored in the cytoplasm until signals to fuse with the plasma membrane are received, resulting in the liberation of their contents outside the cell. Targeting mechanisms exist that direct secretory vesicles to the appropriate cellular location for release. For example, some secretory vesicles are released from the apical plasma membranes of epithelial cells, whereas others fuse with basolateral membranes.

Proteins destined for lysosomes are tagged with mannose-6-phosphate (M6P) groups in the Golgi. M6P receptors are present in Golgi membranes and vesicles containing lysosomal proteins bound to M6P receptors bud off from the Golgi and fuse with endosomes to form mature lysosomes. During this process, M6P receptors are recycled for repeated use by vesicular trafficking from endosome to Golgi apparatus.

Lysosomes

Lysosomes are the digestive organelles of the cell and are filled with acid hydrolases that are most active at a pH of about 5.0. Lysosomal vesicles from the Golgi apparatus fuse with endosomes that have received material from endocytotic vesicles. Endosomes have a moderately acidic pH of about 6.0 that promotes dissociation of ligand from internalised plasma membrane receptors as well as dissociation of lysosomal hydrolases from M6P receptors. Both types of receptors are recycled by being routed back toward the plasma membrane and the Golgi apparatus in membranous vesicles that are pinched off from endosomes. The endosome then matures to form a lysosome by condensing into a spherical or irregular membrane-bound structure. Proton pumps in the membrane of the maturing lysosome lower the pH inside the organelle to maximally activate the acid hydrolases to digest the internalised material. Other transporters exist in the lysosomal membrane to allow digested organic molecules to enter the cytoplasm for use by the cell.

In addition to the confluence of lysosomal and endocytotic vesicles at endosomes, material can be targeted for lysosomal degradation by at least two other mechanisms. Neutrophils and macrophages are cells specialised for the engulfment of bacteria and other large particulate material, which are internalised by phagocytosis. Lysosomes fuse with these large phagocytotic vesicles to deliver their hydrolases, resulting in the formation of phagosomes. Lysosomes also contribute to the breakdown of cellular material that is not needed or should be turned over. Excess, old or malfunctioning organelles can be targeted for destruction by becoming enveloped by cisternae of ER, which then fuse with lysosomal vesicles to form autophagosomes. Recently, evidence has been gathered suggesting that a fourth route to lysosomes may exist that involves the transport of single cytoplasmic molecules through the lysosomal membrane by specific transport proteins.

Membrane Flow

It is apparent that there is a complex, but effective and elegant, flow of membranes and molecules between the various organelles and cytoplasmic compartments of eukaryotic cells. With the exception of mitochondria and peroxisomes, the membranes of all organelles, vesicles and the plasma membrane are initially produced by the ER, modified and packaged by the ER and Golgi, then targeted and delivered via the trafficking of membrane-bound vesicles. A number of different types of signals and targeting mechanisms are used to regulate this flow of the membrane. Between the ER and Golgi, vesicles are coated with coat proteins (COPs), that either direct vesicles from the ER to the Golgi (COPII) or direct vesicles from the Golgi to the ER (COPI). Although no mechanisms appear to exist that restrict the flow of material from the ER to the Golgi, the amino acid sequences KDEL and KKXX (where X is any amino acid) mark lumenal and integral membrane proteins, respectively, for return transport from the Golgi to the ER. Thus, proteins with these sequences are essentially restricted to the ER by being rapidly returned from the Golgi apparatus. The exact mechanism of membrane flow through the Golgi apparatus has been a matter of some debate, but at least part of the flow appears to be carried out by membrane-bound vesicles. The flow of membrane from the Golgi to plasma membrane includes a constitutive, default pathway that operates in the absence of specific targeting signals. However, delivery of material to secretory vesicles and lysosomes requires defined targeting information. Interestingly, clathrin is involved in the formation of lysosomal and secretory vesicles from the *trans* Golgi, but not in the constitutive formation of vesicles destined for the plasma membrane. In addition to the ER and Golgi apparatus, bi-directional membrane flow also occurs between plasma membrane and endosome, and plasma membrane and Golgi. Clathrin-coated endocytotic vesicles from the plasma membrane travel inward to fuse with endosomes and the receptors subsequently return to the plasma membrane via small vesicles formed from endosomal membranes. Endocytotic vesicles formed from caveolae may bypass lysosomes and fuse directly with Golgi or ER. Although the details of vesicular targeting are not well understood, it has been proposed that SNARE (soluble N-ethylmaleimide-sensitive-factor attachment protein receptors) proteins on the surfaces of membrane-bound vesicles (v-SNAREs) and target organelles (t-SNAREs) mediate the correct patterns of docking between vesicles and organelles.

Mitochondria

The primary function of mitochondria is to convert energy sources into forms that can be used to drive cellular reactions. Not surprisingly, they comprise a significant volume of the cell-normally, about 20 per cent of the total cell mass. Mitochondria replicate by a process involving growth and fission of preexisting mitochondria. Interestingly, mitochondria contain their own DNA that resembles the genome of prokaryotes. Based on this and other lines of evidence, it appears that mitochondria (and plastids in plant cells) arose by the colonisation of eukaryotic cells by prokaryotes early in their evolution. Although mitochondria contain DNA and are able to carry out transcription and translation, they only produce about 5 per cent of their protein, the rest being encoded by nuclear genes and synthesised by cytoplasmic ribosomes. They also appear to obtain most of their membrane lipid from the ER, mediated by of phospholipid transfer proteins that shuttle these molecules from the ER to the various organelles, including mitochondria.

Cells use ATP as their primary energy source and the main function of mitochondria is the production of ATP from food sources. Energy is obtained from the oxidation of food by the sequential transfer of high energy electrons to lower energy states; the released energy is used to drive membrane-bound proton pumps, thus establishing an electrochemical gradient. Protons are then allowed to flow back across the membrane down their concentration gradient and the released energy is used to drive the synthesis of ATP from ADP and Pi. The electrons are ultimately transferred to O_2 and the entire process is therefore referred to as oxidative phosphorylation.

Mitochondrial structure

Mitochondria are composed of two membranes, that enclose distinct compartments. The outer mitochondrial membrane is somewhat permeable to small molecular weight compounds (<5000 daltons); conversely, the inner membrane contains a very high ratio of protein to lipid and movement of material past this membrane is tightly regulated. The space between the two membranes is called the intermembrane space and the compartment delimited by the inner membrane is called the mitochondrial matrix. The inner membrane is folded into sheet or tube-like invaginations within the matrix, thus increasing its surface area. The increased surface area of this membrane allows mitochondria to house greater numbers of electron transport enzyme systems and ATP synthase complexes. The intermembrane space resembles the cytoplasm, but the internal matrix is biochemically distinct. The matrix is the site of conversion of pyruvate and fatty acids to acetyl CoA and is the location of the citric acid cycle, where acetyl CoA is oxidised.

Chemiosmotic generation of ATP

With respect to energy production, the pathways of carbohydrate and lipid metabolism converge in the generation of acetyl CoA in the mitochondrial matrix. Carbohydrate is converted to glucose-6-phosphate, which, as a substrate for glycolysis, gives rise to two pyruvate molecules. Pyruvate is transported to the mitochondrial matrix were it is converted to acetyl CoA by the pyruvate dehydrogenase complex. Fatty acids are oxidised in the mitochondrial matrix, releasing acetyl groups that are then linked to CoA. Acetyl CoA derived from carbohydrate and fatty acid metabolism is fed into the citric acid cycle, resulting in the production of CO_2 and NADH. NADH conveys high energy electrons to the electron transport chain, which is located on inner mitochondrial membrane. The electron transport chain is a complex composed of at least 40 different proteins. The actual transfer of electrons is carried out by a number of different heme groups linked to various cytochromes, iron-sulphur centre-containing proteins, ubiquinone, copper atoms and a flavin. These are organised into three large enzyme complexes, with ubiquinone and cytochrome C serving as carriers of electrons between the complexes. The three complexes are the NADH dehydrogenase complex, the cytochrome B-C1 complex and the cytochrome oxidase complex. Electrons shuttled across these complexes move from high to low energy states, with the released energy used to pump H^+ from the matrix to the intermembrane space. Then, H^+ is allowed to flow down its concentration gradient (from the intermembrane space to the matrix) through the ATP synthase complex. This is a large transmembrane complex of about 5,00,000 daltons that contains multiple proteins, and constitutes about 15 per cent of the total inner membrane protein.

The energy that is released is used to couple Pi to ADP to make ATP. Finally, the electrons used to drive the H^+ pumps are combined with O_2 and H^+. Thus, the generation of ATP from high energy electrons by this chemiosmotic mechanism consumes O_2 and produces water.

Other mitochondrial functions

In addition to converting food energy into ATP, mitochondria also are involved in a number of other functions, including Ca^{2+} regulation and apoptotic signalling. Like the ER, mitochondria sequester Ca^{2+} to help keep cytoplasmic levels low. In addition to producing ATP, the H^+ gradient can be used to import Ca^{2+} into the mitochondrial matrix, where it is used in part to help regulate the activity of certain mitochondrial enzymes. Deposits of calcium can be formed in mitochondria in response to high cytoplasmic levels of Ca^{2+}. Mitochondria are also involved in the regulation of programmed cell death or apoptosis. A central mechanism by which apoptosis is carried out involves activation of the caspase family of proteases. Release of cytochrome C by mitochondria facilitates caspase activation by forming a complex with other molecules (e.g. APAF-1) and pro-caspases to activate the caspase cascade. Release of cytochrome C from mitochondria can occur in response to specific membrane signalling events, as well as from cytoplasmic, mitochondrial or nuclear damage.

Peroxisomes

Peroxisomes are membrane-bound vesicular organelles that are involved in various oxidative reactions. They contain high concentrations of enzymes that are able to form H_2O_2 by the transfer of hydrogen atoms from substrates to molecular oxygen. In addition, peroxisomes contain catalase, which breaks down H_2O_2 to oxidise various substrates, including some types of toxins. Like mitochondria, peroxisomes replicate by fission and growth of preexisting organelles. All protein and lipid of the peroxisome is synthesised in the cytoplasm and subsequently imported into the peroxisomal membrane and lumen.

Cytoskeleton

The cytoskeleton of eukaryotic cells is composed of a complex system of proteinaceous filaments that are present in both cytoplasm and nucleus. The three major cytoskeletal systems elaborated by cells are microfilaments, microtubules and intermediate filaments. These different cytoskeletal systems are biochemically and functionally distinct.

Microfilaments

Microfilaments are small solid filaments about 6 nm in diametre, composed of the 45 kDa globular protein actin. Actin is one of the most abundant proteins in cells, composing up to 5 per cent or more of the total cell protein. Microfilaments help support and organise the plasma membrane and are involved in cell motility and the maintenance of cell shape, serving as the muscle of the cell.

A large number of actin-associated proteins mediate the functions of microfilaments, including regulating actin polymerisation (e.g. profilin, WASp and ARP), cross-linking microfilaments to form organised arrays (e.g. filamin, fimbrin and villin), interacting with membrane proteins to establish and maintain distinct membrane domains (e.g. vinculin, catenins and Z0-1 of tight junctions) and functioning as motor proteins (e.g. type I and II myosins) to carry out motility events. Much of the actin in cells is present as soluble monomers (g-actin) bound to profilin. This interaction inhibits the polymerisation actin monomers into filaments (f-actin). Signals from the plasma membrane, mediated in large part by small GTP-binding proteins (e.g. rac and rho), activate WASp and ARP proteins, to promote the dissociation of profilin from g-actin and seed the growth of new microfilaments from the sides of preexisting microfilaments. Microfilament polymerisation is controlled by the addition of capping proteins to the end of growing filaments and turnover of filaments occurs by the actions of microfilament cutting proteins such as gelsolin, followed by depolymerisation of f-actin to g-actin and association of the latter with profilin. Although some cell movements and membrane activities appear to be driven by the polymerisation and depolymerisation of actin, many other types of actin-associated motility require the interaction of microfilaments with myosin motor molecules. Myosin functions as an actin-activated ATPase, undergoing cycles of microfilament attachment and detachment, with associated conformational changes, resulting in power strokes. These events are linked to the binding, hydrolysis and release of ATP, Pi and ADP. Myosin activity can slide microfilaments past each other, transport vesicles and other cargo down microfilaments and deform membranes that are attached to microfilaments.

A number of mutations are known that interfere with microfilament functioning. WASp protein was discovered as the protein mutated in Wiscott-Aldrich syndrome, which results from deficits in the ability of actin to polymerise. Dystrophin is a large linking molecule that interconnects submembrane arrays of microfilaments to integral membrane proteins and ECM proteins in skeletal muscle cells. Mutations in dystrophin that interfere with its ability to link microfilaments with the plasma membrane weaken the plasma membrane, causing the eventual death of the muscle cell and giving rise to some forms of muscular dystrophy.

Microtubules

Microtubules are small hollow proteinaceous tubes about 25 nm in diametre, composed of the protein tubulin. Microtubules function to organise the cytoplasm and mediate intracellular motility events. They are associated with motor proteins that interact with membrane-bound organelles and vesicles to help determine their location and organisation within the cytoplasm. They also carry out crucial functions in cell division, forming the spindle apparatus that segregates replicated chromosomes among the daughter cells. Microtubules also support and power cilia and flagella, which are highly motile appendages produced by ciliated epithelial cells and sperm.

Unlike microfilaments and intermediate filaments discussed below, microtubules are associated with a distinct organising, centre, called the centrosome (or MTOC, for microtubule-organising centre). The centrosome is composed of a pair of centrioles surrounded by an amorphous mass of pericentriolar material. Centrioles themselves are short, barrel-like arrays of microtubules and are associated with the ability of the centrosome to replicate. Pericentriolar material is a biochemically complex layer of amorphous material that surrounds the centrioles, which, both nucleates microtubule growth and anchors the ends of microtubules. Three types of tubulin genes are expressed in eukaryotic cells, including α, β and γ-tubulin. Microtubules are composed of heterodimers of α and β-tubulin; γ-tubulin is a component of the pericentriolar material. Microtubules possess an intrinsic polarity and are all oriented so one end (the minus end) is anchored in the pericentriolar material, with the free end (the plus end) extending into the cytoplasm. Microtubule polymerisation and depolymerisation occurs at the plus end and involves the addition or removal of α-β heterodimers. Heterodimers of α and β-tubulin are associated with GTP or GDP. GTP-containing heterodimers readily polymerise, whereas GDP-containing heterodimers bind much more weakly to each other and tend to dissociate. GTPases that hydrolyse microtubule-bound GTP to GDP are present in the cytoplasm; however, because heterodimer addition and removal occur at just the plus end, as long as the terminal tubulin subunits are associated with GTP, the microtubule will grow by the addition of GTP-containing heterodimers. Occasionally, the GTPase activity catches up with a growing end of the microtubule, hydrolysing GTP to GDP in the terminal subunits. At this point, the microtubule rapidly disassembles, shrinking in size back toward the centrosome. Depolymerising microtubules can be rescued and regrown if sufficiently high concentrations of GTP-containing tubulin heterodimers are present so that the GTP cap can be reestablished. Because of these events, most microtubules in the cell continuously oscillate between slow growth and rapid depolymerisation, a feature that has been called dynamic instability.

Like the microfilament cytoskeleton, the organisation and functions of microtubules are regulated and carried out by associated proteins. Microtubule-associated proteins are generally categorised as either structural proteins or motor proteins. Structural proteins include higher molecular weight proteins called MAPs (for microtubule-associated protein) and lower molecular weight tau proteins. Structural MAPs and tau are thought to help organise microtubule arrays in the cytoplasm. Microtubule-associated motor proteins include dynein and kinesin, both of which, like myosin, undergo cycles of binding, conformational changes and dissociation in an ATP-dependent manner to move microtubules past each other or to move cargo along microtubules. Microtubule-mediated intracellular transport is carried out by multiple members of both the dynein and kinesin families of protein, but ciliary and flagellar motility selectively utilise dynein. The microtubule bundle, or axoneme, supporting a cilium is anchored in a specialised centrosome called a basal body. Unlike regular centrosomes, axoneme microtubules originate as direct extensions from one of the centrioles in a basal body and not from associated pericentriolar material. Axoneme microtubules form circular arrays of doublets surrounding a central pair of microtubules. The outer microtubule doublets are associated with dynein, which spans adjacent microtubule pairs. Dynein motor activity attempts to slide microtubule pairs past each other, which is converted into a bending of the cilium because the bases of the microtubule pairs are attached to the basal body and are not free to slide. In this way, hydrolysis of ATP by dynein powers the rapid, whip-like movements of cilia and flagellae in a microtubule-dependent manner. Other forms of microtubule-mediated motility occur in the cytoplasm, where membrane-bound vesicles, organelles and other cargo associated with dynein or kinesin move along microtubules. Motor proteins exhibit a directionality which allows for vectorial transport of material within the cell. Dyneins move cargo toward the minus ends of microtubules and kinesins generally move cargo toward the plus ends of microtubules (although minus end-directed members of the kinesin family are known).

In dividing cells, centrosomes replicate along with DNA in S-phase and subsequently participate in the formation of the mitotic spindle. Daughter centrosomes move apart and promote the complete reorganisation of the microtubular cytoskeleton prior to and during, nuclear envelope breakdown. The plus ends of microtubules radiating from the centrosomes, now called spindle poles, bind and become stabilised by the kinetochores of chromosomes, forming distinct bundles of kinetochore microtubules. Microtubule-mediated motility events at the kinetochore line chromosomes up on the metaphase plate and are subsequently responsible for the separation of daughter chromosomes in anaphase of mitosis. Pinching the cell into two daughter cells (mediated by bundles of microfilaments in association with the plasma membrane at the cleavage furrow) leads to the inheritance of the correct number of chromosomes and a single centrosome by each daughter cell. Interestingly, other organelles such as mitochondria and peroxisomes appear to be randomly apportioned to each daughter cell by virtue of the fact that they are distributed throughout the cytoplasm, whereas the ER and Golgi apparatus vesiculate and disperse throughout the cytoplasm early in mitosis to be inherited in the same way.

A number of drugs interfere with microtubule dynamics; examples include colchicine, which actively promotes tubulin depolymerisation; and taxol, which stabilises microtubules and inhibits depolymerisation. Both of these drugs are toxic to cells, indicating that the oscillation between polymerisation and depolymerisation is crucial to microtubule function. A number of taxol-based compounds have been developed for use in the chemotherapeutic treatment of cancer, highlighting the importance of microtubule dynamics in cell division.

Intermediate filaments

Intermediate filaments (IF) are solid filaments about 10 nm in diametre, made up of one or more of a large family of intermediate filament proteins. Intermediate filaments are found in both the cytoplasm and the nucleus. They function in strengthening the cytoplasm of cells, as well as in mechanically integrating cells of a tissue by interconnecting desmosomes and hemidesmosomes. The IF family of proteins is the most complex family of cytoskeletal proteins, with over 50 different IF gene products elaborated by cells of higher vertebrates. IF proteins can be divided into five groups: (i) acidic keratins, (ii) neutral/basic keratins, (iii) vimentin-like proteins, (iv) neurofilament proteins, and (v) lamins. Intermediate filament proteins are expressed in tissue-specific patterns, with epithelial cells containing keratins, cells of mesenchymal origin expressing vimentin-like IF proteins and neuronal cells expressing neurofilament IF proteins. Lamins are present in essentially all nucleated cells and form a filamentous network underlying and supporting the inner membrane of the nuclear envelope. There is evidence that lamins help organise chromatin and are involved in some aspects of DNA synthesis, as well.

IF proteins are long, rod-like molecules that contain a central domain rich in α-helices. The rod domain of IF proteins coil around each other to form coiled-coil dimers, which then associate into higher order structures, much like weaving together individual strands to form a rope. The polymerisation state of IF proteins is mediated by phosphorylation and it has been suggested that hyperphosphorylation of IF proteins leads to dissociation of IFs by repulsion of subunits bearing multiple negative phosphate charges. One of the best studied examples is the depolymerisation and repolymerisation of nuclear lamina filaments during cell division. At the onset of mitosis, lamins are hyperphosphorylated and the nuclear lamina depolymerises, facilitating nuclear envelope breakdown. At the end of mitosis, lamins are dephosphorylated and the nuclear lamina and nuclear envelope reforms around the daughter nuclei.

Only a relatively few IF-associated proteins are known and these appear to help organise intermediate filaments and mediate interactions with other cytoskeletal proteins and organelles. Intermediate filaments frequently form a dense basketwork around the nucleus; thus, the nucleus of many cells is supported both by an internal IF lamina, as well as protected by a cytoplasmic network of IF fibres.

Nuclear Organisation

The largest and most prominent structure in most cells is the nucleus. It serves as the repository and organising centre for the genome. In human, chromosomal DNA—of a total length of about two metres when fully extended—is packaged into an average nuclear size of about 10 μM (1/100 of a millimetre) in diametre. The DNA must be packaged in such a way as to allow access to transcriptional and replication machinery and extensive nuclear-cytoplasmic transport must occur. These functions are mediated by the organisation of DNA within the nucleus and the organisation of the nuclear envelope.

The nucleus is bounded by the nuclear envelope, which is comprised of two membranes (the inner and outer nuclear membranes), the nuclear lamina and numerous nuclear pores that span the inner and outer membranes. Nuclear pores are multimolecular arrays exhibiting eight-fold symmetry that are involved in the exchange of material between cytoplasm and nucleus. Material moves through nuclear pores by both passive diffusion and by active transport; molecules smaller than 5000 daltons are freely permeable between nucleus and cytoplasm, but those larger than about 60000 daltons must be actively transported. Molecules between these sizes can move between nucleus and cytoplasm without being actively transported, but take longer to equilibrate with increasing size.

Proteins actively transported into the nucleus contain nuclear localisation sequences that are recognised by the pore complexes. Nuclear localisation signals vary in amino acid sequence, but usually contain a number of lysines and are positively charged.

The first step in DNA packaging involves the winding of DNA around octamers of histone proteins, which are positively charged proteins that closely interact with the negatively charged DNA.

This first order of DNA packing gives rise to a beads on a string appearance, with the beads or nucleosomes, composed of about 200 base pairs of DNA wrapped almost twice around a histone octamer core. Nucleosomes are further coiled to form a 30 nm diametre solenoid fibre, which loops out to form euchromatin (loosely compacted and generally active DNA) or becomes more tightly compacted to form heterochromatin (tightly compacted and relatively inactive DNA). Each chromosome usually consists of a mixture of heterochromatin and euchromatin and occupies a more-or-less defined region within the nucleus. Portions of a number of chromosomes that contain amplified sequences encoding ribosomal RNA and ribosomal protein mRNAs cluster together and associate with a number of other protein elements in the nucleus to form the nucleolus. This is a specialised area where transcription of ribosomal genes and assembly of ribosomal subunits occurs.

Mounting evidence suggests that chromosomes may be organised on a protein or protein-RNA based scaffolding. This scaffolding or nuclear matrix, is biochemically ill-defined, but appears to be composed of filaments that form a three-dimensional meshwork within the nucleus, which is surrounded by the denser filamentous mat of lamin IFs underlying the nuclear envelope. Although the composition of the nuclear matrix is not well-understood, it is possible that lamin IFs are not restricted to the nuclear periphery, but contribute to at least some of the matrix fibres. Certain DNA sequences bind to the nuclear matrix much more tightly than others, leading to the proposal that distinct matrix attachment regions or MARs, periodically link chromosomes to the matrix. These linkages result in the formation of large (20–200 kilobase) loops of DNA tethered to the matrix at MAR domains. MAR DNA sequences do not display a rigid consensus sequence, but have a number of distinguishing features, including being relatively AT-rich, histone-poor and possessing multiple topoisomerase II binding sequences. MAR domain DNA also may confer position independent expression of exogenous DNA incorporated into random sites within the genome. Thus, it has been proposed that MAR domains form long-range regulatory elements helping to control gene expression.

The high concentrations of DNA, RNA and protein in the nucleus make it challenging to study nuclear structure. However, some structural aspects of gene expression and mRNA processing can be visualised by electron microscopy in the form of perichromatin fibres and interchromatin granules. These structures represent sites of RNA processing and include mRNA as well as associated ribonucleoproteins and RNAs that form elements of the splicing machinery, including spliceosomes and splicing islands.

Thus, living eukaryotic cells must carry out and coordinate an enormous number of biochemical reactions in order to obtain and convert energy to usable forms, breakdown and interconvert organic molecules to synthesise needed components, sense and respond to environmental and internal stimuli, regulate gene activity, sense and repair damage to structural and genomic elements, grow and reproduce. This level of complexity requires that biochemical reactions be highly organised and compartmentalised and this is the major function of cell organelles and the cytoskeleton. Cells have elaborated an elegant cytoplasmic membrane system composed of the nuclear envelope, endoplasmic reticulum (ER), Golgi apparatus, and associated endocytotic, endosomal, lysosomal and secretory vesicles. These membrane systems serve to both organise and compartmentalise biochemical reactions involved in protein and lipid synthesis, targeting and secretion. The cytoskeleton facilitates not only cytosolic molecular interactions, but also serves to organise the entire cytoplasmic membrane system. The key to cellular life is organisation and eukaryotic cells display a remarkably rich and elegant architecture to carry out the demands of life.

CELL SIGNALLING

Intercellular communication is essential for development and homeostatic function in multicellular organisms. The language of intercellular communication takes many different forms. These include protein growth factors, e.g. local paracrine, like Fibroblast growth factor (FGF), blood-borne endocrine growth hormone; hydrophobic steroids, e.g. estrogen; lipid mediators, prostaglandins, leukotrienes; modified amino acids, e.g. neurotransmitters such as adrenaline and other metabolites, e.g. nitric oxide. This section will focus largely on small protein growth factors that modulate growth, differentiation, apoptosis and steady state function during development and in the adult.

An essential role of signal-transduction is to coordinate functions of diverse cell types and sets of identical cells within an organ that require close and synchronous activity in the multicellular organism. The speed of intercellular communication is dependent on distance and the mode of delivery of the intercellular signal. Local or paracrine intercellular communication acts within milliseconds over distances less than 10–20 cell diametres (approx 200 microns), but endocrine or blood-borne signalling that occurs over a distance of metres requires minutes. Specialised short distance signalling, like that mediated by gap junctions, allows linked cells to share small intracellular signal-transduction intermediates downstream of receiving cell-surface receptors. Specialised long distance signalling, over a distance of metres, can be expedited to the millisecond range, by increasing the conductance speed. This is accomplished by saltatory movement of signals in neurons coupled with the fast action of neurotransmitters at post-synaptic membranes.

Once the interactor, i.e. the ligand, has bound to its receptor, intracellular signal transduction is initiated. After the receptor is activated by phosphorylation; receptor binding of nonenzymatic docking molecules like IRS-1 (insulin-receptor substrate) peaks within 1 minute. At the end of this signal transcription pathway, phosphorylation of transcription AP-1 factor initiates transcription of c-fos within 1 minute which peaks within 15 minutes. Other hormones, such as estrogen activate transcription over slower time periods, approaching 1 hour. In some signal-transduction processes, such as vision, the complete process of photons activating rhodopsin is computed in one second.

Receptor

If the ligands are the words of intercellular language, the receptors are the ears. *Trans*-membrane plasmalemma receptors are of several types:

1. Receptor tyrosine kinases such as the FGF receptor.
2. Serine-threonine kinase receptors such as the TGF-β receptor.
3. Nonenzymatic transmembrane receptors (e.g. integrins) that are linked to intracellular tyrosine kinases (e.g. focal adhesion kinase [FAK] and proline rich tyrosine kinase tyrosine kinases [PYK2]).
4. Seven transmembrane spanners receptors linked to G-proteins (e.g. Wnt ligand-wingless and int oncogene and its receptor; frizzled).
5. Nonenzymatic receptors that are linked to signalling pathways which are derepressed by allosteric-conformational changes (e.g. smoothened receptor for hedgehog ligand).
6. Receptors which are proteolytically converted to ligand (e.g. the Notch intracellular C terminal domain).

Another class of signalling receptors is located in the cytoplasm. They bind hydrophobic hormones such as steroids (e.g. estrogen), thyroid hormones and retinoic acid ligands. They are then translocated to the nucleus; where they act as transcription factors.

Signal Cascade

Signalling cascades within the cell start as allosteric changes in the receptor or nonenzymatic docking proteins (e.g. the IRS-1 family and FRS-2). These convey the signal by conformational change and by becoming targets for phosphorylation by receptor kinases. In either case, the function of the signal-transduction pathway is to quickly amplify and directionally conduct information reaching the cell by transmitting it through a series of tyrosine and serine-threonine kinases.

The majority of the transmembrane receptors are in the off state until induced by an extracellular ligand. At this point receptors act like allosteric enzymes with the enzyme in the cytoplasmic domain. Many of the tyrosine kinases require multimer formation as there is not sufficient flexibility in the transmembrane alpha-helix to mechanically transduce the ligand-induced conformational change. Multimerisation brings together cytoplasmic enzyme domains that cross-activate and then signal downstream docking and enzymatic signal-transduction proteins.

The receptor is activated for a period of time before it is destroyed (internalised and degraded), desensitised (by phosphorylation by a receptor induced kinase such as β-adrenergic receptor kinase) or dephosphorylated. During the activation period, a single activation event can lead to a highly amplified signal-transduction event. For example, a single quantum of light activating the photoreceptor rhodopsin leads to the hydrolysis of one hundred thousand cGMP signalling molecules for the duration of 1 second. The activated receptor has multiple possible phosphorylation sites on the cytoplasmic domains. These are capable of interacting with large numbers of signalling intermediates that see the activated receptor through the *src* homology domain-2 (SH2) that bind phosphorylated tyrosines (Fig. 2.11).

This branching of pathway choices immediately downstream of the FGF receptor is summarised in Figs. 2.11 and 2.12. The array of these docking proteins distinguishes different cell types that may each express the same receptor and facilitates different signal types in cells with the same receptor. If the activated receptor is the hub of activity, the docking proteins provide the spokes that radiate out to multiple downstream targets. Docking proteins such as IRS-1 and FRS-2 (insulin and FGF receptor substrate) are receptor-binding proteins that can initiate many branches of the signal-transduction pathway. The importance of the additive effect of branched pathways is indicated by recent studies analysing the effects of mutating the phosphorylation/docking sites of the PDGF receptor on the activation of sets of newly transcribed genes. Sets of newly transcribed genes have been analysed for quality and magnitude of the induction using cDNA-based microarrays. The results suggest that more than one phosphorylation/docking site on the PDGF receptor is needed for the full and proper magnitude and breadth of the transcriptional response.

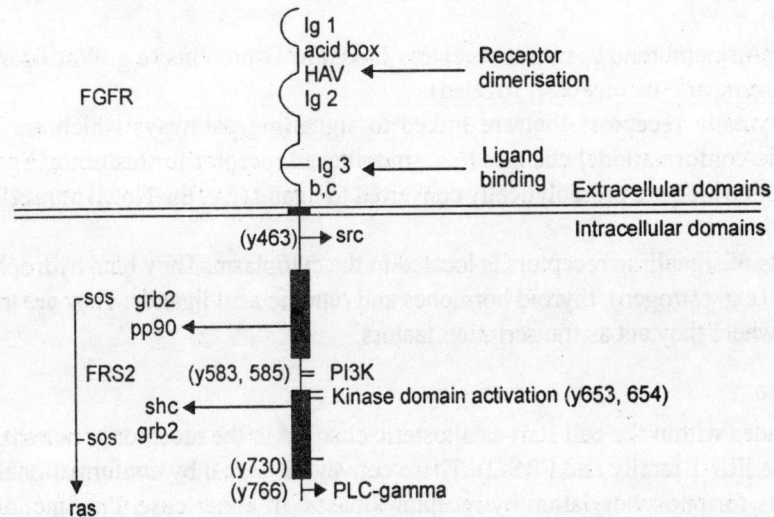

Fig. 2.11. The FGF receptor. The FGF receptor is an allosteric enzyme with the allosteric sites in the ectodomain and the enzymatic tyrosine kinase in the cytoplasm. Many mapped potentially functional and functionally active tyrosine activation sites are known.

There are three MAPK families (Figs. 2.12 and 2.13, Table 2.2), each having its own nonenzymatic signal-transduction intermediate before the G-protein/*ras* signal-transduction intermediate that is itself a GTPase. Thus, *ras* is a key component in mitogenic signal-transduction. There are 4 sequential vertical tiers of serine-threonine kinases (Table 2.2); each can have different horizontal interacting components. In the three MAPK signal-transduction pathways, the first two serine-threonine kinases have only cytoplasmic targets, whereas the last two tiers have both cytoplasmic targets and nuclear targets. Therefore, the activation of these last two tiers of serine-threonine kinases (MAPKs and MAPKAPS) can lead to nuclear localisation, transcription factor phosphorylation (e.g. Elk1 and ATF2 for ERK1,2) and gene transcription.

Other nontyrosine kinase initiated pathways also have homologous cytoplasmic signal transducers. For example, although it is thought that Raf-1 mediates the effects of the FGF receptor (Fig. 2.12, Table 2.2), Raf-1 homologs in the TGF-β pathway (TAK-1; Fig. 2.13, Table 2.2) and seven-spanner G-protein pathway (Raf-B; Fig. 2.13, Table 2.2) also act as cytoplasmic signal transducers. Branching of the pathway can occur at any tier of the vertical cascade (Table 2.2). Regulation of branching also distinguishes cell types and experience of the cell.

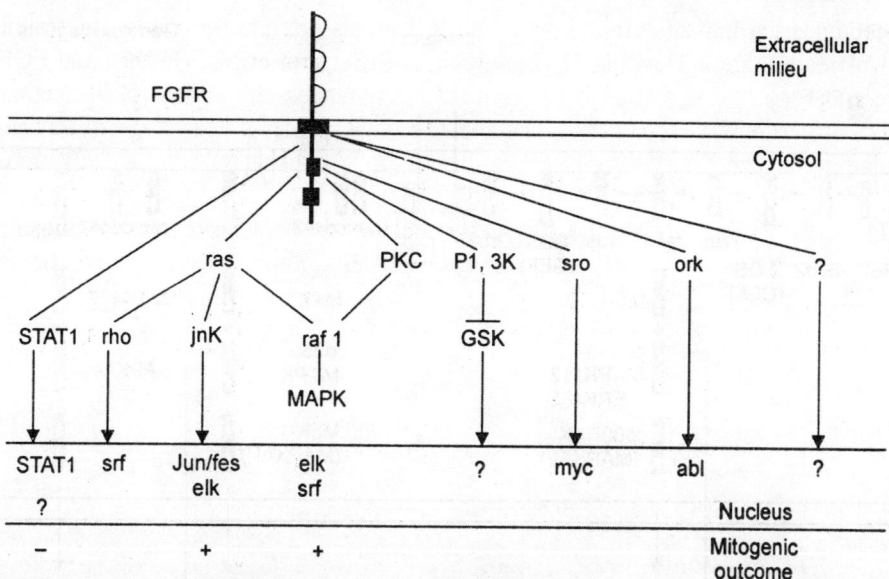

Fig. 2.12. Mitogenic and transcription activating signal-transduction pathways downstream of FGFR. A preponderance of evidence in cell lines suggests that the ras-MAP kinase pathway mediates the mitogenic signal of FGFR. Note that the *src*, crk are only indirectly implicated in FGFR signal-transduction due to sequence homology with other receptors and possible binding sites in the cytosolic domain. Jun kinase and P1,3 kinase can be mitogenic in certain circumstances, but mutation of the P1,3 kinase activating site in an FGFR *in vitro* did not prevent a mitogenic response to FGF. The STAT1 pathway has recently been shown to be anti-mitogenic in FGFR-3 mediated chondrocyte cell division cessation. The + indicate the most likely pathways for FGFR cell-division control.

Turning Off the Response

Signalling requires expeditious and tight control to maintain homeostasis and to ensure proper development. Control is exerted at all tiers of the pathway and at various levels of production and activation of the signal-transduction proteins. The receptor is activated for a period of time before it is destroyed, desensitised or dephosphorylated.

Other tiers of the pathway are regulated in similar ways. Ras is inactivated by GTPase activating proteins (GAPs), MEK family members are dephosphorylated and inactivated by protein phosphatase (PP)-1 and PP2A, ERK family members are dephosphorylated and inactivated by MAP kinase phosphatases MKP-3 and MKP6 and JNK is inactivated by M3/6. The mRNA transcripts for many of the signal-transduction genes have a consensus destruction sequence in the 3'-untranslated region that confers a short half-life. Rapid regulation is achieved at the levels of protein and mRNA stability, protein activation and signal-transduction.

Signal Transduction Pathways

A list of signal-transduction pathway websites is presented in Table 2.3. Information can be obtained on the activation of PKA and PKC, the mechanism of calcium-calmodulin signalling, prostaglandins and leukotrienes and nitric oxide. Other cytostatic pathways mediated by JAK-STAT receptors for the interferon-γ(IFN-γ) receptor and apoptosis pathways through tumour necrosis factor-α (TNF-α) are also included.

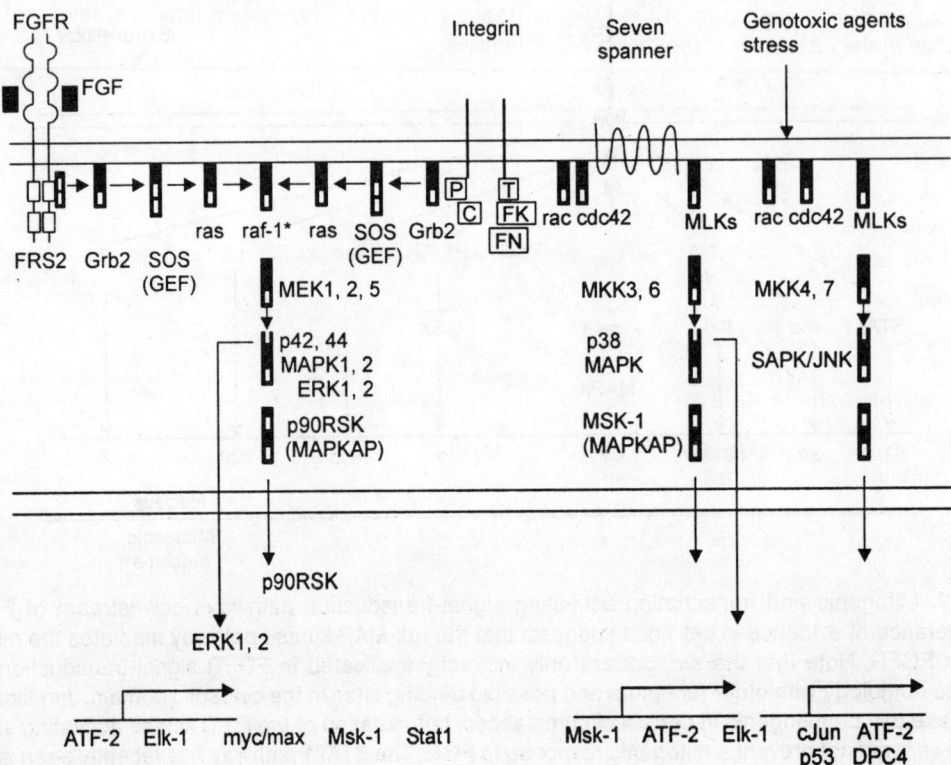

Fig. 2.13. The MAPK family. Each member is embedded in enzymatic cascades of intracellular serine-threonine kinases regulated by tyrosine kinases and allosteric docking proteins. The pathways initiate at the plasmalemma by receptor tyrosine kinases, ECM-binding integrins and G-protein binding receptors. ATF-2-Activating transcription factor 2, CRE-BP1, CREB2; Cas Crk-associated substrate, p130CAS; c-Raf Raf proto-oncogene S/T protein kinase; DPC-4-Deleted in pancreatic cancer locus 4, SMAD4; ELK1-Ets domain transcription factor, ERK-Extracellular signal-regulated kinase, MAPK; FAK-Focal adhesion kinase; FGF-fibroblast growth factor; FGFR-fibroblast growth factor receptor; FRS2-FGF receptor stimulated, lipid-anchored Grb2 binding protein; Fyn-src family tyrosine kinase; GEF Guanine nucleotide exchange factor (example is SOS son-of-sevenless); GRB2-Growth factor receptor-bound protein 2; JNK-Jun N-terminal kinase; Jun-transcription factor; MAPK-Mitogen-activated protein kinase; MAPKAP-MAP kinase-activated protein kinase 2; MEK-MAPK/ERK kinase, MAPKK; MKK MEK kinase; MLK-Mixed lineage kinase; MSK-I-Mitogen and stress-activated kinase 1; p53 Tumour suppressor protein that protects from DNA damage; Paxilin (P in integrin signalling complex); PYK2-Proline-rich tyrosine kinase-2; rac-G-protein; ras-G-protein; RSK-Ribosomal S6 kinase; SAPK-Stress-activated protein kinase; STAT-Signal transducer and activator of transcription.

Noncanonical pathways mediated by serine-threonine receptor kinases (TGF-β receptor) and novel pathways for signalling by derepressing seven spanner receptors (Hedgehog-ligand derepression of patched receptor by smoothened) are also included.

A novel signalling mechanism important in development, signalling by proteolytically cleaved ligand-activated receptor (delta ligand activation of the Notch protein that cleaves and translocates the protein to the nucleus), is at the Science website for signal transduction knowledge environment (website: http://www.stke.sciencemag.org).

Table 2.2. Extracellular to intracellular signal-transduction for three MAPK families: levels of signal-transduction in the cascades of the three MAPK families[a].

Ligand ↓	FGF1–23	Other ligands	
Receptor ↓	FGFR1–4	Other receptors	
Nonenzymatic Docking molecule 1 RTK binding ↓	FRS2	GAB1, 2	IRS1–4
Nonenzymatic Docking molecule 2 RTK binding Docking molecule 1 binding ↓	Grb2	shc	shb
Ras superfamily regulatory molecules ↓	SOS (GEF family)	GRF family rate limiting	GAP family vav
Ras superfamily G-protein family Enzyme ↓	*ras*	Rac	Rho dc42 Rap1
Kinase 1 (MEKK) Enzyme ↓	Raf-1	RafB KSR Tak1	
Kinase 2 ↓	MEK1, 2, 5	MEK3,6 MEK4,7	
Enzyme ↓	MAPK family One	MAPK family Two	MAPK family Three
Kinase 3 ↓	p42, 44 ERK1,2 MAPK1,2, MAPK5	p38MAPK SAPK/JUNK enzyme	
Kinase 4 Enzyme ↓	p90RSK	MAPKAP MNK1,2 MSK1	
Resident or Translocated nuclear Factors	Elkl myc/max pRSK90	MAPK family ATF-2 STAT1 Jun	

[a] FGF signalling is used as an example. See Fig. 2.13 caption for abbreviations.

Table 2.3. Signal transduction websites: Electronic resources for signal-transduction reagents and information.

Website: http://stke.sciencemag.org/

Signal-transduction knowledge environment (STKE). Excellent resource for broad and focused signal-transduction electronic and archival published literature. PDFs and full text articles with JPG figures are available. Requires AAAS membership and an STKE users fee

Website: http://kinase.oci.utoronto.ca/signallingmap.html

Very good focus with map of the 3 MAPK families and clickable short to long descriptions of molecules on the map

Website: http://www-personal.umich.edu/% 7Eino/List/

Good outline of signal-transduction pathways with links to PubMed discovery articles

Website: http://www.grt.kyushu-u.ac.jp/spadindex.html

Good, clickable diagrams, but not recently updated

Website: http://vlib.org/Science/Cell_Biology/signal_transduction.shtml

Good cross-referenced site for information about function and sequence references for signal-transduction genes

Website: http://www.cellsignal.com/

Company site. Short description of signalling intermediates in the literature and available antibodies. Also, check sections under pathway diagrams for other web resources

Website: http://www.cIontech.com/gfp/

Company site for signal-transduction expression transgenes

Website: http://www.scbt.com/

Company site. Short description of signalling intermediates in the literature and available antibodies. Also, check sections under pathway diagrams for other web resources

The Wnt-frizzled-GSK3-β-catenin pathways interaction with E-Cadherin-β-catenin are not discussed in this section. FGF receptor, integrin and G protein-activating receptors and their activation of the three MAPK families (Figs. 2.12 and 2.13) can be used to illustrate the basic principles of signal-transduction pathways.

Receptor Tyrosine Kinases (FGF Receptor) and Mitogenesis

Ligand-dependent autophosphorylation and activation of the FGFRs signals into four pathways leading to new transcription in cell lines (Figs. 2.11 and 2.12). Two of these, p38MAPK and Jun kinase, are generally not mitogenic in cell lines. The major FGFR mitogenic signalling pathway is the *ras*-Raf-1-MAPK pathway, also known as the universal cassette because of the weight of evidence for its mitogenic role in diverse cell lines. FGF activation of MAPK (ERK-1, ERK-2) is necessary and sufficient to activate transcription factors elk and SRF, leading to new transcription and a strong mitogenic response in cell lines.

A second pathway that mediates mitogenesis through the FGFRs leads to binding of phospholipase C (PLC)-γ and Ca^{2+}-dependent PI-3-kinase through phosphorylation of other unique tyrosine residues and the subsequent activation of phosphoinositol turnover, generation of diacylglycerol and the activation of PKC. There are three groups of PKC; conventional (α, β, γ), novel (η, ν, θ and ξ), atypical (λ). The ξ and atypical families are not mitogenic and are brain-specific. Activation of PKC-α, β and γ leads to an increased mitogenic response, primarily through Raf: 1 and MAPK, although this appears to be less important than the *ras*-dependent MAPK pathway. Substitution of the tyrosine on FGFR-1 responsible for PLC-γ binding and activation of PKC does not diminish FGF-dependent mitogenesis, suggesting that PKC is not necessary for mitogenesis. However, in studies with a related PDGF receptor, mutations causing inactivity in all tyrosine sites for mitogenic effects were rescued by the inclusion of the tyrosine that activates the PLC-PKC pathway. This suggested that the PKC pathway can be sufficient for mitogenesis. It is important to note that PKC and ras activate Raf-1 by a separate mechanism and that Raf-1 activates mitogenesis via MAPK activity. Therefore, the FGF receptor can activate Raf-1 through either pathway, although *ras* is most powerful. Recent analysis of the raf-1 null mutant has suggested that *ras* is the most important, but that the Raf-B, not Raf-1 is necessary for growth factor mediated mitogenesis.

As observed in cell lines, activation of *src* is a third possible pathway of FGFR cell cycle activation. The FGFR activation of *src* (Fig. 2.11) has not been found to be mitogenic for FGF, but is mitogenic in other cell lines and mediates functions like cell scattering and activation of nuclear transcription during PC-12 differentiation.

A fourth pathway where FGF activity suppresses cell division through STAT1 has been identified. In the gain-of-function mutation leading to sporadic nonfamilial dwarfism, a single change in a transmembrane amino acid in FGFR-3 results in a gain-of-function enzymatic activity that leads to cessation of the cell cycle in chondrocytes. Recently, suppression of chondrocyte division was shown to require STAT1 activity, but the mode of activation of STAT1 is not understood. The expression of the STAT1 pathway has not been tested in preimplantation embryos. However, STAT1 should be considered when interpreting results after perturbing FGF receptors.

MAPK Families

The structure of the cascading biochemical pathway of the three MAPK family pathways docking proteins and kinases, are very similar (Table 2.2, Fig. 2.13). However, functionally, the MAPK/ERK pathways are more mitogenic and the p38MAPK and SAPK/JNK pathways are cytostatic. The mechanistic basis of the separation of function is not clear, but is based more on the quantity of each type of transcription factor activated than the quality. Each MAPK family activates a large overlapping group of transcription factors (Fig. 2.13), but overexpression of receptors (increasing pathway strength), can change the outcome of mitogenesis to one of differentiation within a single cell type. Early studies examined functionally similar receptors (mitogenic FGF and PDGF) and did not compare receptors that mediate more diverse biological outcomes. In comparison, recent studies using cDNA microarrays have suggested that different factors result in transcriptional activation of similar sets of genes. Differences in strength of transcription is an important difference. The use of cDNA microarrays to analyse intermediate transcriptional outcomes (primary and secondary waves of induced transcription) with respect to upstream receptor signalling capacity and downstream biological outcome, will yield significant insights into the function of signalling pathways. As described in the section 'The Signal Cascade', the three MAPK family pathways go through similar tiers of nonenzymatic docking proteins and serine threonine kinases. Each of these tiers branch to affect cytoplasmic targets, but only the last two tiers of proteins migrate to the nucleus and directly affect transcription factors (Table 2.2, Fig. 2.13).

A long initial phase of research in signal-transduction has focused upon identifying novel signalling intermediates and their roles in the various pathways. The three MAPK families illustrate common features of related and interacting signal-transduction pathways: speed of transduction, amplification via cascading enzymatic activity, branching and interaction with other pathways, and distinct and shared biologic function mediated through shared and distinct and shared transcription factors. The next phases of research will focus on the function of all members within a family of signal-transduction genes as the human and mouse genome projects provide complete sets of family members. Large-scale approaches paint a broader picture of the responses of cells to ligands that induce distinct biological outcomes, such as cell death, mitosis, or motility. In this case, microarrays will be utilised to detect broad changes in signalling quantity and quality of the sets of transcription factors between normal cells and null mutants or cells with receptor mutants with differential signal-transduction capacities. For example, differences in transcriptional quantity and quality of functionally different receptors that activate mitogenesis through FGF receptor-ERK signalling, that block mitogenesis through TGF-β receptor-SMAD (contraction of Sma and Mad [Mothers against decapentaplegic] genes) signalling or induce apoptosis through TNF-α receptor-Fas-associated protein with death domain (FADD) signalling, are sure to be studied.

## Chapter 3

Transcription and Translation

INTRODUCTION

DNA contains the instructions needed to produce and regulate the components of a cell. This information is encoded in the order, or sequence, of the four possible nucleotide bases contained in the DNA polymer. Hydrogen bonding interactions between complementary base pairs bring two linear DNA polymers together to form a double helix. James Watson and Francis Crick not only deduced the double helical structure of DNA but also recognised that hydrogen bonding between complementary DNA bases would provide a mechanism for DNA duplication. Watson-Crick base pairing allows one strand of DNA to serve as a template for synthesis of a new strand by directing the incorporation of adenine opposite thymine and guanine opposite cytosine (Fig. 3.1). This complementary base pairing also provides a mechanism for preserving the code. If one strand of DNA is damaged, the other can be used as a template to regenerate the damaged strand and recover information encoded in its sequence.

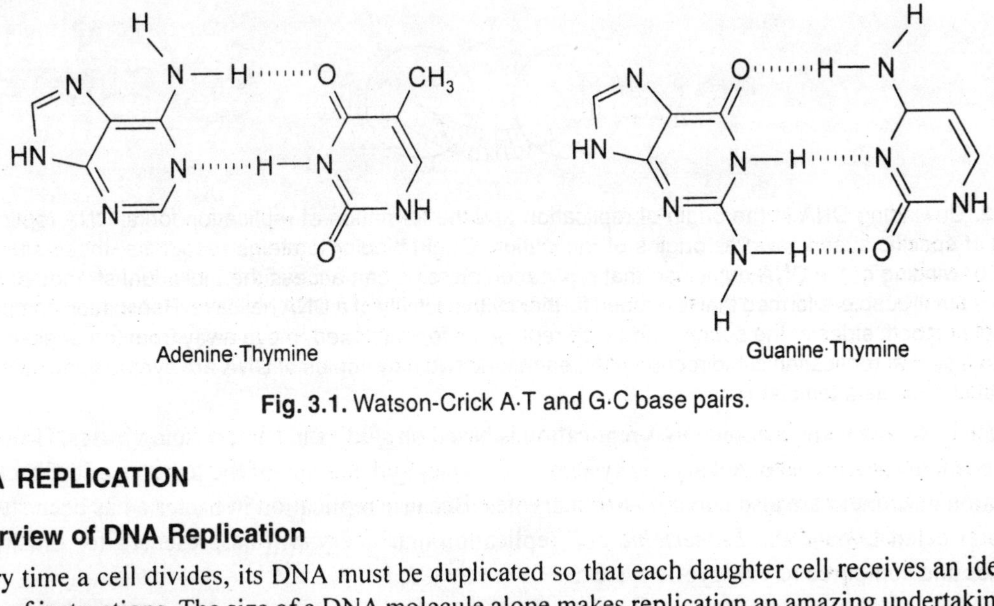

Adenine·Thymine   Guanine·Thymine

Fig. 3.1. Watson-Crick A·T and G·C base pairs.

DNA REPLICATION

Overview of DNA Replication

Every time a cell divides, its DNA must be duplicated so that each daughter cell receives an identical copy of instructions. The size of a DNA molecule alone makes replication an amazing undertaking. For example, human cells contain 3 billion base pairs of DNA divided into chromosomes ranging in size from about 50–250 million base pairs. If they were completely stretched out, these DNA molecules would range in length from about 1.7–8.5 cm. Many enzymes and proteins are required to physically manipulate these large polymers and to catalyse the synthesis of new DNA. These enzymes and the process of DNA replication are regulated by the cell so that replication is complete and genomes are duplicated only once every cell division.

DNA replication begins at a specific time in the cell cycle and at specific sites, origins of replication, in the genome. The DNA duplex is unwound at these replication origins to allow the enzymes that synthesise DNA access to the individual DNA strands (Fig. 3.2). Each strand of parental DNA serves as a template for a DNA polymerase to make a new strand of DNA. Single nucleotide monomers that form Watson-Crick pairs with template bases are incorporated into a new DNA polymer by DNA polymerases. As the new DNA grows, the parental duplex is progressively unwound forming replication forks that move away from the origin. DNA replication is semi-conservative, ultimately forming two DNA double helices that contain one strand of parental DNA and one strand of new DNA. In bacteria, replication forks move at a rate of about 500 nucleotides per second while in eukaryotes they move somewhat slower. Because genomes of eukaryotes are in general larger than bacteria and replication fork movement is slower, replication in eukaryotes is initiated at several origins instead of a single origin so that DNA duplication can be accomplished in a reasonable amount of time.

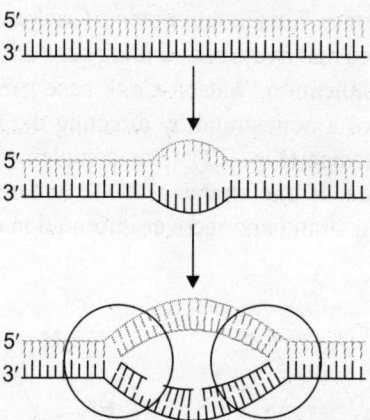

Fig. 3.2. Unwinding DNA at the origin of replication and the formation of replication forks. DNA replication begins at specific sites known as origins of replication. Origin binding proteins recognise, these sites and initiate unwinding of the DNA duplex so that replication proteins can access the individual strands of DNA. Initially a small bubble is formed that is opened further by the activity of a DNA helicase. Replication complexes assemble on both sides of the bubble and these replication forks (circled) move away from the origin in both directions so that replication is bidirectional. At, each fork, two new copies of DNA are synthesised using the parental strands as a templates.

Much of what we know about DNA replication is based on studies in bacteria and viruses. However, more recent investigations of eukaryotic systems are revealing that many of the features of the bacterial replication machinery are also common to eukaryotes. Because replication in bacteria has been studied in greater detail to date, the *Escherichia coli* replication machinery will be presented for illustrative purposes and compared to eukaryotic systems.

Initiation of DNA Replication

Origins of DNA replication contain two general DNA sequence elements, an element that is relatively easy to unwind, and an element that is recognised by initiation proteins. The genome of *E. coli* exists as a single circular DNA molecule of about 4.5 million base pairs and contains a single 245 base pair (bp) origin of replication, oriC. Within oriC are three 13-bp AT-rich regions of DNA that are relatively easy to unwind and four 9-bp regions that are recognised by the *E. coli* initiator protein, DnaA. A complex containing several DnaA molecules binds to oriC in the region containing the 9-bp repeats and bends the DNA. This bending helps to unwind the DNA helix at the 13-bp AT-rich sequences (Fig. 3.3). Many of the steps in DNA replication and repair, such as the unwinding of the origin, require energy to manipulate the structures of macromolecules and disrupt noncovalent interactions such as hydrogen bonding. The enzymes catalysing these changes utilise the chemical energy stored in the phosphate bonds of adenosine-5'-triphosphate (ATP) to do the mechanical work. The DnaA protein utilises the energy gained from ATP hydrolysis to power the unwinding of DNA at the origin. An origin recognition complex also exists in eukaryotes but its mechanism of action has not yet been completely defined.

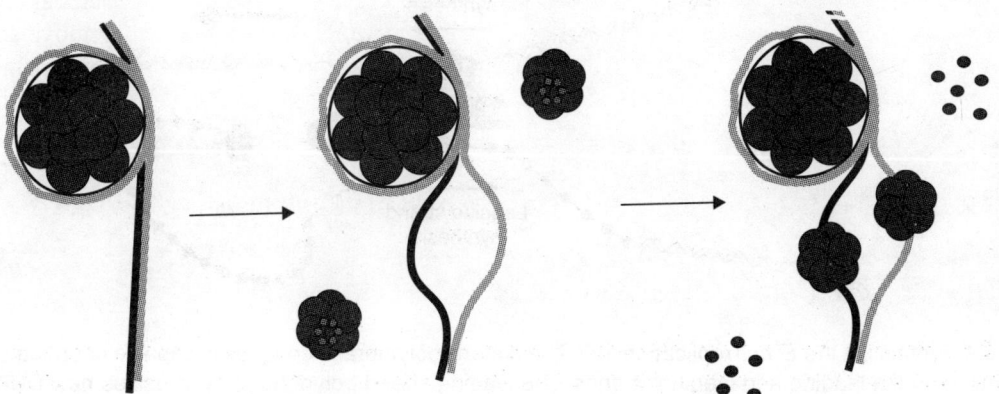

Fig. 3.3. Initiation of DNA replication at oriC in *E. coli*. DnaA protein binds to oriC to form a protein-DNA complex where the DNA is wrapped around several molecules of DnaA protein. DnaA binding induces unwinding of the DNA duplex at the A·T rich segments. DnaC protein binds the ring-shaped hexameric DnaB helicase and assembles the helicase onto the origin. One helicase complex is assembled at each fork of the replication bubble. After assembling the helicase, DnaC is released.

Once the DNA duplex is opened, a DNA helicase can be loaded onto the single-stranded DNA to continue the unwinding process. DNA helicases are enzymes that utilise the energy from hydrolysis of ribonucleoside 5-triphosphates, most commonly ATP, to break hydrogen bonding interactions between complementary DNA strands and unwind nucleic acid duplexes. In *E. coli*, six molecules of the DnaB protein form a ring-shaped hexamer that encircles single-stranded DNA and functions as a helicase. This hexameric helicase structure is common to other organisms including eukaryotes where the MCM (Mini-Chromosome Maintenance) proteins are believed to perform the function of replicative DNA helicase. In *E. coli*, the DnaB hexamer is assembled around DNA by the ATP-dependent activity of DnaC (Fig. 3.3).

Before DNA synthesis can begin, RNA primers must be made. DNA polymerases are unable to synthesise DNA *de novo* and can only extend RNA (or DNA) primers that are already paired with the template to be copied. Primases synthesise these primers using ribonucleoside 5'-triphosphates as building blocks to form a short strand of RNA complementary to the DNA template. The *E. coli* primase interacts with the DnaB helicase and begins synthesis of RNA primers shortly after DnaB has begun to unwind DNA. In eukaryotes, a hybrid RNA-DNA primer is synthesised by an enzyme complex containing both primase and DNA polymerase α. Once primers are formed, they can be extended by a DNA polymerase.

Enzymes at the Replication Fork

Assembly of a *replisome* is complete when the replicative DNA polymerase and its accessory proteins join the helicase and primase at the replication fork (Fig. 3.4). The replisome will then continue to synthesise new DNA, unwinding the parental duplex as it goes. The actual synthesis of new DNA is catalysed by a DNA polymerase contained within the replisome. Cells contain many different DNA polymerases that have different functions in DNA replication and repair. There are 5 known DNA polymerases in *E. coli* and at least a dozen in humans. In *E. coli*, DNA polymerase III catalyses the bulk of DNA synthesis during replication and DNA polymerase δ does so in eukaryotes.

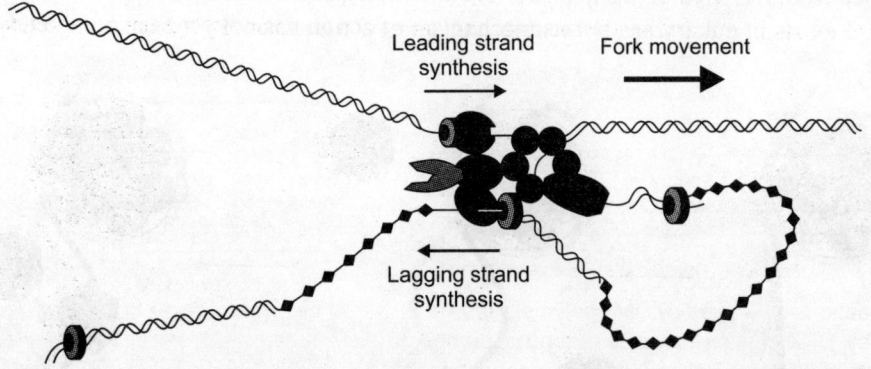

Fig. 3.4. Proteins at the *E. coli* replication fork. The dimeric polymerase complex is capable coordinated DNA synthesis on the leading and lagging strands. The leading strand polymerase synthesises new DNA in the direction of fork movement and the lagging strand polymerase synthesises DNA in the opposite direction. The hexameric helicase (light blue) unwinds DNA ahead of the polymerase and primase (red) makes RNA primers (red lines) on the lagging strand. Single-stranded DNA that forms as the helix unwinds is coated with single-stranded binding protein to prevent reannealing of strands and to remove secondary structure that may form within a single-strand. Sliding clamps (green) are assembled on each primer on the lagging strand by the clamp loading complex (yellow and dark blue).

All DNA polymerases use 2'-deoxyribonucleoside-5'-triphosphates (dNTPs) as monomeric building blocks for making DNA. They catalyse the attack of the 3' hydroxyl group of the nucleotide at the primer end on the α-phosphoryl group of an incoming dNTP displacing pyrophosphate (Fig. 3.5, upper panel). Thus, DNA polymerases extend DNA polymers in the 5' to 3' direction by incorporation of 2'-deoxyribonucleoside monophosphates. Watson-Crick base pairing interactions between the incoming dNTP and the next unpaired template base direct incorporation of correct nucleotides. Frequencies of adding incorrect nucleotides can be as low as one in a million, but even with this low error frequency mistakes will be made. To further reduce error frequencies, the DNA polymerases that function in replication contain a 3' to 5' exonuclease activity that allows them to *proofread* nucleotides that have been incorporated. This exonuclease activity catalyses the hydrolysis of phosphodiester bonds to remove the last nucleotide added to the 3' primer end (Fig. 3.5, lower panel). Thus, a nucleotide that has been added incorrectly can be removed.

The overall efficiency of synthesis by DNA polymerases is enhanced by accessory proteins which increase DNA polymerase processivity or the number of nucleotides incorporated per DNA binding event. These accessory proteins consist of a ring-shaped sliding clamp that binds both DNA and the DNA polymerase and a clamp loader that assembles the clamp on DNA. Sliding clamps, made of identical protein subunits, encircle DNA and are capable of sliding along a DNA duplex (Fig. 3.6). By binding a sliding clamp, a DNA polymerase is effectively tethered to a DNA template so that it is capable of incorporating thousands of nucleotides without dissociating. In the absence of a sliding clamp, DNA synthesis is less efficient because DNA polymerases frequently dissociate from the template and must rebind to continue. Sliding clamps are assembled around DNA by the ATP-dependent activity of clamp loaders.

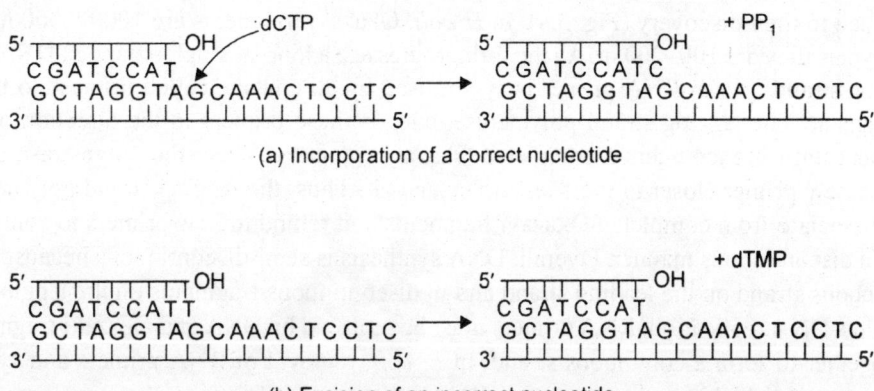

(a) Incorporation of a correct nucleotide

(b) Excision of an incorrect nucleotide

Fig. 3.5. Reactions catalysed by DNA polymerases. (a) 2'-Deoxyribonucleoside 5'-triphosphates are used as substrates by DNA polymerases to extend a primer in template-directed reactions. The net reaction is incorporation of 2'-deoxyribonucleoside monophosphates onto the 3' hydroxyl of a primer with loss of pyrophosphate. (b) DNA polymerases can proofread newly incorporated nucleotides and excise incorrect nucleotides. The excision reaction removes the last nucleoside monophosphate that was incorporated.

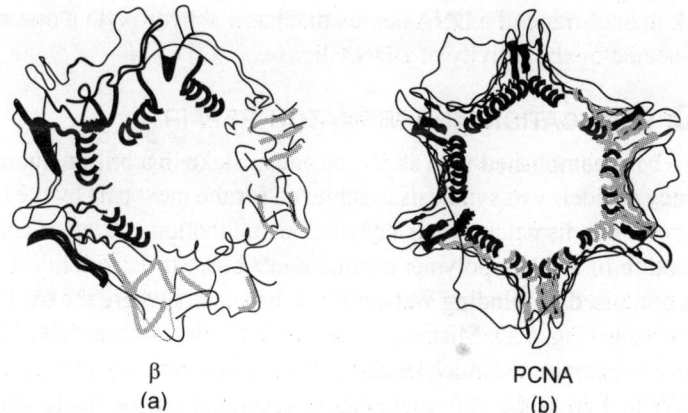

β
(a)

PCNA
(b)

Fig. 3.6. Structures of sliding clamps from *E. coli* and humans. (a) The *E. coli* β sliding clamp is a head-to-tail dimer of identical monomer subunits. (b) The human PCNA sliding clamp is similar in overall structure to the β clamp but is composed of identical trimers. Each ring has a central hole that is large enough to encircle B-DNA.

Leading and Lagging Strand Synthesis

In *E. coli*, a complex containing a dimeric DNA polymerase and accessory proteins interacts with the helicase and primase to form a replisome. This interaction stimulates the activity of the helicase and increases the rate of fork movement. The replisome, which contains two copies of DNA polymerase III, is capable of simultaneously copying both strands of parental DNA at the replication fork. But the two DNA polymerases must work in opposite directions to do this because DNA strands in a duplex are antiparallel and DNA polymerases can only synthesise DNA in the 5' to 3' direction. To accomplish this, one DNA polymerase working on the leading strand, synthesises DNA in a single continuous piece moving in the direction of the replication fork. The other DNA polymerase working on the opposite or lagging strand, synthesises DNA in shorter fragment named *Okazaki* fragments after Reiji Okazaki whose work led to their discovery (Fig. 3.4). In *E. coli*, Okazaki fragments are 1000–2000 nt in length and in eukaryotes they are 100–200 nt. As the fork progresses, a loop of single-stranded DNA is created on the lagging strand and an RNA primer is synthesised by an enzyme called primase to begin each Okazaki fragment. The lagging strand polymerase extends these primers in the direction opposite to fork movement until it encounters a completed Okazaki fragment. Then, the polymerase dissociates and rebinds a new primer closer to the fork and extends it. Thus, the lagging strand polymerase must repeatedly dissociate from completed Okazaki fragments and rebind to new primers to continue DNA synthesis in a discontinuous manner. Overall, DNA synthesis is semi-discontinuous because it is made in one continuous strand on the leading strand and in discontinuous fragments on the lagging strand.

To complete DNA replication, RNA primers must be replaced by DNA and Okazaki fragments must be joined together to form a continuous strand. In *E. coli*, removal of RNA primers and synthesis of DNA can be accomplished by a single enzyme, DNA polymerase I. The 5' to 3' exonuclease activity of DNA polymerase I degrades RNA primers while the 5' to 3' polymerase activity simultaneously synthesises DNA to replace the RNA. In eukaryotes, separate enzymes are responsible for degrading the RNA and replacing it with DNA. Finally, DNA fragments on the lagging strand are joined by a DNA ligase to form one continuous polymer. DNA ligase catalyses the formation of a phosphodiester bond between the 3' hydroxyl group at the end of one Okazaki fragment and the 5' phosphate at the beginning of the next. Any nick in one strand of a DNA duplex that has a 3' hydroxyl on one side and 5' phosphate on the other can be sealed by the activity of a DNA ligase.

FIDELITY OF DNA REPLICATION AND MISMATCH REPAIR

DNA replication can be accomplished with as few as one mistake in a billion nucleotides incorporated. This amazing accuracy or fidelity of synthesis is achieved for the most part by the DNA polymerase but is enhanced by a group of mismatch repair enzymes that function to detect and correct replication errors. One main feature of a DNA polymerase that contributes to its fidelity is the geometry of the active site, which is optimised for binding Watson-Crick base pairs where the overall shape of both A·T and G·C pairs are the same (Fig. 3.1). Mismatches such as G·T deviate from this ideal geometry so that incorrect nucleotides are incorporated much less efficiently. Frequencies of adding an incorrect nucleotide range from 1 in 1000 to 1 in 10,00,000 nucleotides depending on the nucleotide added. In the rare instant when a mistake is made, DNA polymerases have the ability to remove the incorrect nucleotide using the 3' to 5' exonuclease activity contained in the enzymes. This proofreading capability is further enhanced by a reduced efficiency of adding the next correct nucleotide onto a primer that ends with an incorrect nucleotide. Thus, when a mistake is made, the rate of adding more nucleotides is greatly reduced which allows the exonuclease time to remove the incorrect nucleotide. Once an incorrect nucleotide is removed, rapid incorporation of correct nucleotides by the DNA polymerase activity resumes. This proofreading activity increases the accuracy of DNA synthesis by a factor of about 10–100.

Mismatches that escape proofreading by the DNA polymerase can be corrected by the postreplicative mismatch repair process (Fig. 3.7). The net result is the removal of a segment of DNA containing the incorrect nucleotide and resynthesis of DNA to replace the segment that was excised. The key enzymes responsible for mismatch repair in *E. coli* are MutS, MutL, MutH and MutU. Mismatches are detected in double-stranded DNA by MutS which then interacts with the MutL protein. Together MutS and MutL signal where the mismatch is located to MutH and MutU. MutH is an endonuclease that is stimulated by MutL to cut the DNA strand containing the incorrect nucleotide. MutU is a DNA helicase that unwinds the duplex displacing the strand containing the incorrect nucleotide which is then degraded by an exonuclease. New DNA is synthesised to replace the segment that was removed. Homologs to MutS and MutL exist in eukaryotic cells and the overall repair process is similar.

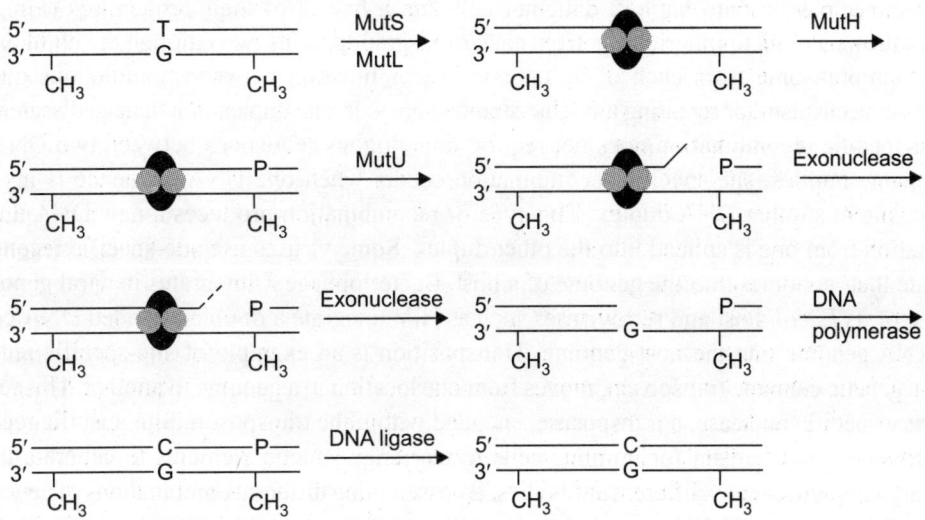

Fig. 3.7. Methyl-directed mismatch repair in *E. coli*. MutS protein recognises and binds mismatches such as G·T in DNA and is joined by the MutL protein. MutL within the MutS-MutL-mismatched DNA complex stimulates the endonuclease activity of MutH to cleave the unmethylated DNA strand at the GATC sequence closest to the protein-mismatched DNA complex. The cut DNA strand is unwound by the activity of MutU helicase and then degraded by an exonuclease until the mismatch is removed. The missing segment of DNA is replaced by a DNA polymerase and the DNA strands are joined together by the activity of a DNA ligase. The letter P indicates a 5' phosphate group.

How do the mismatch repair enzymes recognise which nucleotide of the mismatch is incorrect? In *E. coli*, the methylation status of the DNA allows the mismatch repair enzymes to distinguish between the newly synthesised DNA strand and the parental strand. Adenine is methylated in the *E. coli* genome when it appears in the sequence 5'GATC. This methylation of the genome occurs shortly after replication, so for a short time, the daughter strand is unmethylated while the parent strand is methylated. These 5'GATC sequences are also recognised by MutH which cuts the unmethylated daughter strand. These cut sites can be up to 1000–2000 nt away from the mismatch so a fairly large segment of DNA may be removed and replaced. While the overall process of mismatched repair is similar in eukaryotes, it is not yet clear how the eukaryotic enzymes distinguish between the newly synthesised strand and the parental strand.

DNA RECOMBINATION

Through the process of recombination, two DNA duplexes can exchange information to create hybrid molecules containing sequences from each of the original molecules. Recombination provides mechanisms for generating genetic diversity and for repairing DNA strand breaks. Recombination pathways can be grouped into two major classes, homologous and site-specific. Homologous recombination is the most general mechanism for recombination and plays a central role in both the generation of genetic diversity and repairing DNA. Homologous recombination occurs between two regions of DNA with similar or homologous sequences. Crosses between these two regions produce two new molecules that are hybrids of the original sequences. During meiosis (process of cell division that ultimately produces germ cells containing a single copy of each chromosome), these crosses allow alleles (alternate forms of the same gene) to be exchanged between homologous chromosomes so that chromosomes passed onto haploid daughter cells are a hybrid of their progenitors (Fig. 3.8a). This process allows a child to inherit traits from each of its grandparents even though the child only receives a single chromosome from each of its parents. Recombination between homologous duplexes also provides a mechanism for repairing a double-stranded break in one duplex or a damaged segment of DNA.

Site-specific recombination does not require homologous sequences between two DNA duplexes. As its name implies, site-specific recombination occurs when one DNA sequence is inserted into a specific site in another DNA duplex. This type of recombination produces a new DNA duplex where information from one is spliced into the other duplex. Some viruses use site-specific recombination to integrate their genomes into the genome of a host. Bacteriophage λ integrates its viral genome into the genome of its *E. coli* host and retroviruses such as HIV integrate a double-stranded DNA copy of their viral RNA genome into the host genome. Transposition is an example of site-specific recombination where a genetic element, transposon, moves from one location in a genome to another. This repositioning requires a specific nuclease, a transposase, encoded within the transposon. Site-specific recombination also provides a mechanism for immune cells to rearrange genetic elements to generate the diversity necessary to produce many different antibodies. By assembling different combinations of genetic elements through the process of V(D)J recombination immune cells are capable of producing genes encoding a multitude of different immunoglobulins that recognise different antigens.

Homologous Recombination

Homologous recombination is the most general pathway of recombination and is fairly well-defined. Homology or significant complementarity in DNA sequences is a prerequisite for homologous recombination between two duplexes. In addition, the physical exchange of information requires breaking and rejoining of the DNA molecules. Modern models of homologous recombination propose that recombination is initiated by the formation of a double-stranded break in one of the two duplexes. These breaks can be created by specific enzymes or can result from DNA damage. The broken duplex will serve as a substrate to initiate recombination after it is partially degraded by an exonuclease to generate free single-stranded ends. One of the single-stranded ends will invade the intact duplex and pair with the homologous region to produce a heteroduplex containing strands from two separate DNA duplexes (Fig. 3.8b). The strand invasion and homologous pairing reactions are not spontaneous but require the activity of an enzyme, RecA protein in *E. coli* and its homolog, Rad51, in eukaryotes, to catalyse the reactions. The strand invasion reaction generates a D-loop structure formed by the complementary strand from the intact duplex that was displaced. The invading strand can be extended by a DNA polymerase, which increases the size of the single-stranded region in the D-loop. This opens up a region of DNA homologous to the other single-stranded end of the broken DNA which then pairs with the D-loop. This end can also be extended by a DNA polymerase. Extension of both ends effectively replaces the segments that were removed by the exonuclease to generate single-stranded ends that initiate recombination.

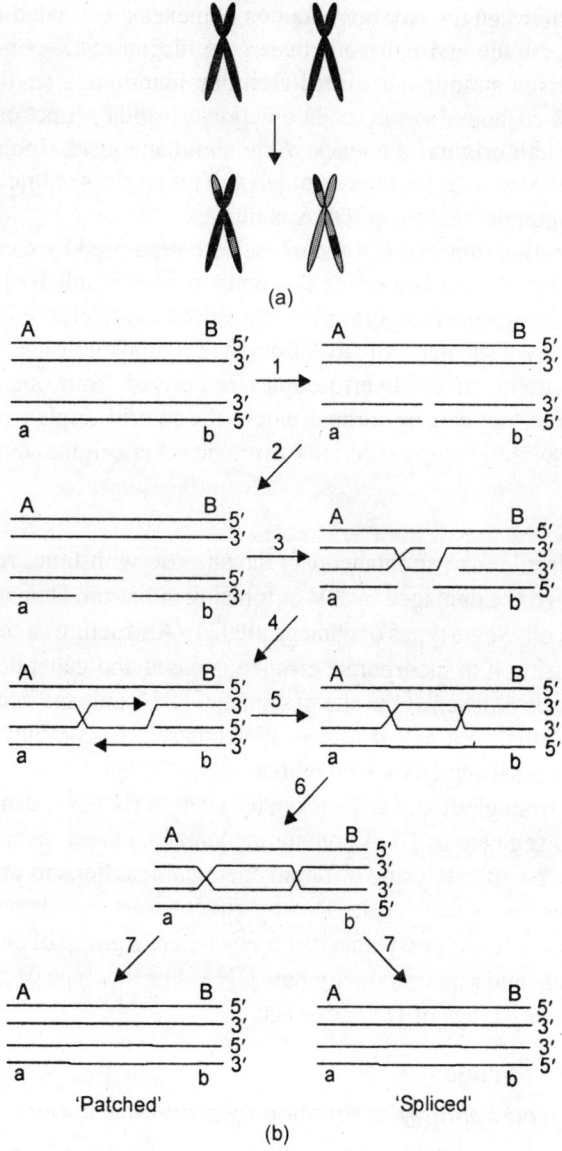

(a)

(b)

Fig. 3.8. Homologous recombination. (a) Recombination between sister chromatids during meosis results in exchange of information to generate two new chromatids that are hybrids of the originals. (b) Double-strand break model for homologous recombination. In this model, recombination is initiated by forming a double-stranded break (step 1) in one of the homologous duplexes. The broken DNA is then processed by partial degradation by an exonuclease to generate single-stranded DNA on the 3' ends (step 2). One 3' single-stranded end invades the homologous duplex forming a D-loop in the intact duplex (step 3). The invading 3' end is extended by a DNA polymerase enlarging the D-loop which can then pair with the remaining 3' single-stranded end (step 4). As the D-loop expands, it can displace the 5' end of the broken duplex which is then free to pair with the intact duplex (step 5). Branch migration enlarges the regions of heteroduplex DNA by unzipping the regions that were originally paired and zipping them onto the homologous duplex (step 6). Finally, the cross-over points or Holliday junctions are resolved by cleavage of the crossing strands (step 7). Two different products, patched and spliced, are formed depending on which of the crossed strands are cleaved.

Two crossover points between the two homologous duplexes are created following strand invasion by one half of the broken duplex and pairing between the displaced D-loop and the other half of the broken duplex. These crossed strands are named Holliday junctions after Robyn Holliday, who first proposed their occurrence in homologous recombination. Holliday junctions can migrate down the DNA duplexes unzipping the original duplexes while simultaneously zipping these strands together with new partners to extend heteroduplex regions of DNA. This process of branch migration can continue as long as homology between the regions of DNA is high.

Following branch migration, the two DNA duplexes are separated by cleaving the DNA strands at the Holliday junctions. This cleavage is catalysed by a nuclease or resolvase that is specific for DNA in Holliday structures. Depending on which strands of the junctions are cleaved, two distinct products can be formed that contain different segments of DNA from the original duplex (Fig. 3.8b). A spliced product can be formed where each end of the hybrid duplex is derived from one of the original duplexes. Alternatively, a patched product can be formed where the hybrid duplex contains a single-stranded segment from one duplex within a duplex derived from the other original duplex.

DNA REPAIR

DNA, like any other molecule, can spontaneously decompose with time, react with other chemicals (naturally present in a cell) or be damaged by UV or ionising radiation. Damage to DNA can have many deleterious effects on the cell. Some types of damage alter DNA structure so that the sequence is misread by DNA polymerases causing it to incorporate erroneous bases and generate mutations. Others are so severe that DNA synthesis is blocked at the site of damage. DNA damage occurs with a frequency high enough that it would be lethal to a cell if it were not repaired. Recombination, as discussed earlier, provides a mechanism for repairing DNA strand breaks.

There are two general strategies that can be taken by a cell to fix DNA damage, direct reversal of the damage, and removal of a segment of DNA containing damage. Direct reversal of DNA damage relies on different enzymes capable of catalysing different chemical reactions to undo the damage. There are two known examples of enzymes that repair DNA by direct reversal of damage. The majority of DNA damage is repaired using an excision/resynthesis strategy where a group of enzymes removes a segment of DNA containing damage and replaces it with new DNA. For this type of process, the same basic set of enzymes can remove many types of DNA damage.

Direct Reversal of DNA Damage

DNA photolyase catalysed splitting of thymine cyclobutane dimers

When exposed to UV light, two neighbouring pyrimidine bases, C or T, in DNA can react with each other to become covalently joined. One reaction that occurs is the formation of thymine cyclobutane dimers (Fig. 3.9). When these thymine dimers are formed, they distort the local structure of DNA and are no longer recognised as a pair of T's by DNA polymerases. In bacteria, the enzyme, DNA photolyase, reverses the formation of thymine dimers. Enzyme-bound cofactors absorb light and initiate an electron transfer reaction that catalyses the splitting of the thymine dimer to regenerate two intact thymine bases.

Removal of methyl groups by O^6-methylguanine methyltransferase

Chemicals that are naturally present in the cell, as well as chemicals in the environment, can react with DNA to methylate bases. One product of this reaction, O^6-methylguanine (O^6-MeG), induces the incorporation of an incorrect base by a DNA polymerase (Fig. 3.9). O^6-MeG is repaired by

O^6-methylguanine methyl transferase (MGMT) by directly removing the methyl group to regenerate a normal guanine residue. MGMT is not an enzyme in the true sense of the word because it does not act catalytically; instead it is a suicide enzyme. The methyl group is transferred from guanine to a cysteine residue on the protein where a covalent bond is formed. Because MGMT cannot be demethylated, it is incapable of catalysing the removal of other methyl groups and becomes inactive. MGMT is found in both bacteria and eukaryotes.

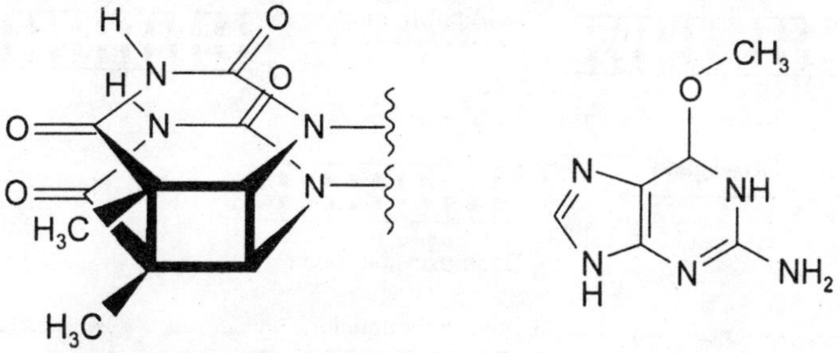

Thymine cylcobutane dimer O^6-methylguanine

Fig. 3.9. Structures of a thymine cyclobutane dimer and O^6-methylguanine.

Repair by Excision/Resynthesis

The process of excision of a section of damaged DNA followed by resynthesis allows cells to use the same basic chemical reaction and a common set of enzymes to repair many different types of DNA damage. The two main pathways responsible for excision repair are base excision repair that usually replaces a single damaged base and nucleotide excision repair that replaces a short segment of DNA containing the damaged nucleotide.

Base excision repair

The base excision repair pathway primarily repairs damage to DNA bases much of which occurs spontaneously in the cell without the influence of environmental hazards. Examples include oxidation, deamination and alkylation of DNA bases. These damaged bases are recognised by damage-specific DNA glycosylases that initiate the base excision repair pathway. DNA glycosylases bind to damaged bases and cleave the C1′-N glycosylic bond between the base and sugar. This leaves a baseless sugar or AP site (for apurinic or apyrimidinic), in DNA that is removed by other enzymes in the pathway (Fig. 3.10a). Several different DNA glycosylases are present in cells and each recognises a specific damaged base or a class of damaged bases. For example, uracil DNA glycosylase recognises and excises only uracil which can be formed in DNA by deamination of cytosine. Formamidopyrimidine (FaPy) DNA glycosylase recognises several different bases damaged by oxidation.

Once a DNA glycosylase has removed a damaged base, the AP site that it leaves must be repaired. An AP *endonuclease* starts this process by cleaving the phosphodiester bond on the 5′ side of the AP site to generate a 3′ hydroxyl and a deoxyribose phosphate. A deoxyribophosphodiesterase then cleaves the 3′ phosphate of the baseless sugar to remove it and leave a one nucleotide gap in the DNA. A polymerase subsequently adds the missing nucleotide and the nick is sealed by the activity of a DNA ligase. In *E. coli*, separate enzymes catalyse the removal of the baseless sugar and the incorporation of the missing nucleotide. In humans, DNA polymerase β contains two enzymatic activities and is capable of both incorporating the missing nucleotide and removing the baseless sugar.

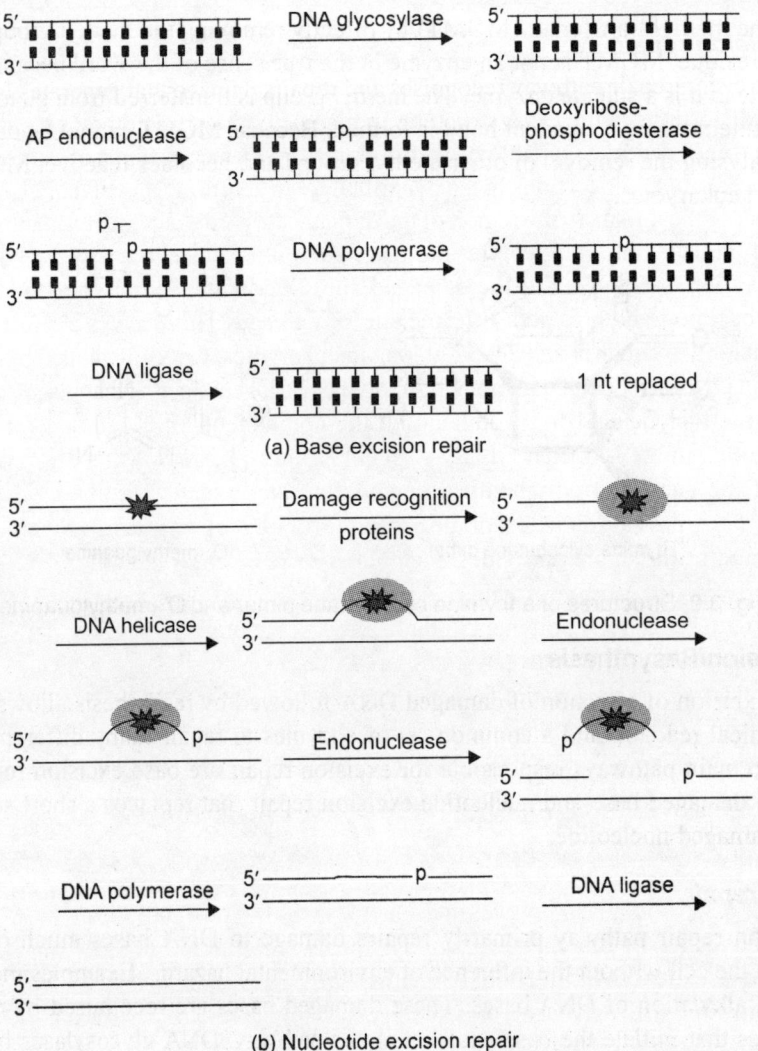

Fig. 3.10. Repair of DNA by excision of the damage and resynthesis of DNA. (a) The base excision repair pathway begins with the removal of a damaged base by a DNA glycosylase. In this scheme undamaged DNA bases are indicated by black squares and the damaged base is indicated by a light square. The Cl'-N glycosylic bond between the base and the sugar is cleaved leaving a baseless sugar residue (AP site) in DNA. The DNA strand is cut 5' to the AP site creating a 3' hydroxyl on one side of the cut and a 5' phosphate ('P') on the other. Deoxyribophosphodiesterase activity is required to excise the sugar-phosphate residue to create a one nucleotide gap that can be filled in by a DNA polymerase. Repair is complete when the strands are ligated by a DNA ligase. (b) The nucleotide excision repair pathway removes a short segment of DNA containing a damaged base (red starburst). The damaged base is recognised and bound by a protein complex. This protein complex serves to direct the other proteins to the site of damage so that it can be repaired. A DNA helicase separates the DNA strands on either side of the damaged nucleotide. Specific endonucleases recognise the forked single-stranded/double-stranded DNA junctions at these sites and cleave the DNA at the junctions. The DNA strand is cleaved 3' to the damaged nucleotide followed by cleavage on the 5' side. The gap created by excision of the damaged DNA segment is filled in by a DNA polymerase and the two strands are joined by a DNA ligase.

Nucleotide excision repair

The nucleotide excision repair pathway recognises and repairs damage that generates larger more bulky lesions and local distortions in the DNA structure. In the nucleotide excision repair pathway, damage is recognised by a protein complex capable of identifying many different types of damage. It is believed that this complex recognises distortions in the overall DNA structure at sites of damage or an increase in the ease of unwinding the duplex in the region of the damage. Regardless of the mechanism, this complex identifies sites of damage and helps recruit the rest of the repair machinery (Fig. 3.10b). This repair complex unwinds the DNA duplex at the damaged site. Endonuclease activities within the complex cleave the DNA backbone both 5′ and 3′ to the site of damage. This creates a short oligonucleotide segment, 12–13 nt long in bacteria and 24–32 nt long in eukaryotes, that is displaced by a DNA helicase. The resulting gap in DNA can be filled in by a DNA polymerase to leave a nick that is sealed by DNA ligase.

Thus, the instructions needed for producing all the components of a cell and for regulating their functions are encoded in the sequence of DNA. Accurate transmission of this information to progeny and protecting of the genome from chemical degradation are essential to life. Complementary base pairing in duplex DNA provides an elegant means for accurate replication of DNA and repair of DNA damage. Each strand of the duplex provides a template for generating the other strand and in essence acts as a 'back-up copy' of the information. The many different proteins and enzymes required to physically manipulate large DNA polymers in replication, recombination and repair, all take advantage of the complementary base pairing between strands to accomplish their tasks. These enzymes are capable of a sufficient level of accuracy to maintain genetic integrity, yet also allow a low level of mutations to generate genetic diversity ultimately allowing a population to adapt to changing conditions. Understanding how the cellular machinery functions to replicate, recombine, and repair the genome is central to understanding evolution of species and the origin of genetic diseases.

TRANSCRIPTION

The processes of transcription, RNA processing (in eukaryotes), and translation constitute the pathway that leads to the conversion of genetic information in the linear sequence of bases in genomic DNA into the linear amino acid sequences of functional proteins. Thus, DNA undergoes transcription to synthesise a primary RNA transcript, which in eukaryotes undergoes RNA processing to produce a mature messenger RNA (mRNA), then mRNAs are translated into functional polypeptides. Each of these cellular processes will be described below.

The process of transcription involves the sequential and enzyme-catalysed polymerisation of ribonucleotide triphosphates into a single-stranded linear RNA molecule that is complementary to, and encoded by, one strand of a DNA template. This process in eukaryotes occurs in the nucleus. The growth of the nascent RNA chain proceeds from the 5′ end to the 3′ end of the chain, elongating by adding nucleotides to the –OH group at the 3′ end of the RNA. As depicted in Fig. 3.11, polymerisation occurs by formation of a phosphodiester bond between the –OH group of the ribose moiety at the 3′ end of the elongating RNA and the 5′ phosphate of the ribonucleotide triphosphate (rNTP) precursor to be added to the growing RNA chain. Thus, unidirectional growth of the RNA chain occurs in the 5′ to 3′ direction. The phosphodiester bond is synthesised by a condensation reaction involving the 3′ –OH group of the sugar and the α phosphate group of the rNTP, with release of pyrophosphate (PPi). As shown in Fig. 3.11, the nucleotide sequence of the elongating RNA chain is specified by the nucleotide sequence of one strand of the duplex DNA template. Following the rules of Watson-Crick base pairing, adenine, cytosine, guanine and thymine in the template DNA sequence direct the addition of uracil, guanine, cytosine, and adenine, respectively, to the RNA sequence. In most cases, only one strand of a given region of double-stranded DNA is transcribed into RNA, though a small but increasing number of eukaryotic genes show transcription from both strands over all or a portion of the gene. In several cases, a gene encodes a functional sense transcript as well as a so-called anti-sense transcript (often of unknown function) that extends over the entire region encoding the sense transcript. Some of these anti-sense transcripts have been postulated to regulate the expression of the sense transcript.

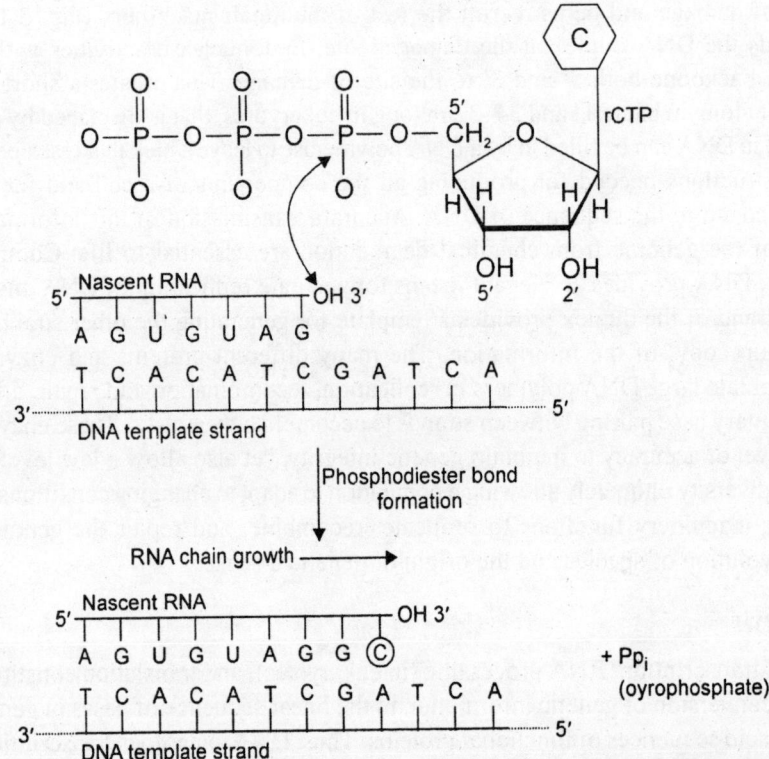

Fig. 3.11. DNA-dependent synthesis of RNA. In this example, a cytidine triphosphate (rCTP) precursor is added to the 3′ end of an elongating RNA chain by forming a phosphodiester bond between the 5′ phosphate of the rCTP precursor and the 3′ OH of the previously added nucleotide. The nucleotide sequence of the nascent RNA is specified by the complementary nucleotide sequence of the DNA template strand according to Watson-Crick base pairing. The circled C residue indicates the position of the newly added nucleotide.

The synthesis of RNA from a DNA template is catalysed by the enzyme RNA polymerase. Most, if not all, RNA synthesis in prokaryotes is directed by a single RNA polymerase, while RNA synthesis in eukaryotes is catalysed by three different RNA polymerases, pol I, pol II and pol III, each of which transcribes a different class of genes. The high-resolution structure of both bacterial RNA polymerase and eukaryotic RNA polymerase II has recently been determined by X-ray crystallography. The amino acid homology of certain subunits in the prokaryotic and eukaryotic polymerases and their many shared structural features are notable though not unexpected due to their similar functions.

The macromolecular complex formed during the process of transcription consists of RNA polymerase, the DNA template and the nascent RNA (Fig. 3.12). The double stranded DNA template is melted to form a transcription bubble (of approximately 12 base pairs) within the bubble the elongating nascent

RNA forms an approx 9 bp RNA:DNA duplex with the template strand of the DNA at its 3' end. As the polymerase moves downstream along the DNA template, the double-stranded DNA helix is unwound at the front of the bubble and rewound behind the bubble. Growth of the nascent RNA occurs by the addition of nucleotides at the 3' end of the nascent RNA within the bubble, with nucleotide triphosphate precursors presumably translocated to the active site of the enzyme via a pore and channel within the structure of the polymerase.

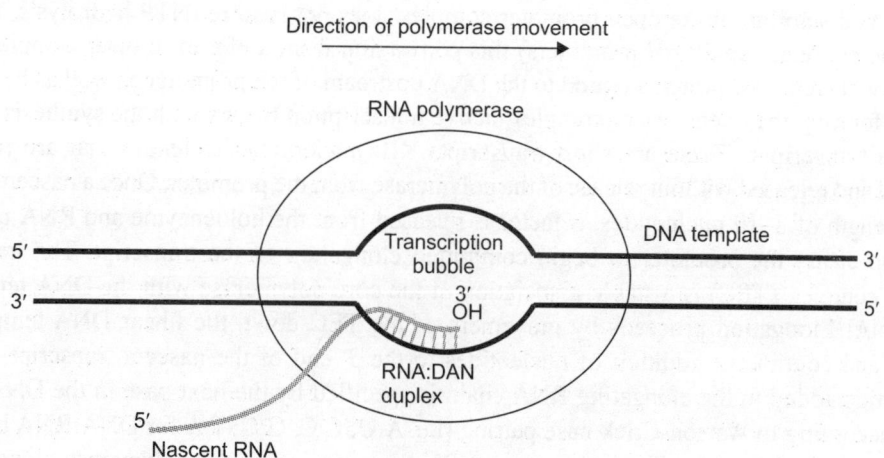

Fig. 3.12. Schematic of the transcription elongation complex.

Regulation of transcription, particularly regulation of transcription initiation, is a major mechanism that regulates macromolecular biosynthesis in the cell. However, the processes by which transcription is initiated and regulated in prokaryotes and eukaryotes are notably different. Therefore, a description of each of these processes in prokaryotes and eukaryotes is presented.

Transcription in Prokaryotes

Transcription of prokaryotic genes is accomplished by a single RNA polymerase. The prototype of the prokaryotic RNA polymerase is the polymerase of *Escherichia coli*. It is composed of four different polypeptide subunits, α, β, β' and σ. The RNA polymerase core enzyme, which functions in transcription elongation, is composed of two α subunits and one each of the β and β' subunits. The RNA polymerase holoenzyme, which initiates transcription, is organised as the core enzyme plus one copy of the σ subunit.

To initiate transcription, RNA polymerase holoenzyme first binds to DNA sequences immediately upstream of a gene. This region upstream of the gene, termed the promoter, contains DNA sequences specifically recognised and bound by the RNA polymerase holoenzyme. The σ subunit confers upon the holoenzyme the ability to recognise and bind to the promoter in a DNA sequence-specific manner, and to initiate transcription at a site specifically from the template strand of the DNA. Different σ subunits, such as σ^{54} and σ^{70}, recognise and bind different subsets of prokaryotic promoter sequences. For example, σ^{70}-containing holoenzyme recognises and contacts (via the σ subunit) specific promoter sequences surrounding positions -10 and -35 (upstream of the transcription initiation site).

Initial binding of the polymerase to the promoter leads to formation of a closed binary complex where the polymerase-bound DNA duplex remains double-stranded. This closed complex is then converted to a more stable open complex where melting of the DNA duplex occurs and the two strands of the promoter DNA undergo separation. The DNA duplex is melted over ~12 bp, from the -10 region to just downstream of the transcription initiation site (i.e. the deoxynucleotide in the DNA, encoding the first ribonucleotide in the RNA transcript). Both the closed and open promoter complexes are composed of multiple intermediate forms, with formation of an open complex accompanied by a major conformation change in the RNA polymerase. Conversion to an open promoter complex is followed by entry of ribonucleotide triphosphates (rNTPs) and binding of the initial (rNTP) to form a ternary complex. For σ^{70} promoters, conversion and stability of the open promoter complex does not require rNTP hydrolysis, though for some promoters (e.g. certain σ^{54} promoters) this conversion from a closed to open complex requires interaction with activator proteins bound to the DNA upstream of the promoter as well as hydrolysis of ATP. After forming the open ternary complex, active transcription begins with the synthesis of a series of abortive transcripts. These are short transcripts <10 nucleotides in length that are repetitively synthesised and released without release of the polymerase from the promoter. Once a nascent transcript reaches a length of 8–10 nucleotides, σ factor is released from the holoenzyme and RNA polymerase escapes and clears the promoter to begin committed elongation of the transcript. The transcription elongation complex (TEC) is a stable association of the core polymerase with the DNA template and nascent RNA. Elongation proceeds by movement of the TEC down the linear DNA template, with sequential and continuous addition of nucleotides to the 3' end of the nascent transcript. The exact ribonucleotide added to the elongating RNA chain is specified by the next base in the DNA template sequence according to Watson-Crick base pairing (i.e. A:U, C:G, G:C, T:A for DNA:RNA base pairs). Misincorporation of a nucleotide in the nascent RNA or pausing of the polymerase along the DNA template during elongation, leads the polymerase to backtrack along a short stretch of the DNA, cleavage of the newly synthesised portion of the nascent RNA at the 3' end and continuation of elongation from the newly truncated nascent RNA (including resynthesis of the cleaved portion of the RNA).

Termination of transcription in prokaryotes occurs at specific sites downstream of the coding region of genes and is accomplished by either of two possible mechanisms. One, termed *rho-dependent termination*, is mediated by the action of the rho termination protein and requires the hydrolysis of ATP. The second mechanism is rho-independent termination and occurs via formation of specific hairpin structures in the nascent RNA that destabilises the ternary complex immediately downstream of the hairpin and leads to dissociation of the ternary complex and transcription termination. Rho-independent termination can also occur via terminators formed by an RNA:DNA hybrid between the nascent RNA and the DNA template just upstream of the elongation complex.

Following termination of transcription and release of the RNA polymerase from the DNA template and the RNA transcript, the free core polymerase is able to rebind another σ factor and reinitiate another round of transcription. Regulation of transcription in prokaryotes occurs by a wealth of different mechanisms that often involve activator and repressor proteins.

Initiation and Regulation of Transcription in Eukaryotes

The three eukaryotic RNA polymerases all synthesise RNA transcripts encoded by a DNA template, but transcribe different subsets of genes. RNA pol I synthesises the precursor of ribosomal RNAs (rRNAs) which is eventually processed into the mature 5.8S, 18S and 28S rRNAs. The bulk of RNA synthesis in a cell is carried out by pol I. RNA pol II primarily transcribes the mRNA encoding genes and therefore is responsible for transcription of the largest and most diverse subset of genes in the cell. RNA pol III catalyses synthesis of an assortment of small RNAs including tRNAs and 5S rRNA. Unlike the prokaryotic RNA polymerase, highly purified eukaryotic RNA polymerases do not recognise promoter sequences by themselves or initiate transcription by binding directly to specific DNA sequences in eukaryotic promoters. Rather eukaryotic polymerases are recruited to promoter regions via protein-protein interactions by both proteins that bind to specific DNA sequences in promoter and other regulatory regions as well as additional proteins that interact with these DNA-binding proteins.

The following description of eukaryotic transcription and regulation will focus on mechanisms of pol II transcription because of the diversity of genes it transcribes and the current intensive efforts to elucidate mechanisms of pol II transcription and regulation.

RNA polymerase II and pol II core promoters

Eukaryotic RNA polymerase II (pol II) consists of 12 subunits totalling greater than 500 kD in size, with all subunits very similar between yeast and humans. Most human subunits can function in place of their yeast homologs and 9 pol II subunits are highly conserved among the three different eukaryotic RNA polymerases. Furthermore, the two largest pol II subunits, Rpb1 and Rpb2, show significant similarity to the β' and β subunits of bacterial RNA polymerase, respectively, while two other pol II subunits show lesser similarity to the α subunit of the bacterial enzyme. The structure of yeast pol II has recently been determined by X-ray crystallography at 2.8 angstrom resolution. The largest pol II subunit, Rpb1, contains a conserved tandem repeat heptapeptide sequence at the C-terminus termed the C-terminal domain (CTD). The CTD and its phosphorylation state play a critical role in both transcription and RNA processing. An unphosphorylated CTD is associated with the pol II initiation complex, whereas a phosphorylated CTD is correlated with the elongation phase of transcription and association of the pol II complex with RNA processing factors.

Promoters transcribed by pol II exhibit a diverse structure. Most consist of a core promoter (sometimes referred to as the basal promoter) located in the immediate vicinity of the transcription initiation site, as well as nearby regulatory sequences that activate or repress activity of the core promoter, usually in response to e.g. cellular conditions, extracellular signals and environment, cell type and stage of development. In addition, the function of many eukaryotic promoters, particularly in higher eukaryotes, is positively and/or negatively modulated by regulatory DNA sequences that can be located within the gene, upstream of the gene and/or downstream of the gene at distances exceeding 50 kb of DNA.

The core promoter contains cis-acting elements (i.e. DNA sequences) that can act as a nucleation site for the formation of the preinitiation complex (PIC) and recruitment of pol II. Core promoter elements in association with the PIC also determine the site(s) where transcription of each gene is initiated. These core elements frequently include the so-called TATA box; however, other core DNA elements can either replace the function of the TATA box in TATA-less promoters or can action conjunction with the TATA box to facilitate transcription initiation. These other cis-acting elements in the basal promoter include initiator (Inr) elements, a downstream promoter element (DPE) and a TFIIB recognition element (BRE). These cis-acting elements function by interacting with sequence-specific DNA-binding proteins that initiate and/or mediate PIC assembly.

Formation of the preinitiation complex

A multi-protein complex, termed the preinitiation complex (PIC) and consisting of a series of general transcription factors (GTFs) as well as pol II, is assembled at the core promoter as the first step of transcription initiation. These GTFs include the transcription factors TFIIA, TFIIB, TFIID, TFIIE, TFIIF and TFIIH, though not all promoters require all of these factors. In vitro studies suggest that the PIC is assembled at core promoters in a sequential fashion (Fig. 3.13). For genes with a canonical TATA box in the core promoter, this sequential assembly is initiated by the sequence recognition and binding of the multi-subunit GTF TFIID to the TATA box; TFIID consists of a DNA-binding subunit termed the TATA box-binding protein (TBP) that recognises and binds the TATA sequence, plus a variety of TBP associated factors (TAFs). TBP appears to be a common component of the PIC formed at pol I, pol II and pol III promoters. Binding of TFIID to the core promoter DNA of pol II genes is followed by binding of TFIIA and TFIIB to the TFIID-TATA box complex, then recruitment of a preformed complex of pol II, TFIIF and TFIIE and finally binding of TFIIH. TFIIA appears to stabilise the binding of TBP to DNA and TFIIB may function in selecting the position of the transcription initiation site. TFIIF bound to pol II suppresses nonspecific binding of the polymerase to DNA and stabilises the PIC. TFIIE may be involved in recruiting TFIIH and melting the DNA duplex when forming the open promoter complex. The multi-subunit complex that comprises TFIIH contains an ATP-dependent helicase activity, a DNA-dependent ATPase and CTD kinase activity. Thus, TFIIH appears to be involved in forming the open promoter complex via its helicase activity, and also, may be required for the conversion of abortive transcription to committed elongation. The kinase activity of TFIIH phosphorylates the CTD of pol II and therefore, may be involved in triggering the functions associated with a phosphorylated CTD. In addition, the observed coupling of transcription and DNA repair appears to be due to the common subunits shared by TFIIH in the transcription complex and the nucleotide excision repair complex.

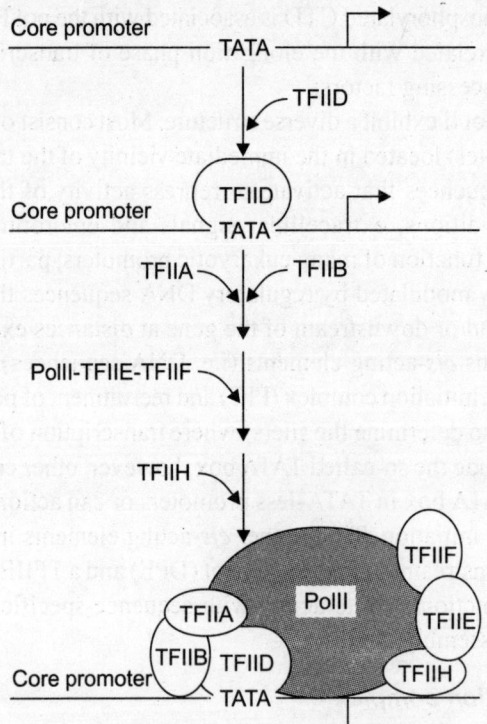

Fig. 3.13. Model for sequential assembly of the general transcription factors (GTFs) and pol II into the preinitiation complex (PIC). The right angled arrow indicates the position and direction of transcription initiation.

However, a significant percentage of eukaryotic promoters lack a canonical TATA box and/or contain other core promoter elements such as an Inr (initiator element), DPE (downstream promoter element), and BRE (TFIIB recognition element). This leads to a diversity of mechanisms for forming the PIC at different promoters and for the activation of basal transcription from the core promoter. TATA-less promoters often contain an Inr element that serves as the nucleation site for assembly of PIC. The Inr is a short conserved DNA sequence spanning the transcription initiation site that acts as the binding site for several different DNA-binding initiator proteins such as YY1, TFIII, USF, $TAF_{II}250$ and $TAF_{II}150$. The Inr (bound by its transcription factors) can function alone in TATA-less promoters or in combination with a TATA box or DPE (if these elements are present) to nucleate assembly of the PIC at core promoters. If present in a core promoter, the DPE is typically located approx 30 bp downstream of the transcription initiation site and is recognised and bound by subunits of the general transcription factor TFIID. The BRE element is located immediately upstream of the TATA box in certain core promoters with TATA boxes and facilitates the interaction and binding of TFIIB to the core promoter. In addition, a subset of promoters, commonly those that lack TATA boxes, do not initiate transcription at a discrete nucleotide, but initiate transcription at multiple sites within the core promoter.

Overall, assembly of the PIC on the various forms of the core promoter serves to recruit and stabilise binding of pol II to the promoter, positioning pol II at the correct site on the gene for initiating transcription. It helps form an open transcription initiation complex by melting of the DNA duplex and in the conversion of the PIC from transcription initiation to the transcription elongation complex. The open transcription initiation complex formed at the core promoter is associated with a melted DNA duplex of 12–15 bp that extends halfway from the transcription initiation site to the TATA box.

Activators, coactivators, enhancers

Transcription from the core promoter is usually augmented by the action of additional transcriptional activator proteins that bind regulatory DNA sequences outside (upstream and/or downstream) of the core promoter. These activator (or repressor) elements serve to increase (or decrease) levels of transcription above the basal activity of the core promoter. They often act in the context of cell type, e.g. cellular conditions, stage of development and response to stimuli such as hormones and growth factors. The combinatorial action of multiple activators and repressors on a given gene under a given set of cellular conditions determines the transcriptional status of the gene and governs its level of expression.

Activator proteins bound to their *cis*-acting regulatory sites appear to function by at least two mechanisms. Some activators bind their cognate site in the vicinity of the core promoter and appear to facilitate recruitment of certain GTFs to the core promoter and assist in formation of the PIC. These activators are presumed to assist PIC formation via protein-protein interactions between the activator and its target component(s) of the PIC. Alternatively, some activators may function by stimulating activity of the PIC and facilitating release of the PIC from the core promoter and/or facilitating transcription elongation. Some activators also appear to act by participating in the recruitment of chromatin modifying and remodelling complexes. In many cases of activator function, contact between the DNA-bound activator protein and the PIC requires bending or looping of the intervening DNA. Thus, some classes of activator proteins function by facilitating the bending of the DNA between the bound activator and the core promoter.

However, not all DNA-binding activator proteins that act on assembly or functions of the PIC can operate by direct contact with components of the PIC. Some activators require the action of an intermediary protein or protein complex between the activator and the PIC. These cocalled coactivators act through protein-protein interactions as a bridge between the DNA-bound activator protein and the PIC at the basal promoter. Thus, the function of many activator proteins are carried out via association with coactivator proteins or protein complexes. A protein complex (of ~20 subunits in yeast) that appears to play an important role in activated transcription is the mediator complex. It functions as a general coactivator of transcription and appears to mediate the action of a variety of activator proteins. The mediator complex is bound to the unphosphorylated form of the CTD of pol II and has been found to be a component of the pol II holoenzyme complex.

In addition to *cis*-acting activator sequences that bind activator proteins in the vicinity of the core promoter, other *cis*-acting activator sequences are found at larger distances from the core promoter (up to tens of thousands of kb) both upstream, downstream and within genes. Some of these distal activator sequences are thought to function by looping the intervening DNA to contact the transcriptional machinery in the vicinity of the core promoter. A subset of these long-range activators, termed enhancers, have been found to act regardless of their distance from the promoter, location relative to the promoter (i.e. upstream and downstream) and either in the forward or reverse orientation of the *cis*-acting activator element. These enhancer sequences have been shown to contain a variety of binding sites for a constellation of DNA-binding transcription factors that are presumed to form large DNA-protein complexes that activate transcription.

A large enhancer-like region spanning several thousand bps in mammals, termed a locus control region (LCR), also activates transcription at a distance, and can regulate activation of multiple coregulated genes within a gene cluster such as the β-globin gene family. The characteristic feature of LCRs is their ability to allow ectopically integrated transgenes to be regulated independent of the effects from the flanking DNA and chromatin at their new integration sites. LCRs also have been postulated to be involved in opening of chromatin structure across entire loci or domains; however, this role for LCRs is currently unclear.

Pol II holoenzyme

Recently, holoenzyme complexes containing pol II have been purified intact from eukaryotic cells. These heterogeneous pol II holoenzyme complexes include pol II, a subset of the GTFs and the mediator complex which is believed to be bound to the CTD of pol II. This finding of a pol II holoenzyme complex suggests that formation of the PIC *in vivo* may not always involve step-wise and sequential assembly of the GTFs and pol II and that much of the PIC, as well as coactivators required for activation of the basal promoter, may be preassembled *in vivo* and brought to the core promoter intact. Nonetheless, the lack of TBP in these pol II holoenzyme complexes suggest that, in part, formation of the PIC with these holoenzyme complexes may still be initiated by TBP binding to the TATA box followed by recruitment of the holoenzyme.

Role of chromatin structure

A major mode of transcriptional regulation in eukaryotes involves altering the chromatin structure of genes and regulatory regions to repress and/or activate transcription. DNA is packaged with basic histone proteins within the eukaryotic nucleus to form chromatin. The basic unit of packaging genomic DNA into chromatin is the nucleosome, a discrete nucleoprotein complex composed of ~200 bp DNA wrapped around a highly structured core of the histone proteins H2A, H2B, H3 and H4. Linear arrays of nucleosomes resembling 'beads on a string' form the first level of packaging DNA in the nucleus; organisation of the linear nucleosomal array into higher-order configurations continue the packaging of genomic DNA into the chromatin found in eukaryotic nuclei. The structures of these higher-order organisations of nucleosomal arrays are still not well-defined.

The formation of nucleosomes over promoters and other regulatory regions generally has a repressive effect on the transcription of genes by blocking or otherwise inhibiting the binding of specific transcription factors to their cognate regulatory DNA sequences. Furthermore, in higher eukaryotes, the higher-order packing of nucleosomal arrays also appears to regulate transcription by governing the general access of an entire locus (with its regulatory regions) to components of the transcriptional machinery. Thus, modulating the higher-order chromatin structure of an entire gene or domain, as well as altering the position and structure of individual nucleosomes over regulatory DNA sequences, constitute critical mechanisms regulating transcription of eukaryotic genes. A number of transcriptional activators (and repressors) appear to act by recruiting and regulating the function of chromatin modifying and remodelling complexes within specific genes.

The position and structure of individual nucleosomes associated with critical regulatory regions of genes has recently been shown to be regulated by ATP-dependent, multi-subunit complexes that remodel or modify nucleosomes or localised nucleosomal arrays (e.g. Swi/Snf, NURD, CHRAC, RSC). Some of these nucleosome remodelling complexes appear to act by repositioning (e.g. sliding and/or transferring) intact nucleosomes from regulatory regions or sites and presumably uncover previously obstructed binding sites in DNA for sequence-specific DNA-binding transcription factors. Furthermore, a number of remodelling complexes also appear capable of subtly altering the structure of individual intact nucleosomes by changing the interactions of the DNA with the histone core. This allows transcription factors access to their otherwise obstructed DNA binding sites within native nucleosomes.

Nucleosome structure is also altered by the activity of various nucleosome modifying complexes. These complexes covalently modify the side chains of amino acids (particularly lysines) in the N-terminal region of histones, thereby altering the structure of the associated nucleosomes and/or nucleosomal arrays. Examples of these nucleosome modifying complexes include histone acetylation and deacetylation complexes, as well as histone methylases. Acetylation of histone H4 has been associated with actively transcribed chromatin, while underacetylation of histone H4 has been associated with transcriptionally repressed chromatin. Presumably, these histone modifiying activities alter chromatin structure and either facilitate or preclude the access of transcription factors to their sites of action. Regulation of higher chromatin structure (i.e. the organisation of nucleosomal arrays into higher-order structure) across entire genes or domains is not well-understood, and mechanisms and regulatory elements that carry out the structural alterations of chromatin have not been definitively identified.

In summary, the opening of higher-order chromatin structure, the modification and/or positioning of nucleosomes to allow transcription factors to bind their cognate DNA binding sites, and the action of activators, enhancers, etc. all facilitate formation of a stable and functional PIC. Assembly of the transcriptional machinery at the promoter is associated with formation of a stable open promoter complex, leading to clearance of the pol II complex from the promoter and elongation of the nascent RNA.

Elongation

As with prokaryotic transcription elongation, the initial phase of RNA chain elongation is associated with abortive transcription, the repetitive synthesis of very short RNA molecules that are synthesised, released, and reinitiated. After the polymerisation of four or more nucleotides into a nascent RNA, the transcript becomes stabilised in the complex. In part, this permits a transition from transcription initiation to promoter release (or clearance) and productive elongation. Conversion of the pol II complex from transcription initiation to elongation is accompanied by phosphorylation of the CTD of pol II, release of certain general transcription factors GTFs and the mediator complex, and association of TFIIS and other elongation factors as well as certain RNA processing factors. However, details of the process that converts the initiation complex to transcription elongation are not well-understood.

Specific factors have been identified that facilitate promoter clearance (e.g. P-TEFb) while other factors act negatively to repress promoter clearance (e.g. NELF, DSIF). Positive elongation factors that facilitate promoter clearance also include the GTFs, TFIIF and TFIIH. Other factors facilitate the processivity of elongation by the pol II complex such as TFIIS, elongin and CSB. The elongation complex appears to contain 9 bp of RNA:DNA hybrid within the transcription bubble, with the front of the bubble positioned 3 nucleotides before the beginning of the RNA:DNA hybrid. As with prokaryotic transcription, the pol II elongation complex catalyses the sequential addition of ribonucleotides to the 3' end of the elongating mRNA.

The exact linear sequence of ribonucleotides in the mRNA is dictated by the nucleotide sequence of the template DNA strand based upon Watson-Crick base pairing.

Termination

Termination of eukaryotic gene transcription differs significantly from termination in prokaryotes. Rather than terminating transcription at discrete sites as seen in prokaryotes, termination in eukaryotes does not appear to occur at specific sites, but appears to occur by loss of processivity or stability of the elongation complex downstream of the gene. Thus, 3' end formation of eukaryotic mRNAs does not occur as a direct result of transcription termination at a specific site, but occurs by post-transcriptional processing of the RNA transcript where sequence-specific cleavage of the transcript at a specific site in the RNA is followed by post-transcriptional polyadenylation of the 3' end of the cleaved transcript. Evidence suggests that the polyadenylation signal and/or the site-specific cleavage of the nascent RNA may be involved in signalling or facilitating transcription termination downstream.

RNA PROCESSING

Generating a mature eukaryotic mRNA molecule from the primary transcript produced by transcription requires a series of post-transcriptional RNA processing steps that include 5' mRNA capping, 3' polyadenylation, RNA splicing, and RNA editing. Alternative sites for polyadenylation and RNA splicing within the same gene also play a significant role in post-transcriptional regulation of gene expression. As discussed in the following, several of these processes appear to be directly coupled to transcription via association with the elongating pol II complex.

5' Capping

After the nascent RNA transcript has reached the ~25–30 nucleotides, the 5' end of the transcript is covalently modified by enzymatic addition of a guanine triphosphate moiety via an unusual 5'–5' covalent linkage (Fig. 3.14a). This novel bond structure between the first and second nucleotides at the 5' end of the mature mRNA protects the mRNA from degradation by a 5' → 3' exonuclease activity in the cell. Formation of this 5' cap structure is catalysed, in part, by guanylyltranferase, an enzyme that is bound to the phosphorylated form of the CTD of pol II. Subsequent to the capping reaction, methytransferases add methyl groups to the N7 position of the newly added guanine to generate the 7-methylguanosine cap and a methyl group to the 2' hydroxl group of the first and second (in vertebrates) ribose moieties of the nascent transcript.

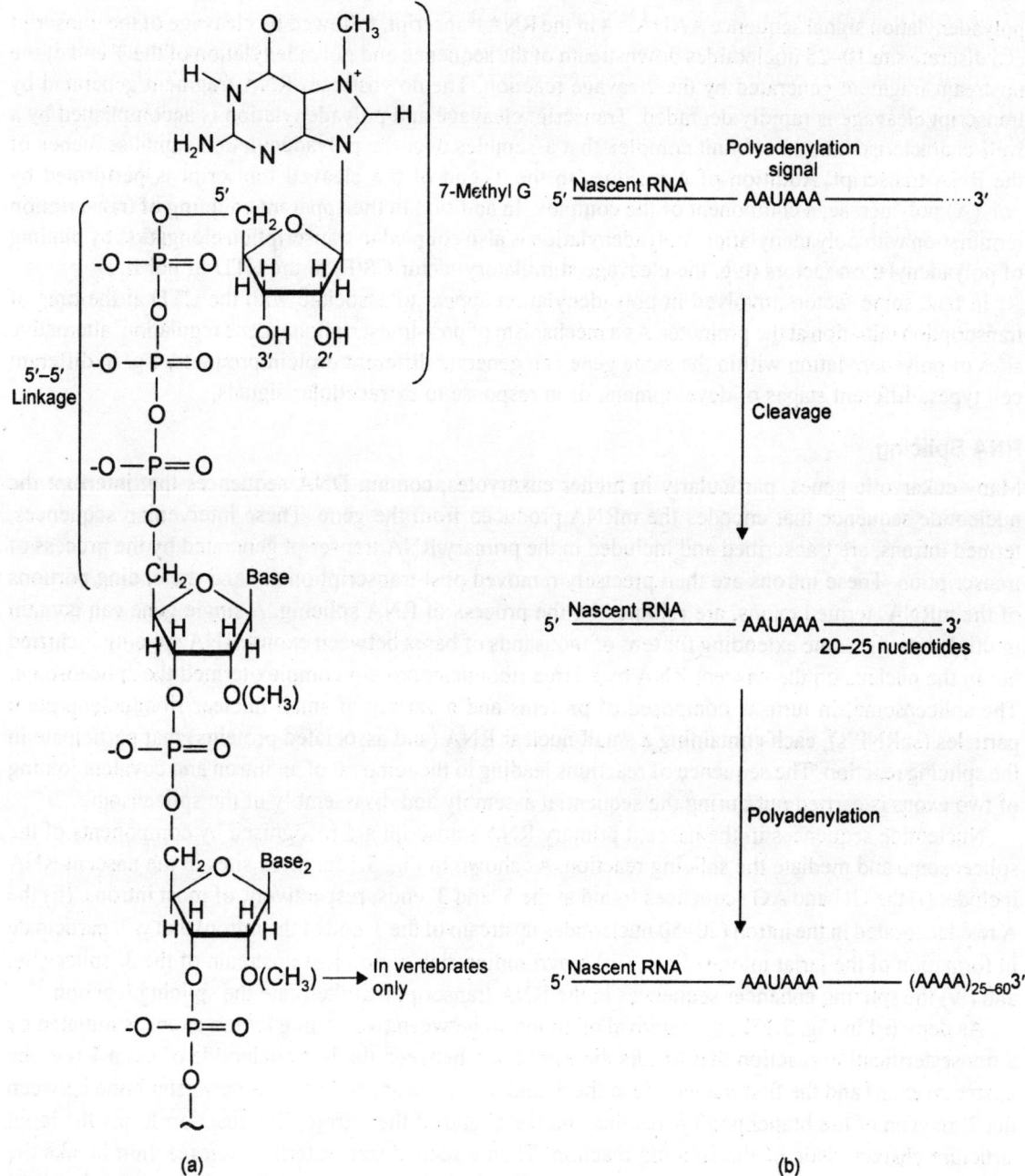

Fig. 3.14. Capping and polyadenylation. (a) The 5' mRNA cap structure; and (b) 3' polyadenylation of mRNA.

Polyadenylation

Formation of the 3' end of eukaryotic mRNAs is accomplished by enzymatic cleavage of the nascent RNA transcript followed by the post-transcriptional enzymatic addition of 100–250 adenosine residues to the 3' end of the mRNA (Fig. 3.14b). Cleavage and polyadenylation is initiated by recognition of the polyadenylation signal sequence AAUAAA in the RNA transcript, followed by cleavage of the transcript at a discrete site 10–25 nucleotides downstream of the sequence and polyadenylation of the 3' end of the upstream fragment generated by the cleavage reaction. The downstream RNA fragment generated by transcript cleavage is rapidly degraded. Transcript cleavage and polyadenylation is accomplished by a well-characterised, multi-subunit complex that assembles over the polyadenylation signal sequence of the RNA transcript. Addition of A residues to the 3' end of the cleaved transcript is performed by poly(A) polymerase, a component of the complex. In addition to the apparent coupling of transcription termination with polyadenylation, polyadenylation is also coupled to transcription elongation by binding of polyadenylation factors (e.g. the cleavage stimulatory factor CStF) to the CTD of pol II.

In fact, some factors involved in polyadenylation appear to associate with the CTD at the time of transcription initiation at the promoter. As a mechanism of post-transcriptional gene regulation, alternative sites of polyadenylation within the same gene can generate different protein products, e.g. in different cell types, different stages of development, or in response to extracellular signals.

RNA Splicing

Many eukaryotic genes, particularly in higher eukaryotes, contain DNA sequences that interrupt the nucleotide sequence that encodes the mRNA produced from the gene. These intervening sequences, termed introns, are transcribed and included in the primary RNA transcript generated by the process of transcription. These introns are then precisely removed post-transcriptionally and the coding portions of the mRNA, termed exons, are rejoined by the process of RNA splicing. A single gene can contain multiple introns, some extending for tens of thousands of bases between exons. RNA splicing is carried out in the nucleus on the nascent RNA by a large ribonucleoprotein complex termed the spliceosome. The spliceosome, in turn, is composed of proteins and a variety of small nuclear ribonucleoprotein particles (snRNP's), each containing a small nuclear RNA (and associated proteins) that participate in the splicing reaction. The sequence of reactions leading to the removal of an intron and covalent joining of two exons is carried out during the sequential assembly and disassembly of the spliceosome.

Nucleotide sequences in the nascent primary RNA transcript are recognised by components of the spliceosome and mediate the splicing reaction. As shown in Fig. 3.15a, these sites in the nascent RNA include: (i) the GU and AG sequences found at the 5' and 3' ends, respectively, of most introns, (ii) the A residue located in the intron (20–50 nucleotides upstream of the 3' end of the intron) that will participate in formation of the lariat intermediate, (iii) a pyrimidine-rich region just upstream of the 3' splice site, and (iv) the splicing enhancer sequences in the RNA transcript that facilitate the splicing reaction.

As depicted in Fig. 3.15b, the removal of an intron between two coding region exons is initiated by a transesterification reaction that breaks the ester bond between the last nucleotide of exon 1 (i.e. the upstream exon) and the first nucleotide at the 5' end of the intron, and forms a new ester bond between the 2' oxygen of the branchpoint A residue and the 5' end of the intron. This reaction forms the lariat structure characteristic of the splicing reaction. Then a second transesterification reaction breaks the phosphodiester bond between the last nucleotide of the intron and the first nucleotide of exon 2 (the downstream exon) and forms a new phosphodiester linkage between the 3' end of exon 1 and the 5' end of exon 2. This results in covalent joining of the two exons into a contiguous uninterrupted sequence in the mature mRNA and release of the intron-containing lariat structure which is then degraded.

The process of RNA splicing is highly precise; any deviation from single-nucleotide accuracy would introduce mutations into the final mRNA leading to the synthesis of defective proteins. The accuracy of the splicing reactions is mediated in part by the SR proteins, a family of structurally related serine and arginine-rich RNA-binding proteins. The SR proteins are required for accurate recognition of exons and splice sites during assembly of the spliceosome and during the splicing reactions. Specific sequences in the nascent RNA, termed splicing enhancers, also are involved in exon definition (i.e. recognition of exons by the spliceosome) and recognition of splice sites, as well as facilitating the splicing reactions. These splicing enhancers do not appear to share an identifiable consensus nucleotide sequence, but are recognised and bound by SR proteins.

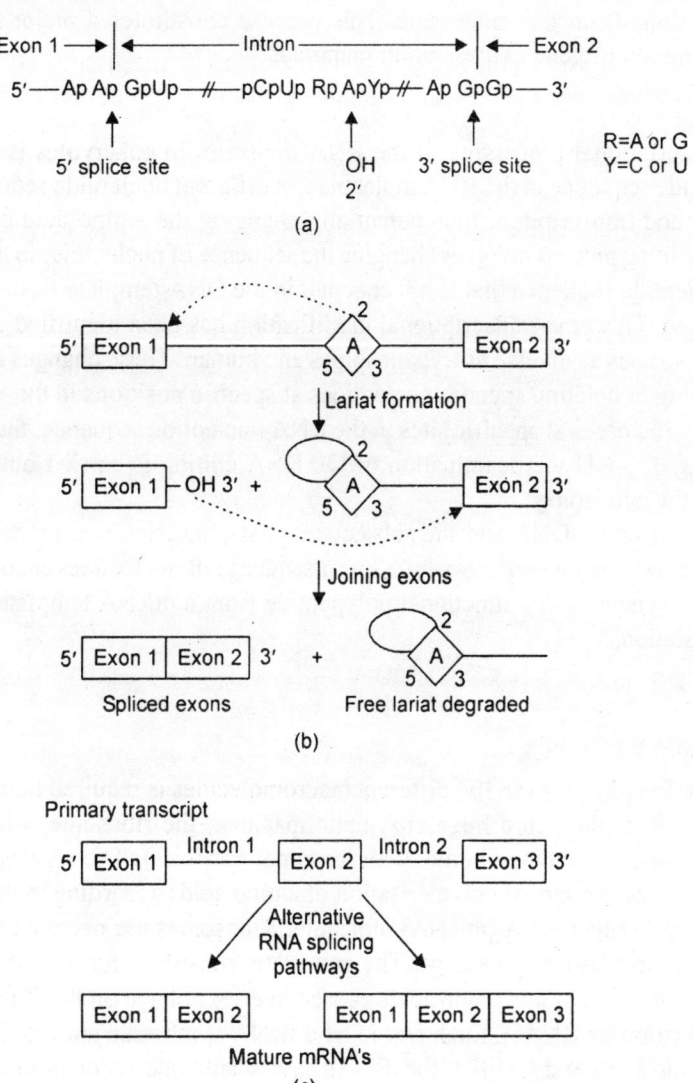

Fig. 3.15. Schematic of RNA splicing. (a) Location of conserved elements involved in RNA splicing; (b) Sequence of reaction in RNA splicing; and (c) Alternative RNA splicing; a gene with three transcribed exons produces two different mRNAs via alternative splicing pathways.

Like capping and polyadenylation, several lines of evidence indicate that RNA splicing also appears to be coupled to transcription. This evidence includes the colocalisation of splicing factors in the nucleus to discrete sites of active transcription and the association of SR-like proteins to the CTD of pol II.

Alternative pathways of splicing exons within the same gene can lead to the formation of different mature mRNAs from the same gene, each of which carries a different subset of exons from the same primary transcript (Fig. 3.15c). Thus, from the same nascent transcript, some spliced mRNAs can skip specific exons that are present in other mRNAs from the same primary transcript or have additional exons that are absent in other mRNAs. This alternative splicing of exons from a single primary RNA transcript is highly regulated (mediated by SR proteins) and often leads to synthesis of different proteins with different functions from the same gene. This process constitutes a major mechanism of post-transcriptional regulation of gene expression in mammals.

RNA Editing

The final post-transcriptional processing of the RNA transcript in eukaryotes is the alteration of the transcribed nucleotide sequence in the RNA molecule to a different nucleotide sequence independent of the DNA template and transcription, thus potentially changing the amino acid coding of the mature mRNA. This RNA editing process involves changing the sequence of nucleotides in the newly synthesised RNA to a new nucleotide sequence that is not encoded in the DNA template from which the RNA was originally transcribed. This post-transcriptional modification has been identified for a relatively small number of genes in species as diverse as trypanosomes and human. These changes in the RNA sequence can occur by inserting or deleting specific nucleotides at specific positions in the RNA transcript or by modification of specific bases at specific sites in the RNA nucleotide sequence, thereby converting one base to another (e.g. $C \rightarrow U$ via deamination of C). RNA editing is carried out by macromolecular complexes termed the editosome.

Transcription of genomic DNA and the subsequent post-transcriptional processing of the primary RNA transcript generate a mature mRNA whose linear sequence of nucleotides encodes a linear sequence of amino acids. The synthesis of a functional polypeptide from a mRNA template is accomplished by the process of translation.

TRANSLATION
Overview of Protein Synthesis

The ordered interaction of well over 100 different macromolecules is required to make a single protein. The entire process takes place in a huge enzymatic machine, the ribosome, which in all life forms consists of two ribonucleoprotein subunits (subribosomal particles). The ribosome provides a large, dynamic platform for the sequential polymerisation of amino acids according to the sequence of triplet codons in a bound messenger RNA (mRNA) molecule. Ribosomes are necessarily large, in excess of 2.5 MDa, because their substrates are large. The enzymatic substrates for protein synthesis are amino acyl-tRNAs, activated forms of the amino acids carried in ester linkage on the 3′ terminal nucleotide of the various tRNAs (transfer RNAs). Each amino acyl-tRNA synthetase enzyme is specific for one of the 20 different amino acids and for all of the tRNAs having anticodons corresponding to the particular amino acid. The amino acyl-tRNAs are escorted to the ribosome as ternary complexes with initiation (IF-2) or elongation factors (EF-Tu) and GTP. The selection of particular amino acyl-tRNAs on the ribosome is made on the basis of tRNA anticodon base-pairing interactions with triplet codons that are exposed in a limited region of mRNA within the decoding centre on the small ribosomal subunit. The peptidyl transferase activity of the large subunit catalyses peptide bond formation between amino acids carried by amino acyl-tRNAs (or peptidyl-tRNAs) that are juxtaposed at specific sites (A, aminoacyl; and P, peptidyl) in the intersubunit space. After each peptidyl transferase reaction, the peptidyl-tRNA and the uncharged tRNA which has donated an amino acid to the growing peptide chain are moved (translocated) with the aid of elongation factor EF-G, along with the mRNA, to maintain the reading frame and present the next codon in the A site of the decoding centre. Next an amino acyl-tRNA having an anticodon complementary to the A site codon enters the A site and this process is repeated until a termination codon is encountered in the decoding centre. Then, with the aid of protein termination factors, the protein is released from peptidyl tRNA and another protein, RRF, ribosome-recycling factor, promotes disassembly of the translation complex.

Given the wealth of information about protein synthesis in bacterial systems and the recent advances in bacterial ribosome structure, it is appropriate to review protein synthesis in prokaryotes.

Elements of Translation in Prokaryotes

Genetic Code

The 20 natural amino acids are each specified by one or more triplet codons in the mRNA. Four bases in mRNA, taken three at a time, results in 64 different triplet combinations (Fig. 3.16). Some of the amino acids (identified here by their three letter abbreviations) are specified by single codons (AUG, for Methionine), while others are specified by as many as six different codons (Leucine, for example).

		U	C	A	G
U		UUU Phe	UCU Ser	UAU Tyr	UGU Cys
		UUC Phe	UCC Ser	UAC Tyr	UGC Tyr
		UUA Leu	UCA Ser	UAA End	UGA End
		UUG Leu	UCG Ser	UAG End	UGG Trp
C		CUU Leu	CCU Pro	CAU His	CGU Arg
		CUC Leu	CCC Pro	CAC His	CGC Arg
		CUA Leu	CCA Pro	CAA Gln	CGA Arg
		CUG Leu	CCG Pro	CAG Gln	CGG Arg
A		AUU Ile	ACU Thr	AAU Asn	AGU Ser
		AUC Ile	ACC Thr	AAC Asn	AGC Ser
		AUA Ile	ACA Thr	AAA Lys	AGA Arg
		AUG Met	ACG Thr	AAG Lys	AGG Arg
G		GUU Val	GCU Ala	GAU Asp	GGU Gly
		GUC Val	GCC Ala	GAC Asp	GGC Gly
		GUA Val	GCA Ala	GAA Glu	GGA Gly
		GUG Val	GCG Ala	GAG Glu	GGG Gly

Fig. 3.16. The genetic code, as used by most organisms. The first base of the codon (5' end) is shown in the first column and the second base is shown in the top row. AUG (and sometimes GUG and UUG) usually serves as the initiation codon, when it occurs at the beginning of the open reading frame. The three termination codons (end) are recognised by termination factors.

mRNA

Messenger RNAs may contain one open reading frame (monoscistronic), bounded by initiation and termination codons, or several (polycistronic). The mRNAs often have a nontranslated leader sequence at their 5' end preceding the initiation codon. Some mRNAs have short regions of four to six bases, which are complementary to sequences in the 3' end of 16S RNA exposed on the platform of the small ribosomal subunit. These sequences, called Shine-Dalgarno sequences, lie 10 or so bases upstream of the initiation codon, serving to bind and orient the mRNA, placing the initiation codon within the decoding centre on the small subunit. The greater the region of complementarity, the stronger the binding and consequently the particular mRNA will be translated more frequently, relative to those with weaker ShineDalgarno interactions.

Transfer RNAs (tRNAs)

All organisms use tRNAs as so-called adaptor molecules to convert the sequence of nucleic acid codons into a sequence of amino acids. These are a family of small RNA molecules, 70–80 nucleotides long, which fold into a series of stem-loop structures, usually depicted as a characteristic cloverleaf structure (Fig. 3.17). They typically contain unusual or modified bases, such as dihydrouracil (prominent in the D loop, so named because of the dihydrouracil content), pseudouracil and ribothymidine. The sequences of the various tRNAs are different, but they contain an invariant CCA, added posttranscriptionally at the 3' end of the amino acid acceptor stem, as well as a sequence, TψCG, in the TψC loop. As its name suggests, the variable loop is highly variable, both in sequence, as well as size. The anticodon and the amino acid that it specifies are separated by about 70 Angstroms, at opposite ends of the L-shaped molecule (Fig. 3.18a) which forms when the D loop and TψC loop fold further, stabilised by additional, tertiary base pair interactions.

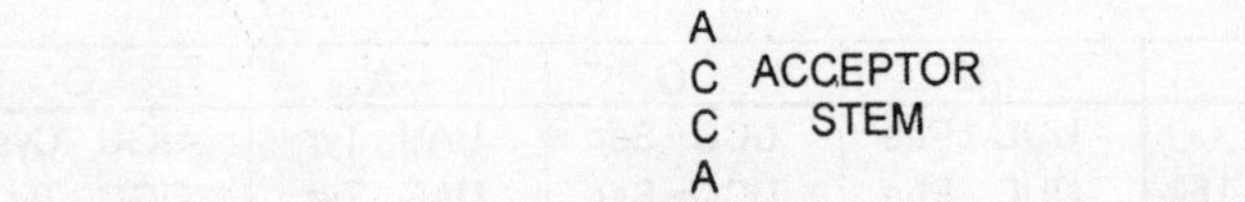

Fig. 3.17. Transfer RNA structure. Shown here is the secondary structure of phenylalanyl-tRNA (Phe-tRNA), in the familiar cloverleaf diagram characteristic of most tRNAs. The anticodon, 5'GAA, is complementary to one of the two codons for Phe (5'UUC) in Fig. 3.16. D, dihydrouridine; ψ, pseudouridine; T, ribothymidine.

Amino acyl-tRNA synthetases

Amino acids are activated through coupling in ATP-dependent reactions to the appropriate tRNAs by amino acyl-tRNA synthetases specific for each amino acid and for the corresponding tRNAs. There are two general classes of synthetase enzymes, I and II, which tend to function as monomers or dimers, respectively. The enzymes recognise key identity elements at various locations in the cognate tRNAs.

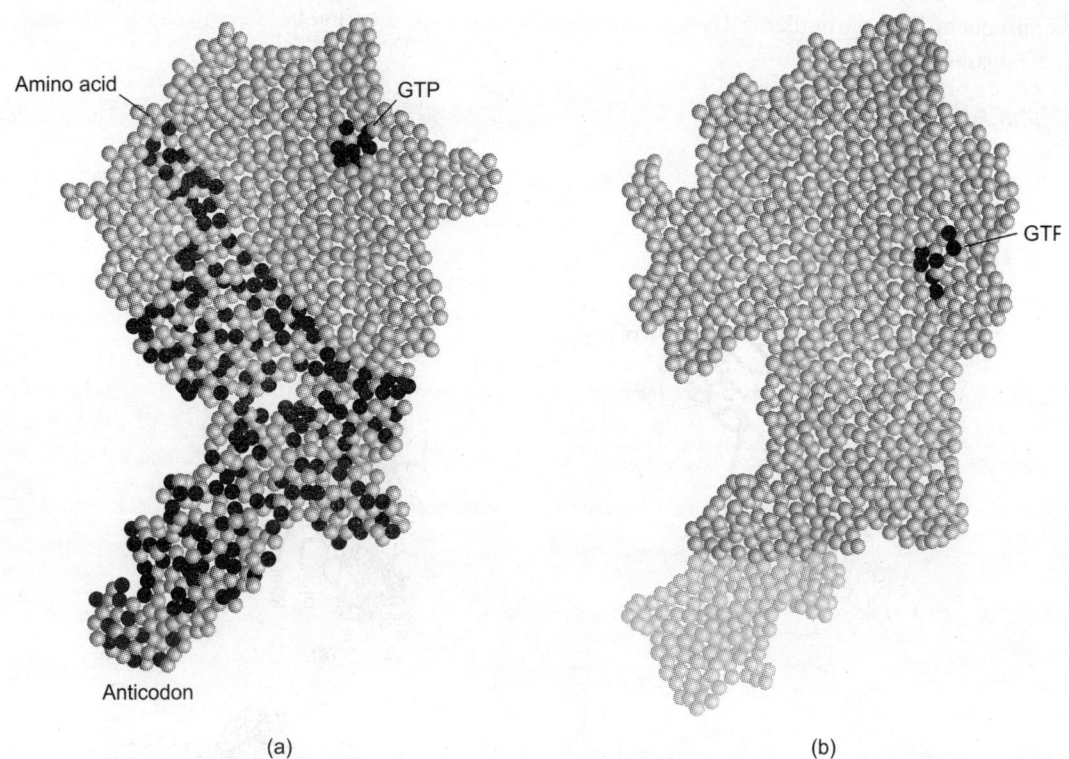

Fig. 3.18. Elongation factors EF-Tu and EF-G. (a) EF-Tu (lighter gray) is shown as a ternary complex with bound amino acyl-tRNA and GTP; (b) EF-G resembles the complex of the protein EF-Tu and amino acyl-tRNA. This is an example of macromolecular mimicry where similar binding sites accommodate the different species.

Ribosome

The small subunit (30S) of prokaryotic ribosomes contains one 16S RNA molecule and about 21 proteins. The RNA molecules are generally characterised by their sedimentation coefficient (S) as an indication of their size or mass. The larger and more compact the RNA molecule is, the higher the sedimentation coefficient. The 16S rRNA (ribosomal RNA) of *E. coli* is 1542 nucleotides long and the molecule is folded into a rather compact shape (Fig. 3.19a). Adjacent complementary regions along the molecule result in the formation of a series of stem-loop structures. This has the effect of bringing together distant complementary regions to form additional stems, resulting in the formation of distinct domains through these long distance interactions. The 21 proteins are distributed around the periphery, mainly on the back or solvent side. Only one protein, S12, is located on the interfacial side, near the decoding centre.

The large subunit (50) contains two rRNA molecules, a 5S RNA, forming the central crown structure (Fig. 3.19f) and a larger 23S RNA, forming the body of the subunit. The 33 proteins of the large subunit are located mainly on the periphery and the backside of the subunit. One of the ribosomal proteins, L12, is present in four copies. These proteins form two L12-dimer structures (Fig. 3.19f). The L12 dimer stalk is the site where the elongation factors (EF-Tu and EF-G) first engage the ribosome. The 30S and 50S subunits associate during the initiation phase of protein synthesis to form a roughly spherical 70S ribosome.

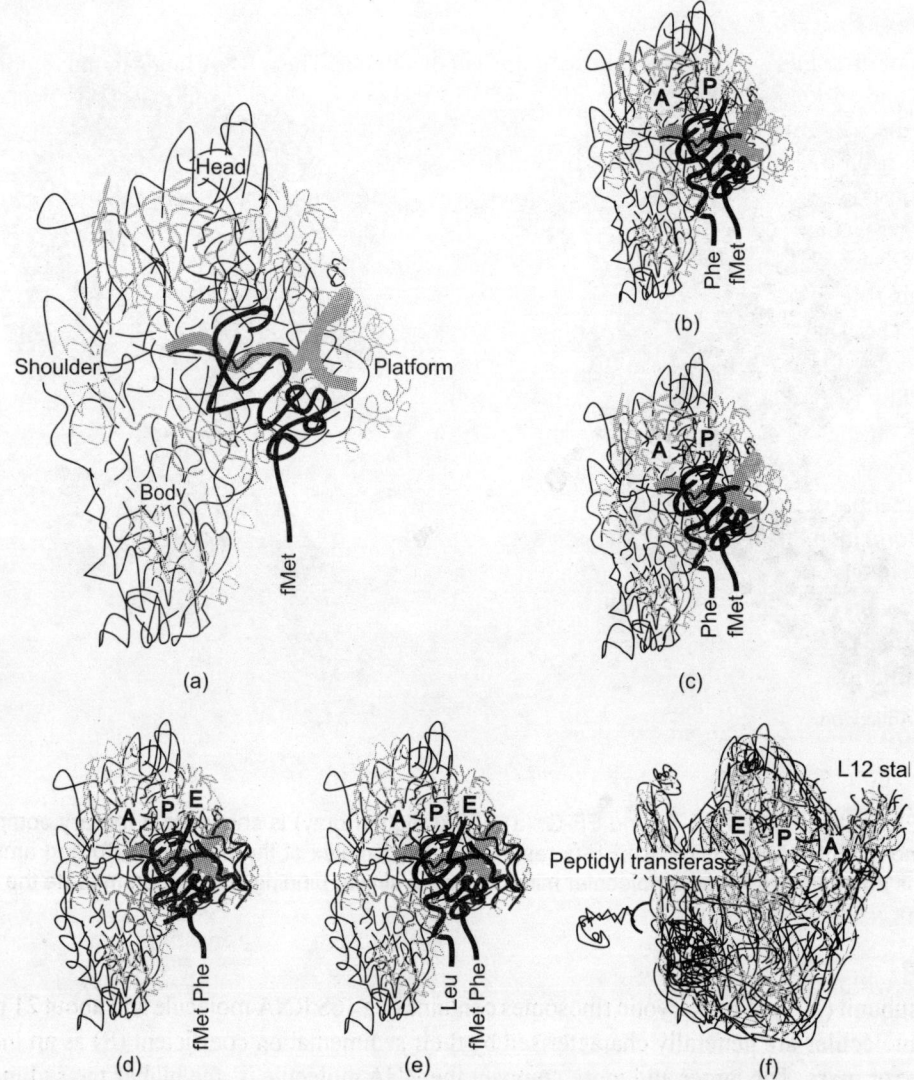

Fig. 3.19. Structure of the small and large subunits of the bacterial ribosome. (a) Interfacial aspect of the 30S subunit, showing the 16S RNA backbone (thin dark tracing) and associated proteins (alternatively shaded). A section of bound mRNA (thick bright backbone) includes the Shine-Dalgarno region (5' helical structure on the right), the initiation codon and an adjacent Phe codon. The anticodon of the initiator tRNA, fMet-tRNA (thick dark backbone) is base paired with the initiation codon in the P site. (b) Same as (a) with the addition of Phe-tRNA at the adjacent codon in the A site. (c) Peptidyl transferase catalysed transfer of the fMet to the Phe-tRNA, resulting in a dipeptidyl-tRNA in the A site. (d) Post translocation state of the ribosomal small subunit. Through the action of EF-G with bound GTP, the uncharged initiator tRNA, fMet-Phe-tRNA and the mRNA are moved, in register, into the E and P sites. (e) Entry of the third amino acyl-tRNA into the A site, in advance of the ejection of the E site tRNA and peptide transfer (peptidyl transferase reaction). (f) Interfacial aspect of the 50S subunit, showing the 5S and 23S RNA (thick backbone) and associated proteins (variously shaded). The peptidyl transferase activity lies deep within a cleft in the 23S RNA, an area entirely devoid of protein. The coordinates for the 30S subunit, mRNA fragment, A, P and E site tRNAs are available at the RCSB database with PDB accession numbers 1GIX and 1JGO.

Initiation of Protein Synthesis

Initiation of protein synthesis takes place on the small subunit. The mRNA binds in the region between the head and the body, tracking from the platform through a downstream entrance channel formed between the head and the shoulder of the subunit (Fig. 3.19a). If the mRNA has a Shine-Dalgarno sequence, it binds more efficiently, stabilised by base pairing with the complementary region of 16S rRNA exposed on the platform. This interaction places the initiation codon in the vicinity of the decoding centre, where it can base pair with the anticodon of the initiator tRNA. The initiator tRNA in prokaryotic systems is fMet-tRNA, a special tRNA that carries a methionine modified by formylation on its amino group. This fMet-tRNA is escorted to the small subunit in a ternary complex with initiation factor 2 (IF-2) and GTP. The fMet-tRNA is the only amino acyl-tRNA to bind directly and initially to the P site, where the initiation codon will be able to form base pairs with the anticodon (Fig. 3.19). This interaction is facilitated by two other initiation factors, IF-1 and IF-3. IF-1 is a protein mimic of tRNA and it binds to the A site on the small subunit, forcing the IF-2 ternary complex to enter at the adjacent P site. IF-3 binds between the head and the platform, where it serves a dual role. It acts as an anti-association factor, ensuring a supply of free 30S subunits for initiation complex formation and it promotes the fidelity of initiation complex formation by favouring the dissociation of noncanonical complexes, such as base pair interactions between elongator tRNAs and the initiation codon. Upon proper recognition of fMet-tRNA by the initiation codon in the P site, the IF-2-bound GTP is hydrolysed to GDP, causing a conformational change allowing IF-2 GDP to leave after depositing the initiator tRNA in the P site. The 50S subunit then joins the 30S initiation complex to form the 70S initiation complex, setting the stage for the elongation phase.

Elongation Phase of Protein Synthesis

The elongation factor EF-Tu (Fig. 3.18a) escorts the various amino acyl-tRNAs to the ribosomal A site as ternary complexes with GTP. They engage the ribosome first at the Ll2 stalk and if the codon exposed in the A site (UUC, in Fig. 3.20b, for example) is complementary to their anticodon, the amino acyl-tRNA is deposited and the EF-Tu-bound GTP is hydrolysed, favouring the exit of EF-Tu-GDP. Note that the mRNA is kinked between the adjacent codons in the decoding centre. This kinking allows the A and P site tRNAs to read adjacent codons. In this manner the amino acyl ends of the A and P site tRNAs are placed within 5 Angstroms of each other (Fig. 3.19b), in the peptidyl transferase centre of the 50S subunit (Fig. 3.19f) where they await peptide bond formation. Peptidyl transferase activity of the 50S RNA catalyses the transfer of the fMet to the Phe-tRNA in the A site (Fig. 3.19c). At this point in the elongation cycle the peptidyl-tRNA (fMet-Phe-tRNA, in the example of Fig. 3.19c) and the P site tRNA must be moved to open the A site for entry of the next amino acyl-tRNA able to base pair with the third codon brought into the A site. Elongation factor G, EF-G with bound GTP (Fig. 3.18b) engages the Ll2 stalk on the large subunit and proceeds to carry out this translocation event, while maintaining the mRNA reading frame fixed by the A and P (E) site tRNAs. During translocation, the uncharged tRNA is moved into the E site while the A site peptidyl-tRNA moves into the P site (Fig. 3.19d). EF-G is a striking example of tRNA mimicry by protein. Note the structural resemblance of EF-G (Fig. 3.18b) and EF-Tu-amino acyl-tRNA (Fig. 3.18a) which bind to similar sites on the ribosome. After hydrolysis of the bound GTP, EF-G leaves to make the A site available for entry of the next amino acyl-tRNA (Fig. 3.19e). The growing peptide chain will emerge through a tunnel traversing the body of the 50S subunit. Upon entry of the next cognate amino acyl-tRNA the affinity of the E site for the uncharged tRNA is lowered, allowing for release of the E site tRNA. This cycle is repeated until a termination codon appears in the A site, setting the stage for the termination of protein synthesis.

Termination of Protein Synthesis

Termination codons exposed in the A site are recognised by protein release factors. RF1 recognises UAA and UAG and RF2 recognises UAA and UGA. After binding of either release factor in the A site, peptidyl transferase activity transfers the C-terminal residue of the polypeptide to a water molecule, resulting in release of the protein. The departure of RF1 and RF2 is facilitated by a third release factor, RF3, which is another example of mimicry in translation systems. RF3 is a GTP binding protein that resembles EF-G.

Translation in Eukaryotes

The fundamental process of protein synthesis in eukaryotes resembles that of prokaryotes, with the introduction of additional complexity and regulatory features. The ribosomes are larger and the initiation factors are more numerous. Eukaryotes do not employ a Shine-Dalgarno-like mechanism to promote mRNA binding, but rather, use a collection of initiation factors that recognise a uniquely eukaryotic decoration of the 5′ end of mRNAs, the 5′-methyl-G cap structures. In addition, most of the mRNAs are further decorated by a poly(A) tail at their 3′ end, which recruits poly (A)-binding proteins (PABPs). The 40S ribosome small subunit contains 18S RNA. The large subunit contains three molecules of RNA, a large, 28S RNA, 5S RNA and a species unique to eukaryotes, a 5.8S RNA. The 80S ribosome contains about 80 different proteins, some of which are homologs of bacterial ribosomal proteins, but many of them unique to eukaryotes.

The initiation phase of protein synthesis employs at least 12 initiation factors, containing as many as 28 protein subunits. These protein factors interact with the initiator Met-tRNAi, the mRNA, the 40S and 60S subunits to promote formation of the 80S initiation complex. The factor names are preceded by 'e' to denote their eukaryotic nature. The factor eIF1A is homologous to the bacterial IF1 and it aids in positioning the initiation codon in the decoding centre. The homolog of IF2, eIF2 escorts Met-tRNAi to the P site of the ribosomal 40S subunit. The large factor eIF3, which contains 11 protein subunits, binds to the platform region of the 40S subunit. The eIF4F factor is a heterotrimeric factor; in addition to its central component, eIF4G, its eIF4A component is an ATP-dependent RNA helicase and its eIF4E subunit binds to the 5′ cap structure on the mRNA. The versatile factor eIF4G serves as a bridging factor that binds to eIF4E, as well as the PABPs [on the poly(A) tail], which has the effect of bringing the 5′ and 3′ ends of the message together. The message is then brought to the 40S subunit when the loaded eIF4G binds to eIF3 already on the subunit. The initiation AUG codon is as many as 100 or more nucleotides downstream of the 5′ cap structure. This necessitates an ATP-dependent scanning search for the downstream initiation codon, recognisable by its ability to base pair with the waiting anticodon of Met-tRNAi. After selection of the initiation codon, eIF5 is recruited to aid in the dissociation of eIF2-GDP, eIF3 and eIF4 factors in preparation for the joining of the 60S subunit to form the 80S initiation complex. Some mRNAs, such as the polycistronic genomic RNA of the poliovirus, have no 5′-methyl-G cap structures, but contain internal ribosome entry sites (IRES) where initiation of protein synthesis can take place without the need for the initiation factors required for most cellular mRNAs.

SECTION III

MOLECULAR GENETICS AND THEIR DATABASE

## Chapter 4

Genomics—Basic Concepts

INTRODUCTION

Bioinformatics is basically database mining—the extraction, sorting and analysing of sequence information about genes, genomes and proteins. Simply put, genes have to be sequenced; in order to do that, they must be isolated and cloned into the appropriate form which will allow them to be manipulated in the laboratory. Therefore, cloning and sequencing are not part of bioinformatics per second. Cloning and sequencing, combined with bioinformatics, however, are interwoven activities. The technical advancement of one activity greatly impacts the other two. The increasing numbers of sequences improve the quality of statistical analysis, while the development of new bioinformatics software allows for the identification of biological functions associated with sequence patterns, thus allowing faster detection and cloning of novel genes.

DNA CLONING AND PCR

DNA sequences are often found based on predictive tools, meaning that sequence similarities of newly discovered genes yield information about their physiological functions and structures, PCR (polymerase chain reaction), finding sequence fragments of significance (how is significance judged? By predictive biology, once again), finding distribution of genes or mRNAs (often an indicator of gene activity in an organism) and amplifying the amount of DNA for purification, sequencing and mutational analysis.

Analysing the rapidly accumulating sequence and structure information must be done with accuracy if the underlying methods of obtaining this information are to be evaluated in a critical and timely manner. Therefore, it is helpful to understand the biological background of how DNA and protein sequences are obtained.

DNA Cloning

Cloning is commonly known as the process of asexually producing a group of cells (clones), all genetically identical, from a single ancestor. Here, it refers to the use of DNA manipulation procedures to produce multiple copies of a single gene or segment of DNA through recombinant DNA technology. A desired gene or DNA fragment is cut out of its chromosomal location and inserted into vector DNA that is used for replication (amplification) in a host organism. Such cloning vectors are DNA molecules originating from viruses, bacteria or yeast that contain proper strings of promoter sequences to control gene expression independently of DNA amplification in the host cell. Thus, a bacterial promoter is used on vectors for mammalian expression systems (cell lines). The bacterial RNA polymerase will specifically control the vector DNA, while the cell's genome is unaffected. Unrelated DNA fragments are integrated without loss of the vector's capacity for self-replication in its natural cellular environment, allowing foreign or recombinant DNA to be reproduced in large quantities in host cells. Examples of cloning vectors are plasmids (bacterial origin), cosmids (viral origin), yeast and bacterial artificial chromosomes. Vectors are also called expression vectors when they contain the elements necessary for gene regulation. This feature is used to synthesise large quantities of mRNA or proteins in host organisms that normally do not contain or express these genes.

Behind every sequence stored electronically in a computer database (electronic sequencing) is a physical library of tissue samples and cloned DNA. When originating from genome projects, they are often random collections of genomic DNA obtained through shotgun techniques such as mechanical shearing or *in vitro* radiation-induced chromosome fragmentation. Chromosomal fragments are recombined into expression vectors. The collection of those cloned fragments constitutes a library. A vector DNA contains genes that make possible their functional expression and transformation into cell lines.

Transcriptional Profiling

How is a gene of interest selected? A gene is a sequence of base pairs and despite the ability to predict a protein's function, experimental work to study the biochemistry and physiology of the actual protein is necessary. Yet before proceeding to laborious cell biology and biochemistry, the activity pattern of a gene (i.e. within which cells in a body and at what time of development or life stage a gene is expressed and a protein synthesised) is often the first piece of information used to select an 'interesting' project or to identify a useful 'target' for drug discovery. Specifically, some genes may be restricted to certain cell types, tissues or organs; their activity patterns may change from healthy to diseased (like tumours) or may differ among young and old people.

How can the functional significance of a gene for a specific cell type, tissue or organism be evaluated? First, cells where a gene is expressed (Northern blotting) must be found. This is done by finding the corresponding messenger RNA that serves as the intermediary template for protein synthesis (the m in mRNA stands for messenger, meaning that the RNA sequence is used to translate or forward the DNA sequence information into an amino acid sequence). Cytoplasmic levels (concentrations) of mRNA are good indicators for gene activity. High levels of mRNA are in many, but not all, cases indicative of the presence of a protein. The presence of protein levels must be demonstrated independently, if it is to be established as fact.

Identifying mRNA is done by hybridising (binding) radio-active labelled oligonucleotides in a sequence-specific manner to isolate target mRNA. Obviously, some sequence information must be obtained in advance. This information could have been derived from short amino acid sequences obtained from protein fragments or peptides or by searching the DNA databases for sequences with desired properties such as a human homolog to a known gene from a mouse or rat or simply a similar, but not homologous sequence representing a potential novel gene and so forth. Comparing the hybridisation pattern of different samples at varying times during the life cycle of an organism or cell, before or after differentiation during development or under varying conditions (resting vs. hormone-induced state), can be used to construct a time-space map of where in the body a specific gene or groups of genes are actively expressed.

Once the presence of a gene of interest has been verified, DNA fragments containing the gene need to be isolated and amplified. One strategy is to use enzyme reverse transcriptase (RT) which produces a

DNA copy of the mRNA fragment. The gene that codes for the mRNA can be synthesised *in vitro* and is known as complementary DNA or cDNA. The cDNA represents the coding sequence of a gene including short noncoding or flanking, regions on either side that contain regulatory sequences.

It is imperative to understand the importance of the coding sequence of eukaryotic genes because of the particularity of how most eukaryotic genes are organised on the chromosomes in the cell nucleus, which differs from the sequence found on the mRNA. A cDNA sequence of an eukaryotic gene is normally shorter than the genomic version due to the organisation of genes into coding (exons) and noncoding (introns) regions. Although the entire gene (intron plus exon plus control sequences) is transcribed into an mRNA, the mRNA will be catalytically modified in order to eliminate the introns or intervening sequences. This leaves a shortened mRNA—a combination of all exon fragments found at the genome level. This is why the use of mRNA for the synthesis of cDNA yields synthetic genes that differ from their genomic origin and can be cloned into vector DNA for easier use in the laboratory (such as *in vitro* biosynthesis of proteins, transformation of DNA into new cell lines and transgenic animals).

Positional Cloning

An alternative strategy used for the detection of hereditary disease genes is positional cloning. Here, a gene that causes a disease or contributes to the development of one, is first located on the chromosome using genetic markers, which are short, easily detectable sequences preferentially on noncoding parts of the genome. For this method, family histories must be available for analysis of the population genetics for those genes that contain mutations and appear at a specific frequency in the human population (alleles). An allele refers to a particular gene within the genome of every individual in a population. The actual sequence of the gene, however, may vary from individual to individual due to the random occurrence of mutations. While many mutations have no visible effect on the phenotype (i.e. the function of the protein), occasional mutations can cause the malfunctioning of this protein. Once a chromosomal location has been identified, clones with large inserts are identified by physical mapping, with subsequent identification of the gene(s) by sequencing. Finally, a mutation analysis compares the identified gene(s) in affected and unaffected members of a population.

Once the entire genome sequence is known, the human genome projects promise much faster identification of mutations related to diseases. Of course, the chosen sequence representing the human genome contains only one of two loci of any given gene within a population. The human genome sequence will, in fact, be the sequence of an individual revealing little information about allelic variants in a population. This will be achieved by a phenotypically selective partial genome comparison. Thus, mutation analysis of different members of the population is still a necessary step in the positional cloning approach, since no individual's genome can possibly be sequenced in its entirety. Polymorphism databases are specifically constructed to yield this information.

In addition, medical databases for every disease, susceptibility for infection, cancer and possibly psychological traits can be envisioned for the future. NCBI provides the OMIM (Online Mendelian Inheritance in Man) database (http://www.ncbi.nlm.nih.gov/Omim/). This database is a 'catalog of human genes and genetic disorders. The database contains textual information, pictures and reference information' (NCBI).

Polymerase Chain Reaction (PCR)

The technique that revolutionised DNA amplification is polymerase chain reaction (PCR). This technique is used in virtually every biomedical laboratory in the world. The process has been automated and machines that amplify DNA from small quantities into large ones are commercially available. The process, from template design (oligonucleotide to find a target gene sequence in the genome library) to mapping an organ for gene expression, is done by computer program.

The increasing numbers of sequences allow the search for functional units of unknown genes. Large-scale identification of gene expression by measuring messenger RNA levels allows researchers to keep pace with the sequencing results of genome projects (public and proprietary libraries and databases). DNA sequences can be used to generate short search sequences to screen for mRNA. In an effort to increase the efficiency of finding good drug targets, the pharmaceutical industry is developing multiarray plate and microchip assays where hundreds, even thousands, of gene fragments or cell types can be screened in a single assay.

DNA chip technology developed by Affymetrix in Santa Clara, California is leading the technology push to determine tissue distribution of expressed genes and so-called expression sequence tags (ESTs). The importance of PCR to bioinformatics—and the genome projects in particular—is its ability to amplify DNA without any biological information attached. This means that both coding and noncoding regions can be analysed as long as short stretches of sequence (between 10 and 20 nucleotides long) are known. The technique is also extremely sensitive to initial sample quantity because of the enzymatically controlled DNA amplification process in noncellular test tube solutions.

Monitoring Sequencing Progress

Many web sites contain information and links to various genome projects and databases; they all focus on specific programs and are relatively complete. It is still, however, up to the interested scientist to validate the amount and timeliness of data contained in a database. A good example of monitoring the sequencing progress of a human DNA clone can be found at the Sanger web site (www.sanger.ac.uk/). The site also provides links to FTP sites through a FASTA sequence format so that a status summary for a clone or a sequence (i.e. is the protein or gene of interest cloned? Is it homologous to other species?) can be obtained.

The monitoring of progress is a fascinating activity. It is really overwhelming to see how fast the numbers of sequences are added to the many databases. For an overview, 'progress statistics' (http://www.sanger.ac.uk/info/statistics/) can be accessed and will give the unfinished and finished numbers of nucleotides sequenced at the Sanger centre of the British medical research council. Unfinished clones provide updated information on incomplete sequences. This allows rapid access to new genes of potential interest. Such sequence information must be dealt with cautiously, as it may contain erroneous sequences and therefore, must be considered unpublished. It is important to note that the clone information pertains only to those obtained at the Sanger Centre and does not reflect the total number of sequences for any given organism. Finished clones are annotated and submitted to GenBank, EMBL and DDBJ (DNA Database of Japan), unfinished ones are not.

The Internet information is as varied as the people who are interested in particular projects. Unlike the three main public databases—the National centre for biotechnology information, the european bioinformatics institute and the national institutes of genetics in Japan (http://www.nig.ac.jp/home.html) an individual organisation's web site generally reflects only the scope of work done there. Some people focus on the individual chromosomes of specific organisms. Some are interested in mapping entire genomes or developing resources, while others focus on automation, data handling and analysis. Still others are involved in developing new tools to analyse sequences, compare genomes, study the structure and expression of genes, identify polymorphism and study chromatin structure in relation to function. All these studies put together will help generate new insights into the biological function of genomes.

COMPUTATIONAL TOOLS FOR DNA SEQUENCE ANALYSIS

Classical examples of the roles of computers in life sciences are sequencing, sequence analysis, comparison, evolution, tracking mutations, finding similarities for drug design, predicting the function of proteins and predicting the roles of genes in cellular mechanisms and pathogenesis. The usefulness of centralised databases is not only in their availability to scientists who want to learn about other researchers, cloning efforts, but also in the ability to use them as a basis for comparative genetics. Understanding the evolution of life is impossible without an understanding of the relationship between DNA sequences of different proteins and organisms.

Database Submissions

The main sources of sequence information in central databases are scientists themselves. The current development of the Internet has made the process of submitting information to NCBI, EBI or DDBJ very easy. BankIt (World Wide Web direct deposit) or Sequin (a stand-alone program) are provided by NCBI to send sequence information and biological annotation to GenBank's staff scientists who assign them accession numbers for immediate release to the public (usually within 48 hours). Daily exchanges of new submission data between GenBank, EBI and DDBJ ensure that the information submitted by the researcher is nonredundant (submitted only once).

The genome projects, however, require specialised submission procedures for sequence information originating from ESTs (expressed sequence tags), STSs (sequence tagged sites) and GSSs (genome survey sequences). These sequences differ from traditional sequences of functional genes or proteins in their relative short length and large number.

Data Retrieval

Sequence analysis includes four major biologically relevant topics: (i) comparison of gene sequences for similarities and defining homologies from phylogenetic analysis; (ii) identification of the gene structure, including reading frames, exon-intron distribution and regulatory elements; (iii) prediction of protein structural elements; and (iv) genome mapping, the linear arrangement of genes on chromosomes and its assessment within the context of metabolic pathways.

The data currently available for DNA and protein sequences is so enormous that searching for information is dubbed 'biological data mining'. Search engines perform two basic tasks: simple string searches for information retrieval of stored data (GenBank: nucleotides and proteins; and PubMed's MEDLINE: 3-D structures, genomes and taxonomy databases) and similarity searches (e.g. BLAST) to retrieve, align and compare sequences or structures.

The first step in sequence analysis includes retrieving sequences based on specific criteria (one of which is similarity or identity between sequences) that can be obtained through a search tool such as BLAST. If no sequence is known or available, the NCBI's search engine can be screened at either the nucleotide or protein level by typing in a keyword referring to the name of a protein, the names of authors doing research on the protein of interest or the proper accession number. These searches will retrieve reports showing the number of entries in the selected database containing the keyword anywhere in the data file.

For example, consider a researcher who is looking for bacterial proteins called porins. On the Entrez search site for 'nucleotide sequence query' (http://www3.ncbi.nlm.nih.gov/Entrez/nucleotide:html), he simply types in the keyword 'maltoporin' using the search field 'all fields' and the search mode 'automatic'.

Sequence Alignment

Studying a gene means understanding its variations within population and across taxonomic groups. Sequence alignment, the pairwise comparison of sequences, is the first step in assessing the property of a newly sequenced gene, finding homologs in other organisms or identifying a new sequence as novel. NCBI allows us to compare two sequences using a 'BLAST 2 sequences' tool. This is a specialised version of the general BLAST algorithm to search for similar sequences and to retrieve them from databases. The BLAST 2 algorithm allows nucleotide (BLASTn) or amino acid sequences (BLASTp) to be compared. Several different matrix algorithms can be selected. Sequences can be entered by accession number (GI) or in FASTA format.

For multiple sequence alignment, the program ClustalW is available at many bioinformatics web sites. The European Bioinformatics Institute (EBI) can be accessed for this purpose.

Several sequences can be submitted and different output settings can be selected. The results include information about the identities from pairwise alignments and the order of most-identical to least-identical sequence pairs. An output description for creating a graphical representation (phylogenetic tree) is also included. Programs that create trees can be downloaded as stand-alone versions and ClustalW output files can be saved on the local hard drive for later reference, analysis and representations.

What a Sequence Reveals About the Biological Function of a Gene

NCBI's website is an example of a matrix database for biological knowledge. To understand a gene or its sequence, its context must be known. The context for a gene means all associated biological information that defines its function, its structure, its cellular (chromosomal) location, the structure and function of its product—protein or RNA and its taxonomic ranking. The following is a list of the biologically important annotations that may come with a DNA sequence:

1. Related sequences in database.
2. Structure prediction/comparison with X-ray structure.
3. ORF (open reading frame) if function is unknown.
4. Domain structure.
5. Transmembrane segments.
6. Signal sequence.
7. Consensus site for glycosylation, phosphorylation, lipid anchors.
8. Alternative nomenclature.
9. Genetic information such as regulatory sequences.
10. Translation.
11. 2-D gels, pI (charge), molecular weight.
12. Bibliography.

A recurring challenge stemming from the genome projects is identifying a DNA sequence representing or containing a gene. A gene is a functional unit in the genome of an organism. It includes regulatory sequences and a reading frame between a start and a stop codon, which defines the sequence corresponding to the amino acid sequence of a protein. The structure of a gene can differ dramatically from organism to organism and there are two major types: those with a continuous reading frame and those with an interrupted reading frame (exons and introns; all exons together represent the reading frame with the introns being enzymatically cut out at the mRNA level—so-called RNA splicing). The latter are typical for higher organisms (eukaryotes) and are not found in bacteria or archaea.

How to Identify a Gene: ORFs and URFs

If a gene has been sequenced in the absence of any information about the protein, no biological function will be associated. This is an intrinsic outcome of genome projects, where long contiguous sequences of DNA have to be analysed for the presence of genes. This requires software that identifies ORFs (open reading frames) or often URFs (unidentified reading frames) by searching for long stretches of sequence between a start and a stop codon.

The length of the ORF is directly related to the size or molecular weight of the coded protein and is a useful indicator for a putative ORF. In eukaryotic genes, the signature of splice sites (i.e. the sites delineating exons and introns) provide additional help in identifying a gene. For a gene to be a functional unit, the presence of transcription consensus sequences close to a start codon must be found.

Databases provide functional sites to analyse a DNA sequence for the presence of an ORF. They allow the prediction of the associated amino acids and potential structural features of the protein. If related sequences are found and if a related sequence already contains a gene sequence, sequence alignment—the comparison of the similarity of two or more sequences—is a good indicator for the potential biological function of the gene.

The ORF finder is a graphical analysis tool that finds all open reading frames of a selectable minimum size in a user's sequence or in a sequence that is present in the database. This tool identifies all open reading frames using the standard or alternative genetic codes. The deduced amino acid sequence can be saved in various formats and searched against the sequence database using the www.BLAST server. The ORF finder should be helpful in preparing complete and accurate sequence submissions.

The ORF finder screens a cDNA sequence for appropriate stretches flanked by a start and stop codon. 'Appropriate' refers to the size of a gene and thus the size of a protein for which no function is known or may be inferred from homolog sequences. In the latter case, the ORF finder is a tool for reliable confirmation of the identification of novel genes for known, predicted protein functions. It provides the means to ensure that the investigated cDNA sequence contains a functional version of the gene. The ORF finder is useful for screening bacterial genomes, cDNA libraries and EST databases, but not the raw sequence of an eukaryotic organism. Therefore, the proper gene fragments, exons and introns, must first be identified, cloned, sequenced and put together into a contiguous sequence which then may contain the continuous coding sequence of a gene.

Genes are working units on chromosomes containing ORF fragments and noncoding regions that are important for the regulation of gene expression. Eukaryotic gene structures can often be very complex, allowing for recombinatorial processes such that a gene complex can recombine its exons in different ways (splice variants) resulting in different gene products. Entire gene clusters can form the basis of hypervariable domains in proteins of the immune system.

A Word About Redundancy

Scientists work independently, which often results in repetitive naming of identical genes and proteins. This is typical in the submission of data for new, emerging fields; in this case, DNA sequences occur more than once and under different entries, names and annotations. Only a specialist in the field would be able to recognise that seemingly different entries refer only to one subject. Obviously, redundancy can be useful; for handling DNA sequences in databases, it is actually an unintentional quality control. It sometimes happens that two competing laboratories publish the sequence of the same gene, but with one or more base differences. Does this represent a true mutant coming from different strains of mice or a sequencing error? If the source of the gene is the same organism, a sequencing error is usually the case.

GENOME ANALYSIS

Genome analysis can determine locations of genes on chromosomes and give information on heritability and linkage to other genes, genetics (classical), medical importance, gene therapy, tracking autosomal mutations and X-linked diseases. The yeast protein database (YPD) links information of DNA sequences, protein structure and function, cellular localisation and pathways and cell-cycle information into one coherent database with links to literature information, a commercial approach with the intention of selling database access to companies, proteomics as compared to genomics, 2-D gel electrophoresis, image processing, storage, retrieval and pattern recognition.

Genome Organisation

Bioinformatics tools and databases are slowly becoming an integrated system that reflects the complexity of organisms. With genome projects of small organisms being completed one by one, an understanding of the differences of genomes from the three urkingdoms (eubacteria, archaea and eukaryotes) and the relationship of genome organisation to the form and function of an organism may be just around the corner. Prokaryotes have very different genome structures compared to eukaryotes. While their names refer to the absence or presence of a nuclear compartment within the cell, the differences do not stop there. The relative frequency of coding vs. noncoding regions differs as do the arrangements of genes on the chromosomes. While bacteria have a compact genome with little noncoding DNA, eukaryotic chromosomes are often extremely large and found in great numbers, especially in plants. The genes of eukaryotes and the prokaryotic archaea are often fragmented into noncontinuous 'exons'.

Special databases containing entire genomes of organisms provide information such as relatedness of genes within the genome, closeness in space, coregulation, etc. For example, metabolic pathways in different bacterial species may vary because of an additional enzymatic step in one species but not another. The way to find out is to see if specific proteins belong to a cluster of genes (this structure is an operon) that is often aligned along the micro-organism's genome such that an entire pathway for the synthesis of an amino acid is upregulated in a coordinated fashion, avoiding the individual regulation of every enzyme needed for a pathway. The existence of pathways and multiple genes coding for the enzymes of pathways has important consequences on how mutations affect cellular physiology. Mutations affecting an enzyme that is part of a pathway may affect this entire pathway because it, as such, constitutes a phenotype. The progress in sequencing entire genomes of both prokaryotic and eukaryotic organisms will undoubtedly help in determining the physiological role of organisational structures of genomes and its importance for metabolic processes.

Although genes are important because they code for all the proteins and RNA existing in a cell, these structural genes often constitute a fraction of genomes, particularly in eukaryotic organisms—fungi, plants and animals. For example, an estimated 90 per cent of the human genome constitutes noncoding regions. It was not that long ago that these noncoding regions were casually dismissed as junk DNA, reflecting a lack of understanding and knowledge of their function. More and more, the DNA that does not code for proteins or RNA (regulatory, structural and enzymatic) is being recognised as important in how cells have access to the coding 10 per cent of DNA. Essentially, this noncoding DNA is important in replication and control of cell-specific gene expression. It seems to contain information that is 'read only' (short sequences that function as specific binding sites for proteins involved in gene expression and replication). Such proteins are growth factor or hormone receptors. These protein-binding elements are crucial for cells and play a role in cell differentiation, morphogenesis and pattern formation during embryogenesis.

The implications of noncoding regions in DNA on evolution is tremendous. Because mutations are random events, the noncoding parts of chromosomes absorb most of these changes in base composition and serve as a 'playground' for chromosomal recombination and accumulation of silent mutations. Polymorphic markers (the markers used in DNA fingerprinting technology) are found in this portion of the DNA. A surprising finding of genetic analysis of clusters of genes from different individuals reflects the high frequency of nucleotide sequence differences between individuals (restriction fragment length polymorphism: reflects sequence variations in DNA sites that can be cleaved by DNA restriction enzymes). This genetic polymorphism has recently been used in forensic science. This so-called genetic 'fingerprinting' yields information unique to one individual in several billion. Genetic fingerprinting has changed our court system. The use of PCR has been successful in identification since very tiny tissue samples from blood stains, dead skin or a single hair found at a crime scene are enough to amplify DNA for analysis.

To understand the relationship between the 'blueprint' of life and life itself requires information about the relative position of genes within the genome, as well as the relationship between sequence and structure in proteins. Since proteins are not isolated entities and multiple protein-protein interactions are the basis of cellular activity, selection pressure on individual genes is likely to be coupled over several genes whose proteins work together. This makes sequence-to-structure and structure-to-function relationships extremely complex. The multitude of interactions is too complex. New technologies such as genomics and proteomics, where the simultaneous expression levels of RNA or proteins are determined, are starting points to address the complex molecular interactions involved in cells.

How do we measure independence and interdependence of inheritable properties? We can refer to Gregor Mendel and his study of independently inherited traits on the colour and consistency of peas. At the molecular level, two independent traits (phenotype) are coded for by genes (or alleles) located on physically separated chromosomes. If they are located on the same chromosome they are regularly— but not necessarily—inherited together (because the distance between genes on the same chromosome is also crucial), i.e. they are said not to segregate.

The importance of genome structures and chromosomal stability can be demonstrated in studies of the molecular evolution of histone proteins—the proteins responsible for the packing and storage of DNA into high-density forms of our chromosomes. During cell division, chromosomes condense into the well-known, double-arm structures (pairs of chromosomes; see karyotype), but during the normal resting state of a cell, these chromosomes are loosely packed and amenable to the proteins that transcribe genes into RNA (polymerase) and others which control access to DNA (transcription factors). This is the essence of gene regulation (transcription or expression). It is a balance of access to DNA strands among structural proteins (or histones), the nucleic acid synthesising proteins (or polymerases) and DNA binding proteins (or transcription factors) which control accessibility of polymerases to the DNA molecule.

The importance of gene transcription in the viability of organisms is obvious, since genes code for proteins and proteins control every process within a cell. The importance of chromosome structure, however, is less clear, but evidence indicates that interfering with the structure of chromosomes is lethal for cells. Analysing the amino acid sequence of histone proteins has provided one line of evidence. Histone genes are highly conserved across all species within the eukaryotic kingdom. They are a key feature of the genetics of animals, plants and fungi. Their conserved sequences also indicate a single evolutionary ancestor cell or organism from which all modern eukaryotes are derived. Indeed, histone proteins are used as molecular docks, molecular rulers to measure the phylogenetic distance (time since separation of two species) between distantly related organisms. The survival of an organism (or a population) is linked to its phenotype and hereditary changes in phenotype (mutations) occur and are stored exclusively at the DNA level by random changes in the base composition (DNA sequence). Mutations are 'rejected' if the phenotype confers a lethal trait. The organism either dies before reaching reproductive age or becomes infertile, thus losing the chance to pass its genome to the next generation. The rate of mutations accumulating in a gene (nucleotide sequences which are not rejected) over time is a direct measure of the importance of the phenotype (the protein) to the viability of the individual, but not of the population. Allelic variations within a population, however, are indicators of the susceptibility of specific genes to mutations. Histone genes show an extremely low mutation rate over hundreds of millions of years indicating that the structure of these proteins is essential for all eukaryotic organisms. This means that besides gene replication and transcription, differential DNA packing in chromosomes during different states of the cell cycle is crucial for survival.

Genomics, the attempt to catalog the gene content, organisation and temporal expression patterns of a genome, will give detailed information about the evolution of cellular function. It is therefore not surprising that the Internet has become an essential tool for scientists because of the many databases containing information about the genomes of thousands of species, their taxonomy and evolutionary relationship in the form of phylogenetic trees or 'the tree of life'. Phylogenetic trees are visual ways of understanding evolutionary relationships.

The tree of life is a figurative representation of the diversifying life forms on earth originating from a common ancestor. It is believed that there is only one such tree (e.g. a single progenitor 'cell') and that life is not of multiple origin. Although reasonable and consistent with the findings of molecular biologists, this is speculative and corroborates the notion of the slim chance of life having arisen by chance out of nonliving matter. That this event happened is not disputed here, but it is astounding since scientists agree that the spontaneous generation of new life from (in-) organic material is highly unlikely.

The tree of life project at the University of Arizona (http://phylogeny.arizona.edu/tree/life.html) provides a visual overview of the phylogeny of all life on earth. It is not a molecular evolution type of tree, but a classical taxonomy tree. This is a very useful tool for molecular biologists who often have no formal training in evolution, zoology, botany and ecology. The project contains information about the diversity of organisms on Earth, their history and characteristics. It is a multi-authored website coordinated and created by David R. Maddison at the University of Arizona.

Proteins can be found as part of larger protein complexes and only within the context of these complexes can the activity of these proteins be studied. They are not independent, thus their genes cannot be independent, yet some proteins linked through functional complex formation are coded by genes found randomly, without any apparent linkage on different chromosomes. Is there significance for such an apparent lack of organisation of certain groups of genes in the human genome? The red blood cell protein haemoglobin, the transport molecule in our blood that helps carry oxygen from the lungs to target muscles or organs like the brain, is made of four tightly packed protein subunits coded for by two different genes. The genes are called alpha and beta globin genes and the functional haemoglobin protein complex contains two copies of each gene product. Although these two genes always need to be expressed together for the proper complex formation (there is no functional haemoglobin made of four alpha subunits or four beta subunits), the globin gene coding for the alpha subunit is actually a cluster of alpha globin genes with slightly different sequences and is differentially expressed during subsequent embryonic stages. Thus, only one gene copy of the alpha cluster is expressed at any given time during development. While clusters are located close to each other, the alpha subunit cluster is found on chromosome 16, while the cluster for beta globin subunits is found on chromosome 11.

Anatomical and physiological phenotypes are multi-trait phenotypes, meaning that several gene products constitute the genotype. Besides the obvious visual characteristics of an individual's appearance, cellular metabolism is the best example for studying multi-enzyme pathways. The synthesis and degradation of metabolites such as sugars, fats, amino acids and lipids are part of these complex, interdependent pathways. The organisation of genes that constitute a pathway for individual metabolites in genomes is different for different organisms. As a rule, there is no strict correlation between proteins that functionally and structurally interact with each other and the position of their genes on chromosomes. Sometimes such genes are closely grouped into functional units in gene expression and are often loosely scattered all over the genome. Functional genomics may help shed some light on this problem.

There is a definite relationship between a particular DNA sequence and the chromosomal morphology of the organism. The following distinct morphological (structural) features have been established:

1. Telomeric regions (tandemly repeated sequences, ageing related).
2. Centromeric regions (tandemly repeated sequences).
3. Nucleolar organiser (genes for ribosomal RNA; relate to Fig. 4.1 of metacentric chromosome pair).

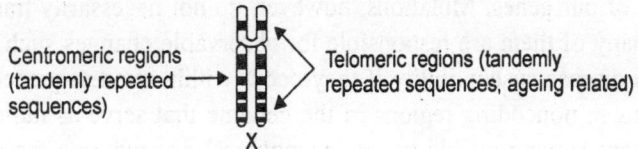

Centromeric regions (tandemly repeated sequences) → X ← Telomeric regions (tandemly repeated sequences, ageing related)

Fig. 4.1. Chromosome pair; G-banding and chromosome identification.

Because of the relationship between gene function and chromosome structure, the physical mapping of genomes is essential to gaining an understanding of the uniqueness of an organism and its developmental plan (stages of life cycle). The uniqueness of an organism lies not only in its gene composition, but also its chromosome structure. Mammalian chromosomes come in metacentric and acrocentric form. It has been shown that one reason members of different species (although closely related in their gene sequences) are reproductively incompatible is that their chromosomal structures (the superstructure of DNA which is also dependent on histone proteins) are incompatible during cell fusion and division (mitosis, meiosis). Here we can see the emergence of a loop where genes coding for histone proteins are regulated by how these proteins interact with each other and DNA to form the superstructure of chromosomes and which determines the viability of the cell because of its importance during cell division. Nucleotide changes (mutations) in histone genes affect their amino acid composition, which affects chromosome structure, which affects histone gene inheritance (replication) and expression (transcription).

Mapping the Genome

Genome databases play an increasingly important role in understanding novel genes whose functions have yet to be determined. Yet by analogy to a gene's location and association to chromosomal location, its function might be inferred and be useful in the design of future experiments. Chromosome locations, like DNA sequences, are subject to changes (e.g. mutations) and can change from generation to generation. In eukaryotes, rearrangements of chromosomal fragments (homologous recombination, reciprocal crossing over, meiosis and mitosis) is an important part of genetic variability among individuals. Genetic polymorphism, as mentioned above, based on chromosomal rearrangements, also makes individuals genetically unique, although the overall genomic contents (the whole of all genes inherited) remain constant. Rearrangements can influence and alter gene expression in an orderly and programmed fashion.

Many of these rearrangement processes also cause diseases, an additional motivation to understand the relationship between gene expression and chromosomal morphology. This is reflected in the growing size of genome databases related to medical issues, as well as information sites about inheritable diseases and their relationship to genetics (NIH health information at http://www.nih.gov/health/).

Genetic linkage maps

Genetic linkage maps depict the relative chromosomal locations of DNA markers (genes and other identifiable DNA sequences) by their patterns of inheritance. Are they inherited together or not? The distance between markers on the map indicates the frequency of how often they are inherited together (inverse relationship). This is the field of population genetics and in human is the study of family history of autosomal and sex-linked traits. DNA markers must be polymorphic to be useful. Polymorphisms (mutations) are variations in DNA sequence that occur, on average, once every 300 to 500 bp, representing the lower end of length distribution of genes. This means that polymorphism is a fairly common feature of our genes. Mutations, however, do not necessarily translate into an altered phenotype, although many of them are responsible for observable changes such as differences in eye colour, blood type and disease susceptibility if they occur within exon sequences. It is precisely the occurrence of mutations in noncoding regions of the genome that serve as molecular markers at the level of the DNA without leaving visible traces (phenotypes) or rendering the organism less viable. Because they commonly reside in noncoding parts of the genome they can be considered hidden mutations and can only be seen at the level of DNA analysis. In short, genetic linkage maps are constructed by observing how frequently two markers are inherited together within a family tree (from generation to generation). Mendel's pea colours constitute such markers and although some are obviously inherited independently (not linked on chromosomes) while others are linked, they reside on the same chromosome. Genetic maps have been used to find the exact chromosomal location of several important disease genes, including cystic fibrosis, sickle cell disease, Tay-Sachs disease, fragile X syndrome and myotonic dystrophy (Fig. 4.2).

'One short-term goal of the genome project is to develop a high-resolution genetic map (2 to 5_cM [centimorgan]; Two markers are said to be 1_cM apart if they are separated by recombination 1 per cent of the time. A genetic distance of 1_cM is roughly equal to a physical distance of 1 million bp [1 Mb]); recent consensus maps of some chromosomes have averaged 7 to 10_cM between genetic markers. Genetic mapping resolution has been increased through the application of recombinant DNA technology, including *in vitro* radiation-induced chromosome fragmentation and cell fusions (joining human cells with those of other species to form hybrid cells) to create panels of cells with specific and varied human chromosomal components. Assessing the frequency of marker sites remaining together after radiation-induced DNA fragmentation can establish the order and distance between the markers. Because only a single copy of a chromosome is required for analysis, even nonpolymorphic markers are useful in radiation hybrid mapping.' [In meiotic mapping, described above, two copies of a chromosome must be distinguished from each other by polymorphic markers.]

Physical maps

Physical maps describe the molecular organisation of genes or markers within a genome or chromosome. Depending on the technique available or used, the resolution of the map can vary widely. Early methods relied on microscopic techniques analysing banding patterns on condensed forms of chromosomes. Bands often correlate to differently active regions of genomes. While light microscopy needs DNA preparation in a fairly organised form (such as during mitosis), electron microscopy provides higher resolution and can thus detail finer structures.

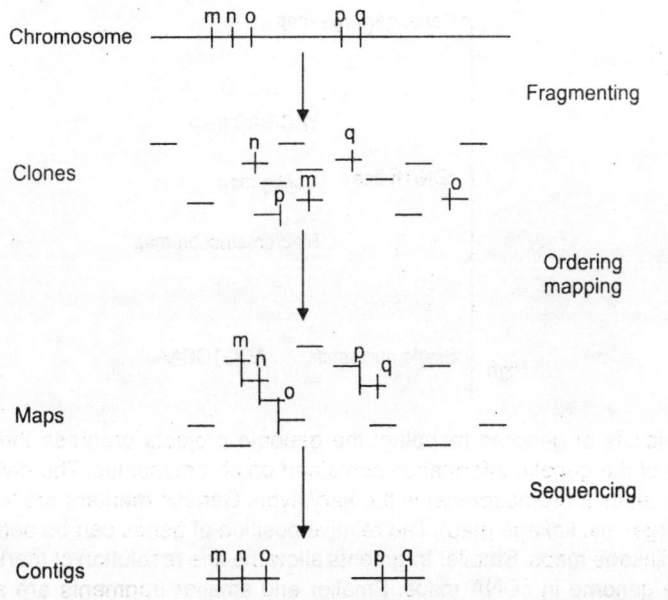

Fig. 4.2. Mapping and sequencing of chromosomes: a chromosome containing five markers (m,n,o,p,q) is fragmentised and the fragments (clones) identified by markers. These clones are ordered and mapped by comparing overlapping strings of sequences. As long as fragments show such overlapping sequences, they can be linked to continuous segments (contig 1 mno and contig 2 pq). If some fragments are missing, the entire chromosome cannot be reproduced, but is rather represented by several contigs. Since fragments have been sequenced in full, the corresponding contig sequences are known and can be stored in the database (e.g. GenBank).

High-resolution physical maps (Fig. 4.3) make use of the increasing sequence information available, combining microscopic data with genetic linkage maps and DNA sequences around those markers (genes). The ultimate physical map, then, will be the entire, contiguous DNA sequence of the (human) genome or its chromosome. Since genetic linkage maps measure distances of markers based on recombinatorial activity of chromosomes, the relative distances between marker on physical and genetic linkage maps can be quite different. This is based on the fact that recombination during meiosis and mitosis has different frequency at different locations within chromosomes.

The mechanism of this behaviour is not understood. It could be 'simply' sequence dependent or related to chromosome structure, which actually may be determined by sequence patterns. This difference between physical and functional maps, therefore, is also of interest and genome projects will contribute information that could ultimately answer their questions.

The Sanger web site (http://www.sanger.ac.uk/) shows examples of human chromosomes and the hierarchical organisation where the user interested in a clone and its localisation on a particular chromosome can zoom into an incrementally detailed map until the nucleotide sequence level is reached.

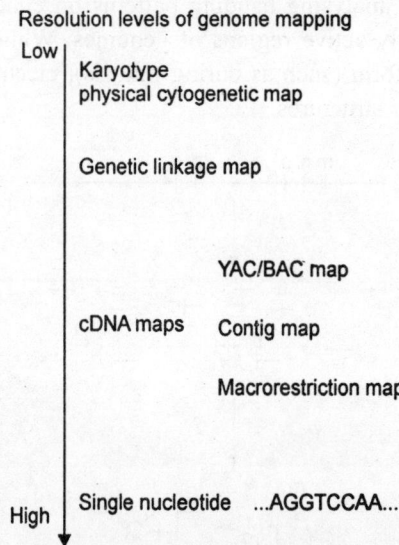

Resolution levels of genome mapping

Low
Karyotype
physical cytogenetic map

Genetic linkage map

YAC/BAC map

cDNA maps   Contig map

Macrorestriction map

Single nucleotide   ...AGGTCCAA...

High

Fig. 4.3. Resolution levels of genome mapping: the genome projects progress through several levels of increasing resolution of the genetic information contained on chromosomes. The division of the genome in physically individual pieces (chromosomes) is the karyotype. Genetic markers are linked if they are on the same chromosomes (genetic linkage map). The relative position of genes can be determined by correlating physical and genetic linkage maps. Smaller fragments allow the fine resolution of markers located very close to each other on the genome in cDNA maps. Smaller and smaller fragments are amenable to complete sequence analysis at the single nucleotide level.

Expression maps

The identification of structural genes has been driving the human genome project from the beginning and is also characteristic of the major cloning efforts in drug discovery. The reason for this is simple: structural genes are easy to identify because they can be activated and inactivated. In fact, the problem is reduced to the identification of mRNA in cells. The resulting sequence tags have been instrumental in identifying novel eukaryotic genes. Instead of waiting for complete genome sequences, very short fragments are being selected and sequenced for the construction of so-called expression maps. Because genes are composed of both coding and noncoding flanking regions containing regulatory sequences, both expressed sequence tags and sequence-tagged sites have been instrumental in creating linkage and high resolution maps of human chromosomes.

The identification of ESTs is a short-cut for identifying human genes since they are derived from active genes. ESTs can be obtained without any knowledge of their function. Since genes are not expressed all the time and often in a cell type-specific manner (as well as being dependent on different states of the development of an organism), the entire life cycle and all physiologically relevant tissues have to be probed for the presence of mRNA and its subsequent sequencing. This approach misses a major portion of an eukaryotic genome, but reveals interesting physiological and medical conditions.

Noncoding DNA is sequenced fragment by fragment through PCR technology. The creation of the dbSTS depository includes specific sequence tags which can be used to uniquely identify chromosome locations (they serve as markers for genes when cosegregating). By using electronic PCR, STS with known chromosomal positions can be searched and compared with new sequences and the genomic position of the latter can be determined. In this way, e-PCR can be used for the creation of various types of genomic maps.

All in all, the rapid pace of sequencing often results in partial or unfinished sequences. The high-throughput genome division of GenBank (http://www.ncbi.nlm.nih.gov/HTGS/) tries to accommodate this fact and coordinates submission of such fragments not only to GenBank, but also to the Japanese and European depositories. This is an effort coordinated among the three international nucleotide sequence databases: DDBJ, EMBL and GenBank.

Elimination of Redundancy

As the genome projects develop into an organised enterprise, the elimination of redundancy is a major concern in streamlining and optimising the databases. Redundancy not only comes from the fact that different researchers are interested in the same protein or gene, but that different techniques of cloning and sequencing random genomes creates fragments with little biologically relevant annotation.

Redundancy, of course, is beneficial for certain aspects of genome mapping and quality control and redundancy and homology are closely related concepts with homology actually referring to two (or more) different genes with great similarity. Those are likely to be alleles in a population or the homologs of a specific gene in different species or taxonomic groups.

FUNCTIONAL GENOMICS

With over 3,00,000 DNA sequences stored in databases around the world, the potential is tremendous for identifying 'interesting' novel genes for medical and biological studies. It is evident from the twenty-something completed microbial genome projects that as many as 40 per cent of structural genes are novel. This means that they have never been studied experimentally for their biochemical and physiological properties. Therefore, annotation of structure and function for those sequences which show some resemblance to known proteins relies on automated, statistical analysis.

This method of predicting structure and function represents a crude, first run to gather biological information. These annotations, however, are increasingly based on previously predicted information. The biology behind the sequences, the phenotype-protein structure and function—still the systematic annotation of what is known biochemically about proteins—often falls behind. This means that even after the completion of a genome, project, years of investigation are needed to understand the full complexity of the organism at the physiological level. One of the first tasks after genomes are completely sequenced is to understand their content, i.e. to relate phenotype and genotype. In other words, the task ahead consists of assigning function to sequences based on the organisation of genes within genomes and comparing these structures to distantly related genomes.

The task of extracting and analysing the large amount of genomic data is made possible through public domain software that allows the analysis and characterisation of all kinds of properties associated with DNA, RNA and proteins. Tables 4.1 and 4.2 show the most common goals in studying genome structure, the identification of novel genes and their related protein structures and the major Internet addresses where these programs can be accessed.

Table 4.1. Public domain software analysis tools for DNA and RNA.

Goal	Program	Internet address
Sequence similarity	BLASTn and tBLASTx and BLASTx	www.ncbi.nlm.nih.gov/BLAST
Finding open reading frames (ORF)	ORF finder	www.ncbi.nlm.nih.gov/gorf/gorf.html
Finding PCR-based sequence tagged sites (STSs) in DNA sequence	Electronic PCR	www.ncbi.nlm.nih.gov/STS/
Translating DNA or RNA → Protein	Translate and Protein machine	www.expasy.hcuge.ch/tools/dna.html and www.ebi.ac.uk/translate.html
Comparison of genomic DNA and protein sequence	GeneWise	www.sanger.ac.uk/Software/Wise2/genewiseform.shtml
Finding genes	Gene recognition and Assembly Internet Link (GRAIL) and PROCRUSTES	www.compbio.ornl.gov/Grail-1.3/ and www-hto.usc.edu/software/procrustes

Table 4.2. Public domain software analysis tools for proteins.

Goal	Program	Internet address
Sequence similarity	BLASTp and tBLASTn	www.ncbi.nlm.nih.gov/BLAST
Automated structural modelling	SWISS-MODEL	www.expasy.ch/swissmod/SWISS-MODEL.html
Identification and characterisation	Protein identification and characterisation programs	www.expasy.ch/tools/#proteome
Finding patterns and profiles	Pattern and profile search programs	expasy.hcuge.ch/tools/#pattern
Structure analysis	Primary structure analysis, secondary structure prediction and tertiary structure programs	www.expasy.ch/tools/#primary www.expasy.ch/tools/#secondary www.expasy.ch/tools/#tertiary
Sequence alignment	Sequence alignment programs	/www.expasy.ch/tools/#align
2-D page analysis	Melanie II	www.expasy.ch/melanie/

The first step in understanding the relationship between genotype and phenotype is to look at the function of the entire genome. This is reflected in the cellular expression pattern of mRNA. Novel genes can thus be identified as being expressed in relation to a cellular activity for which we have some biologically significant information. The study of expression patterns then allows us to assign spatio-temporal information to unknown genes. Such a simple procedure can be used to structure a database according to perceived correlations. Databases are subdivided to reflect different levels of function ascribed to proteins and genes. Hierarchical, structures of databases are practical ways for biologists to quickly find information about a protein, gene, metabolic pathway, enzymatic activity or evolutionary relationships. Current databases are constructed using information of related sequences, proteins, taxonomic information, predicted secondary structures or domain organisation of proteins.

It is also necessary to understand structure and function of protein families from organisms that are evolutionarily distant (i.e. they belong to different groups or kingdoms), like bacteria and human. Sequence comparisons of distantly related organisms fall into three major classes. The first group comprises highly similar sequences and is observed for proteins of cell replication and information-storage processes. These proteins are true homologs, they share a common ancestral gene and form a protein family. The second group includes proteins with similar structure and function, but dissimilar sequence. Their relationship can be inferred from structural and functional similarity, but lack significant sequence similarity. They may or may not be related evolutionarily and may be examples of convergent evolution. The third group shows no similarity for sequence function or structure.

Local sequence patterns that code for nucleotide binding pockets are valuable in assessing evolutionary relatedness because structural features of catalytic sites are better conserved than DNA or amino acid sequences of entire genes or proteins. This relationship conceptually allows us to search for conserved patterns in sequences and it is those patterns that are significant in establishing evolutionary relationships among genes. Even when the full-length (gene) sequence shows little or no similarity to other proteins, functional domains show a high degree of structural conservation. Because only selected stretches of fragments of genes show high similarity, these patterns can point out evolutionary mechanisms like gene duplication and recombination events leading to 'chimeric' structures.

Adam Godzik of the Scripps Research Institute in La Jolla, California develops and applies novel algorithms to address some of the problems associated with identifying proteins with similar structure, but dissimilar sequence. The genome analysis page (http://cape6.scripps.edu/leszek/genome/) offers the comparison of sequence information of the genomes of *Mycoplasma genitalium*, *Escherichia coli* and *Helicobacter pylori* with the protein structures in PDB. The program compares the predicted structures of all ORFs of an entire genome with all known crystal and NMR structures in the protein database. Comparing structural motifs allows us to identify weak relationships that are routinely missed by BLAST, but still fails to predict the function for a large portion of bacterial genomes. As an example, the genome of *Escherichia coli* contains a total of ~4300 genes coding for 1500 hypothetical proteins (40 per cent of all known genes or ORFs). From these, 30 per cent (or ~500 ORFs) could not be predicted reliably as to what protein structure they encode or what the putative function of these proteins would be. An additional 30 per cent could not be predicted at all, meaning they are completely novel proteins with no known counterparts in bacteria, archaea, plants or animals.

Unidentified Reading Frames: URFs

The genome projects completed thus far have identified approximately 30 to 40 per cent completely new and unidentified gene sequences. They are referred to as URFs (unidentified reading frames) and no biological information is associated with them. No homologies are known, so they must be coding for new proteins that have not been found by biochemists or functionally identified by microbiologists. Structure prediction algorithms like that of Adam Godzik are of tremendous help here, but often do not help in understanding the function, indicating the big gap in knowledge of relating structure to function. Often it is a rationalisation vaguely based on experimental evidence. Many structure prediction methods are statistical methods and rely on information obtained from known structures. The limited sample size (i.e. the number of known structures), limits the accuracy of predicting folds.

An alternative tool used to explore evolutionary relationship for novel genes is direct genomic comparison by studying the 'behaviour' of a genome. What is the mutation rate of known proteins of an organism? This information may help predict the uniqueness of a new gene in an organism that shows no sequence similarity to any known protein. Assuming that the mutation rate is even in the entire genome of an organism (an assumption which is not necessarily true), the sequence dissimilarity of a URF sequence is an indicator that it may belong to a new class of proteins that define the uniqueness of the organism.

Take as an example the enzymes that link amino acids with a small class of RNA molecules called transfer or tRNA. In all mammalian organisms there are at least 20 different enzymes, one each for each of the 20 amino acids used to synthesise proteins (a universal fact of life). From the completed genome project of the archaea *M. jannaschii*, for four of these amino acyl tRNA synthetase no corresponding gene has been identified, although they must exist, since all tRNAs are linked properly with their respective amino acids.

One possibility explaining the lack of genes is to assume a totally new mechanism for amino acyl tRNA synthesis: chemical modification of amino acids linked to tRNA molecules. One of the unidentified genes codes for the *lysyl*-tRNA synthetase. However, it has been demonstrated by functional cloning in a research project unrelated to the genome project, that this synthetase responsible for linking the amino acid lysine to its tRNA partner has a sequence totally unrelated to any known lysine-tRNA syntheses. Indeed, this is an example of an entirely new family of proteins. The conclusion is that two entirely unrelated proteins, as judged on the bases of their DNA sequence, perform the same enzymatic activity. This has been shown for other classes of enzymes such as the serine protease chymotrypsin and subtilisin. They catalyse the same chemical reaction using structurally conserved active sites albeit with different substrate specificity.

The existence of evolutionarily unrelated but functionally similar proteins demonstrates that in the complete absence of functional data, the interpretation of what kind of protein DNA sequences code for can be difficult and sometimes impossible. The use of data from functional cloning efforts was necessary to assign a biological function to URFs. To understand the relationship between structure (sequence) and function of the amino acyl tRNA synthetases requires a great deal of familiarity with the topic. Scientists unfamiliar with tRNA metabolism are not likely to find the apparent relationship.

Cluster of Orthologous Groups: COGs

Finding functional relationships between genes across taxonomic groups (orthologs) as well as within a population or the same organism (paralogs) provides the true potential of genome projects. Comparing protein sequences encoded in eight complete genomes, representing six major phylogenetic lineages delineated clusters of orthologous groups. This is an effort to use databases to generate new information by linking sequence information from various complete genomes. Any two proteins from different lineages that belong to the same COG are orthologs according to the functional definition used by NCBI to construct COGs and are assumed to have evolved through speciation. COGs also contain paralogs, which arise through gene duplication events.

Using the completed genomes of eight organisms (*E. coli, H. influenzae, M. genitalium, H. pylori, M. pneumoniae, Synechocystis, M. jannaschii,* and *S. cerevisiae*), a total of 864 COGs have been identified belonging to information storage and processing (groups J, K, L), cellular processes (groups O, M, N, P), metabolism (groups C, G, E, F, H, I) and predicted or unknown functions (groups R, S). This group of poorly defined proteins comprises a total of 180 COGs (out of 864) with 1828 proteins and domains associated to predicted function (R) and 271 uncharacterised proteins and domains (S). The analysis of COGs allows for the understanding of evolutionary relationships and the identification of related functions across taxonomic divisions.

Group N contains 20 COGs, one of which represents the signal peptidase family of proteases involved in protein secretion in eubacteria and eukaryotes, but not archaea (COG ID 0681;). Signal peptidase I is a small, membrane-bound protein that cleaves off the N-terminal signal sequence of proteins transported across the endoplasmatic reticulum membrane of eukaryotes and inner membrane of bacteria and mitochondria (the current members of completed genomes include seven bacterial and one eukaryotic organisms). Signal peptidase I COG consists of eight members, one *E. coli* protein LepB, the *H. influenzae* protein HIN1152, *Synechocystis* sp. paralogs slr1377 and sll0716, *M. jannaschii* protein MJ0260 and three yeast paralogs, proteins YMR150c, YMR035w and YIR022w.

The COG demonstrates the complexity of searching for phylogenetic relationships among proteins of distantly related organisms. One of the yeast paralogs (YMR035w) shows best-hit similarity to three different, bacterial species (*E. coli, H. influenzae* and *Synechocystis* sp.). YMR150c and YMR035w are inner-membrane proteases of yeast mitochondria, responsible for removal of signal peptides from some proteins of the inter-membrane space, but with different substrate specificity. YIR022w is the yeast signal sequence processing protein in the endoplasmatic reticulum, required for signal peptide cleavage and normal rate of protein secretion.

The cluster dendrogram shows the close relationship of mitochondrial proteases with bacterial orthologs and the relationship of the ER protease paralog with the archaea ortholog of *M. jannaschii*. This is consistent with the proposed common ancestral single-cell organism of eubacteria and mitochondria (endosymbiotic theory). That the *M. jannaschii* protease shows an orthologous relationship to both yeast and cyanobacteria, stresses the taxonomic classification of archaea as different from both eukaryotes and eubacteria. This COG analysis indicates that of the three yeast peptidases, the two mitochondrial subtypes are true paralogs with a common eubacterial origin, whereas the ER subtype evolved independently or originates from an older ancestral gene that precedes split into eubacteria and archaea. This split may be the event behind the paralogs in *Synechocystis* sp.

The COG database lists related genes in patterns indicating their occurrence in different organisms. One such pattern reads *eh—cmy*, which excludes the two Gram-positive, pathogenic mycoplasmodia and the ulcer-inducing *H. pylori*, but includes the Gram-negative pathogen *H. influenzae*. Thirty-nine other COGs with this pattern have been identified, including the one for signal peptidase I. The COG which represents the most commonly found phylogenetic pattern, including all eight genomes in this analysis, contains 110 clusters, most of which belong to functional group J relating to translation, ribosomal structure and biogenesis. Other groups of enzymes belong to such central metabolic pathways as glycolysis, pentose phosphate pathway, RNA polymerases, protein folding and secretion.

The importance of identifying such patterns where different organisms share sets of enzymes or pathways can bring about information on the biochemical requirements necessary for survival in different environments.

The group of pathogens well suited for study of the minimal genetic requirements for host infection and replication is viruses. Viruses are less complex systems because they make use of the cellular machinery of the host organism. Their genome appears to have adapted and streamlined presence of necessary genes. Viruses are the best adapted, but so are host-dependent minimal organisms containing minimal genomes. Because of their small size, viral genomes have been sequenced long before that of the first pathogenic bacteria *H. influenzae*.

Chapter 5

Molecular Genetics

INTRODUCTION

Molecular genetics is the field of biology which studies the structure and function of genes at a molecular level. The field studies how the genes are transferred from generation to generation. Molecular genetics employs the methods of genetics and molecular biology. It is so-called to differentiate it from other sub-fields of genetics such as ecological genetics and population genetics. An important area within molecular genetics is the use of molecular information to determine the patterns of descent and therefore the correct scientific classification of organisms—this is called molecular systematics.

Along with determining the pattern of descendants, molecular genetics helps in understanding genetic mutations that can cause certain types of diseases. Through utilising the methods of genetics and molecular biology, molecular genetics discovers the reasons why traits are carried on and how and why some may mutate.

EPIGENETIC MECHANISMS REGULATING GENE EXPRESSION

Epigenetic mechanisms regulate gene function in a heritable manner, but do so without modulating the DNA sequence of the affected gene. Many different genetic functions are influenced by epigenetic mechanisms in various species. These include regulation of gene expression, DNA modification and restriction, genomic imprinting, X-chromosome inactivation, paramutation, position effect variegation, mating type, cell determination, transposable elements and mutator and suppressor genes. This chapter will focus on epigenetic mechanisms that regulate gene expression and the manner in which they accomplish this in mammalian species.

Nuclear DNA acts as the repository of genetic information in eukaryotic cells. In mammals, and many other animal species, a complete representation of the genome is maintained in essentially every nucleated cell. However, only a subset of this collection of genes is expressed in any particular cell type. Thus, it is not the presence of specific genes, but rather the expression of specific genes, that leads to the unique identity and function of any particular cell.

For protein-encoding genes, two primary steps are involved in gene expression: transcription of DNA into RNA and translation of that RNA into a polypeptide. This affords two levels of regulation of gene expression: transcriptional regulation and translational (or post-transcriptional) regulation. For tissue-specific genes (those expressed in only a subset of tissues or in a single tissue or cell type), regulation is primarily manifest at the transcriptional level. Extensive studies of this process have revealed a consensus mechanism whereby the promoter region, typically located at the 5′-end of the gene, acts to bind specific proteins called transcription factors which, in turn, attract (or prevent) binding of the RNA polymerase that is required to initiate transcription.

Binding of transcription factors to specific gene promoters and to specific sites within those promoters is regulated by the ability of a DNA binding domain within each protein factor to recognise a unique three-dimensional structure of double stranded DNA. This unique structure is imparted by a specific nucleotide sequence, typically 5–15 base pairs (bp) in length. Thus, this mechanism does rely on the DNA sequence and is therefore not a truly epigenetic mechanism. However, because these transcription factors can be either ubiquitous or tissue-specific, and can either promote or inhibit transcription, this mechanism can modulate tissue, cell-type or developmental-stage specificity of transcription, as well as controlling the relative level (or frequency) of transcription. Nevertheless, protein-DNA interactions between transcription factors and promoter sequences, respectively, are not the only mechanism by which gene expression is regulated in eukaryotic cells.

In mammals there are several examples in which genes are regulated by mechanisms other than transcription factors. For example, in female somatic cells, genes on the active X-chromosome are transcribed, whereas homologous genes on the inactive X-chromosome remain transcriptionally silenced. This is despite the fact that both the active and inactive copies of these genes share identical nucleotide sequences and reside within the same nucleus.

Thus the presence of identical promoter sequences and cognate transcription factors alone does not ensure identical regulation of genes. Similarly, in mammals, the phenomenon of genomic imprinting results in the expression of only one of the two copies of a particular gene within a single diploid cell. In this case the choice of which allele is expressed is dictated by the parental origin of that allele. However, the mechanism that regulates such monoallelic expression cannot be based solely on transcription factors and promoter sequences, because the former are present throughout the nucleus in which both alleles reside, and the latter are often identical on both alleles.

The unavoidable conclusion from these observations is that there must be additional mechanisms by which gene expression is regulated in eukaryotic cells, and these mechanisms must function in a manner that does not depend on differences in nucleotide sequence or the cell-type specific presence or absence of transcription factors. Yet, as exemplified by the examples noted earlier for X-chromosome inactivation and genomic imprinting, these mechanisms must function in a heritable manner, such that the same alleles remain expressed or silenced, even after replication of the DNA and division of one cell to produce two daughter cells.

We now know that there are multiple mechanisms that meet the criteria of epigenetic mechanisms in that they regulate gene expression in a heritable manner that does not rely on differences in DNA sequence. Examples of mechanisms that either have been shown to operate in this manner or have the potential to operate in this manner include: DNA methylation, chromatin structure and/or composition, DNA loop domains and association with the nuclear matrix and DNA replication timing.

DNA Methylation

In mammals, methylation of DNA is found only on cytosines present in a 5′-CpG-3′ dinucleotide sequence. Because cytosine and guanine are complementary bases, wherever there is a CpG dinucleotide in one DNA strand, there will be a complementary CpG on the opposite strand. This double-stranded structure can exist in three different states with respect to methylation (Fig. 5.1). It can be fully methylated, meaning that both cytosines are methylated (Fig. 5.1b) or it can be completely unmethylated if neither cytosine is methylated (Fig. 5.1a). When a fully methylated site is replicated by semi-conservative replication, the resulting structure is hemimethylated (Fig. 5.1c). This is typically a transient state because it forms a template for a ubiquitously functioning DNA maintenance methyl transferase that recognises the hemimethylated structure and returns it to a fully methylated state. Thus, fully methylated and unmethylated sites are maintained (and/or reestablished) throughout replication of DNA and cellular division. In this way methylated and unmethylated states of DNA are heritable.

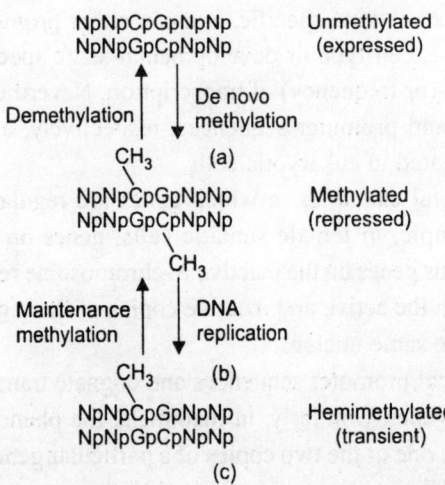

NpNpCpGpNpNp
NpNpGpCpNpNp   Unmethylated
(expressed)

Demethylation | De novo
methylation

CH₃   (a)

NpNpCpGpNpNp
NpNpGpCpNpNp   Methylated
(repressed)

CH₃

Maintenance
methylation | DNA
replication

CH₃   (b)

NpNpCpGpNpNp
NpNpGpCpNpNp   Hemimethylated
(transient)

(c)

Fig. 5.1. Alternate states of DNA methylation in mammalian DNA. Methylation occurs only on cytosines present in CpG dinucleotides in mammalian DNA. A CpG dinucleotide sequence in one DNA strand mandates the presence of a complementary CpG dinucleotide in the other strand of double-stranded DNA. (a) If both cytosines in such a site are unmethylated, the site is said to be completely unmethylated. This structure is often found in actively expressed or potentiated genes, especially in the 5' regulatory region. (b) An unmethylated site can undergo *de novo* methylation to form a fully methylated site in which both cytosines are methylated. This structure is often found associated with repressed genes. Conversely a demethylase activity can convert a fully methylated site to a fully unmethylated site in the absence of DNA replication. (c) Upon semi-conservative replication of a fully methylated site, a hemimethylated site is formed. This structure is typically transient as a maintenance DNA methyl transferase rapidly recognises a hemimethylated site and returns it to a fully methylated state. The function of the maintenance methylase provides a mechanism to heritably maintain DNA methylation patterns. C, cytosine; G, guanine; N, any base; p, phosphate bond; CH₃, methyl group.

It is possible for an unmethylated site to be directly converted to a fully methylated site and *vice versa*. Methylation of an unmethylated site is achieved by a *de novo* methylase, whereas a direct transition from a fully methylated to an unmethylated structure in the absence of DNA replication is accomplished by a demethylase activity. The function of these enzymatic activities and the manner in which they are regulated are not as well-characterised as that of the maintenance methylase activity. However, there is ample evidence that such activities do indeed exist. Shortly after fertilisation in the mouse, nearly all of the methylation that is brought into the zygote by the gametic genomes is lost, such that the blastocyst genome is nearly devoid of DNA methylation except for that at a few imprinted sites. This may occur either by dilution of methylated strands as replication proceeds in the absence of maintenance methylase activity or by direct demethylation or by some combination of these two mechanisms. Subsequently, at about the time of gastrulation, there is a *de novo* methylation event at numerous different sites throughout the genome. This must be accomplished by a *de novo* methylase because completely unmethylated sites become fully methylated. Following gastrulation, many different cell lineages become allocated and begin to develop and differentiate. Coincident with this, selective demethylation of many tissue-specific genes is often observed within the cell lineage in which these genes will ultimately be expressed. In most cases this appears to occur via a demethylase activity, because in at least some cases demethylation occurs in the complete absence of DNA replication or cellular division.

In addition to tissue-specific genes that are expressed in a limited tissue, cell-type or developmental-stage specific pattern, another set of housekeeping genes is widely expressed in a ubiquitous and constitutive manner. These genes, which do not require as complicated transcriptional regulation as that needed for tissue-specific genes, often bear a CpG island, most commonly in the 5'-portion of the gene. A CpG island has been defined as a region in the mammalian genome of > 100 bp with a GC content of > 50 per cent that lacks the typical underrepresentation of CpG dinucleotides seen in other regions of the genome. Generally, CpG islands remain constitutively unmethylated throughout development and differentiation of cells. Exceptions to this rule include CpG islands associated with genes on the inactive X-chromosome or with nonexpressed, inactive alleles of imprinted genes, as well as those associated with certain genes in cancerous tumours (e.g. tumour-suppressor genes). In these cases, the island associated with the nonexpressed allele or gene is typically methylated.

For both individual CpG dinucleotides located in non-CpG island regions and CpG dinucleotides within CpG islands, a general correlation has been observed between the presence of DNA methylation and inhibition of expression, and between the absence of DNA methylation and active transcription. This is especially true for sites in the 5'-flanking region or in the 5'-half of transcribed portions of genes. At least two types of mechanisms have been proposed by which DNA methylation or the lack thereof, might contribute to regulation of transcription. In one case, the presence or absence of methylation on key cytosines within a particular transcription factor binding site may modulate the ability of the factor to bind to that site. In a second scenario, the presence or absence of methylation at sites either within factor binding sites or in regions adjacent to factor binding sites may inhibit factor binding indirectly by affecting chromatin structure. A direct mechanistic connection has now been established between DNA methylation and chromatin structure. In this case, it is suggested that the presence of methylation stabilises a condensed (closed) chromatin structure that is, in turn, refractory to binding by transcription factors and/or RNA polymerase. Conversely, an absence of methylation leads to a less condensed (open) chromatin structure that is accessible to transcription factors and RNA polymerase. Effects of DNA methylation on chromatin structure appear to be mediated by methylated DNA-binding proteins that bind to methylated DNA on the basis of the presence or absence of methylation, rather than on the basis of a particular binding sequence as is the case for transcription factors.

Two methylated-DNA binding proteins were originally identified, MeCP1 and MeCP2. MeCP1 is a large protein complex that binds best to regions of DNA containing >10 methyl-CpGs and has been shown to be involved in repression of transcription from densely methylated promoters. It also binds to, and represses transcription from, more sparsely methylated promoters, although this is a much weaker interaction. MeCP2 is a single polypeptide that can bind to as few as a single fully methylated CpG site. *In vivo* it appears to bind predominantly to highly methylated satellite DNAs adjacent to centromeres in the mouse genome, but shows a more dispersed binding pattern in the genomes of human and rats, which do not contain highly methylated satellite DNA.

Recently, screens for cDNAs encoding methyl-CpG binding domains (MBDs) have revealed at least four such genes, MBD1–4. The MBD1 protein is a component of the MeCP1 protein complex. The MBD2–4 encode methylated DNA binding proteins that are distinct from those associated with either

MeCP1 or MeCP2, but bear a striking similarity to the MBD of MeCP2. The products of MBD2 and MBD4 bind to methylated CpGs both *in vitro* and *in vivo* and are thus considered to be additional candidates for mediators of mechanisms associated with methylated DNA.

The manner in which tissue, cell-type and/or gene-specific patterns of DNA methylation are established or modulated remains to be fully elucidated. However, there appears to be a combination of general and specific mechanisms that contribute to this process. The general mechanisms include those that result in genomewide loss or gain of methylation, especially during early embryogenesis, along with the maintenance methylase activity that reestablishes full methylation at hemimethylated sites following replication of DNA. Cell-type, developmental-stage and gene-specific demethylation have been shown to be regulated by signal sequences within the promoter region of at least one tissue-specific gene. Regulation of CpG island methylation has also been shown to be dependent on signal sequences within certain imprinted genes. However, it appears that different methylases and demethylases may be responsible for *de novo* methylation/demethylation of CpG dinucleotides within or exclusive of CpG islands, respectively.

Chromatin Structure and Composition

Although DNA exists in a double helix structure within eukaryotic cells, this structure alone, otherwise known as naked DNA, is rarely found in cells *in vivo*. Rather the nuclear DNA is typically complexed with proteins to form chromatin. At a primary level, chromatin structure commonly involves double-stranded DNA wrapped periodically around protein structures called nucleosomes (Fig. 5.2a). Approximately 150 bp of double-stranded DNA are wrapped in two superhelical turns around each nucleosome and nucleosomes are typically separated by approx 10 bp of double-stranded DNA.

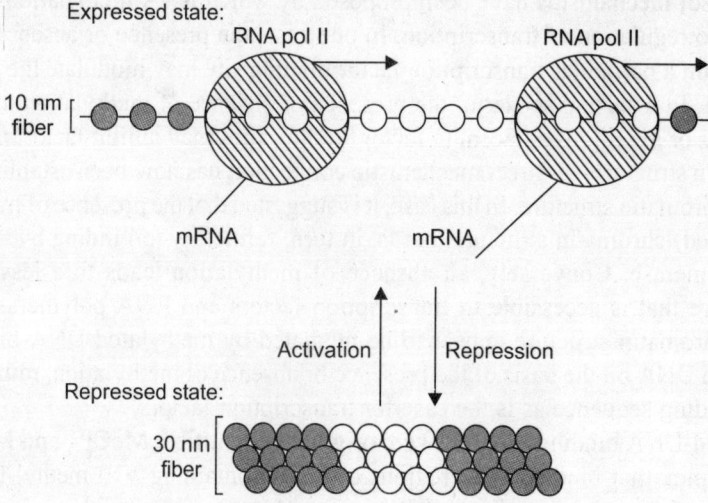

Fig. 5.2. Alternate states of chromatin structure. (a) In eukaryotic cells double-stranded DNA is typically complexed with clusters of histones called nucleosomes to form a beads on a string structure. This structure, which forms a fibre of approximate 10 nm in diametre, is typically found in genes that are undergoing active transcription as shown in the Expressed state in this figure. The RNA polymerase II complex is able to traverse and transcribe portion of this structure to produce mRNA transcripts. (b) Long-term repression of gene transcription is accomplished by condensation of chromatin to form a 30 nm fibre as shown in the Repressed state in this figure. This condensed structure is refractory to binding by transcription factors and/or RNA polymerase II inhibiting initiation of transcription. Open circles, nucleosomes within the transcribed portion of the gene; filled circles, nucleosomes between genes; hatched oval, the RNA II polymerase complex.

This forms what has been termed a beads on a string structure that is approx 10 nm in diametre. This is also known as an open or potentiated chromatin structure, and is the structure, most commonly found in genes that are undergoing active transcription. In this structure the nucleosomes are typically evenly spaced at regular intervals of approx 10 bp, however, as necessary, nucleosomes can be displaced, eliminated or newly formed to facilitate initiation of transcription from a promoter region. Such modifications may be required to permit or even promote access to specific factor binding sites in the double-stranded DNA.

Changes in chromatin structure at the level of nucleosome positioning can be modulated by ATP-dependent chromatin remodelling complexes. The SWI2/SNF2 complex originally discovered in *Drosophila*, is the best characterised of these. It is also conserved in mammals where it functions in a similar manner. The primary function of chromatin remodelling machinery is to remodel nucleosomal arrays to enhance accessibility to transcription factors. Once the necessary transcription factors and then the RNA polymerase complex have become bound to the gene promoter, transcription can proceed through the entire gene as it exists in the 10 nm diametre chromatin structure.

An alternate chromatin structure is achieved when the 10 nm chromatin fibre becomes supercoiled to form a 30 nm structure sometimes referred to as a solenoid (Fig. 5.2b). This structure is typically found in transcriptionally repressed genes. This highly condensed structure is refractory to nucleosome displacement and/or factor binding. Thus, if transcription factors cannot gain direct access to their cognate binding sites in the double-stranded DNA, they will not bind and hence will not promote initiation of transcription. The option to exist in this repressive chromatin structure reconciles how a gene that contains all necessary factor-binding sites can reside in a nucleus in which all the necessary transcription factors are present and still not be transcribed.

The composition of chromatin has been shown to vary in a manner that correlates with the different structures described earlier. A primary component of nucleosomes are histones. Each nucleosome consists of an octamer of two molecules each of histones H2A, H2B, H3 and H4, plus one linker histone H1 or H5. When chromatin is present in the 10-nm open or potentiated configuration most often associated with active transcription, the histone H4 in that region is often hyperacetylated. Conversely, when chromatin is present in the 30 nm repressed structure, histone H4 is typically hypoacetylated. Acetylation of histone H4 is believed to inhibit condensation of the 10 nm chromatin fibre and thus contribute to the maintenance of an open or potentiated chromatin structure, whereas the absence of acetylation on histone H4 contributes to chromatin condensation to form the repressive 30 nm structure. The acetylation of histones is regulated by a dynamic balance of histone acetyl transferases (HATs) and deacetylases (HDACs). The recruitment of these enzymes to specific loci can be regulated by transcription factors located by specific protein-DNA interactions or by the methylated DNA-binding proteins. The latter are particularly associated with histone deacetylases. This provides a mechanistic basis for the frequently observed correlation between hypermethylation of DNA and a condensed, repressed chromatin structure.

DNA Loop Domains and Association with the Nuclear Matrix

Regulation of chromatin structure and transcriptional activity can occur over relatively large distances within the mammalian genome. While this affords significant advantages for coordinate regulation of gene expression, it also poses potential disadvantages in that it raises the possibility that controlling influences targeted to one locus could inadvertently affect other loci, resulting in ectopic and/or inappropriate gene expression or suppression. This potential problem is mitigated in mammals by an additional level of regulation that results in segregation of chromatin into essentially independent loop domains (Fig. 5.3). Delineation of these domains is believed to be achieved by the presence of boundary elements and/or by anchorage of the boundaries of each loop to a three-dimensional proteinaceous structure in the nucleus called the nuclear matrix. This arrangement affords multiple additional opportunities for control of gene expression. First, each loop is essentially insulated from adjacent loops and can thus be regulated independently. Second, it has been proposed that many factors and enzymes that regulate DNA replication, transcription and post-transcriptional processes may be embedded in the nuclear matrix, so that proximity of individual genes to the matrix may influence the rate at which these processes occur in a gene-specific manner.

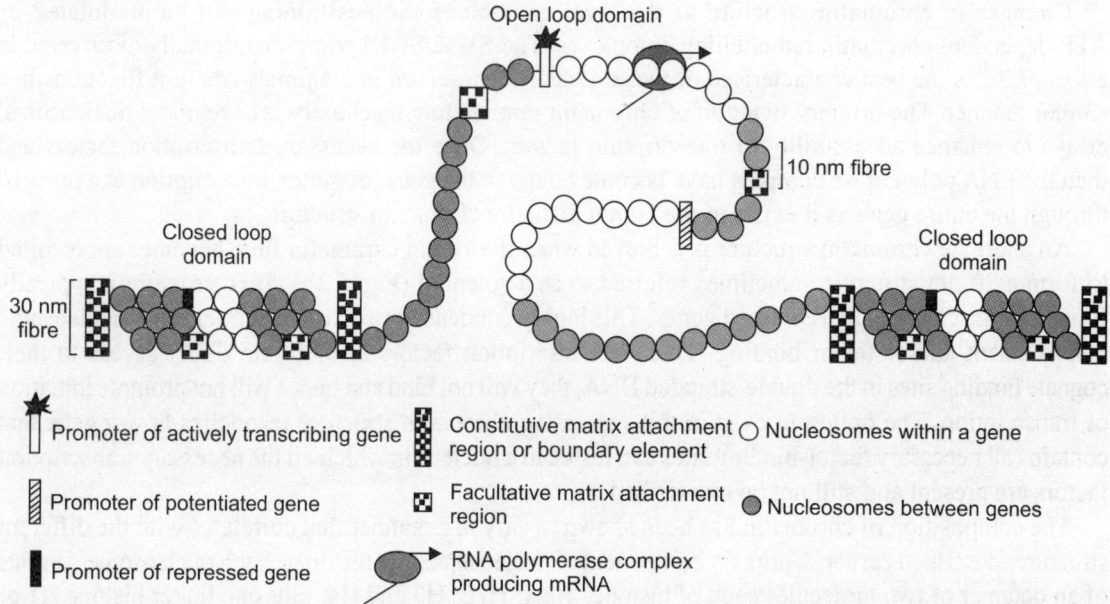

Open loop domain

10 nm fibre

Closed loop domain

Closed loop domain

30 nm fibre

Promoter of actively transcribing gene

Promoter of potentiated gene

Promoter of repressed gene

Constitutive matrix attachment region or boundary element

Facultative matrix attachment region

RNA polymerase complex producing mRNA

Nucleosomes within a gene

Nucleosomes between genes

Fig. 5.3. Organisation of DNA Loop Domains. Adjacent chromatin Loop Domains can exist in alternate states of condensed (closed) or decondensed (open) structure. Genes within closed Domains are typically repressed. Genes within open domains are potentiated for transcriptional activation. Activation of transcription requires transcription factor binding and initiation of RNA synthesis by RNA polymerase II.

Specific sequences in chromosomal DNA have been shown to have nuclear matrix-binding capacity. These regions are known as matrix attachment regions or MARs (the nuclear matrix is also known as the nuclear scaffold and so these attachment regions are also known as scaffold attachment regions or SARs). MARs/SARs can be A/T-rich sequences that are often found at the boundaries of transcription units or in the vicinity of transcriptional enhancers. There appear to be at least two classes of MARs, constitutive and facultative. Constitutive MARs are believed to remain bound to the matrix in all cell types at all developmental stages. Thus, constitutive MARs would define a primary loop domain structure. Facultative MARs are believed to be differentially associated with, or disassociated with the matrix in a gene, cell-type, and developmental-stage specific manner. Thus, facultative MARs would have the potential to form a secondary loop structure and/or to regulate tissue or stage-specific associations between individual genes and the nuclear matrix. The extent to which boundary elements and MARs represent identical or distinct structures remains to be clearly elucidated.

Chromosome loop domains show both developmental-stage and tissue-specificity. These loops are generally small in nuclei of sperm and early embryonic cells, but become larger in differentiating somatic cells. Although the germ cells also undergo significant differentiation during gametogenesis, the loop sizes appear to remain generally smaller than in somatic cells. This difference in loop size could be produced by differential activity of facultative MARs, such that more of these are functional in germ cells and early embryonic cells leading to an increased incidence of DNA-matrix interactions in these cells and hence, delineated loops of smaller average size. It is tempting to suggest that small loop size is characteristic of a state of genetic/developmental pluripotency. This is consistent with the observation that genes that are actively transcribed or in a state of readiness or potentiated for transcriptional activation and are typically found more closely associated with the nuclear matrix than are transcriptionally repressed genes. Thus, in the gametes and early embryonic cells, maximum use of facultative MARs could maintain a maximum number of genes in a potentially expressible state. However, as specific cell lineages become committed to a particular differentiated phenotype, many unneeded genes could become terminally repressed by selective disassociation of facultative MARs from the matrix to sequester the repressed genes away from transcription factors and RNA polymerase complexes associated with the matrix.

Replication Timing

The entire genome is duplicated during S phase of the cell cycle. However, the order in which gene loci are replicated varies among cell types and at different developmental stages. Typically, genes that are actively expressed in a particular cell type are replicated relatively early during S phase, whereas repressed genes are replicated later. For example, the same tissue-specific gene that is replicated early in the expressing cell type may be replicated later in nonexpressing cell types.

For most genes, both alleles are replicated simultaneously during S phase. However, in cases of monoallelic expression as seen for imprinted genes or genes on the active and inactive X-chromosomes, the two alleles replicate asynchronously. In the case of X-linked genes, expressed alleles on the active X-chromosome tend to be replicated earlier than their nonexpressed homologues on the inactive X. Interestingly, while imprinted genes also show asynchronous replication, the paternal allele is always replicated earlier than the maternal allele, regardless of which allele is expressed and which is repressed.

Differential replication timing has been demonstrated by direct fluorescence *in situ* hybridisation (FISH) and by DNA hybridisation using cells separated according to DNA content by fluorescence-activated cell sorting (FACS). It is not clear whether this is a cause or effect of related epigenetic mechanisms. It has been suggested that key chromatin remodelling and/or transcription factors may be limiting within individual nuclei and that following disassociation of these factors from the DNA during replication, early replicating genes or alleles might be afforded a preferential opportunity to reassociate with these factors immediately following replication (Fig. 5.4). If so, this could then contribute to subsequent differential transcriptional activity of these genes or alleles. However, this theory is not supported by the observation that for certain imprinted genes, the maternal allele is preferentially expressed even though the paternal allele is replicated early. An alternative hypothesis is that early replication might simply be a reflection of the presence of DNA replication enzymes associated with, and/or embedded in the matrix, since actively expressed or potentiated genes tend to be more closely associated with the nuclear matrix. In either case, replication timing is indicative of epigenetic differences among gene loci and/or between alleles of the same gene.

Interactions Among Epigenetic Mechanisms

The epigenetic mechanisms discussed earlier represent additional levels of gene regulation that are available to mammalian cells beyond that afforded by direct protein-DNA interactions between transcription factors, the RNA polymerase complex and gene promoters. An important question is how these multiple levels of gene regulation are orchestrated by the cell to achieve proper patterns of expression of batteries of housekeeping and tissue-specific genes. Clearly a variety of strategies are employed depending on the particular regulated gene and/or the particular cell type in which the regulation takes place. An example cascade of epigenetic and genetic mechanisms is presented below to demonstrate how these different mechanisms could interact to facilitate transcriptional activation of a tissue-specific gene.

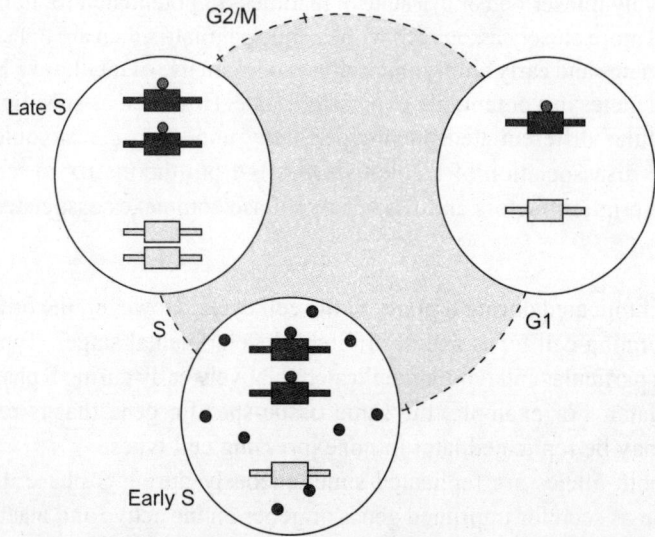

Fig. 5.4. Distinction of genes or alleles based on differential replication timing. The potential for, differential timing of replication during S phase to maintain an epigenetic distinction between different genes or between different alleles of the same gene is depicted in this figure. The model is based on the concept that protein-DNA interactions become disrupted during DNA replication. These interactions must be reestablished following replication. If certain proteins are present in limiting quantities, those genes or alleles that replicate earliest during S phase will gain preferential access to bind these proteins. In this way one gene or allele will bind a disproportionate quantity of a specific protein(s) and become distinguished from another gene or allele, even if both genes or alleles share similar protein-binding sequences.

Activation of transcription of a tissue-specific gene requires a derepression process that takes the gene from a transcriptionally repressed state first to a potentiated state, and subsequently to a transcriptionally active state (Fig. 5.5). The transcriptionally repressed state of a gene is typically characterised by a condensed chromatin structure in which histones are deacetylated, DNA is hypermethylated and complexed with methylated DNA-binding proteins, and the gene is disassociated from the nuclear matrix and replicates relatively late during S phase. In the scheme depicted in Fig. 5.5, an initial tissue and gene-specific demethylation event leads to a loss of binding of methylated DNA-binding proteins and their associated histone deacetylase activity (Fig. 5.5a, b). The histones then become acetylated and this facilitates a transition from the condensed, 30 nm chromatin structure to the decondensed, 10 nm structure, a process that has been termed gene potentiation (Fig. 5.5b, c). Once the gene is in this open configuration, chromatin remodelling complexes can rearrange or displace nucleosomes to provide direct access for interaction between transcription factors and their cognate binding sites in the promoter region (Fig. 5.5c-e). The bound transcription factors then attract the RNA polymerase complex to the proper transcriptional start site to initiate synthesis of RNA (Fig. 5.5e-g).

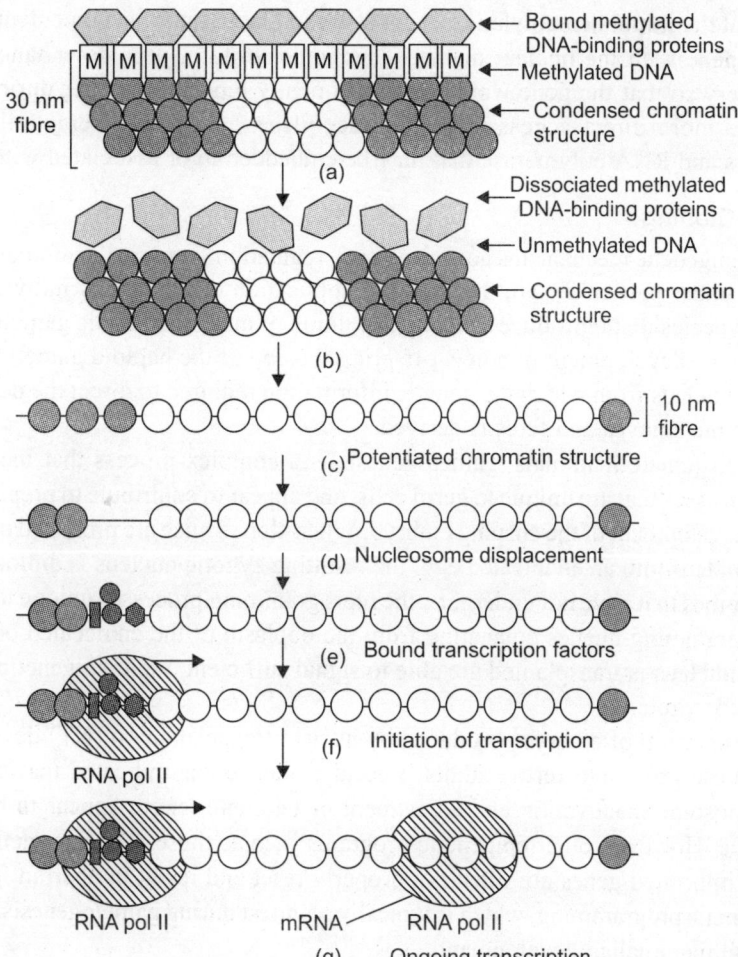

Fig. 5.5. Interactions among epigenetic mechanisms to regulate gene expression. Multiple epigenetic mechanisms contribute to regulation of transcriptional activity in mammals. An example of how this may occur is presented in this figure. (a) A fully repressed gene is often found to be hypermethylated, complexed with methylated-DNA binding proteins, comprised of deacetylated histones and in a condensed chromatin structure characterised by a 30 nm structure that inhibits binding of transcription factors or RNA polymerase. (b) Derepression leading to transcriptional activation begins with demethylation of the gene, which in turn leads to dissociation of methylated-DNA binding proteins and acetylation of histones. (c) Potentiation of chromatin structure is marked by decondensation of the chromatin fibre from the 30 nm structure to the 10 nm beads on a string structure. (d) Displacement of nucleosomes creates an assayable DNase I hypersensitive site which marks the presence of naked DNA that is available for binding by transcription factors. (e) Binding of ubiquitous transcription factors to the core promoter region and tissue-specific transcription factors to enhancer regions attract the RNA polymerase II complex to the gene promoter. (f) Binding of the RNA polymerase II complex initiates transcription. (g) Ongoing transcription is characterised by sequential binding of multiple RNA polymerase II complexes to facilitate synthesis of multiple RNA transcripts. Open circles, nucleosomes within the transcribed portion of the gene; filled circles, nucleosomes between genes; squares containing Ms, DNA methylation; hexagons, methylated-DNA binding proteins; small filled hexagons, circles and rectangles, bound transcription factors; large, hatched oval, RNA polymerase II complex.

It is possible that the initial demethylation event also facilitates and/or is coincident with, enhanced association of the gene with the nuclear matrix. This could, in turn, provide enhanced proximity to replication machinery so that the gene would be subsequently replicated earlier during S phase. This could also provide more direct access to histone acetylases, chromatin remodelling complexes, transcription factors and RNA polymerase that may be embedded in or associated with the matrix.

Epigenetics and Cloning

The critical role of epigenetic mechanisms governing gene regulation for normal mammalian development has recently come under particular scrutiny with the application of cloning of individuals by nuclear transplantation. In species that reproduce sexually, the union of male and female gametes at fertilisation is the initial step in the development of a new offspring. Fusion of the haploid gametic genomes forms the diploid zygotic nucleus from which the genetic information required to direct the development of all subsequent cells of the embryo and fetus is derived.

In both male and female mammals, gametogenesis is a complex process that includes epigenetic reprogramming processes that are unique to germ cells, and appear to contribute to preparing the gametic genomes to direct development of the ensuing embryo. When cloned mice are produced by transplantation of a somatic cell nucleus into an enucleated egg, the resulting zygotic nucleus is diploid, but it consists of two haploid genomes that have not undergone the reprogramming processes unique to gametogenesis. Presumably, reprogramming queues emanating from the ooplasm of the enulceated oocyte into which the somatic donor nucleus is transplanted are able to signal sufficient, rapid epigenetic reprogramming in the newly formed zygote.

Only a small proportion of embryos produced by nuclear transplantation (NT) develop to birth and only a subset of these grow into fertile adults. Recent evidence has indicated that certain processes including X-chromosome inactivation and adjustment of telomere length appear to become properly reset in cloned mice. However, other epigenetic programs such as those affecting methylation patterns and expression of imprinted genes are often not properly reset and result in aberrant gene expression. Thus, proper epigenetic programming, which is typically manifest during gametogenesis, is indispensably required for normal mammalian development.

Interestingly, epigenetic reprogramming appears incomplete and/or unstable in cloned mice. If these mice are able to subsequently participate in natural breeding they produce offspring that appear relatively normal. Thus it appears that genetic and epigenetic programming is largely restored in the gametes of cloned mice by mechanisms that function uniquely in the germline. In as much as the oocyte is a product of gametogenesis in the female, it is not surprising that it contains signalling factors that can potentially contribute to reprogramming of a transplanted somatic cell nucleus. However, those epigenetic mechanisms that normally function uniquely during spermatogenesis are not represented in a zygote produced by NT and this deficiency may contribute to the very low success rate of full-term development of clones produced by NT.

Thus, when considering the process of differential gene expression and the mechanisms which regulate this, it is important to bear in mind that there are various levels of control and that these are based on a combination of genetic and epigenetic mechanisms. A great deal of emphasis has been placed on the genetic mechanism of protein-DNA interactions between transcription factors and promoter binding sites for regulating gene expression. Although this mechanism is indeed critical to transcriptional regulation, it can only function if it is preceded by the proper functioning of the epigenetic mechanisms described in this chapter.

GENE FAMILIES AND EVOLUTION

Gene families refer to two or more genes that come from a common ancestral gene in which the individual members of the gene family may or may not have a similar function. The idea of gene families implicitly invokes a process in which an original gene exists, is duplicated and the resulting gene products evolve. The most common result of gene duplication is that mutation renders one of the products nonfunctional and in the absence of conserving natural selection, one of the members becomes no longer recognisable. Gene families may be clustered or dispersed and may exchange with each other through the mechanisms of gene conversion or unequal crossover. Therefore, understanding the processes of molecular evolution are essential to understanding what gene families are, where they came from and what their function might be. In a sense, duplicate genes allow for more evolutionary potential. At first glance this could be beneficial; if one gene incurred a lethal mutation the other gene simply takes over, there is some protection from mutation based on redundancy. Having two identical genes could result in twice as much product; this may or may not be beneficial in a cell where the integration of thousands of gene products must be coordinated and slight concentration differences can alter biochemical pathways.

Antiquity of Gene Families

Almost all genes belong to gene families. Evidence from sequence or structural similarity indicates that all or at least large parts of genes came from ancestral genes. Analysis of the human genome has shown that over half of the human genome is comprised of clearly identifiable repeated sequences. Although much of this is owing to self-replicating transposons, i.e. mobile genetic elements, over 5 per cent of the genome has been involved in large segmental duplications in the past 30 million years. If we look further into the past using evidence from protein similarity of three or more genes that occur in close proximity on two different chromosomes, we find over 10,310 gene pairs in 1077 duplicated blocks contain 3522 distinct genes. Because our observations are based on genes that retain similarity, only a small fraction of the ancient duplications can be detected by current means. What is clearly evident is that a very large part of the human genome has come from duplications and that duplication is a very frequent event.

   With the evidence showing that gene duplication plays a major role in modern genomes, the question is where did it all begin? How many genes did life start with? Various estimates of the minimal gene set suggest that as few as 250 genes could provide the minimal number of components necessary to sustain independent life. The number of genes in mycoplasms ranges from 500–1500 genes and in bacteria from 1000–4000 genes. Yeast (*S. cervisiae*) has ~6000 genes, worms (*C. elegans*) have ~18,000 genes, the fruit fly (*D. melangaster*) has ~13,000 genes, a plant, *Arabidopsis*, has 26000 genes, and humans have at least 30000 genes. The difference between 250 or 1000 genes and 30,000–40,000 genes is only two orders of magnitude yet the difference in the complexity of life forms seems far greater than could be explained by a simple gene count. Certainly with the increased number of genes comes the opportunity for more complexity in terms of gene interaction. But can synergy alone explain the differences in morphological complexity? Partial explanations invoke more complex differential splicing to account for a higher proportional number of protein products stemming from only 30,000 genes, but one wonders if this observation is merely an artifact of the few numbers of whole genomes available to us.

Origins

Gene duplications can come from a variety of sources including whole or partial genome duplication. Polyploidy results from a failure of chromosome segregation during the cell division of gametes. The most distinguishing feature of polyploidy is that it effects all of the genes simultaneously so that the relative proportion of genes within cells remains the same. Among plants and invertebrates, polyploidy is quite common and in many species it has little effect on phenotype. Ohno has argued that whole genome duplications are the most important events in evolution yet others have suggested that polyploidy has no effect on phenotype. More recent discussions: acknowledge the potential that polypoidy brings to gene family evolution but also appreciate the role of complexity of gene interactions in determining the impact of whole genome duplications. In vertebrates, polyploidy is quite rare. Most of the 188 examples of genome duplication have been found in amphibians, reptiles and some fish (salmon). In these instances, polyploid species have undergone dramatic changes to reestablish diploidy through chromosome loss, mutation and rearrangement. Tetraploid genomes have no trouble going through cell division as long as chromosomes remain very similar. But as mutations arise and duplicated chromosomes begin to differ, cell division can no longer insure equal division of genetic material to germ cells and severe imbalances can occur during chromosomal segregation. The initial transition phase from tetraploid to diploid results in huge losses of gametes and developing young. In salmon it is estimated that approx 50 million years after a polyploid change, only 53 per cent of duplicate genes remain. The result of duplication by whole or partial genomes can result in large changes in gene number but there are major difficulties in cell replication that must be overcome.

The rapid increase in genome size through polyploid events has been used to explain the increased size of mammalian genomes. Ohno suggested that two rounds of genome duplication occurred early in vertebrate history. This may explain the Cambrian explosion in which vertebrates appeared in paleontological records quite rapidly. Evidence for two rounds of genome duplication comes from vertebrates having four times the number of developmental regulator genes (Hox, Cdx, MyoD, 60A, Notch, elav, btd/SP...) as *Drosophila*. While this concept has become very popular in the literature, recent studies examining expected phylogenetic relationships among genes have called into question whether the number of genes was a result of two genome-wide duplications or simply a result of ongoing, frequent genome segment duplications. While the primary support for quadruplicated genomes comes primarily from chromosomes 2, 7, 12 and 17, which contain the Hox gene clusters, a more extensive examination of the number of homologous genes within human as compared to genes within Drosophila was unable to resolve the question of whether two whole genome duplications gave rise to modern vertebrate genomes.

Mechanisms

Duplication of large blocks of DNA cannot be explained by chromosomal segregation errors. Mechanisms of large segmental duplication are varied and the role of transposable elements in gene duplication is often cited as a primary cause. Transposable elements and in particular retrotransposable elements are highly repetitive dispersed sequences that can replicate independent of nuclear division. In human they comprise over 45 per cent of the genome. While there are a number of instances where retroposons have been found at the junctions of duplicated segments, there are also a number of instances where they have not. To understand why gene segment duplications appear common, it is perhaps important to look at the DNA molecule itself. DNA is composed of duplex strands held together by hydrogen bonds whose strength varies. In a fluid environment, various local salt concentrations, temperatures, physical torsion forces and local nucleotide compositions (e.g. levels of G + C, simple repeats) can result in temporary separation of strands of duplex DNA. If similar sequences are found in the same physical location, unstable heterologous duplexes can form. Heterologous pairing or single-strand conditions are prone to stress and breakage. These situations are repaired correctly in the vast majority of cases but occasionally mistakes are made that result in new gene neighbours. The possibility of error is particularly high during cell division when DNA is being replicated and when similar sequences are in close proximity. The potential impact of highly repeated transposable elements as a destabilising factor and a potential focal point for rearrangement becomes clear in our genome. It is, therefore, somewhat surprising to find that many of the duplications are not flanked by repeat elements. What is clear is that duplication involves local chromosome instability that results in breakage and aberrant repair of the ends.

Factors that promote segmental duplication include close proximity and high sequence similarity. It then follows that duplications resulting in adjacent genes would be more susceptible to further changes than duplications resulting in dispersed genes. Furthermore, adjacent duplications create far fewer chromosomal segregation problems during cell division and therefore, should be found more often in the genome. What is observed is that large segmental duplications involving multiple genes are dispersed throughout the genome whereas duplications involving single gene segments are both dispersed and in close proximity. There are many instances of clustered gene families (globins, Hox, Ig, Tcr, Mhc and rRNA). Among tandemly duplicated gene segments there is the possibility of extensive gene conversion and unequal crossing over (Fig. 5.6). The later is the predominant mode of change. Unequal crossing over between dispersed genes results in extreme difficulties in chromosomal segregation in cell division but gene conversion does not.

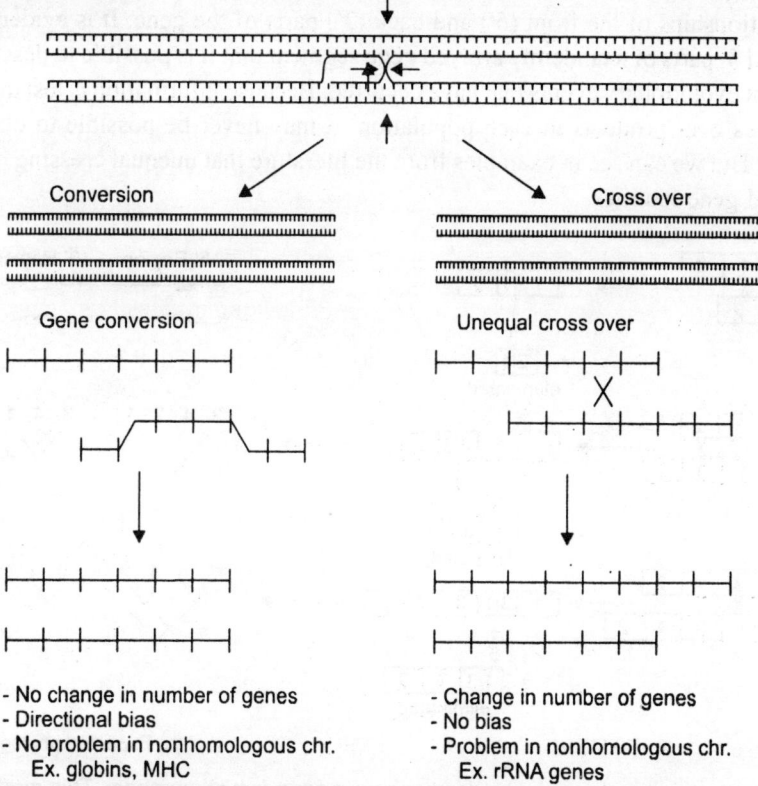

Fig. 5.6. Gene conversion and unequal crossing over mechanisms of communication among gene family members. The arrows indicate possible break points that would result in either conversion or cross over results.

Gene conversion replaces the sequence of one family member with the sequences of another close (> 90 per cent similarity) member but it does not effect the total number of genes. Gene conversion requires DNA strand breakage followed by strand migration to a similar gene and the formation of a heteroduplex. DNA repair mechanisms then repair differences in the heteroduplex often using one strand corresponding to the unaffected homologous chromosome as a template. The heteroduplex then resolves and may go back to its original location carrying with it DNA changes. Heteroduplex formation is often temporary and most often occurs between alleles of the same gene though occasionally it may affect paralogous genes in which more than 100 bases are greater than 95 per cent similar. Depending on the resolution of the heteroduplex and biases in mismatch repair, adjacent base differences may both reflect one or the other parental strand or they may reflect a combination of parental strands. The end result is that the total genetic variation is reduced but a particular gene may increase its number of alleles. Genetic variation at one gene can increase over a single conversion event, but over multiple conversion events variation is reduced.

The resolution of heteroduplexes formed from the invasion of a DNA strand from one gene segment into the duplex of a similar, adjacent duplicate can also result in unequal crossing over. Unequal crossing over changes the number of genes. For example, in a tandem arrangement, unequal crossing over results in one chromosome with one duplicate and the other chromosome with three duplicates where the front and the back parts of the single duplicate and the middle duplicate of the triplicated segment reflect different origins. Figure 5.7 shows three successive unequal crossing-over events and shows the expected phylogenetic relationships of the front (5') and back (3') parts of the gene. It is evident from the final trees for the 5' and 3' parts of a tandemly arrayed gene segment that it is possible to describe some of the major, more recent evolutionary events that have occurred. Because information is lost due to the fixation of one of the cross over products in each population, it may never be possible to obtain a complete historical picture. But we can see in examples from the literature that unequal crossing over is the major factor in clustered gene families.

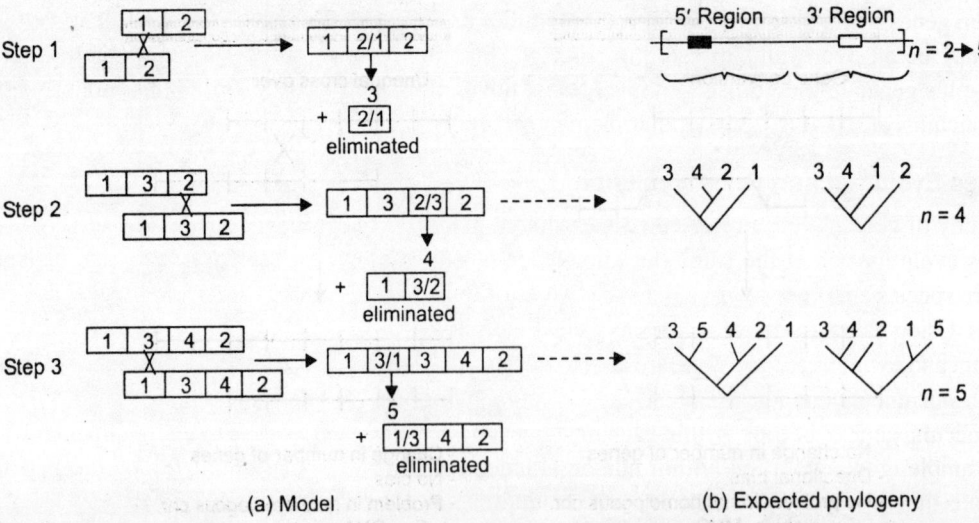

(a) Model   (b) Expected phylogeny

Fig. 5.7. Unequal crossing over between tandemly arrayed gene family members. This model (a) assumes a break-point near the middle of the duplicated segments. The expected phylogeny (b) represent sequence relationships between the 5' and 3' regions of the duplicated gene segments.

Variation

Genetic variation increases when the number of duplicates increases but it is decreased when the number of duplicates decreases. It is important to remember several tenets of unequal crossing over. First, the ultimate fate of duplicates undergoing multiple unequal crossing overs is to return to a single copy unless selection maintains multiple copies. Second, while the overall variation may increase over a single event, the result over multiple expansions and deletions is homogenisation of duplicates (example rRNA genes). Third, unequal crossing over between dispersed gene segments often results in fatal problems in cell division. Lastly, unequal crossing over is the predominant mechanism that increases or decreases the number of gene family members in clusters. It appears that the factors that promote duplication include proximity, high similarity, larger numbers of existing duplicates and internal sequences that are prone to breakage. Given these factors, it is perhaps surprising that we do not see more evidence of repetitive elements playing a larger role in gene duplication. At the same time it becomes easy to see the complex evolution and interactions among both dispersed and clustered gene families.

Genes and Domains

Duplication can involve very large stretches of DNA, whole genes or even parts of genes. Of 1077 duplication blocks containing three or more genes in the human genome, 159 contained 3 genes, 137 contained 4 genes and 781 contained five or more genes. At the same time we often see clusters of gene family members. This indicates that duplications often involve one gene or even parts of genes. Clearly the mechanisms of duplication outlined earlier play a major role at all levels of gene family evolution. However, it is important to remember that the events that are most evident are those that are fairly recent or those that involve conserved genes. Sequence similarity for older duplications of noncoding DNA rapidly fades. It is our focus on function that draws us to study genes. As mentioned, several genes within larger segments can be duplicated but perhaps just as interesting, parts of genes (introns and groups of introns) can be duplicated. This is particularly interesting because genes are composed of functional domains. Remarkably, there may be fewer than 1000 classifications in existence. Domains can be mixed, matched, duplicated and modified to provide novel functions within genes as well as between genes. Only 94 of the 1278 protein families in our genome appear to be specific to vertebrates. That may be an overestimate resulting from our inability to recognise similarity. It appears that the 30000-plus genes in the human genome are not novel but simply products of duplications and mixing and matching of existing genes and domains to create new genes and new functions.

Species Evolution and Gene Evolution

The study of gene evolution is incomplete without the study of species evolution. Gene evolution and species evolution is not the same but knowledge of one greatly benefits our knowledge of the other. Modern species are the result of a dense network; of transient species that occasionally give rise to other species. Using paleontological records as well as morphological, physiological and developmental studies of extant and extinct life forms, we are able to trace some of the origins of modern species. But numerous gaps in our understanding remain. Gene evolution can occur within a species but when a speciation event occurs, gene evolution within each new lineage is independent of gene evolution in other lineages. For example, gene evolution within human is independent of gene evolution within chimpanzees. To illustrate this point, Fig. 5.8a shows a gene duplication in a common ancestor of species A and B followed by a speciation event and separate A and B lineages. Below Fig. 5.8a is the corresponding gene phylogenetic tree. Note that the timing of speciation events can be used to time major events in gene evolution. In Fig. 5.8a, gene duplication occurred before the speciation event. In Fig. 5.8b, a more complex gene evolution is shown. Within each species one of the genes has been eliminated and the other has been duplicated so that each species has two genes, which appear to have arisen after the speciation event. While many other scenarios can occur, these two illustrations show how even in relatively simple cases, one must be cautious when interpreting gene trees. A number of studies have used these methods to identify new gene family members. Slightom was one of the first to use combined gene and species studies to examine genetic mechanisms of change. What is clear is that the use of both gene trees and species trees can be a very powerful method of studying species evolution and gene evolution.

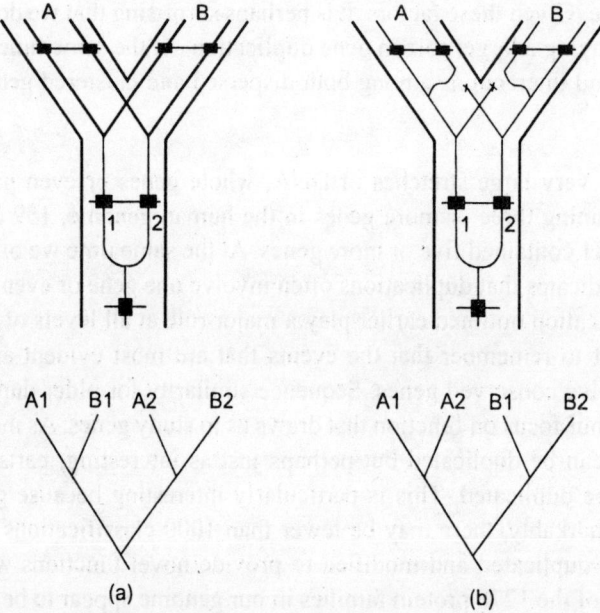

Fig. 5.8. Species evolution (in bold outline) and gene evolution (light lines). (a) Shows a gene duplication in a common ancestor of species A and B followed by a speciation event and separate A and B lineages. (b) A more complex gene evolution is shown. Within each species one of the genes has been eliminated and the other has been duplicated so that each species has two genes, which appear to have arisen after the speciation event.

Examples

The globin gene family offers one of the most studied and widely discussed examples of gene family evolution. Globin proteins function to transport oxygen and are found in bacterial, plant and animal kingdoms. In vertebrates, a series of gene duplications (Fig. 5.9) correspond to major events in the evolution of man. A monomeric globin gene duplicated 600–800 million years ago to give rise to myoglobin (functional in muscle) and haemoglobin (functional in blood). 450–500 million years ago another duplication gave rise to an α form and a αβ form. About this same time haemoglobin changed from a monomeric form to a tetrameric form (2α subunits and 2β subunits), which permitted oxygen transport in a much broader range of physiological conditions. The time frame for this event is supported by molecular clock estimates and by the fact that fish, amphibians, birds and mammals all have a tetrameric haemoglobin with 2α and 2β subunits. Over the next several hundred million years homeothermy evolved. Prior to the separation of mammals and marsupials (~150 million years ago), the β gene duplicated and gave rise to a form (ε) that is only found expressed in embryo's and a form (β) that is expressed in adults. Subsequent to the separation of marsupials and true mammals (eutherians), the embryonic form again duplicated into three separate genes. At this same time, major changes in the placenta made it possible to hatch eggs inside the body and allow for prolonged development prior to birth. In most eutherians there are also two adult forms (δ and β). In primates as well as cows (artiodactyls) the γ gene is found expressed in juveniles. In the α lineage, a similar chain of events occurred giving rise to embryonically expressed genes and genes expressed in the adult. What is clear from the study of globin gene evolution is that duplication allowed subsequent specialisation, which in turn allowed for greater physiological complexity within species. The study of globin gene evolution within and between species also provided evidence for mechanisms of change which helps us to understand several globin-related diseases (thalasemia).

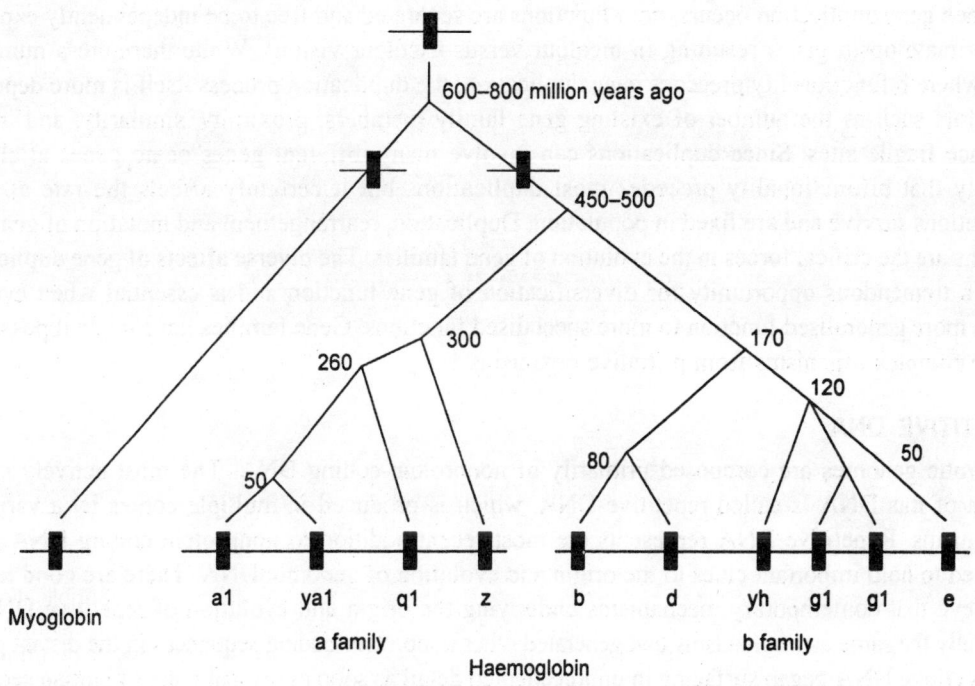

Fig. 5.9. Vertebrate globin evolution.

Over the past three decades, many other gene families have been studied and in each case these studies have provided important information about the numbers of gene family members, distribution, and functional specialisation as well as information about the rates, modes, and mechanisms of change within each family. There is a tremendously diverse array of gene families with their own story. Some of the gene families such as the immunoglobulin super gene family incorporate evolutionary mechanisms of change into their function. In T-cell receptor genes, recombination, and alternative splicing of up to a hundred different gene family members results in the production of up to 10^{15} different receptors. This capability greatly facilitates the ability of T-cell receptors to recognise foreign proteins in the body and is a critical component in the overall function of the immune system. The rRNA genes also incorporate mechanisms of change into their overall functionality. In human ~300 tandemly arrayed rRNA genes undergo extensive unequal crossing over to maintain several hundred nearly identical genes. In most cases, duplication of genes results in new and better control of physiology, growth and development.

Significance

Evolutionary biologists have suggested that gene duplication followed by modification is the most important mechanism for generating new genes and biochemical processes. This has made it possible to evolve complex organisms from primitive ones. Based on traditional models, once duplications occur, one of the two genes is redundant and thus freed from functional constraints. All mutations, even missense or nonsense mutations, occurring in a redundant gene will be neutral unless by chance a mutation or combination of mutations results in a modified gene with some novel function. There are problems with this model because both gene products may still be subject to selection. Altered gene duplicates often result in products that can compete with each other for limited *cis*-acting promoter/enhancer molecules, or can produce altered products that can interfer with biochemical processes and molecular interactions. Furthermore there are examples (primates, opsins) where alternative alleles code for different functions and when gene duplication occurs, both functions are separated and free to be independently expressed (e.g. primate opsin genes resulting in bicolour versus tricolour vision). While there are a number of cases where bifunctionality precedes gene duplication, the duplication process itself is more dependent on factors such as the number of existing gene family members, proximity, similarity, and internal sequence fragile sites. Since duplications can involve many different genes or no genes at all, it is unlikely that bifunctionality precedes most duplications but it certainly affects the rate at which duplications survive and are fixed in population. Duplication, rearrangement and mutation of genes and domains are the critical forces in the evolution of gene families. The diverse affects of gene duplications offers a tremendous opportunity for diversification of gene function and is essential when evolving from a more generalised function to more specialised functions. Gene families have made it possible to evolve complex organisms from primitive organisms.

REPETITIVE DNA

Eukaryotic genomes are composed primarily of nonprotein-coding DNA. The most actively studied portion of this DNA is called repetitive DNA, which is produced in multiple copies by a variety of mechanisms. Repetitive DNA represents the most recent addition to nonprotein coding DNA and is expected to hold important clues to the origin and evolution of genomic DNA. There are good reasons to believe that contemporary mechanisms underlying the origin and evolution of repetitive DNA are essentially the same as mechanisms that generated other nonprotein-coding sequences in the distant past.

Repetitive DNA began surfacing in unprecedented detail as soon as critical mass of human sequence data permitted comparative analyses. This set the stage for a new era of repeat studies dominated by computer-assisted sequence comparisons. Currently, 42 per cent of the human genome is recognisable as being derived from repetitive DNA. This proportion may vary from species to species in a seemingly arbitrary manner and the exact reasons why some eukaryotic species preserve more DNA than others are not well understood.

Studies of repetitive DNA are important not only *per se*, but also in the context of genome biology, including its structure, stability and evolution. Repeats often obscure proteins and other regions of biological significance and for this reason they need to be identified and filtered out of the sequence data to facilitate such studies. Identification of repeats is also necessary for probe and primer design in DNA-DNA hybridisation and polymerase chain reaction (PCR) studies, respectively. Inevitably, they are increasingly being studied in various biological contexts including but not limited to phylogenetic analysis, population studies, gene polymorphism and chromosomal organisation.

Simple Sequence Repeats (SSRs)

There are two basic classes of repetitive DNA sequences: (i) those expanded spontaneously on-site; and (ii) those transposed from somewhere else as copies of transposable elements (TEs). These two classes are not totally independent because TEs can initiate or stimulate on-site expansion of repetitive DNA. The most common repeats generated on site are tandem repeats, often referred to as simple sequence repeats or SSRs. Typically, tandem repeats with a unit size of 10 bp or less are referred to as microsatellites. Tandem repeats with a unit size over 10 bp are called minisatellites. There is a significant twilight zone between micro- and minisatellites, usually applicable to repeats with unit size 7–14 bp, which is listed in either category in the scientific literature.

The number of units, i.e. overall length of micro and minisatellites, can vary from generation to generation and this property makes them very useful in studies of sequence polymorphism in eukaryotic population. Growing evidence indicates that micro and minisatellite expansion occurs by different mechanisms: the former mostly due to polymerase slippage and the latter due to an illegitimate recombination process stimulated by double-stranded breaks. Tandem repeats are often transformed to a cryptically simple DNA composed of various sequence motifs rearranged, and often obscured by mutations. Tandemly repeated sequences include satellite DNA. Satellites are primarily located in centromeres, whereas other tandem repeats, tend to be interspersed within genomic DNA. Like other tandem repeats, satellites; are quite variable and even closely related species may carry completely unrelated satellites. Satellite variability may be fueled by mechanisms similar to those involved in minisatellite variability.

Transposable Elements (TEs)

The major source of interspersed repetitive DNA are transposable elements (TEs). There are two major classes of TEs in the eukaryotic organisms: class 1, retro-elements; class 2, DNA transposons; including rolling-circle transposons, which was recently discovered in plants and nematodes (Fig. 5.10).

Retroelements include long interspersed nuclear elements (LINEs) and elements related to retroviruses, including some domesticated endogenous retroviruses. All retroelements use reverse transcriptase to copy their RNA to DNA as a part of their reproduction process. LINEs generate a variety of retropseudogenes including SINE elements. In the case of mammalian LINE1 (L1) element, reverse transcription is initiated (primed) by a reverse transcriptase-generated nick in host DNA. A second nick is generated on the opposite strand leading to target site duplication (TSD) where the duplicated target is represented by a short, ~15 bp long DNA fragment delimited by the nicks. The final integration is probably completed by the host replication system. Unlike LINEs, retroviruses appear to be inserted in a separate step after they are reverse transcribed to DNA. There is no specific mechanism for excision of retroelements although integrated retroviruses can be deleted due to homologous recombination between long terminal repeats (LTRs), leaving behind a single (solo) LTR repeat.

DNA transposons (class 2) encode transposase, which is involved in insertion and excision of these elements to and from host DNA. The transposase recognises terminal inverted repeats (TIRs). Replication of a DNA transposon is accomplished by the host replication system. If excision does not occur, the transposon becomes permanently integrated usually as an inactive repetitive element.

The third class of eukaryotic TEs is represented by complex rolling-circle (RC) transposons. In addition to a cleavage and replication transposase, RC transposons use enzymes such as helicases and the single-strand DNA-binding protein, probably adopted from the host. RC transposons integrate at AT dinucleotides without target site duplication.

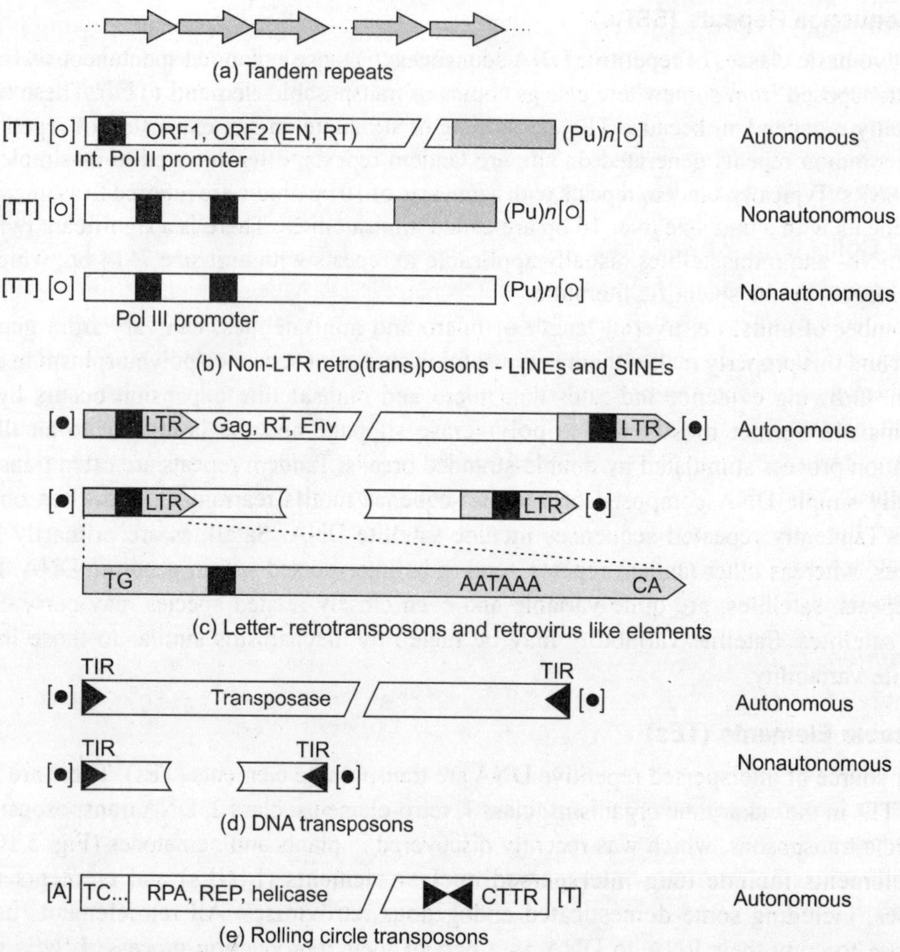

Fig. 5.10. Basic categories and biological characteristics of repetitive elements. (a) Tandem repeats including minisatellites, microsatellites and satellites. (b) Structure of LINE (autonomous) and SINE (nonautonomous) retroelements; black boxes show transcription promoters and (Pu)n indicate purine (A or G) tails. Target site duplications (TSDs) and other target components throughout the figure are indicated by brackets. (c) LTR retrotransposons and retrovirus-like elements. Characteristic sequence features of LTRs: 5′ TG, 3′ CA and polyadenylation signal AATAAA are indicated in the enlarged long terminal repeat. (d) Autonomous and nonautonomous DNA transposons. Black triangles at both ends indicate terminal inverted repeats (TIRs). (e) Autonomous and nonautonomous rolling-circle transposons. Characteristic 5′ TC, 3′ CTTR and hairpin-like structures (inverted black triangles) are indicated.

All classes of autonomous TEs in eukaryotes are associated with nonautonomous elements that do not encode any active enzymes. They depend on their autonomous relatives for reproduction and insertion into the genome. In this context, autonomous TEs can play a role of mutator genes that must be restricted or tightly controlled by the host. In general, only few active TEs at a time appear to find favourable circumstances for proliferation in any given population. They produce a discrete genomic fossil record of repetitive families/subfamilies derived from a limited number of actively expressed source genes or active TEs. Both autonomous and nonautonomous elements have their actively expressed source genes. Source genes can be active for millions of years but are eventually replaced by their variants or become extinct. Interestingly, copies of nonautonomous elements, particularly short ones, tend to predominate over the autonomous ones. It appears that all eukaryotic genomes integrated a patchwork of TEs inserted at different times from the beginning of their evolutionary history. As indicated earlier, the human genome is among the best repositories of repetitive DNA going back over 200 million years. Unlike human, all repetitive elements in plants and insects appear to be relatively young. This may indicate rapid turnover of TEs in plant and insect genomes.

Reference Collections of Repeats

A practical approach to identifying and masking repetitive DNA began with creating comprehensive reference collections of repeats that could be compared against newly sequenced DNA. Prior to whole-genome sequencing projects, only human sequences were available in sufficient quantities to reveal a significant variety of human repeat families. These studies laid the foundation for the first collection of 53 representative human repeats. It was followed by collections of other mammalian repeats and placed in a database named Repbase. Since 1997, Repbase was succeeded by Repbase update and over time it included repeats from other eukaryotic species as they became available. Originally, Repbase update (RU) played the role of a database and an electronic journal releasing newly discovered repetitive families that were not published elsewhere. This arrangement is designed to facilitate proper referencing and documentation of the original data deposited in RU.

Current content of repbase update

The current release of RU contains around 2400 unique entries from all sequenced eukaryotic species. The primary release of RU is in the EMBL format. A sample entry is shown in Fig. 5.11. Simultaneously, RU is also released in fasta format (without annotations) as well as in preprocessed, software-specific RepeatMasker format. The major files in the current release include repeats from human (humrep.ref), rodents (rodrep.ref), other mammals (mamrep.ref), Zebrafish (zebrep.ref), other vertebrates (vrtrep.ref), *Caenorhabditis elegans* (celrep.ref), *Drosophila melanogaster* (drorep.ref), other animals (invrep.ref). *Arabidopsis thaliana* (athrep.ref), other plants and fungi (plnrep.ref) and simple repeats (simple.ref). Some sections can be merged together, pending specific needs. For example, the reference collection of plant repeats used by CENSOR server (Website: http://www.girinst.org) includes two RU files: athrep.ref and plnrep.ref.

Sequences deposited in RU continue to be updated over time and the record of modified entries is preserved in appendix files accompanying the active files. For example, changes in the active file of human/primate repeats humrep. ref are documented in humapp. ref; changes in rodrep. ref are documented in rodapp. ref. Appendix files are for documentation purposes only and they should not be used for annotation. Most repetitive elements deposited in RU have been assigned to general biological categories discussed earlier. For practical reasons, some of these categories are expanded within the framework of the original classification. For instance, mammalian retroviruses include true retrovirus-like elements and a distinct category of retroelements called MaLRs, distantly related to retroviruses. Moreover, long terminal repeats (LTRs) are listed separately from internal protein-coding retrovirus sequences. LTRs often represent the only known fragments of retroviruses in RU because they are by far more abundant and more readily identifiable than the internal sequences. Finally, except in the case of LINEs and SINEs, separation between autonomous and nonautonomous elements is not always possible because many elements in RU are reconstructed from inactive genomic copies. Therefore, nonautonomous and autonomous LTR-retroelements and DNA transposons are listed together.

```
ID    LOOPER    repbase; DNA; HUM; 1460 BP.
CC    LOOPER DNA
XX
AC    ;
XX
DT    01–APR–1998   (Rel. 6.4, Created)
DT    13–May–1999   (Rel. 6.9, Las update, Version 2)
XX
DE    Molecular fossils of autonomous DNA transposon—a consensus sequence.
XX
KW    Putative autonomous DNA transposon; TTAA–superfamily; LOOPER.
XX
OS    Homo sapiens (consensus)
CC    consensus
OC    Eukaryota; Animalia; Metazoa; Chordata; Vertebrata; Mammalia;
OC    Theria; Eutheria; Primates; Haplorhini; Catarrhini; Hominidae.
XX
RN    [1]
RP    1–1460
RC    [1]   (bases 1 to 1460)
RA    Kapitonov V.V., Jurka J.
RT    ;
RL    Direct submission (March 31, 1998)
XX
RN    [2]
RP    1–1460
RC    [2] (bases 1 to 1460)
RA    Kapitonov V.V., Jurka J.
RT    ;
RL    Direct submission (May 12, 1999)
XX
CC    LOOPER encodes 278 aa–long protein (position 480–1313) similar
CC    to the transposase-like protein encoded by ORF1 in IFP2
CC    (PiggyBac) DNA transposon from cabbage looper see IFP2 transposon
CC    In the invrep.ref section of Repbase.
CC    There are about 200–500 copies of LOOPER preserved in the human
CC    genome. Most of them are severely damaged by mutations since LOOPER
CC    is relatively old element. There is 80 per cent average nucleotide identity
CC    between LOOPER's copies and the consensus sequence.
CC    LOOPER belongs to the TTAA superfamily of DNA transposons in mammals.
CC    Hallmarks of this superfamily are TTAA target site duplication and
CC    short terminal inverted repeats, including 5'- and 3'-terminal
CC    CCY and GGG, respectively.
CC    Activity of the protein encoded by the LOOPER-like elements could be
CC    related to multiple transpositions of non-autonomous elements MER75
CC    and MER85 identified recently in the human genome.
CC    The consenus sequence may be incomplete.
XX
CC    [2] (consensus)
XX
SQ    Sequence 1460 BP; 521 A; 199 C; 240 G; 465 T; 35 other;
      ccttyagaay aycatcaggt cttgnannnn nttttatttt tgagtttta httgtaacta      60
      ...
//
```

Fig. 5.11. This is a sample entry from RU that describes a new class of human DNA transposons, related to PiggyBac transposon in cabbage looper. Its sequence has been reconstructed from the genomic fossil record (see subheading 'identification, reconstruction and classification of new TEs'). The entry includes: a unique sequence identification name (ID); definition (DE), date of creation and of the latest update (DT), keywords (KW), biological classification of the species in which it was found (OC), reference (RN, RA, RL), basic commentary (CC), source of the sequence data (DR) and base composition of the consensus sequence (SQ). This particular consensus sequence led to identification of a PiggyBac-like gene in the human genome.

Nomenclature

Each repetitive element listed in RU carries a unique name. Originally, standard names such as medium reiteration frequency repeats or MERs were assigned to unclassified sequence fragments discovered at the time. As more sequence information became available the nomenclature has evolved. For example, MER37 was later classified as a DNA transposon and became Tigger, MER115 and MER118 led to identification of Zaphod (see Repbase update). The evolving nomenclature has been preserved in the keyword KW sections of RU entries (Fig. 5.11) and in the appendix files. Unfortunately, new names usually are not any more informative than the old ones, as there are no standards that would systematically relate particular names to biological classification. Entire genomes have been sequenced and annotated based on Repbase update. The value of such annotation depends to a large extent on the ability of nonspecialists to rapidly classify particular repeats based on their names. This requires comprehensive indexes linking individual names, or groups of names from RU to the corresponding classes of repeats. Because repeat annotation in the human genome is based exclusively on RU and the reference collection of repeats is among most complete in RU, the first such index was prepared for human TEs. This index is expanded here (Table 5.1) to include the nomenclature of other mammalian repeats from RU. Table 5.1 includes three columns. Column 3 summarises individual and group names of repetitive families/ subfamilies as used in RU. Column 1 lists major biological categories discussed in the previous section. Column 2 reflects further subdivision of TEs based on biological attributes as well as on their occurrence in different mammalian species. It must be noted here that many repetitive elements are shared among different mammals (e.g. MIR, MIR3) or are closely related (e.g. L1 elements). For practical purposes, the shared elements are listed only once in Table 5.1. For example, MIR, MIR3 and L3 present in all mammals, are listed only under human/shared category. This category also contains human-specific sequences such as Alu, SVA and SVA2.

Table 5.1. Major categories of mammalian repetitive families from repbase update and their family/subfamily loci names.

Major categories	*Subcategories*	*Family/subfamily loci names*
LINEs	Human/shared	IN25, L1*, L2A, KER2, L3, CR1_HS
	Rodent/shared	LINE3_RN (LI_RN), LX*, LLME
	Other mammalian	ARMER 1, ART2*, BDDF*, BOV2, BTALU2, LINE1E_OC, LINE_C, THER2
SINEs	Human/shared	Alu*, FLA*, HAL1*, L2B, MIR, MIR3, SVA, SVA2
	Rodent/shared	B1*, B2*, B3*, BC1, FAM, ID_B1, MUSID* (IDI-6), PB1*, RDRE1_RN (ID_RN), RNALUIII, RSINE1, RSINE2*(B4*), SQR2_MM
	Other mammalian	BCS, BOVA2, BOVTA, BTALU1, BTCS, C_OC, CHR-1, CHR-2, D_CH, DREI, MAR1, MON1, MVB2, NLA, PRE1_SS, SINEC*, THER1
Retroviruses and retrovirus-like elements (*internal sequences*)	MaLRs-human/ shared	MLT1R, MLT1AR (MLT-int), MLT1CR (MLT1-int), MLT1FR (MLT1F-int), MSTAR (MST-int), THE1BR
	MaLRs-rodent/ shared	MTA1 (MT-int), ORR1-AI (ORR1-int), ORR1BI (ORR1B-int).
	Other rodent/ shared retroviruses	ERVL, HARLEQUIN, HERV*, HRES1, HUERS-P*, LOR1I, MER4I, MER4BI, MER21I, MER31I, MER41I, MER50I, MER51I, MER52AI, MER57I,

(Contd...)

Major categories	Subcategories	Family/subfamily loci names
		MER57A_I, MER61I, MER65I, MER66I, MER70I, MER83AI, MER83BI, MER84I, MER89I, MER110I, PABL_AI, PABL_BI, PRIMA4_I, PRIMA41
	Other rodent/ shared retroviruses	ETNERV, IAPA_MM, IAPEY1, IAPEZI, MERVL, MMETN, MMLV30, MULV, MYS1_PL (MYSPL), MYSERV
Long terminal repeats (LTRs)[a]	MaLR LTRs-human/shared	MLT1*, MST*, THE1*
	MaLR LTRs-rodent/shared	MTA, MTB, MTC, MTD, MTE, MT2*, ORR1A*, ORR1B*, ORR1C, ORR1D
	Other human/ shared retroviruses LTRs	HARLEQUINLTR, LTR*, LOR1, MLT2*, MER4*, MER9, MER11*, MER21*, MER31*, MER34*, MER39*, MER41*, MER48, MER49, MER50*, MER51*, MER52*, MER54*. MER57*, MER61*, MER65*, MER66*, MER67*, MER68*, MER70*, MER72*, MER73, MER74*, MER76, MER77, MER83*, MER84, MER87, MER88, MER89, MER90, MER92*, MER93*, MER95, MER101*, MER 110*, PABL_A, PABL_B, PRIMA4_LTR, PTR5
	Other rodent/ shared retrovirus LTRs	BGLII, LTRIAPEY, LTRIS, MERVL_LTR, MYS1_LTR, NICER_RN, PMR89, RAL, RLTR*, RMER2, RMER3, RMER4, RMER5, RMER6*, RMER10, RMER12, RMER13*, RMER15, RMER16, RMER17*, RMER19, RMER20
	Other mammalian retrovirus LTRs	ALTR2, BTLTRI, ECE1LTR, FCLTRI, MTV9LTR1_SM
DNA transposons	Human/shared	BLACKJACK, CHARLIE*, CHESHIRE*, GOLEM*, HSMAR*, HSTC2, LOOPER, MADE1, MARNA, MER1*, MER2*, MER3, MER5*, MER6*, MER8, MER20*, MER28, MER30*, MER33, MER44*, MER45*, MER46, MER53, MER63*, MER69*, MER75, MER80, MER81 MER82, MER85, MER91*, MER94*, MER96*, MER97*, MER99, MER 103, MER104*. MER105, MER106*, MER107, MER113, MER115, MER116, MER117, MER119, ORSL, PMERI, RICKSHA*, TIGGER*, ZAPHOD, ZOMBI*
	Rodent/shared	URR1
Minisatellites satellites	Human	IVR, R66
	Human/shared	ALR*, BSR, CER, (GGAAT)n, GSAT*, HSATI*, LSAU, MER22, MER122, MSRI, REP522, SAR, SATR*, SN5, TAR1
	Rodent/shared	CENSAT, GSAT_MM, ISAT_RN, R91ES8_RN, SATI_RN, SATMIN, ZP3AR_MM
	Other mammalian	BMSATI, BTSAT*, F ASAT(?), OOREP1(L1?), OSSAT*, SSRS2, RTREPI, SATIA_MM
Composite/simple	Human	MER120
	Rodent	SQRI_MM
	Other mammalian	MRSATI, SSRS1
Unclassified/ incomplete	Human	HIR, MER35, MER109, MER112, MER121
	Rodent	ALSAT_RN (LI?), C573, CYRA11_MM, DRB_RN, LPKR_RN, MREP_MC, PMR89 (HERVL?), RMER1*, SQR4_MM, YREP
	Other mammalian	LMER1

[a] This list does not include the internal sequence names listed above.

* Indicates multiple names starting with the same theme name. For example, RMER1* represents three subfamilies named RMER1, RMER1A and RMER1B. The theme name RMER1 is shared among the three.

The current release of RU contains 835 mammalian repeat families and subfamilies, many of which share variants of the same name (e.g. MT2A, MT2B, MT2C). Such variants are grouped together and the variations are indicated by asterisks (MT2*, see column 3). For example, RLTR* stands for 27 different long terminal repeats (LTRs). For historical reasons LTRs also carry other unassuming names such as BGLII, PMR89 and RMER. The corresponding internal retroviral sequences, if available, are listed in a separate section above the LTR section in Table 5.1. The application of Table 5.1 to the interpretation of repeat annotation is discussed in the next section.

Analysis of Repetitive DNA

Identification and annotation of known repeats

The basic routine underlying identification and annotation of repetitive DNA remains essentially unchanged since it was first implemented in the Pythia server and reimplemented in XBLAST and CENSOR. Since 1996, major progress has been achieved in terms of speed and sensitivity of repeat detection based on dedicated hardware used in CENSOR server (see Website: http://www.girinst.org/ CensorServer.html) and an efficient implementation of Smith-Waterman algorithm used in RepeatMasker (see Website: http://repeatmasker.genome.washington.edu).

Detection and annotation of repetitive DNA is based on comparing a query sequence against representative collections of repeats as schematically shown in Fig. 5.12. To avoid nonspecific matches, it is first advisable to filter out simple repeats from the query or reference sequences prior to the analysis by replacing sequence letters with neutral characters such as 'N' or 'X'. There are several ways to identify simple repeats based on their similarity to a reference set or on their nonrandom base composition. Another program, particularly useful for analysing cryptically simple repeats, has been implemented as a part of repeat analysis on the CENSOR server (see Website: http://www.girinst.org/Censor_Server.html). After simple repeats are masked, complex repeats can be detected by sequence comparisons using the FASTA, BLAST or Smith-Waterman algorithms. FASTA and BLAST are significantly faster but less sensitive than Smith-Waterman-based programs. The latter are essential to detect very old repetitive elements such as the extinct human MIR3 and LINE3 elements that are related to CR1 elements from birds. Conversely, relatively young repeats such as most Alu subfamilies can be detected using a less sensitive approach. Therefore, dividing repeats into detectable categories and the selective application of different algorithms may facilitate the detection process. Apart from these knowledge-based improvements, there are algorithm-based attempts to accelerate repeat detection without sacrificing the sensitivity of the process. It must be noted, the major determinant of speed, sensitivity, and accuracy is the quality of reference collections as discussed in the next section.

There are several types of output files generated by repeat annotation program (examples are listed in Fig. 5.12). They include maps of repeats summarising location and basic characteristics of individual elements, query file(s) with masked repeats, sequences and coordinates of the identified repeats and alignment to reference sequences for detailed inspection. A sample of repeat maps generated by CENSOR (see Website: http://www.girinst.org/Censor_Server.html) is shown in Fig. 5.13. The top part of the figure (Fig. 5.13a), illustrates a human endogenous retrovirus HERV3 flanked at both ends by long terminal repeats (LTR61). It also contains a MER11A element inserted in opposite orientation. All MER11 elements are classified as LTRs different from LTR61 (Table 5.1). Therefore, MER11A most likely represents a remnant from a different retrovirus inserted at that spot. The internal portion of the retrovirus (HERV3) and the 5' LTR are chopped by the program into smaller fragments separated by blank regions without any identified repeats. Because the blank regions are relatively short (< 50 bp), the fragments can be combined into a single LTR (see the bottom part of the figure). If the blank regions are much longer in relative terms, additional testing may be required. For example the first two 5' fragments of the internal sequence HERV3 are separated by 457 bp. A corresponding, gap of similar size can be seen in the reference sequence from RU (see columns 4–6). This suggests that the nucleotide sequence at positions 54059–54515 represents another homologous fragment of the same retrovirus not detected by the algorithm. In such cases a separate test may be needed to verify whether or not such a spot does not represent any unknown element(s) inserted in the retrovirus. In this case, additional alignment has shown that this region is most similar to HERV3 and therefore, it can be incorporated in the internal portion of the retrovirus pictured below the map.

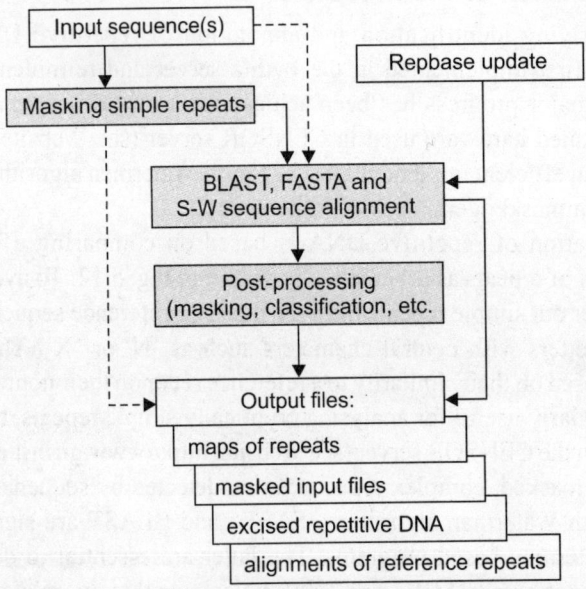

Fig. 5.12. A scheme for automated identification and annotation of repetitive DNA. Continuous arrows indicate critical steps, whereas broken arrows show major variants of the process. Typical output files include: maps of repeats (Fig. 5.13), masked query file(s), a list of masked sequences and alignments against the reference sequences as described in the text.

The bottom example (Fig. 5.13b), shows a more complicated pattern of insertion into another endogenous retrovirus (HERVK22I), flanked by LTR22. This retrovirus contains two independent L1 elements (LlPA2 and L1PA3) inserted in its internal sequence. LlPA2 appears to be complete or nearly complete whereas LlPA3 is represented only by a short 419 bp 3' fragment and its orientation is opposite to LlPA3. Due to this opposite orientation, and typical 5' truncation, it is likely that L1PA3 represents a separate integration event of an incomplete L1 element.

Identification, reconstruction and classification of new TEs

Interspersed repetitive DNA seldom contains complete copies of TEs. It is believed that from the start many retro (trans)posons generate 5' truncated copies of themselves (e.g. L1PA3 in Fig. 5.13b). Even if the inserted copies are originally complete, over time they can undergo genetic rearrangements or partial to complete deletion. Furthermore, copies of TEs undergo base-substitution mutations, accelerated by methylation of CpG dinucleotides, due to conversion of the 5-methylcytosine to thymine by spontaneous deamination.

GB Acc.	Beg.	End	RU locus	Beg.	End	O	S
AC007379	53088	53232	LTR61	74	233	d	0.74
AC007379	53260	53333	LTR61	234	311	d	0.76
AC007379	53368	53661	LTR61	299	595	d	0.77
AC007379	53671	54058	HERV3	10	393	d	0.74
AC007379	54515	54846	HERV3	794	1126	d	0.69
AC007379	55021	55802	HERV3	1302	2081	d	0.73
AC007379	55925	56582	HERV3	2161	2826	d	0.71
AC007379	56638	57091	HERV3	2863	3305	d	0.72
AC007379	57108	57996	HERV3	3334	4221	d	0.77
AC007379	58043	58767	HERV3	4268	5005	d	0.73
AC007379	58861	59905	MER11A	1126	1	c	0.86
AC007379	60087	61081	HERV3	5278	6313	d	0.72
AC007379	61173	61305	HERV3	8287	8418	d	0.74
AC007379	61316	61829	LTR61	72	595	d	0.74

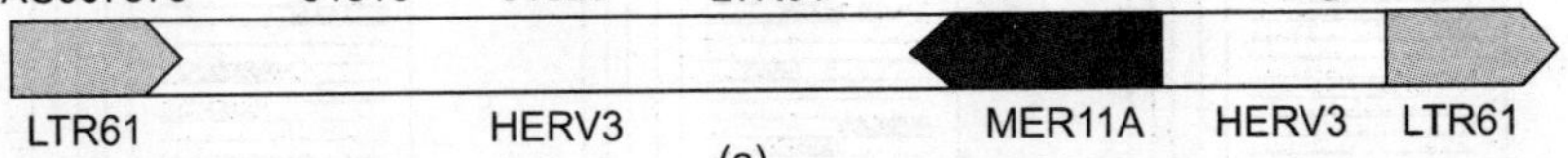

LTR61   HERV3   MER11A HERV3 LTR61

(a)

GB Acc.	Beg.	End	RU locus	Beg.	End	O	S
AB045363	38248	38745	LTR22	1	580	c	0.70
AB045363	38748	40067	HERVK22I	5514	6835	c	0.89
AB045363	40075	40494	L1PA3	483	902	c	0.98
AB045363	40495	42621	HERVK22I	5527	2327	c	0.86
AB045363	43041	43432	HERVK22I	339	741	c	0.85
AB045363	43434	48611	L1	1	5303	d	0.95
AB045363	48612	49463	L1PA2	51	902	d	0.97
AB045363	49492	49842	HERVK22I	3	350	c	0.88
AB045363	49845	50338	LTR22	1	580	c	0.69

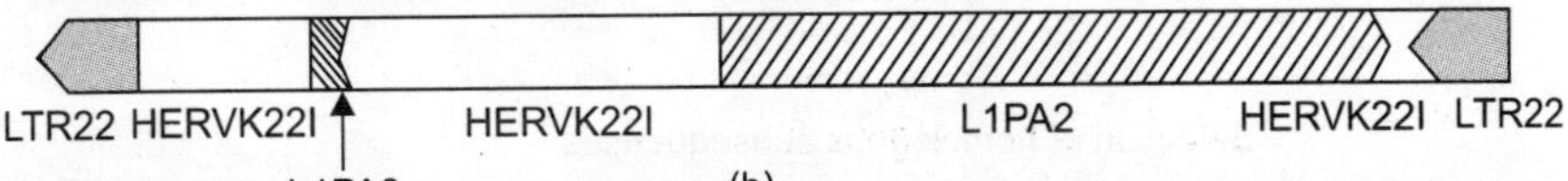

LTR22 HERVK22I   HERVK22I   L1PA2   HERVK22I LTR22

L1PA3   (b)

Fig. 5.13. Sample maps of repetitive elements generated by CENSOR (see Website: http:// www.girinst.org) and their graphic interpretation. Column 1 lists the GenBank accession numbers of the query sequences, followed by coordinates of the repeats. Column 4 lists repeat names and coordinates relative to RU sequences. Column 7 shows the orientation of the repeats (direct or complementary), and the last column shows similarities to sequences from RU. Graphic interpretations are given below the maps. (a) HERV3 flanked by LTR61. (b) HERVK22I flanked by LTR22.

As a result methylated CpG doublets mutate to CpA or TpG at a rate about a factor of magnitude higher than the average mutation rate. Thus, fragmented and mutated copies usually represent the only source of information about complete and active TEs. For this reason most TEs deposited in RU represent consensus sequences reconstructed from scattered partial sequence information. Consensus sequences are not only more complete, but also more similar to individual repeats than individual repeats to each other. The relationship between similarity to the consensus (y) and average pairwise similarity between individual repeats (x) is given by the Equation 5.1:

$$y = \frac{1 + \sqrt{12x - 3}}{4} \qquad \qquad \dots (5.1)$$

For example, individual repeats that are on average 50 per cent similar to each other will be 68 per cent similar to their quality consensus sequence (i.e. for $x = 0.5$, $y = 0.68$). This significantly facilitates the identification of highly diverged repeats.

The reconstruction process is usually, but not necessarily, associated with discovering new repetitive elements. There are many different ways in which previously unknown repetitive elements can be identified. For example, the coordinates of potential new repeat sequences can be determined from blank spot in the maps similar to those described above. A routine approach, presented in Fig. 5.14, takes advantage of the same computer software as used in annotating known repeats. It starts with masking the existing repeats from a GenBank file or other large data set.

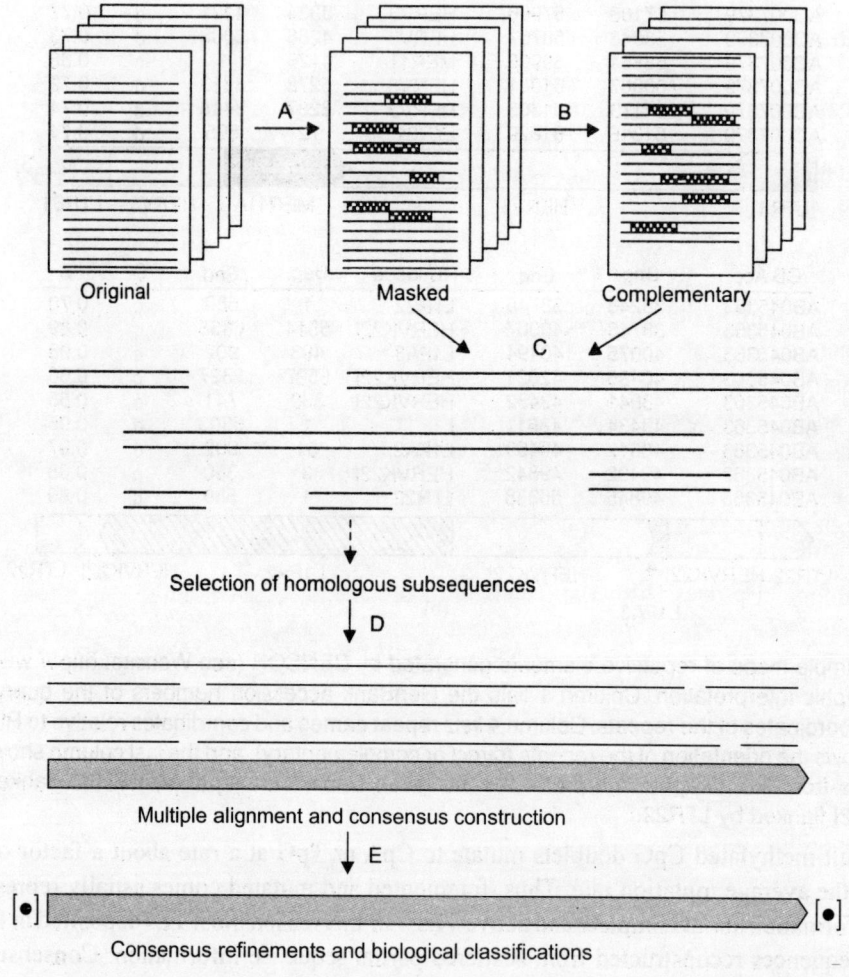

Fig. 5.14. Identification and reconstruction of TEs. The steps involved are: (a) masking known repeats in the query database; (b) generation of a complementary database; (c) comparison of direct and complementary databases in search of homologous regions, followed by selection of potential repeats; (d) multiple alignment and consensus building; (e) evaluation of consensus and determination of target sites as detailed in the text.

The masked sequence data is then compared against itself, preferably in opposite orientation to minimise obvious matches from known multi-copy genes. The resulting output file will contain homologous sequence fragments including repeats. These repeats need to be tested to exclude matches between duplicated genes or other obvious similarities not related to repetitive DNA. The next critical step is the generation of a multiple alignment as a basis for developing a consensus as summarised in

Fig. 5.14. Multiple alignment of partial sequences can be carried out using CLUSTALX program, but it usually requires refinement using sequence editors. A partial consensus sequence may be used to realign sequence fragments in order to verify and improve the original alignment. This iterative approach is particularly useful in the case of highly diverged sequences.

Prior to consensus building it is important to subdivide repetitive elements into meaningful subfamilies if the number of repeat sequences is sufficient. In most cases it can be done using a standard phylogenetic analysis package (e.g. PHYLIP; see Website: http://evolution.genetics.washington.edu/phylip.html). In the past, constructing phylogenetic trees proved to be unsuccessful in determining Alu classification and alternative approaches were necessary. Retrospectively, most difficulties encountered using tree-based classification for repeats were due to interference between rapidly mutating CpG doublets and other sequence positions containing critical information. Therefore, in the case of at least CpG-rich repeats, it may be important to exclude CpG doublets and their common derivatives (TpG, CpA) when constructing phylogenetic trees.

Initial reconstruction almost always leads to partial consensus sequences. To determine exact boundaries, it is important to obtain maps of repeats that would include the newly built consensus sequence. The best way to determine exact ends of the new repeat is to study its insertions into other repetitive elements. This is also the best way to determine target site duplications that are often essential for proper classification of the repeat.

Systematic analysis of sequence data during the last decade has revealed a large variety of transposable elements in eukaryotic genomes. This has led to the creation of specialised databases and tools essential for eukaryotic genome analysis during the sequencing era. Some approaches outlined in this chapter are relatively straightforward. However, much of the analysis still relies heavily on human judgement and creativity that have not yet been encoded in computer software. Transposable elements are intrinsically involved in biological processes that still remain to be understood. Therefore, repetitive DNA is no longer viewed as a troublesome junkyard but rather as a gold mine of information underlying biology of eukaryotic genomes.

MOLECULAR GENETICS OF DISEASE AND THE HUMAN GENOME PROJECT

The haploid (n) human genome contains approx 3 billion nucleotides (or bases) of DNA strung amongst 23 chromosomes. The diploid ($2n$) complement, which consists of a haploid genome inherited from each parent, therefore comprises 46 chromosomes of 6 billion nucleotides of DNA, all contained within the cell nucleus. The same complement of DNA is found in every cell (except red blood cells) in the body. Mitochondrial DNA, which is a circular molecule of genetic material, 16,000 nucleotides long, is also part of the human genome.

It is located outside the nucleus in the cytoplasm of the cell and encodes a small but important subset of human genes. Mitochondrial DNA is only transmitted from mothers to their offspring. On average, the human genome is 99.9 per cent identical between any two individuals, with nucleotide differences existing only about 1 in every 1000 bases. Less than 5 per cent of the genome contains genes or protein-coding regions.

The remaining 95 per cent (noncoding part) contains repetitive elements and other sequences whose functions are not completely understood and is often referred to as junk DNA. These regions may play a role in maintaining the structural integrity of chromosomes. There at least 30,000–40,000 genes in the human genome, ranging in size less than 1 to 200 kilobases (kb), with the average size of a gene being 50 kb. General information on the human genome is provided in Table 5.2.

Table 5.2. Components of the human genome.

The genome is the total genetic material in a cell

The nuclear genome is comprised of 46 chromosomes, which come as 23 pairs; one of each pair comes from either parent

Mitochondrial DNA is also part of the genome. It is always inherited from the mother and is found in the cytoplasm

Chromosomes are made of deoxyribonucleic acid (DNA)

DNA is made of four chemical units (nucleotides) called adenine (A), guanine (G), cytosine (C) and thymine (T)

The genome is comprised of about 3 billion A, C, G and Ts

Genes are the portions of DNA that encode functional RNA molecules or proteins

There are approx 30000–40000 genes in the genome

Proteins provide the structure for the cell and are involved in biochemical reactions (enzymes)

Genes are comprised of exons-regions that code for mature mRNA- and introns-intervening segments of DNA that are transcribed, but then cut out from the transcript during mRNA processing (Fig. 5.15). There is no uniformity to the number or size of introns; this is the main reason why there is a vast range of gene sizes.

Genes contain promoter sequences at their start (5' end). Typical promoters contain several DNA sequence motifs that bind regulatory proteins and control the level of transcription and the start position of the mRNA. Expression of tissue-specific genes are unique to individual or sets of tissues (muscle, brain, liver, etc.) in our bodies. There are also housekeeping genes that are expressed in all cell types because their products provide basic functions (Table 5.3).

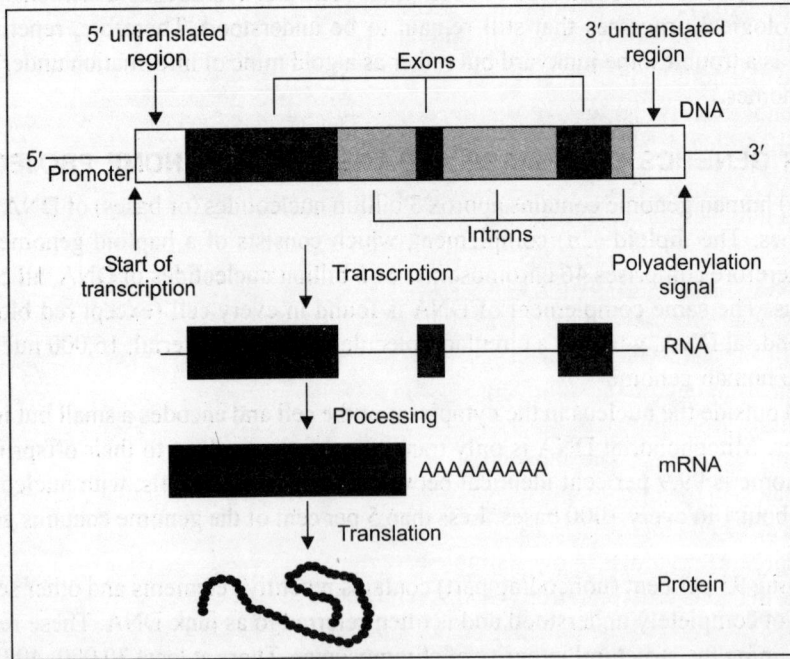

Fig. 5.15. Anatomy of a gene. Information flows from DNA to RNA (transcription) to protein (translation).

Table 5.3. Gene expression.

Transcription	The synthesis of a single-strand RNA molecule from a DNA template in the cell nucleus
	This process is controlled by the interactions between proteins and DNA sequences near each gene
RNA processing	
Capping	Addition of a modified nucleotide chain to the 5' end of a growing mRNA chain. This is required for the normal processing, stability and translation of mRNA
Splicing	The process of removing introns and joining exons into a mature mRNA molecule
Polyadenylation	Addition of 20–200 adenosine residues (poly A tail) to the 3' end of the RNA transcript
Transport	The fully processed RNA is taken to the cytoplasm where translation takes place
Translation	The synthesis of a protein from its mRNA template
Housekeeping genes	Expressed in all cell types because their products provide basic functions in cells
Tissue-specific genes	Expressed in only certain cell-types because their products have specific functions

Simple and Complex Patterns of Inheritance

Every individual has two copies of each gene, one on each of the chromosomes. Owing to DNA sequence variation, there can be two or more alternative forms of a gene (called alleles), that result in different gene products. This variation contributes to the uniqueness of individuals. The term genotype is defined as the complete heritable genetic composition of an individual. Phenotype is the physical or biochemical manifestation of that genotype, and in some instances this can be associated with disease. However, in most cases, different alleles contribute to physical characteristics such as height, hair colour and other nondisease related cellular functions. The dominant and recessive forms of a trait in any given person are governed by which alleles (dominant or recessive) are inherited from the parents (Fig. 5.16). Only individuals with two recessive alleles will show the recessive form of a trait (e.g. blue eyes). However, in the presence of a dominant allele (e.g. brown eyes), the trait associated with the recessive allele is not expressed phenotypically. Recessive alleles are not lost in a population; they can be passed on to subsequent generations where in the presence of another copy of the allele, the recessive trait reveals itself again.

There are a number of diseases that are manifested owing to this simple dominant/recessive pattern of expression. Sickle cell anemia and cystic fibrosis are common examples of when the disease (termed autosomal recessive) develops owing to the presence of two copies of the recessive gene. A person with only one copy of the recessive allele does not develop the disease, but remains a carrier, because the normal copy of the gene predominates. Autosomal dominant disorders like Huntington's disease are produced when a single mutated dominant allele is present even if the other copy of the allele is normal. Diseases resulting from mutations in genes on the X-chromosome are known as X-linked disorders. Since males only have one X-chromosome, these diseases (e.g. hemophilia) act like dominant mutations in males. Females on the other hand, act as carriers and in the next generation their male offspring may or may not be affected (Fig. 5.16).

Not all disorders and traits follow a simple pattern of inheritance as described earlier. One gene can influence more than one trait (pleiotropy) and several genes can affect only one trait (polygenic disorders). Although genes may determine whether or not a person will have heart disease or be predisposed to cancer, many traits can be triggered or influenced by the environment as well as in the case of complex multifactorial diseases such as schizophrenia and alcoholism.

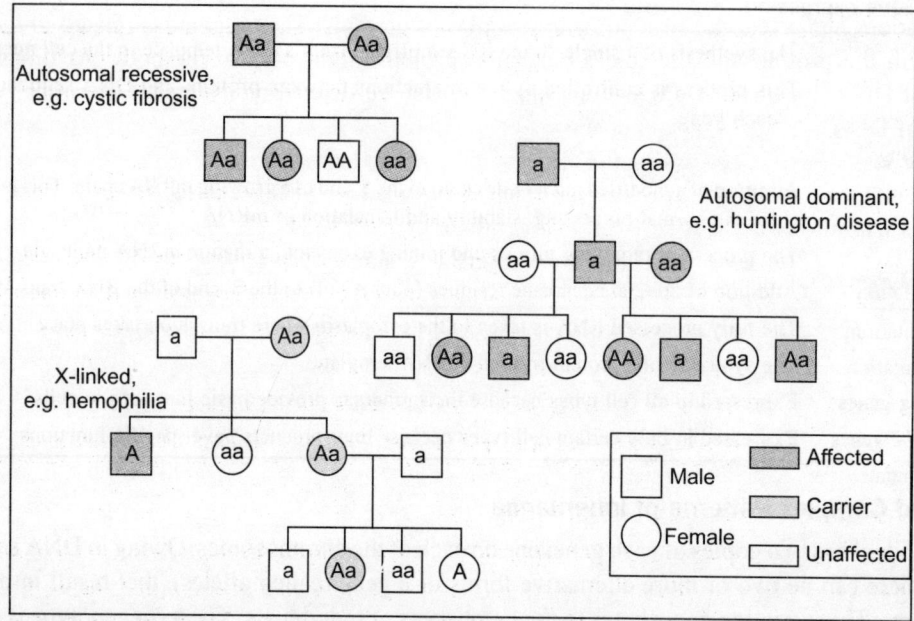

Fig. 5.16. Patterns of inheritance for autosomal recessive, autosomal dominant and X-linked disorders. Recessive alleles are indicated by 'a' and dominant alleles by 'A'. Males only have one X-chromosome, therefore only one allele is shown for X-linked inheritance.

DNA Sequence Variations and Gene Mutations

The human genome is predominantly stable and does not vary significantly between individuals. As described earlier, the genome of two individuals is only 0.1 per cent different. Some parts of the genome are more prone to variations than others, based on properties inherent to the DNA sequence. Most of these variations are found outside the coding regions of genes and are thus not harmful. These variations include mutations and polymorphisms.

A mutation is any permanent, heritable change in the DNA sequence that in some cases can result in disease. There are different kinds of genetic mutations. Gene mutations can be inherited from a parent or acquired during an individual's lifetime. The former, known as germline mutations, exists in the reproductive cells and can be passed on to later generations. This type of mutation is present in every cell that descended from the zygote to which the mutant gamete contributed. Somatic mutations are changes that occur in nonsex cells in the body (e.g. bone marrow or pancreatic cell) and are not passed on to the next generation. Whatever the effect, the ultimate fate of that somatic mutation is to disappear when the cell in which it occurred, or the individual, dies. On average, approx. 200 somatic mutations accumulate within the genome during each of our lifetimes.

Genes can be altered in many ways (Table 5.4). An incorrect base may be incorporated into the DNA sequence (point mutations) or a nucleotide or more may left out (deletions) or added (insertions). In some diseases like cystic fibrosis, different mutations in the same gene can produce different effects in different individuals (Fig. 5.17), but mutations in several different genes can also lead to the same clinical consequence, as in some forms of Alzheimer's disease. In some cases, the effects of mutational changes may not be critical to the proper functioning of proteins and these are called silent mutations.

Other mutations can affect the structure and function of proteins. The outcome is related to the degree of change in the protein and the role a particular protein might play in the body. At times, longer stretches of DNA, millions of nucleotides long, can also be deleted or inserted. Occasionally, longer segments of DNA are doubled (duplications) or interchanged between chromosomes (translocations). The gain or loss of entire chromosomes or chromosomal segments can also occur. Common disorders associated with these kinds of chromosomal changes include Down's syndrome, trisomy 18 and trisomy 13. Patients with these diseases carry an extra chromosome 21, 18 or 13, respectively, in their cells.

Table 5.4. Types of mutations and their effects.

Missense mutations	Single-nucleotide changes resulting in the substitution of an amino acid in the protein
Nonsense mutations	Single-nucleotide changes that create one of the three termination codons (TAA, TGA or TAG) resulting in a shortened, dysfunctional protein
Silent mutations	Have no detectable phenotypic effect
Splice-site mutations	Altered sequences at the ends of introns (5′ donor or 3′ acceptor) during RNA processing, that affect gene splicing and function
Insertions	Addition of extra DNA sequences of varying sizes
Duplications	Doubling of DNA sequences
Translocations	Interchange of segments of DNA between two different chromosomes
Inversions	Occur when a region of DNA inverts its orientation with respect to the rest of the chromosome
Trinucleotide repeats	Expansion of triplet repeat sequences
Deletions	Loss of part of a DNA sequence (could be loss of a single nucleotide or millions of nucleotides)
Deletion of:	Effects:
A gene	No protein product
An exon	Truncated protein
An intron	Usually no phenotypic change
Promoter	Gene nonfunctional
Splice-site	Protein nonfunctional
Many genes	Chromosomal abnormalities and usually a heterogeneous phenotype

Polymorphisms are differences in the genetic make-up of individuals that can be observed at the chromosomal, gene or even single base-pair level. They were originally considered to be genome variations that were neither harmful nor beneficial. However, there is evidence that polymorphisms can sometimes influence an individual's risk to disease. A single nucleotide polymorphism (SNP), which is a DNA point mutation, comes from variations in single nucleotides where any four of the bases may be substituted at a particular position. Most SNPs tend to have only two alleles instead of four. Considering that the human genome contains more than 3 million SNPs that make up 90 per cent of polymorphisms and most of the genome variations, the trend towards genome-wide screening for insights into disease mechanisms is increasing.

Microsatellites (also called short tandem repeats, STRs) represent another class of genetic polymorphism. These are tandemly repeated sequences, where the repeating unit is 1–4 nucleotides long. The number of times the unit is repeated in a given STR can be highly variable, a characteristic that makes them useful as genetic markers. The majority of microsatellites occur in gene introns or other noncoding regions of the genome. Generally, the microsatellite itself does not cause disease;

rather it is used as a marker to identify a specific chromosome or locus. When being used as a marker, the specific number of repeats in a given STR is not critical, but the difference in the number of repeats is of importance. There are other genetic markers that vary in length from 2–60 nucleotides; these are called variable number tandem repeats (VNTRs).

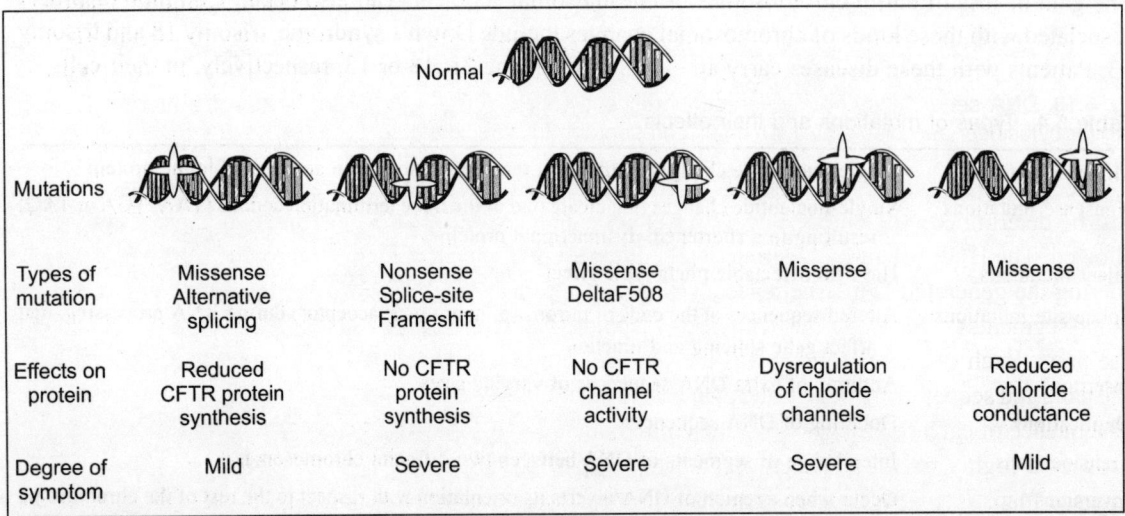

Types of mutation	Missense Alternative splicing	Nonsense Splice-site Frameshift	Missense DeltaF508	Missense	Missense
Effects on protein	Reduced CFTR protein synthesis	No CFTR protein synthesis	No CFTR channel activity	Dysregulation of chloride channels	Reduced chloride conductance
Degree of symptom	Mild	Severe	Severe	Severe	Mild

Fig. 5.17. Different mutations in the same gene (e.g. CFTR in cystic fibrosis) can produce different clinical outcomes. The clinical symptoms (severe/mild) correlate to the pancreatic function of the patients.

Human Genome Project and DNA Sequencing

The Human Genome Project (HGP) was formally initiated in the early 1990s, as an international effort to determine the complete DNA sequence of the human genome and all of the genes it encodes. The most immediate benefit of this information was to facilitate disease gene research.

DNA sequencing is the process of determining the specific order and identity of the three billion base pairs in the genome, with the ultimate goal of identifying all of the genes. Mapping is the process of identifying discrete DNA molecules of known position on a chromosome; which are then used for sequencing. Mapping is a crucial step for proper reconstruction of the genome. It usually precedes sequencing but is also necessary at the postsequencing stage.

Sequencing is now carried out through a process called fluorescence-based dideoxy sequencing. Fragments of DNA are first cloned in bacteria; they are then put into a polymerase catalysed reaction with free nucleotides, some of which are tagged with fluorescent dyes. Nucleotides attach themselves to the DNA fragments in a particular order. Similarly, dyed nucleotides can attach themselves to the DNA fragments, but other nucleotides will not adhere to the dyed nucleotides. Thus the enzymatic reaction generates DNA fragments of varying lengths that terminate at fluorescently labelled A, T, C or G nucleotides. An automated sequencing machine then determines the underlying sequence for the range of DNA fragments created in the chemical reaction (Fig. 5.18). The fluorescently tagged bases at the ends of the fragments are detected with a laser and a computer collects the resulting information. The order in which the particular tagged nucleotides are read reflects their order on the stretch of DNA that has been replicated. Each reaction reveals the sequence of at least 500 letters (G, A, T, C) of DNA before the process runs its course.

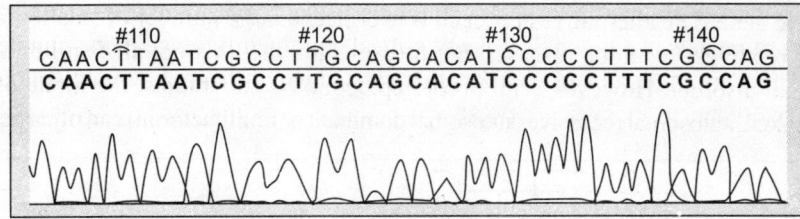

Fig. 5.18. DNA sequencing. Four different fluorescently tagged dyes (red for thymines, green for adenines, blue for cytosines, and black for guanines) represent the four nucleotides.

Once these relatively tiny sequences are obtained, their place in the overall genome DNA sequence must be determined. To achieve a working DNA sequence draft of the genome, two approaches were followed. The HGP began by creating detailed genetic and physical maps, to provide a framework for ordering the generated DNA sequences. Using this approach, the HGP divided the genome into about 30,000 segments (a technique called physical mapping), each containing an average of 1,00,000–2,00,000 base pairs. Each of these sections was then broken down into even smaller fragments, of about 2000 base pairs and sequenced. Initially, the plan was to put the fragments in order and systematically determine the sequence of each fragment so that the entire human DNA sequence would be revealed. This method produces a highly accurate sequence with few gaps. However, the up-front process of building the sequence maps is costly, time-consuming and therefore, determines the speed at which the project is completed.

A second approach used by the HGP to generate a draft sequence of the human genome is what is called the whole genome shotgun or WGS (an approach that bypasses the need to construct physical maps). In WGS, sufficient DNA sequencing is performed at random so that each nucleotide of DNA in the genome is covered numerous times, in fragments of about 500 base pairs. Determining where those individual fragments fit in the overall DNA is accomplished through the use of powerful computers that analyse the raw data to find overlaps. A working draft of DNA sequence usually covers 95 per cent of the genome (maintaining 99 per cent accuracy) but it is divided into many unordered gapped segments. Additional sequencing is required to generate the finished DNA sequence, such that there are no gaps or ambiguities. The final sequence has an accuracy of greater than 99.99 per cent. Only partial data was collected from each DNA fragment. This was then assembled to generate a working or rough draft.

Positional Cloning

Positional cloning is the process by which disease-causing genes are identified on the basis of their chromosomal location, with limited or no prior knowledge of the gene's function (Fig. 5.19). Positional cloning can be divided into the following three steps.

Step 1: Family studies

The first step in the positional cloning process is the collection of information on families who have the disease. Family trees (pedigrees) are established and DNA from blood is used for genetic analyses. Critical to this step is the diagnosis and assignment of proper phenotypic features to family members affected by the disease. Finding suitable families can be rate-limiting, particularly when the disease is rare or for disorders in which affected individuals die at a young age. Two general approaches are used when collecting families for studies. A small number of very large families can be studied, where all affected members of the pedigree are known to have the same genetic disease, presumably caused by a mutation in a single gene. The alternative approach is to collect a large number of smaller families. This is easier to do for relatively common diseases, but it carries the risk that not all families may have the genetically identical disorder. However, with proper epidemiological studies, the mode of inheritance of the disease (X-linked, autosomal recessive, autosomal dominant or multifactorial) can often be determined.

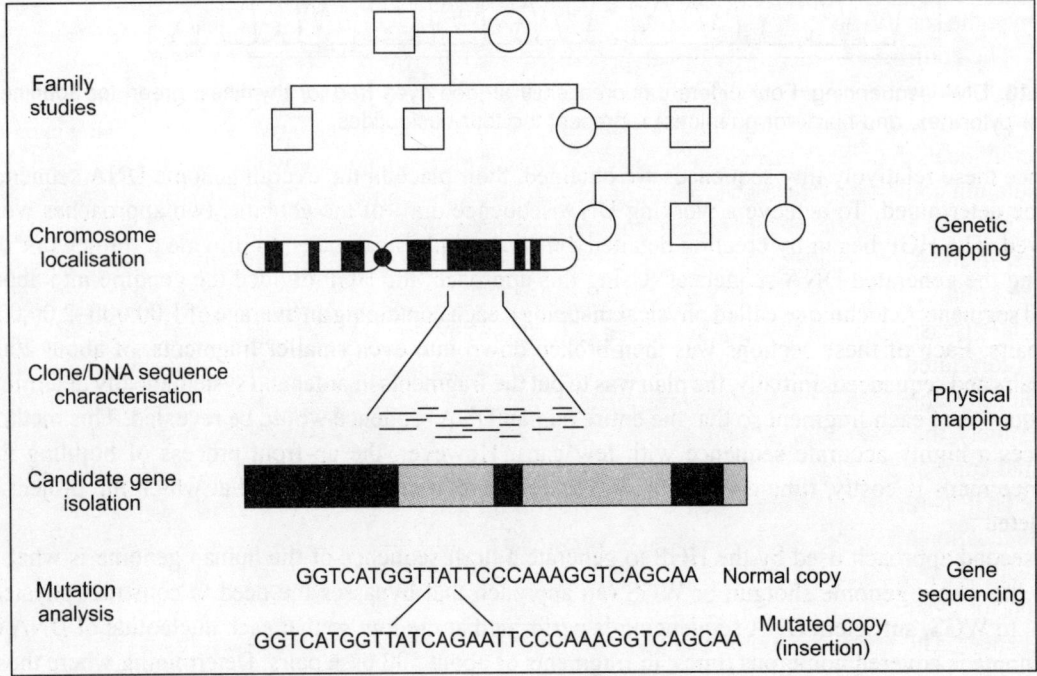

Fig. 5.19. Disease gene identification by positional cloning using mapping and DNA sequencing techniques.

Step 2: Mapping and sequencing

The next step in positional cloning is to identify informative chromosomal rearrangements or genetic markers that are always found in family members affected by the disease. In the simplest case, the disease gene might be closely associated with a chromosomal anomaly, which helps define the position of the causative gene on the chromosome. Unfortunately this is a rare event and not the case for most genetic disorders. In the remainder of cases, genetic mapping is performed to determine the chromosomal region containing the disease gene being sought. This is accomplished by examining genetic markers that have already been mapped to particular chromosomes across the genome, to determine which ones are linked to the disease. If each family member that has the disease also has a particular DNA marker, it is likely that the gene responsible for the disease is in close proximity to that marker, thus defining where the gene search should be focused.

Step 3: Candidate gene isolation and mutation analysis

The last step in positional cloning is to identify the genes within the candidate region. Historically, mapping the disease gene was followed by the construction of physical maps by ordering overlapping fragments of DNA along the region of interest and determining the nucleotide composition of the clones.

Now that most of the human genome has been sequenced, candidate genes from the chromosomal region of interest are usually available for further study. However, a complete gene catalogue is not yet established. Therefore, at times, one must scan the DNA sequence to look for features characteristic of genes. Since the coding sequence of genes is usually not continuous, this is not always simple. Looking for exon-intron boundaries of coding and noncoding regions, amino acid encoding DNA sequences to determine the start and end of the gene or evolutionarily conserved DNA segments, all help to focus this search. The confirmation that a candidate gene is causative in the disease requires a direct association between a mutation in that gene and expression of the disease phenotype. The identified mutation should be present only in affected individuals and not in unaffected relatives or controls. However, in some individuals the mutation may not cause the disease, a phenomenon known as incomplete penetrance. The mutation could also cause a variation of the disease, a phenomenon known as reduced penetrance. In the case of a late-onset disorder like Huntington's disease, the mutation may not have had time to manifest itself. A key issue while looking for mutations in a disease gene is the ability to discriminate between nondisease-causing sequence polymorphisms that may just be linked to the disease gene and the actual disease-causing mutations. Various bioassays can be designed to show that a particular gene defect (correlated to an altered amino acid in the protein) can cause the phenotype in question. For example, the abnormal gene can be introduced in an animal model to see if it causes the disease. Alternatively, the normal form of the gene can be introduced and tested to determine if it can replace the abnormal copy of the gene.

The HGP is rapidly identifying all of the genes in the human genome. The goal of this effort is to find the location and pinpoint the function of the at least 30,000–40,000 human genes by the year 2008 (Fig. 5.20). Positional cloning has thus far been used to identify hundreds of disease genes, including the gene for cystic fibrosis, Huntington's disease, some types of Alzheimer's disease and early-onset breast cancer. The identification of a gene prior to the HGP is described in the following.

Identification of the Gene Causing Cystic Fibrosis

The gene for cystic fibrosis (CF) was identified in 1989, providing a paradigm for dozens of future disease gene discoveries using HGP data. CF is the most common fatal, autosomal recessive disorder in the Caucasian population. It is characterised by chronic lung disease and pancreatic insufficiency, and affects 1 in 2500 individuals. The severity of the disease can often be correlated with the mutations present (Fig. 5.17).

In order to locate the CF gene, researchers tested DNA from CF families with a large number of genetic markers. A total of 211 families were pooled and analysed and eventually two markers located on chromosome 7 were found to flank the gene. This key finding, published in 1985, indicated that the CF gene must be inherited along with the markers on chromosome 7. Next, a combination of genetic techniques, including chromosome walking and jumping, was used. In walking to either direction of a known marker, an initial clone containing the marker gene is used to isolate another clone that contains overlapping information from the genome. The DNA segments can then be placed in an order corresponding to that on the chromosome and the process is repeated. A complimentary approach to this technique, called chromosome jumping, utilises only the ends of cloned segments, making jumps over uninformative or repetitive regions of DNA. In the search for the CF gene, each DNA fragment isolated was compared to DNA from animal species in order to determine whether any of these fragments were conserved during evolution. A match was found with a sequence from chicken, mouse and cow, suggesting that this gene was also encoded in these animals.

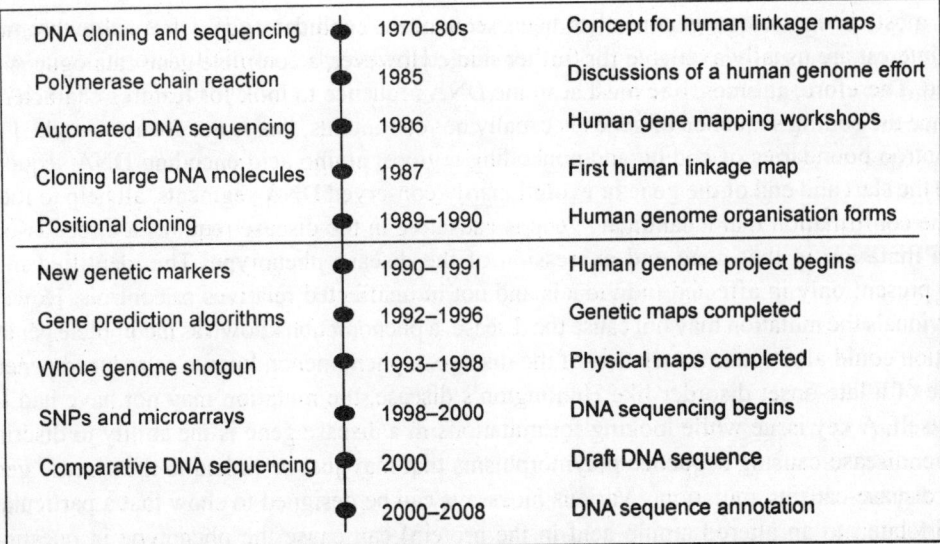

DNA cloning and sequencing	1970–80s	Concept for human linkage maps
Polymerase chain reaction	1985	Discussions of a human genome effort
Automated DNA sequencing	1986	Human gene mapping workshops
Cloning large DNA molecules	1987	First human linkage map
Positional cloning	1989–1990	Human genome organisation forms
New genetic markers	1990–1991	Human genome project begins
Gene prediction algorithms	1992–1996	Genetic maps completed
Whole genome shotgun	1993–1998	Physical maps completed
SNPs and microarrays	1998–2000	DNA sequencing begins
Comparative DNA sequencing	2000	Draft DNA sequence
	2000–2008	DNA sequence annotation

Fig. 5.20. Timeline of the human genome project (HGP). A historical summary of some of the enabling technologies (on the left) and the achievements (on the right) leading up to and including the HGP are shown. Other aspects of the HGP are the study of model organisms, analysis of genome variation, and the development of bioinformatics. Establishing training and public education programs, as well as the study of the ethical, legal and social issues of genetics research in society, are also important priorities.

This fragment of DNA represented the start of the CF gene and was used to identify the remainder of the gene. Since no chromosomal abnormality was evident in the patients, researchers then began searching for a difference between DNA from normal and CF patients. In 1989, a small deletion was found in a particular DNA fragment that appeared in 70 per cent of the chromosomes from CF patients, but was absent from normal chromosomes. The gene was found to be 250 kb long, comprised of 24 exons, encoding a trans-membrane protein, 1480 aa long. This gene located on chromosome 7 was called CFTR (cystic fibrosis trans-membrane conductance regulator), which encodes a chloride channel protein. In the majority of patients, the error that causes CF is minute, only three of the base pairs are missing. This principal mutation, DeltaF508 (deletion of phenylalanine amino acid at position 508 in the protein), is found in approx 70 per cent of carriers of European ancestry and is enough to radically disrupt the function of patients lungs, sweat glands and pancreas. The CF gene is also associated with mutational heterogeneity. Over 550 other mutations have been identified. Many of these are extremely rare, but a few reach frequencies of 1–3 per cent in CF carriers.

Human Genome Project and Disease Gene Identification

With the development of new mapping resources and technologies and massive amounts of DNA sequence generated by the HGP, the ability to clone rearrangement breakpoints and map disease genes has been greatly simplified. This has also accelerated the pace of discovery of new disease loci and the underlying mutational mechanisms. For example, the gene for Parkinson's disease (alpha synuclein) on chromosome 4q21–q23 and the gene for speech and language disorder (FOXP2) on chromosome 7q31, were identified within only a few months of determining their chromosomal location.

After a decade of experience in positional cloning, and with the HGP DNA sequence now well-advanced, it has become possible to dissect the molecular genetics of multifactorial diseases such as cancer and cardiovascular disease. These involve multiple combinations of genes and strong environmental components. Scientists will continue to work on the HGP with an emphasis on annotating the DNA sequence to find new genes, determine the function of the gene products (functional genomics) and apply all of this information to the study of common diseases.

GENE PREDICTION

In this section overview of gene finding techniques, with a software and the method it utilises are discussed.

General Principles

In considering the problem of gene prediction, we must be aware of the structure of a gene. It consists of promoter sequences as well as regulatory sequences upstream of gene. The gene itself is not continuous and is composed on introns and exons. The promoters are generally composed of consensus sequences, like TATA box in almost 70 per cent of cases. The presence of an open reading frame (ORF) is also somewhat indicative of the presence of an exon, although this is not definitive. There are 6 different reading frames, 3 on each strand starting at 1, 2 and 3rd position. The first codon must be a Methionine (MET). One can also use certain preferred codon usage to find genes, coupled with GC bias in the third codon in organisms that have high GC content in their genomes. Thus, gene prediction strategies vary widely in prokaryotic and eukaryotic genomes. Many algorithms utilise codon usage frequencies and then information theory based on log likelihood plots, are used to plot the presence of a gene. The presence of AATAAA within 5 kb of stop codon is also used for detection. There is also a 5' splice site signal as well as a 3' splice site signal to indicate the intron-exon and exon-intron boundaries. Gene finding strategies can be grouped under three categories:

1. Content based methods: Characteristics like periodicity of repeats, codon usage, compositional complexity are used.
2. Site based methods: These are used to detect donor and acceptor sites as well as tf-binding sites, start-stop codons, etc.
3. Comparative methods: Sequence homology is used to detect gene structure based on other known genes.

Thus, in totem, the gene prediction is not as such straightforward. It is hoped that the combination of these tools provided by Genemachine will help us ascertain if a given sequence has putative genes, exons, introns or a combination of them. In prokaryotes the ORF simply consists of start codon ATG and the stop codon(s) TAA, TAG and TGA. In eukaryotes this is further complicated since one has to take into account not only a start codon at the beginning of each exon, but also successive splice site signals between the end of an exon and the start of an intron. There is also a definitive poly A signal to signal the termination. Thus, given a set of sequence, one has to find the underlying sequence of a putative gene in any gene finding exercise. For this, we use state probabilities within an exon and intron as well as transition probabilities between an exon and intron to compute the most likely underlying sequence to predict the presence of a gene using the Viterbi approach.

Mathematical Foundations

We have discussed HMMs in our search for pattern finding, as well as briefly stated about machine learning. Figure 5.21 shows this concept and is well illustrated by signal P a program that has been trained on eukaryotes and that uses HMMs (Fig. 5.22) as well as Neural Nets to predict cleavage sites in proteins. Before we do that we will give a brief primer on protein signal motifs whose discovery resulted in a Nobel prize quite recently to Gunther Bl ö bel. It has been found that proteins carry internal leader signals in the form of sequences internal to them that are used as recognition sites while these proteins are recognised and taken inside a cell. Yet, how do we find them.

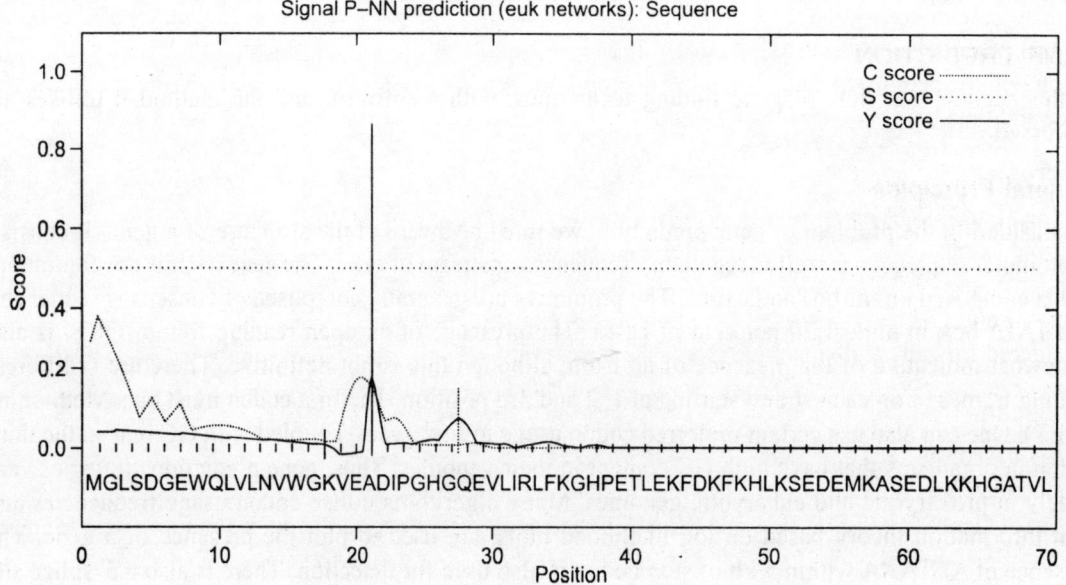

Fig. 5.21. Signal P results to find cleavage site.

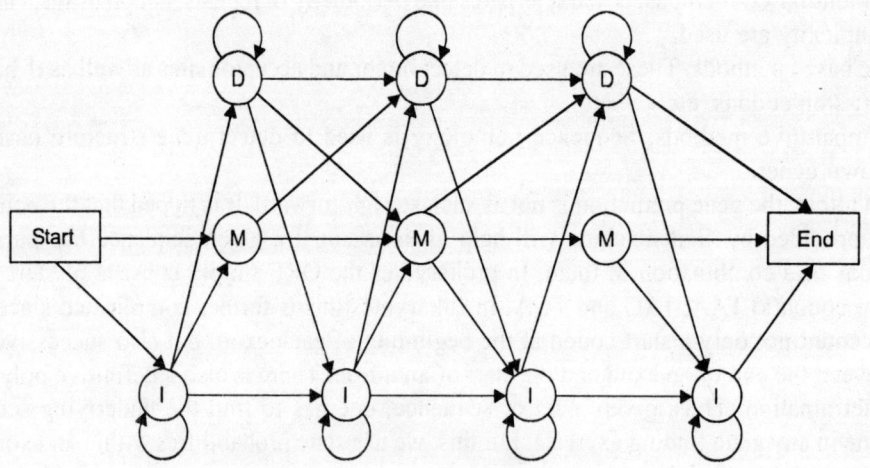

Fig. 5.22. Hidden Markov Model (HMM).

Searching for and locating these motifs is very similar to searching for and finding putative exons, although these leader sequences have a particular motif, positive-hydrophobic-polar, further at the −3, −1 site from the cleavage point, the amino acids are small and neutral. This is the basic theme. As we have covered HMMs, we will only talk about Neural Networks here before we move on to display the results from Signal P[44][45][46].

Grail

This is a free product of Oak Ridge National Laboratories in Tennesse, USA. It utilises methods like GC content calculation, splice junction recognition. It utilises neural network method and training sets to evaluate genes, exons and introns within a given set. The program Xgrail provides a windows environment for grail. Grail also uses log-odds ratio of the presence of say a particular nucleotide at first position of codon with respect to the 2nd, 3rd, etc. This log-odds score can be used to predict say the presence of a *6mer* and thus being indicative of a codon.

Procrustes

The ideas are based on similarity principles with a target protein. It can detect small exons as well as multiple exons based on spliced alignment algorithm. The input is a long genomic sequence, while a number of protein sequences should also be given for similarity searching. The search is started off from AG and GU di-nucleotides to search for internal exons. Further, AUG and UAA, UAG, UGA are considered for start and stop codons to ascertain the intermediate blocks of sequences respectively.

Genescan

This is based on a probabilistic fifth order Markov model. It assumes the presence of multiple genes, promoters genes, and partial-genes, in the given sequence. Dr. Burge of MIT has developed an improved variant of GeneScan, called Genome Scan that makes use of BlastX results in combination with Markov process.

Fgenes

This was developed by Victor Soloveyev and predicts internal exons by seeking acceptor/donor splice sites and finds matches in regions 5' and 3' to putative exon. Linear discriminant analysis is used along with dynamic programming (Viterbi type) to give not just one gene in a given sequence, but multiple genes in a particular stretch.

MZEF

It is based on quadratic discriminant analysis devised by Dr. Zhang's laboratory at cold spring harbour. variables like 3' and 5' splice sites, branch sites, intron-exon transitions to give information about internal coding exons.

Chapter 6

Genome Mapping

INTRODUCTION

In biology the genome of an organism is its whole hereditary information and is encoded in the DNA (or for some viruses, RNA). This includes both the genes and the noncoding sequences of the DNA. The term was coined by Hans Winkler, of Germany, as a portmanteau of the words gene and chromosome.

More precisely, the genome of an organism is a complete DNA sequence of one set of chromosomes; for example, one of the two sets that a diploid individual carries in every somatic cell. The term genome can be applied specifically to mean the complete set of nuclear DNA (i.e. the 'nuclear genome') but can also be applied to organelles that contain their own DNA, as with the mitochondrial genome or the chloroplast genome. When people say that the genome of a sexually reproducing species has been 'sequenced', typically they are referring to a determination of the sequences of one set of autosomes and one of each type of sex chromosome, which together represent both of the possible sexes. Even in species that exist in only one sex, what is described as 'a genome sequence' may be a composite from the chromosomes of various individuals. In general use, the phrase 'genetic makeup' is sometimes used conversationally to mean the genome of a particular individual or organism. The study of the global properties of genomes of related organisms is usually referred to as genomics, which distinguishes it from genetics which generally studies the properties of single genes or groups of genes. Both the number of base pairs and the number of genes vary widely from one species to another, and there is little connection between the two.

Most biological entities more complex than a virus sometimes or always carry additional genetic material besides that which resides in their chromosomes. In some contexts, such as sequencing the genome of a pathogenic microbe, 'genome' is meant to include this auxiliary material, which is carried in plasmids. In such circumstances then, 'genome' describes all of the genes and noncoding DNA that have the potential to be present. In vertebrates such as sheep and other various animals however, 'genome' carries the typical connotation of only chromosomal DNA. So although human mitochondria contain genes, these genes are not considered part of the genome. In fact, mitochondria are sometimes said to have their own genome, often referred to as the 'mitochondrial genome'.

Note that a genome does not capture the genetic diversity or the genetic polymorphism of a species. For example, the human genome sequence in principle could be determined from just half the DNA of one cell from one individual. To learn what variations in DNA underlie particular traits or diseases requires comparisons across individuals. This point explains the common usage of 'genome' (which parallels a common usage of 'gene') to refer not to any particular DNA sequence, but to a whole family of sequences that share a biological context. Although this concept may seem counter intuitive, it is the same concept that says there is no particular shape that is the shape of a cheetah. Cheetahs vary, and so do the sequences of their genomes. Yet both the individual animals and their sequences share commonalities, so one can learn something about cheetahs and 'cheetah-ness' from a single example of either.

COGNATE MODIFICATION ENZYMES

Each Type II R.enzyme has a cognate Modification Enzyme: DNA methylase. This enzyme recognises the same nucleotide sequence as does the R.enzyme and methylates specifically one of the bases in each strand in the nucleotide sequence.

Example: *EcoRI methylase* (GAA*TTC) methylates the inner A in both strands.

Function: This methylation renders this R.site resistant to cleavage by the R.enzyme.

Hence, a cell encoding a restriction enzyme also encodes the modification enzyme; the latter will methylate the cell chromosomal DNA, thereby preventing the R.enzyme from digesting the cellular DNA.

GEL ELECTROPHORESIS OF DNA FRAGMENTS

Digestion of a well-defined DNA molecule, e.g. viral DNA, with a R.enzyme yields a set of well-defined DNA Restriction Fragments (R.frags).

Example: EcoRI cleaves phage lambda DNA (linear dsDNA, 49 kb) at 5 sites, yielding 6 fragments. BamHI cleaves Adenoviral DNA at 12 sites, lambda DNA at 5 sites.

The sizes of these R.frags can be determined using Gel Electrophoresis and the fragments can often be isolated from each other.

Gel Electrophoresis

When 'loaded' as a 'band' at top of a gel matrix and subjected to an electric field, DNA migrates through the gel at rate inversely proportional to its size.

Rough exponential dependence of migration rate with size. Thus,

1. Can separate and purify individual R.frags from a gel.
2. Can analyse for presence and size of R.frags.

Use DNA Markers for size determination avoid variation between gel runs.

Methodology: Slab gels used: several DNA samples in adjacent 'lanes' analysed in same gel.

Agarose gels used for R.frags of size 500 bp or larger.

Polyacrylamide gels used for smaller fragments, e.g. sequencing gels.

'Pulsed gel' electrophoresis used for very large DNA, e.g. entire chromosomes.

Visualise the DNA

1. Using radio-activity: place X-ray film over gel, expose to decaying P^{32}.
2. Fluorescence: Ethidium Bromide (EtBr), a dye, which intercalates between bases; EtBr fluorescences is visible when irradiated with UV light.

PHYSICAL MAP OF GENOME

Restriction Map as a Physical Map

Given a large DNA molecule:

1. Digest it with R.enzyme, measure sizes via Agarose Gels. Repeat with additional R.enzymes.

2. But only get sizes; don't know which fragments are adjacent to each other.
3. Do double digests with the same enzymes as above, 2 at a time.
4. Purify singly digested R.frags and digest with the 2nd R.enzyme (can often avoid this or purify only a few of the first R.frags).
5. Get Ordering of both enzyme set of fragments.
6. Can also do PARTIAL DIGESTS with single R.enzyme. This is particularly useful for END LABELLED DNA assay P^{32} added at 5' ends of DNA with polynucleotide kinase.
7. Can also use hybridisation of a radio-active 'probe' ssDNA or oligonucleotide to one end or the other of the DNA in a Southern gel analysis of the partial digests.
8. Physical maps based on R.sites are now available for most 'model' organisms, e.g. Kohara map for *E. coli*, Sau3A mapping of *C. elegans* as well as ultimate nucleotide sequence for several bacteria, archae and yeast. Level of 'resolution' depends on 8 vs 6 vs 4 bp 'cutter' vs DNA sequence.

PHYSICAL MAPPING USING HYBRIDISATION

Properties of conversion of dsDNA into ssDNA and the reverse, can also be used for physical mapping and other purposes. These properties have to do with DNA Hybridisation.

DNA HYBRIDISATION—MELTING CURVES

Denaturation: Conversion of dsDNA to two Strands of ssDNA

1. When the H bonds break that join the 2 strands in dsDNA, they all tend to break simultaneously thus, the dsDNA 'melts' into two strands. This is like a phase transition similar to the melting of ice into water.
2. Agents which 'denature' DNA:
   (a) Increase the temperature past the 'melting' temperature: Tm.
   (b) (i) Increase the pH to above about 11.3; and (ii) decrease the ionic strength to below 10(–5): repulsion of negative charge.

Assay or Measurement of Denaturation/Renaturation: UV Light Absorption

1. The bases (mainly Pyrimidines) absorb UV light (260 nm) that impinges vertically on the base.
2. Free bases absorb more than ssDNA; ssDNA absorbs more than dsDNA due to this requirement of vertical impingement of the UV light: bases most exposed when free; least exposed when in dsDNA; only partially exposed in ssDNA due to 'stacking' of the bases (hydrophobic interactions).
3. Can measure this denaturation via change in UV absorption. This is an assay, or measurement method, for this process.
4. The Tm is the 'midpoint' in the melting reaction, Tm is proportional to %(G + C), due to 3 H-bonds between C and G but only 2 H-bonds between A and T.
5. The curve of Assay (here: UV absorption) vs Melting Agent (here: temperature) is called a melting Curve.

Renaturation

Joining of two DNA strands of complementary sequence to form dsDNA.
1. Reverse of denaturation: but requires that the two DNA strands have complementary sequence, i.e. permit A joining to T, C joining to G, along the entire length of both DNA strands or chains.

2. Renaturation is also called Hybridisation.
3. Can also occur between DNA and RNA, to form a DNA: RNA hybrid or between two RNA strands of complementary sequence.

DNA Labelling

DNA probes used in hybridisation experiments must be labelled in order to assay their association with a ssDNA substrate in a hybridisation experiment. DNA labels are most often either radioactive labels or fluorescent labels.

Radioactive labelling

Radioactive labels used are radio-active isotopes: H^3, C^{14}, P^{32} or P^{33} the most often used isotopes are H^3 and P^{32}.

Methods of radioactive labelling

1. H^3-labelled thymine or thymidine is often used to label DNA uniformly in appropriate thy-mutant organisms.
2. Deoxyribonucleocide triphosphates, the substrates used by DNA polymerase enzymes for DNA synthesis, can be obtained labelled with P^{32} in the alpha-phosphate position. These substrates can then be used with an appropriate DNA polymerase to label DNA, for example, in the *E. coli* PolI nick translation reaction.
3. Polynucleotide kinase can be used to label the 5'-end of dsDNA with P^{32} using ATP labelled with P^{32} in the gamma-position and a dsDNA substrate with no 5'-phosphates. This is often done for the Maxam-Gilbert chemical method for DNA sequencing, for partial digest restriction mapping, and for other purposes.

Fluorescent labelling

Primarily, radio-active labelling suffers from the obvious problem that people are exposed to radio-activity. This requires specific and special environmental safeguards. Such safeguards do not however solve the problem of long-term isotopes: isotopes that take thousands or millions of years to decay away, how does one dispose of these? This is an unsolved issue.

Radio-active labels are not simultaneously of high sensitivity and of high resolution are given below:

1. High sensitivity: High signal to noise ratio/decay from the label is high compared with cosmic rays and other background 'noise'.
2. High resolution: Ability to pinpoint precisely in the experiment the position of radio-active decay of the radioactive atom.
3. P^{32}: High sensitivity, low resolution, Beta decay, half-life = 14.2 days (half of the atoms have decayed in two weeks), maximum energy of the beta particle (high energy electron): ~1.3 Mev this is high energy; will pass through one or more cm of human tissue.
4. H^3: Low sensitivity, high resolution, Beta decay, half life ~1100 years, maximum energy of the beta: ~ 0.01 Mev low energy (low sensitivity), doesn't go far (high resolution).
   Other radio-isotopes are in between.

Fluorescent labels

Fluorescent labels are by comparison of high sensitivity and high resolution. These are used routinely in automated DNA sequencing reactions and now in DNA micro array experiments. One can purchase fluorescent labelling nucleotide triphosphates and substrates for oligonucleotide (probe) synthesis. Fluorescent labels of different wavelengths, green and red particularly, are available and can be used simultaneously in a given experiment, e.g. in DNA micro array experiments.

Fluorescence *In situ* Hybridisation—FISH

FISH is used to detect the position of a marker on a chromosome via fluorescence. The marker is a fluorescent-labelled ssDNA probe of complementary sequence to that of the position on the chromosome.

Methodology: Metaphase chromosomes (or other DNA substrate) is immobilised on a glass slide. The chromosomes or DNA are denatured, e.g. with formamide. The fluorescent-labelled probe is hybridised to the denatured DNA.

The DNA is visualised via microscopy or other method and the position of the hybridised fluorescent probe is visualised via its fluorescent signal: assay.

Example: Fly DNA probed with centromeric sequences.

Single R.frag identification: Southern hybridisation often use a short DNA oligonucleotide probe to partially purify R.fragments for further cloning, or to identify a given R.fragment, or other DNA fragment containing specific DNA sequences.

One can do this via a combined agarose gel electrophoresis with hybridisation against a radio-active probe that has a complementary DNA sequence to the desired specific DNA sequences.

Can also use hybridisation of a probe to a gene in order to:
1. Detect DNA spotted and denatured on filter paper: dot blots.
2. Disrupted Lambda phage from a Lambda cDNA library on plates.
3. Lysed cells on a plate with DNA transferred to a nitrocellulose membrane.

In situ hybridisation

Methodology
1. Run DNA fragments out on an Agarose Gel.
2. Float Agarose gel on an alkaline solution in a trough. Alkali denatures the DNA, yielding ssDNA fragments in the Agarose gel.
3. Place a nitrocellulose membrane on top of the Agarose Gel and then several layers of absorbent paper (towel paper often used) on top of the nitrocellulose membrane.
4. Let capillary action transfer DNA to the nitrocellulose membrane during transfer of fluid from the trough to the absorbent paper.
5. Dry nitrocellulose membrane and fix DNA to the nitrocellulose membrane: 80°C, under vacuum.
6. Hybridise the radio-active probe to the denatured ssDNA on nitrocellulose membrane-hybridisation conditions in small liquid volume in a 'Seal-a-Meal' sac often used.
7. Dry nitrocellulose membrane and expose radio-activity to film.
8. Develop and examine the film.

Such gels can be used analytically to provide final information such as:
1. Identify whether DNA in a lane contains the probe sequences.
2. See how many such bands are there.
3. Determine their size from position in the gel.

Southern gels can also be used preparatively to purify DNA fragments. Cut the band out of the gel and elute the DNA from the gel slice such partially purified fragments that can then be cloned.

VARIANTS OF SOUTHERN GELS

Northerns

Same as Southerns but with RNA, e.g. mRNA, run out on the Agarose gels.

Westerns

Proteins run out on a polyacrylamide gel polyacrylamide gel electrophoresis—PAGE; generally under protein denaturing conditions, e.g. use of detergent: SDS gels (assay presence of a given protein using an antibody to the protein).

Names here are 'take-offs' on Southern gels not named for scientist named Northern, etc.

Other variants also exist, e.g. South-Westerns run SDS protein gel; attempt to renature proteins in gel; transfer to nitrocellulose as in southerns; probe the proteins so transferred with radio-active oligonucleotide probes assay DNA binding proteins.

GENOME FRAGMENT IDENTIFICATION: DNA MICROARRAYS

One of the profound technological advancements that is a product of this third revolution in molecular biology is that of DNA microarray technology.

DNA microarrays are similar to southern gels in that labelled oligonucleotide probes are used to identify specific DNA sequences from among many, e.g. an entire genome. However:

1. Southerns (and northerns) are one gene at a time technology.
2. DNA microarrays permit simultaneous assay of all genes in a genome. DNA microarrays thus can be thought of as 'the southerns of genome-based molecular biology'.

Methodology: DNA Microarrays are 2D solid surfaces to which have been immobilised ssDNA molecules. They are used by hybridising labelled ssDNA molecules to the DNA on the microarray and assaying for the labelled ssDNA molecules, thereby determining the positions on the microarray where hybridisation occurred.

Current DNA microarray technology includes two rather distinct methodologies:

1. Immobilised single-stranded cDNA molecules: long, nonsynthetic substrates, at low density.
2. Immobilised short oligonucleotide ssDNA: short, synthetic substrates, at high density.

cDNA Microarrays: ssDNA from a cDNA library is used and immobilised to a 2D solid surface, usually either a glass side or a nylon membrane. Individual cDNA species are 'spotted' in a 2D-grid on the solid surface. The number of spots is relatively small, at most about 80 × 80 or 6400 spots.

These individual cDNA species might for example be obtained from separate Lambda Phage in a lambda cDNA library.

Experimentally, such arrays can be prepared at relatively low expense. They are then used to detect expression of cognate mRNAs (or via cDNAs from these cDNAs) by hybridising the cDNAs obtained from some given experimental condition to the cDNAs immobilised on the surface. Since each of the 6400 spots represents expression of a different gene, one can assay expression of 6400 genes simultaneously. Further, using different fluors to label the experimental cDNA, e.g. lissamine-labelled vs fluorescein-labelled, one can assay in the same experiment two different experimental conditions.

Example: cDNA microarray and stage-specific gene expression in the malaria parasite *Plasmodium falciparum*.

Second Example: cDNA microarray of 10 *Arabidopsis* and 1046 human cDNA species.

Oligonucleotide microarrays: To get really high densities of substrate ssDNA molecules on DNA microarrays, companies such as AffyMetrix build DNA microarrays using 'silicon valley' chip technology.

Oligonucleotides (short ssDNA molecules, e.g. 25 bp long) are synthesised on the chips. Synthesis technology is similar to that found in the organic chemistry technology associated with oligonucleotide Synthesisers such as purchased from ABI/Perkin-Elmer via their Gene Chips.

Masks are used such that synthesis occurs only with light radiation and light can only pass through regions in the mask where there are spaces this technology permits synthesis of a high density of oligonucleotides (80000 spots), each of a different sequence, on a chip much like a silicon chip.

cDNA species or mRNA species are then hybridised to such DNA chips or total DNA from an individual appropriately restriction digested, to determine SNP information about the individual.

Usually, several oligos are used per gene, e.g. 5 oligos per gene. Thus, if the gene is expressed, mRNA or corresponding cDNA, should hybridise to all 5 oligos. This provides controls: some oligos hybridise better than others one learns which oligos work best, for the next generation of oligo microarrays and at the same time some hybridisation should occur to all 5 oligos.

This technology then permits automated analysis of the type for which DNA microarrays provide information.

For example, one can automate analysis of individual human beings for their heterozygosity as determined by their single nucleotide polymorphisms (SNPs).

Given that specific SNPs as associated to some degree with a given genetic disease, one can in automated fashion determine the propensity of any given individual for a given genetic disease. The pharmaceutical companies would, will you believe, that given such knowledge, they can better design drugs and treatments for you, taking into consideration all of your genetic disease propensities. This includes when in your lifetime to start treating you for a disease you might get.

That is: individual, cradle to grave, prescriptive life care.

Example of Oligoarray to analyse single nucleotide polymorphisms (SNPs): for SNP microarrays, oligos corresponding to the two alleles are placed in two rows, one below the other.

GENOME FRAGMENT ISOLATION: CLONING AND HIGH RESOLUTION PHYSICAL MAPPING OF GENOMES

Outline:
1. Genome types of cloning experiments:
    (a) Gene isolation—reverse genetics.
    (b) Genome cloning—genome libraries.
    (c) Mapping from cloning: sequence tagged sites (STSs).
    (d) cDNA cloning—expressed sequence tags (ESTs).
    (e) Radiation hybrids.
    (f) Mapping from radiation hybrids: STSs.
2. Other types of cloning experiments:
    (a) Site specific mutagenesis.
    (b) Protein production—bacterial factories.

Genome Types of Cloning Experiments

Gene isolation—reverse genetics

Assays
1. Complementation of host mutant deficient in gene activity.
2. Probe with radio-active short DNA molecule of sequence from the gene.

Obtain short DNA sequence, e.g. from amino acid sequence of purified protein.

Thus go from protein to gene with no previously isolated mutations.

Reverse genetics

This is the reverse of standard genetics, in which mutants are isolated and characterised (gene -> protein). Often use such a short DNA oligonucleotide probe to partially purify R.fragments for further cloning.

Southern gels: Run R.fragments out on a gel transfer DNA from gel to nitrocellulose membrane. Hybridise the fragments in bands on the gel to the probe detect correct bands via radio-activity and film purify R.fragments from this region of the gel to use in cloning.

Characterise gene physically: Restriction map sequence.

Genomic cloning—genome libraries

Purpose

1. Obtain library of complete genome.
2. Usually use phage lambda.
3. Use of Isoschisomer R.enzymes: same sticky ends from cleavage.

Example: BamHI and Sau3A; Sau3A is a '4-cutter' and hence has many more sites in a genome than does Barn HI, which is a '6 cutter'. Partial restriction with Sau3A yields large fragments, whose ends are from sites at many locations on the genome thus get overlapping fragments—much less likely to get good overlapping fragment pattern with BamHI due to lack of sufficient restriction sites.

Mapping from cloning

Sequence tagged sites (STSs): Sequence tagged sites (STSs) are short DNA sequences (usually < 500 bp) determined from unique sequences in a given genome and then mapped to that genome.

These then provide methodology for high-resolution physical mapping of a genome.

Sources of DNA for STSs

Expressed sequence tags (ESTs): These are DNA sequences determined from expressed regions of the genome or genes.

If a given expressed gene is present uniquely on the genome, the sequences of the EST is a good STS sequence.

Genomic sequences

Any genomic sequence that is present uniquely on the genome can be used as an STS. Examples of such are DNA sequences previously determined and deposited in a DNA database such as GenBank.

Mapping of STS sequences

Once one has a set of DNA sequences to be used as STSs, they must be mapped to the genome. This can be done in many ways, including the following two general procedures: (i) cloning and use of a clone library, and (ii) radiation hybrids and use of a radiation hybrid panel.

The STS markers, DNA sequences of length 500 bp or less, are nearly always assayed using Polymerase chain reaction (PCR) amplification of the STS region. PCR is amenable to automation can be used and hence so-called 'high throughput (HTP)' methodology (highly automated, robotic methodology).

cDNA cloning—expressed sequence tags (ESTs)

Purify a messenger RNA of interest. 'Reverse transcribe' the RNA into DNA, get a 'complementary DNA strand':

cDNA

Degrade the mRNA and synthesise the second DNA strand. Clone the DNA so synthesised.

Often use lambda-cloning vehicles for cloning cDNA species can thereby maintain an entire cDNA library as lambda phage in liquid at high density: $> 10^{12}$ phage per ml.

cDNA library

Same thing but with all mRNAs from given tissue. This provides a library of all mRNA sequences expressed in this tissue. Such cDNA libraries can provide the DNA for sequencing to map sequence tagged sites (STSs) to a given genome or chromosome from a genome.

Radiation hybrids

Radiation hybrids provide a methodology for high-resolution mapping of DNA physical markers such as STSs on chromosomes of higher organisms such as human and mouse.

For human chromosomes, radiation hybrid panels are created by:

1. Irradiating human cells with X-rays, thereby fragmenting the chromosomes in these cells into fragments. The fragments are smaller when the X-ray dose is higher.
2. Creating a human-hamster fusion cell by fusing the irradiated human cells with mutant thymine requiring hamster cells. Fusion can occur between these cells when mediated with chemicals or Sendai virus.
3. Creating a hybrid cell line by growing the fused cells in HAT media, selecting for human chromosome fragments containing a thymine gene. Cells in this fused cell line contain the hamster chromosomes plus some human chromosome fragments (as much as about 35 per cent of the human genome).

The radiation hybrid panel consists of several such hybrid cell lines, all created in one fusion experiment. Typically, such a panel has 50–100 different cell lines.

Specific radiation panels, e.g. the G3 panel, have been used to construct a high resolution STS map of the human genome.

Mapping STSs from radiation hybrids

Radiation hybrids can be used similarly to clones in a clone library for high resolution mapping of STS markers. The principles for doing this are as follows:

1. Each hybrid cell line in a given radiation hybrid panel contains many fragments of human chromosomes.
2. STSs that are close together will tend to be present together in the same human chromosome fragment in a given hybrid cell line; those that are far apart or on different chromosomes will not tend to be found in the same hybrid cell lines.
3. This tendency is quantitated by recording what per cent of the time two markers are found in the same cell line. This is almost always the same as the two markers being present on the same human chromosome fragment.
4. Doing this yields the following type of data: data from human chromosome 21q: S16(8) S48(9) S46 (22) S4. With S16 (19) S46 and S48 (29) S4.

Thus, STS markers S16 and S48 appear on the same human chromosome fragment 92 per cent of the time, i.e. the distance between the markers is 8 units. Similarly, STS markers S16 and S46 appear on the same human chromosome fragment 81 per cent of the time, i.e. the distance between the markers is 19 units.

Note that the distance between S16 and S48, i.e. 8 units, plus the distance between S48 and S46, i.e. 9 units, is close to the distance between S16 and S46, i.e. 19 units.

Radiation hybrid and clone mapping of STS markers are widely used to provide high-resolution physical maps of chromosomes and genomes. These STS markers also provide a framework of mixed markers on the genome for complete genome sequencing.

Other Types of Cloning Experiments

Site specific mutagenesis

Introduce specific point mutations (single base changes) into CloneGene. Move back into chromosome via generalised recombination.

Protein production

Overexpress gene product, e.g. insulin, in bacteria.

GENOME MAPPING: GENETIC –> PHYSICAL

Genetic Maps vs Physical Maps

Comparison of genetic and physical maps

Genetic map is colinear with physical placement of genes on DNA but quantitation is difficult due to variations of recombination processes between organisms (more rare in eukaryotes than in prokaryotes) and due to dependence on DNA sequence (hot spots for recombination).

Physical map of genome: Placement of genes and sites on nucleotide sequence of DNA, i.e. on the physically real genetic material.

The ultimate physical map is the nucleotide sequence. Note: to serve as a marker in either a genetic map (genes, map via recombination frequency) or a physical map (sites on DNA, map via locating the site on the DNA), a gene or site must occur in more than one state. Such states are called Alleles.

In classical genetics, the results or manifestations of one state or another, i.e. one Allele or another, of a given gene are called the phenotype associated with a given Allele. Such might be eye colour or pea shape. The differences in the gene itself associated with a given Allele are called the genotype. In modern genetics, the genotype is a change in the DNA sequence encoding the given gene.

The classical phenotype such as the examples just given arise from changes in the amino acid sequence of the protein expressed by the given gene, resulting in change in activity of the protein (perhaps no activity for one allele of the gene), resulting in change in a metabolic pathway, resulting in change in eye colour or pea shape.

In modern genetics, the phenotype can also be defined at the DNA level. The phenotype is any measure of the results of one allele or another. Thus, the phenotype can also be the change in the DNA sequence associated with the change from one allele of a gene to another, because with appropriate sequencing one can determine this change in DNA sequence.

This ability to define the classical genetic concept of genotype in terms of specific molecular changes in the genetic material or DNA molecules, coupled with ability to measure these specific molecular changes via DNA sequencing, bring the concepts of genotype and phenotype into close proximity to each other.

DNA Markers for Genetic Mapping—Polymorphisms

Genetic marker: mutant vs 'wild type', compare 2 phenotypes alleles based on mutation eliminating (or creating) a R.site.

Polymorphisms: individuals in a population have different alleles or variants of a given gene marker. What is an Allele? Some change in a gene or site that can be assayed, that is phenotype.

In principle, any DNA base change is now an allele, can 'assay' any such change via DNA sequencing.

Uses

1. Markers for genetic mapping: pedigree analysis.
2. Markers for physical mapping: restriction mapping.
3. Genetic disease: compare diseased vs nondiseased individuals.
4. Forensic purposes: compare DNA from blood from victim and suspect, compare with blood at 'scene of the crime'.
5. Identification purposes: compare DNA from blood at some site with DNA stock.
   → military, accidents, etc.
6. Parentage identification 'who's the father?' Dogs, horses, other animals.

Restriction Fragment Length Polymorphisms (RFLPs)

R.sites as DNA markers can serve as genome sites for genetic mapping.

Change in a R.site: assay via cleavage or not by R.enzyme bands on gels. A change in a Restriction Site: one allele the R.site can be cleaved another allele the R.site cannot be cleaved. These two alleles yield two different sizes for R.fragments i.e. changes in the restriction fragment length. Thus: restriction fragment length polymorphisms.

Simple Sequence Length Polymorphisms (SSLPs)

These arise from repeated sequences present in DNA genomes of higher organisms.

Repeated sequences are of two general types:

1. MiniSatellites or variable number of tandem repeats (VNTRs): These are regions of DNA containing tandem repeats where the repeats are in the size range 25 bp to a few hundred base pairs in length.
2. MicroSatellite or simple tandem repeats (STRs): These are also tandem repeat regions of DNA, but where the repeat sizes are smaller, generally 2 to 7 bp in length.

Polymorphisms arise in population of the organism either by variations in:

1. The precise sequence found in each repeat.
2. In the number of repeats found in a region of the repeat.

The latter type of polymorphism is currently used more often than the former. Each such naturally occurring polymorphism in a population of the organism is an Allele for the site on the DNA at which the repeat region occurs. Such a polymorphism arising from variations in the number of repeats results in a change in the length of the repeated region, and is called an SSLP.

Measurement of SSLPs—Allelic phenotypes: determine the length of the SSLP in a given DNA sample via its size using gel electrophoresis.

Single Nucleotide Polymorphisms (SNPs)

These are polymorphisms or alleles occurring naturally in a population resulting from point mutations or changes in single nucleotides in the DNA in individuals in the population. They usually are changes within a gene, resulting in a change in an amino acid of the encoded protein, resulting in a change in a pathway, yielding a phenotype such as a genetic disease in human.

Note: That SNPs that occur in a R.site, resulting in Alleles that can be cut or not by the R.enzyme, also result in RFLPs.

## Chapter 7

Gene Identification

INTRODUCTION

Gene identification and functional classification start with the determination of coding sequence. Basically, an open reading frame (ORF) is determined from start codon to a stop codon. This is relatively easy for prokaryotic genomes, where the gene density is high and introns are absent. Usually, ORFs longer than a certain Threshold (300 + 500) are considered a potential genes. Genes that is longer than the threshold and genes on the opposite strand of longer ORF (shadow genes often lead to ambiguities), but can be resolved by analysing the computational differences between coding regions, shadow genes and noncoding DNA. Predictions of coding sequences in eukaryotes is more difficult. The available gene finding programs generate prediction on the basis of transcriptional signals (transcription starts sites, TATA boxes, polyadenylation sites, etc.).

Translational signals (transcription initiation and termination sites) and splicing signals (donar and acceptor splice site positions). Among these programs are GENMARK GRAIL and GENEPARSER. These programs are continuously improved and more advanced programs like GENESCAN take into account reading frame compatibility of adjacent exons and compositional properties of introns and exons. Further increase in sensitivity can be obtained by including different sequences similarity functions for comparison to gene and protein sequences in available databases.

As a complement to the gene identification programs, comparison of complete genomic sequence (20 ± 100) kb of homologous loci between closely related organisms (mouse and human) can reveal most exons and regulatory regions by identifying the regions of particularly high conservation. EST sequences represents spliced genes and are therefore valuable tools for determination of coding sequences in the genomic DNA. Comparison between ESTs and genomic sequences immediately reveals the splice sites. However, among the drawbacks are that inconsistencies might occur due to low quality sequence, alternative splicing presence of pre-mRNA sequences and that the ESTs represents only partial transcript sequences, even after gene indexing by assembly. Gene annotation techniques based on EST and gene prediction algorithm complement each other in the sense that ESTs are often effective in identifying 3-Prime ends of genes where the gene finders often falls, while gene finders relatively well determine the 5-Prime ends which the oligo (dT) primed cDNA clones often fail to reach. This confirms the fact that full understanding of a genome will only be reached by a combination of genomic and cDNA sequencing.

When is a predicted gene a gene? How many encoded in the human genome? This is a simple question without as yet a straightforward answer. The density of genes in human genome is much lower than for any other genome sequenced so far, making it particularly difficult to predict where genes are. Both Celera and the public sequencing consortium used computational algorithms to model genes and make predictions, but such methods are far from perfect. Not only can the start and positions of a predicted gene be wrong but exons (the coding parts of a gene) can be missed entirely or wrongly predicted to exist. To reduce this later effect, the public sequencing consortium required the exons of predicted genes to be confirmed, by showing sufficient similarity to a known sequence (DNA or protein) in a database. But this requirement might be too conservative, making it difficult to predict the presence of new gene families. Celera has required similar confirmation of predictions, but its Mouse; Genome sequencing project may have provided evidence for further vertebrate specific genes. Spurious prediction is also a problem. All genes are expressed by being copied (transcribed) into messenger RNA; most messenger RNA are then translated into proteins. But even evidence that a stretch of DNA is transcribed does not definitely show that stretch to be a gene. We do not know how well the cell identifies transcripts that cannot be translated into a functioning protein. Moreover, proteins that cannot serve any useful function (for example because they cannot fold correctly) could be made, but rapidly removed. To arrive at a true set of protein encoding genes, we cannot rely on computational techniques alone, but must continue to characterise proteins and their functions. These problems provide scope for estimates of human gene to vary widely. Although recent estimates are converging in the 30,000–40,000 range (as opposed to earlier estimates of 1,00,000 or so), it could be in years before we have the final answer.

SEQUENCE FEATURE EXTRACTION/ANNOTATION

Because of high throughout sequencing technologies and automated sequencers now biologists are generating huge amount of sequences. The increasing number of availability of this raw sequence constitutes a complex problem for biologist. Without Transcript sequences a genomic sequence cannot be directly used and whereas the genes is the first of a long list of questions. Furthermore, the public data release policies force the sequencing centres to deposit as quickly as possible the raw sequences in the databases. To meet the scientific communities expectations together with the massive sequence production the first step is to extract rapidly a maximum of biological information from the sequences to establish a basis for further functional studies. This information has then to be associated with the sequences in order to label the genes, allowing biologist to find sequences of interest. This is the goal of genome annotation.

GENE ANNOTATION

Annotation is extraction of useful information from raw sequence. Identification of coding regions and genes in a genome and determination of what they do, a combination of comments, notations, references and citations, either in free format or utilising a controlled vocabulary that together describe all the experimental and inferred information about a gene or a protein.

Classically scientists carry out annotations of sequences by using information linked to experiments. Indeed, in contrast to sequences obtained through individual gene cloning experiments, in turn we should also be able to update annotations and to apply to genes the results of experimental analysis performed later on. This notion of integration is essential from a genomics point of view. Bench work cannot follow the release pace of thousands of new potential genes and experimentally documented genes represent a minor fraction of genes. In order to compensate for this transitional lack of secure data, prediction tools are extensively used to analyse the sequences and extract putative information. By merging statistics, computer science and biological sciences bioinformatics have developed many prediction tools. The analysis of the anonymous sequences combining different prediction programs and the results obtained by bioanalysts are the starting points of the annotation process. For this reason, the annotation work is mostly a predictive work and the result has to be considered as such.

Whole genome annotation should not be taken as definitive and proven, but rather as indication to help biologist in the sequence jungle and to derive future experimental approaches. This point is often forgotten when annotations are used. When in front of a large genomic sequence, the first problem is to localise all the genes on both the strands and more precisely, the different structural elements of these genes. This step is called the structural annotation, to clearly distinguish it from the following one, the Functional annotation, which tries to find signs of function from the deduced protein sequences, as described below, deep and detailed annotation implies numerous complementary analysis and checking. Unfortunately, because of the cost in time and money of this human expertise, genome annotation is generally restricted to the prediction of coding exons to deduce the protein sequence of potential genes and to label it with the functions of the closest homologue. We will compare and discuss the fast high throughout annotation used in the systemic sequencing programs and the possibilities of a deeper but slower annotation with two objectives to highlight the dangerous traps when automatic annotations are blindly used and to present a few novel approaches and applications in genome annotation.

Structural Annotation

The very first information needed when analysing an unknown genomic DNA sequence is where the protein coding regions are located in this sequence. Where are the regulatory sequences? This is very important in genome sequencing projects where a lot of sequences are generated automatically but where only the protein coding sequence may be an interesting to the majority of researchers. Gene structure prediction is not an easy task in prokaryotes and is an even more difficult task in higher organisms, where genes are split into exons and introns, which can be difficult to detect. Modern gene detection software makes use of very involved artificial intelligence methods and still far from being completely accurate, even for prokaryotic genes. DNA sequence, which does not code for protein may still be important in the regulation of genes. They may contain recognition sequences for transcription factor. Identifying these patterns may provide a clue to the function of the sequence.

The prediction of the gene elements is a complex problem and its issue is primordial because of its consequences on all the following analysis. Eukaryotic genes with their mosaic structure are more difficult to find than prokaryotic ones, which are simple open reading frames. The presence of introns complicates the problem, although the binding sites of the spliceosomes may be used to predict the exact position of the exon borders. According to the prediction tools, the results of the prediction concern the splice sites, the exons or the whole gene (gene modelling software). These prediction programs are based on two different approaches. The first version is called intrinsic based on the features of the genes and the genomes. Therefore, significant and representative sets of only experimentally characterised genes are necessary to develop such efficient prediction programs. Furthermore, the origin of the training set has to be species specific because each genome has its own features and style. The second approach to find genes and exons, named extrinsic, uses the similarities detected in homologous genes (in general at the protein level to increase the sensibility of the search) or even better, identities with cognate transcript sequences. Only in this ideal last situation is the resulting gene structure asserted and not merely putative. The performance (sensitivity and specificity) of the annotation softwares differing a lot and consequently, the final prediction are not identically reliable. The structural annotation is generally semiautomatic because human intervention is necessary to integrate the results of the different predictions, in the final gene structure. Although a fully integrated annotation platform is still lacking, some annotation centres use an interactive method to visualise the output of the prediction tools and sequence similarity searches to help in this critical decision step.

Functional Annotation

At the present time, the functional genome annotation is based on the idea that some sequence similarities detected between two proteins means that they are homologous, i.e. that they come from the same ancestor and share the same biochemical function. Therefore, for each predicted gene, the protein is deduced from the coding region and is compared through BLASTP with the protein databases. If the similarities detected are considered relevant, the name (function of the putative homolog protein is associated with the prediction). This minimum approach allows, in the best cases, the biochemical function of the gene product to be suggested. The high-throughout annotation realised by the annotation centres is too basic and quick to extract reliable information on the biological function. Some annotators confirm and complete the BLAST results by full-length alignment between the query protein and the closet homolog detected and by looking for motifs and family signatures. This approach appears to be the best to attribute one or several biochemical functions to a predicted protein. The name attributed to the predicted genes/proteins depends on the results of the homologous sequence research. Four categories of genes have been defined, but the associated nomenclature is not very homogenous. The tendency is nevertheless the following when a predicted gene product is 100 per cent identical to an already characterised protein; it receives the same name, whereas sequences with stringent similarity to known proteins are called putative proteins of the same name. The sequences for which only similarities to ESTs are detected are named unknown proteins. Finally, genes without similar sequences and hence only deduced from intrinsic prediction programs are labeled hypothetical.

Limits

The annotation of a genomic sequence is never perfect and always inevitably incomplete. Classical errors and limits inherent to the annotation will be discussed here. The multinational and fragmented organisation of genome annotation allows the scientists to follow the daily huge sequence production, but sets the problem of the heterogeneous character of the results. All annotated genes do not have the same reliability. The validity level of each prediction is rarely specified in the feature section of the sequences, making it necessary to consult the annotation centres Web site. The ideal case is when the different prediction software are in agreement with each other and with the detected conserved regions. In this too rare situation, the final prediction is very reliable. More frequently, the similarities found are too low and small to influence a choice between different predictions and the validity of the annotation is extremely difficult to estimate. The rebuilt gene has little chance of being true. As shown by the graphical interfaces of the Web sites, the data at the origin of annotations can be very different in terms of quality and quantity and the resulting genes have to be considered with caution. Classical errors in the structural annotation, as a result of prediction failure, are gene splitting (two genes are predicted instead of one) and gene merging (the opposite situation). Even with exon prediction tools becoming more and more efficient, it is still difficult to predict whether the exons are internal or external.

Indeed the gene extremities are not easily predicted for many reasons. The nucleotide content of the introns and intergenic regions is very similar and at least in Arabidobsis, very long introns (up to 4 kb) and very short or even rarely no intergenic regions (overlapping genes) can be found. Consequently, gene-modelling programs have difficulties in making the distinction. Furthermore, very few experimental data on plant promoter sequences and translation initiation sites are available to help the 5' prediction. In the 3' extremity, the canonical polyadenylation may occur and hence cannot be used to predict final exons. As in the case for mammals and yeasts, sometimes only the detection of similarities with only one or two different proteins allows the discrimination between one or two genes. For this reason gene merging is more frequent in genomic regions that contains gene clusters. Prediction softwares evolve very rapidly but it may take sometime to recognise which is the most efficient. For example, gene mark has been evaluated as the best genome-modelling program for Arabidobsis but surprisingly not used by the AGI Annotation centres. To give an idea of the prediction efficiency, this program can find 80 per cent of the actual exons although the modelling of perfect genes is only approximately 40 per cent. An obvious but important limit is that prediction are based on previously known data and consequently the rare and novel gene features splice sites, overlapping genes, a typical translation start, alternative splicing, etc. cannot be found in the annotation. The systemic sequencing of full-length cDNA will probably be the unique long-term solution for structural annotation. In functional annotations, the major problem occurs when an erroneous function is attributed to a predicted gene and spread by recurring references in numerous other annotations. The automatic interpretation of a BLAST result is very dangerous because it increases the background noise of high scoring but biologically irrelevant matches.

In several cases, the similarities detected by local alignments have to be more deeply analysed to avoid giving importance to a no significant match. The additional use of full-length alignments between the predicted protein and the best hits detected by BLAST reduce the error rate but is not systematically done. Because the databases TrEMBl and GenPep are used to find similarities with each novel predicted protein, a false function can be used as a reference and so be propagated afterwards. This kind of problem is very frequent in the case of MultiDomain Protein, to which wrong functions attributed by crossed references are spread even when the similarities detected by BLAST are significant. By a snowball effect, annotations and databases that exploit them (for instance PFam and PRODOM) are really polluted.

Transitively assigning function to a series of closely related sequences appears to be a risky issue. To estimate the consequences of these different difficulties, the automatic annotation of a 400-kb region from arabidiopsis chromosome 4 has been compared to a manual annotation carried out by an expert in sequence analysis. The two annotation methods are in totally in agreement (at structural and functional levels) for only 23 genes out of 106. At present time, the fully automatic annotation methods are not satisfactory and the integrated annotation platforms managed by bioanalyst and regularly actualised seems to be the solution. The nomenclature of genes, proteins and their function is also a source of ambiguities. There is a clear lack of controlled vocabulary both in the literature and the databases. This problem linked to the sequence redundancy in the databases, which can contain several times the same genes under different names. The resulting loss in time for the search and the annotation is very serious. Furthermore the multi origin of the annotation amplifies the diversity of the nomenclature. For example, the AMERICAN Annotators named as putative or like a function deduced from similarities, whereas the Japanese centre and MIPS use potential and similar respectively. For the latter putative applies to unknown proteins tagged by EST the annotations of bacterial genome suffer from the same kind of problems.

The ephemeral feature of some annotations, especially the number of ESTs matches and the closet homolog has to keep in mind when they are used and imposes a regular update. The last important general problem is the lack of accuracy in the annotation sources. It is not always easy to know where the reality ends and where the prediction begins. Predicted and actual genes are considered identical for statistical analysis or definition of motifs and signature of families. The heterogeneity of the annotations can introduce a significant bias in such studies. Once more the consultation of the annotator/web sites is necessary, but is not optimised for automatic works. Biologists have to consider all these weaknesses to optimise their searches and to be capable of exploiting fruitfully genome annotations.

ANALYSIS OF GENE FUNCTIONS AND METABOLIC PATHWAYS FROM DATABASES

The availability of the complete genomes allows many new types of experiments and analysis. The new approaches and question that the genomes make possible are usually referred to as functional genomics. The task is to define the function of a gene (or its protein) in the life processes of the organism, where function refers to the role it plays in a larger context. But what are these life processes? The most obvious example is the metabolism of an organism, the basic chemical system that generates essential components such as amino acids, sugars and lipids and the energy requires to synthesise them and to use them in creating proteins and cellular structures. This system of connected chemical reactions is a metabolic network.

An important emerging field in bioinformatics is to understand metabolic and signalling networks in term of their function in the organism and in relation to the data we already have. This requires combining information from a large number of sources: classical biochemistry, genomics, functional genomics (e.g. micro array experiments), network analysis, life process descriptions, functional genomics and simulations. A theory of the cell must combine the description of the structures in it (genome, proteome, subcelullar structures, etc.) with a theoretical and computational description of the dynamic of the life process. One of the most important future challenges to the bioinformatics is to how to make all this information comprehensible in biological terms. This necessitate in order to facilitates the use of the information for predictive purposes. We want to do more than just describe what is going on in an organism; we also wish to be able to say what will happen in given some specific set of circumstances. This kind of predictive power will only be reached if the complexity of biological processes can be handled.

COMPUTER ASSISTED ANALYSIS OF TRANSCRIPTION CONTROL REGIONS

Identification of all of the genes in the genome is a major objective of the genome projects. Recently as the genome project has entered the phase of large scale sequencing, computational approaches to gene finding have begun to draw significant attention from the molecular biology and genomics community. In addition, significant advances in gene finding methodology have taken place in the past two years and the current methods are significantly more accurate, reliable and useful than those available in the past. Gene discovery in prokaryotic genomes is a quite different problem from that encountered in eukaryotic sequences, owing to the higher gene density typical of prokaryotes and the absence of introns in their protein coding gene.

These properties generally imply that most open reading frames (ORFs) encountered in a prokaryotic sequence that are longer than some reasonable threshold, such as 300 and 500 base pairs will likely corresponds to genes. The primary difficulty arising from this simple approach are that very small genes will be missed and that the occurrence of overlapping long ORFs on opposite DNA strands (genes and shadow genes) often leads to ambiguities. To resolve these problems several methods have been devised that use different types of Markov Models in order to capture the compositional differences among the coding regions, shadow coding regions (coding on the opposite DNA strand) and noncoding DNA. Some degree of caution must be exercised in using such statistically-based methods in view of the relatively high frequency of genetic transformation, the occurrence of lateral gene transfer in many bacteria and other factors that lead to heterogeneity in gene composition.

TRANSLATIONAL SIGNALS

The principal translational signals that have been used in gene finding are the Kozak signal [(GCC) GCCGCCATGG)], proposed by Kozak located immediately upstream of the initial ATG and the termination codon, used primarily for its absence (in frame) in coding exons. Since these signals contain far too little information to allow discrimination in bulk genomic DNA, reliable prediction of translation start and stop sites may not be possible until more progress has been made towards predicting the sites of transcription initiation and termination, which would dramatically reduce the amount of sequence that needs to be searched. Using simple weight matrix description of the Kozak and translational termination signals in the context of the integrated gene finding program GENSCAN, about two-third (66 per cent) of translation initiation sites and about three quarter (78 per cent) of termination codons have been correctly predicted, with specificities of 84 and 91 per cent respectively. Although these levels of accuracy are high enough to be useful they are significantly lower than those achieved for splicing signals and leads to poorer prediction of initial and terminal exons that has been achieved for internal exons.

SPLICING SIGNALS

Even if one could reliably predict promoter and polyadenylation signals and translation start and stop sites in genomic sequences, this knowledge would generally help only in predicting the location of the first and last exons of a gene. Since most vertebrates, invertebrates and plant genes contains several exons, accurate prediction of gene structure in these organisms is much more dependent upon the ability of predictions to pinpoint splice signals. Nuclear Pre-mRNA introns are excised from the primary transcript by a large ribonucleoprotein complex known as the spliceosome, which recognises sites at the 5' and 3' ends of the intron (the donar and acceptor splice sites respectively), as well as an internal site known as the branch point. With a few interesting exceptions, virtually all spliceosomal introns begins with GT and end with AG and this nearly invariant rule is used by the majority of gene finding programs to narrow the search space of possible exon and intron boundaries. Many early gene-finding methods used simple weigh matrix independent models of the position specific compositional biases present in the 5' and 3' splice sites and of the bias towards pyrimidine nucleotides upstream of 3' splice sites. More recently several scientists have observed statistically significant dependencies between positions within both the donar and acceptor splice sites. Certain observed dependencies between donor splice sites positions can be interpreted in terms of the thermodynamics of RNA duplex formation between U1 small nuclear RNA (snRNA) and the 5' splice site region of the pre-mRNA. Of the dependencies observed for human acceptor splice sites, some appears to result simply from the compositional heterogeneity of the human genome, whereas others probably relate to the specificity of pyrimidine track binding proteins.

The development of more complex splice signal models that are capable of capturing such dependencies has been a significant recent trend in the gene finding literature: example includes the Maximal dependence decomposition (MDD) and windowed weight array (WWAM) models, Hidden Markov Models, decision tree methods and multilayered neural networks. These more complex models typically yield significant but not dramatic improvements in splice site discrimination over the simpler models, which assume independence between positions. The final level of accuracy achieved depends critically on whether prediction is measured in isolation or in the context of an integrated gene finding methods.

COMPARATIVE SEQUENCE ANALYSIS

DNA is a very dynamic molecule that undergoes a wide variety of alterations and modifications and gene duplications occur naturally and frequently. With two copies of a gene available in a genome, one copy could provide the necessary original function while the other could accumulate mutations that may alter its function, if this altered copy evolved eventually to serve a new function, it would be retained in the genome and passed on to later generations. It is plausible that most modern genes originated from one or a few ancestral genes, but this is difficult to prove or disprove because the amount of change that would have occurred since then will have obscured any similarities among their modern descendants. Many genes and proteins of an organism are homologous are obviously the products of gene duplication. The genes of such homologous proteins in a genome are said to comprise a gene family. As the number of known protein and gene sequences increases, more and more gene families have been found.

The most studied one family and the most striking for the similarities among its polypeptide chains, is that of globins of higher organisms; this family includes single, chain myoglobin and the various polypeptides of tetrameric haemoglobins. The globins have related functions in that they store oxygen; myoglobin store oxygen in muscle and haemoglobin in erythrocytes, while transporting it. The various polypeptides chains of haemoglobin function at various stages of life and they associate to form comparable tetrameric molecules.

EUKARYOTIC GENE PREDICTION

The aim of this practical is to get hands-on experience running some Web Servers for eukaryotic gene prediction on an 'unknown' sequence. We will use coding prediction programs together with promoter, splice and poly-A site prediction programs. All the information gathered has to be combined to find the coding regions of the gene. There is no time to go into the theory behind the prediction methods.

As anyone who has looked at automatically annotated genome sequence data will know, automatic gene prediction in higher eukaryotes does not work very well. Perhaps this is not surprising, considering that differential and tissue-specific splicing, genes within genes, TATA-less promoters, the rare class of U12-dependent (AT-AC) splice sites, the need for species-specific parametres, all complicate the problem.

In practice, the bench biologist is best advised to inform themselves of the species-specific signals (e.g. mammals tend to have a looser splice site consensus than the worm) that they should expect and then run several servers and synthesise the results, looking (in part) for consistency between different servers. As there is a lot of activity in gene prediction (even though much of it is 'reinventing the wheel') we may hope for better predictions and better presentation in the future.

Step 1: WWW Servers Used in the Gene Prediction Practical

We will use:

1. NetGene2 and HMMgene to predict coding exons and splice sites in eukaryotes.
2. The LBL Promoter prediction service and TSSG, TSSW from the sanger centre.
3. The POLYAH server for the prediction of the poly-A site.
4. GeneWise (from the Wise2 package) for aligning protein vs. spliced DNA sequence.

Note: You now have the sequence available in a form that can be cut and pasted into the query forms we are going to use. Or else get the sequence from the NCBI.

1. Net gene

2. HMM gene
3. LBL promoter   For all these just type 'gene prediction programs'
4. TSSG   in google search option window.
5. TSSW
6. POLYAH
7. GeneWise

Step 2: Looking for a Promoter Candidate

Promoter prediction is heavily dependent on finding good matches to the TATAAA motif. CCAT-Box, CpG islands and other transcription factor binding sites may provide further clues. But if you run MatInspector with the TRANSFAC DB on our query, you will be astonished at the profusion of candidate sites throughout the sequence—so we won't bother. We will run two promoter prediction programs and tentatively assume that the best intersecting promoter is the correct one.

1. Load the LBL Promoter query submission page.
2. It is worth familiarising yourself with the layout and note the on-line help.
3. Cut and paste the query sequence into the sequence box and submit the job.
4. When the result arrives look at the set of predicted promoters:
   (a) Can you see matches to the TATA box consensus tATA$^A/_T$A$^A/_T$.
   (b) Which promoter has the silliest TATA-box?
5. Open a new navigator window and load this page into it.
6. Load the TSSG query submission page.
7. Toggle on the TSSG button.
8. Don't use the sequence paste box (it can't strip out numbers from the sequence).
9. Type (or paste)/home/seqanal/public_html/courses/spring99/seq.fasta in the load box and then perform search.
10. When the result arrives look at the set of predicted promoters:
    (a) How many TATA boxes were found?
    (b) Are the listed transcription factors binding sites informative?
    (c) How well do the two searches agree on candidate promoters?
    (d) How many candidates do they both find?
    (e) Is there a single best candidate from combining the searches?

Note: These outputs are rather terse to say the least. Doing this for real, you should look at the web site helps to get some idea of what is being done and be willing to go to the literature if need be.

Step 3: Poly (A) Site Prediction

In mammalian genes, polyadenylation sites are usually preceded by AATAAA or ATTAAA ~20 bases before the cleavage site and followed by a more weakly conserved GT-based motif. While these motifs are trivial to find, they only function in the right context which is harder to define and includes regulation by upstream splicing factors. An important rule to remember is that there must not be an in-frame stop codon in an internal exon, i.e. the true translation termination will be in the last exon. (Violations to this rule suppress mRNA production, to the cost of many experimentalists and is occasionally used for differential mRNA regulation, e.g. for certain Ig splice variants.)

1. As needed, open a new navigator window and load this page into it.
2. Load the POLYAH query submission page.

3. Toggle on the POLYAH button.
4. Look at the POLYAH help and note the quoted prediction accuracy.
5. Don't use the sequence paste box (It can't strip out numbers from the sequence).
6. Type (or paste)/home/seqanal/public_html/courses/spring99/seq.fasta in the load box and then perform search.
7. When the result arrives, look at the predicted poly(A) sites:
   (a) How many candidate sites were found?
   (b) If one or more of these sites are false is the prediction accuracy as good as claimed?
   (c) How many over prediction of poly(A) sites be avoided?

We can't assess the context of these sites properly until we have the coding/splicing predictions to hand.

Note: If in case you do not get the result by typing the above mention sequence file, then paste the sequence in sequence paste box.

Step 4: Predicting Splice Sites and Coding Exons

There are a number of servers that separately predict splice sites and coding sequence bias but this information needs to be analysed together. We found that the CBS site in Denmark could provide all the information, though from two different servers. The NetGene2 server provides graphical postscripts output that we could print out and mark our predictions on. From the same group, the HMMgene server (using different algorithms) provides list output including potential Start and Stop codons. Both servers over predict splice site candidates. In case you need reminding, classical splice sites look something like:

Donor Consensus: $^c/_aAG \wedge GT^A/_gAGt$

Acceptor Consensus: $(T>C)_nN(C>T)AG \wedge gt$

1. As needed, open a new navigator window and load this page into it.
2. Load the NetGene2 query submission page.
3. Paste in the sequence and submit the job, which takes a few minutes to run.
4. The output provides a list of candidate splice sites (on both strands) and a graphical coding/ splicing prediction.
5. However it is not clear which translation frame is supposed to be coding.
6. It is worth printing this figure out and using it to summarise our prediction attempts!
7. Click on Direct strand and save the compressed postscript output (has a .Z suffix).
8. Open a UNIX X-window (terminal from the desktop).
9. Uncompress the file by typing UNIX command.
   Gunzip filename.ps.Z.
10. Print the file to the printer outside by typing:
    1pr-Plw-v 1 1 1 filename.ps
11. Now load the HMMgene query submission page.
12. Paste/home/seqanal/public_html/courses/spring99/seq.fasta in the local file box.
13. Select 5 best predictions and toggle on predict signals.
14. Submit the job.
15. Click on the Explanation link to understand the output format.
16. We can now begin to assemble a complete gene prediction.

Step 5: Combining the Server Outputs into an Overall Prediction

We now have predictions for all the components needed to assemble the gene, rather inconveniently spread over many separate web outputs. We have to manually assemble all this into one prediction. This can be done on the Netgene2 and DNA sequence outputs using biro and fluorescent marker. The following guidelines may help:

1. Start from a strong point such as.
2. A well-predicted internal coding exon with good splice borders.
3. Work forwards and backwards toward the promoter and poly(A) boundary signals.
4. Reported splice site quality is not a completely robust guide to usage:
   (a) Context dependence is also important.
   (b) Splice sites tend to be over predicted.
   (c) Some (true) splice sites might be better predicted by the HMMgene algorithm than by NetGene2.
5. The terminal exon should be partially coding, including the stop codon and the poly(A) signature.
6. The initiation codon should obey the Kozak rules:
   (a) It is normally the first methionine from the 5' end of the mRNA.
   (b) At least one of the underlined residues should be present in the consensus APuXXAUGG.
7. Once the prediction is completed, we can check it in the next exercise.
8. Good luck!

Step 6: Gene Prediction by Homology Using Genewise

Usually nowadays, related sequences are already present in the databases. When available these may be the fastest way to get a good gene prediction. Often this prediction will be more reliable than the coding bias predictions though one should be aware of the possibility of sequence error, differential splicing, etc. and of course finding the coding exons is not a complete gene prediction. The genewise program has an exhaustive (slow) algorithm to align a protein to a DNA sequence, allowing for splice site recognition. (In a real situation, BLAST programs would be useful for first picking up the matches in a DB search.):

1. Open an X-window (or terminal on Tau's desktop).
2. Type prepare wise2 in the window.
3. We've prepared files with the human DNA and a homologous chicken protein to compare.
4. Now you can type or cut and paste the following command into the UNIX window:
   (a) genewise/home/seqanal/public_html/courses/spring99/kad 1_chick/home/seqanal/public_html/courses/spring99/hsak1.dna
5. The program will run with default parametres and after a couple of minutes will print out the matched exons.
6. Now compare the results to the predictions so far:
   (a) How many Exons are found?
   (b) Are the splice sites between or within codons?
   (c) Did you find all these coding regions earlier?
   (d) Have we now found all the coding exons (the chicken homolog has 194 AA)?
7. Now let's look at the annotated genomic sequence entry for our test sequence, HSAK1.
8. Note that no cDNA has been sequenced for this gene: gene structure was inferred by some transcript mapping and by protein homology.

9. Most of the elements of the gene are listed in the feature table:
   (a) Did you get the promoter?
   (b) Did you get the starting methionine? Does it obey Kozak's rules?
   (c) How many amino acids are in the first coding exon?
   (d) If you made any errors in the prediction, can you see where you went wrong?
10. There is a problem with the annotation of the first intron's acceptor.
    Do you think this is:
    (a) An unusual splice site?
    (b) An annotation error made by the authors?

Take Home Lessons

There seems to be no single high quality tool for doing eukaryotic gene prediction work. The variations in the results from prediction servers indicate that there is scope for improving the algorithms. Graphical presentation of the results is patchy for example we need to know start, stop codons and which frame has the coding potential, information that we did not get from the graphical plot. To do this for real, we would need to assemble results from many servers and work with a hard copy of the DNA sequence and it would take longer than the morning we set aside today, to do the job properly. In fact the Staden package has for many years been able to produce a plot with all this information, although it was clumsy and old fashioned to use and some of the prediction methods may be more sensitive now.

Current gene-finding programs are complex integrated systems that incorporate a number of different methods for gene finding. The set of methods used and the way they are integrated vary between individual programs. It has been observed that these different techniques often correctly predict different elements of the gene, suggesting that programs could complement each other, yielding better predictions.

In order to test this hypothesis we explored different methods for combining predictions from two gene-finding programs. After extensive evaluation of current eukaryotic gene-finding programs, Genscan and HMMgene were chosen for their high prediction accuracy and their reliable estimates of the accuracy of the exon prediction. The predictions were combined on the exon level, using three separate techniques: decision trees, modified set operations and probabilistic networks.

Some of these methods yielded notable improvements in the prediction accuracy especially at the exon level: the sensitivity increased from 0.76 to 0.79 (4.0 per cent) and the specificity increased from 0.77 to 0.86 (11.7 per cent), compared to the best exon level accuracy measures achieved by any single program. The successful methods were tested on three independent datasets, each time outperforming any individual gene-finding program. The results were especially good for the dataset containing sequences with several genes, where exon accuracy measures were improved by 30 per cent compared to Genscan's results.

Chapter 8

Proteome Analysis

INTRODUCTION

Most databases are built from sequences of genes, genomes and proteins. However, little is understood about how macromolecules—nucleic acids, proteins, lipids and carbohydrates—work together to give structure and function to a cell, be they single-cell organisms like bacteria and yeasts or multicellular organisms like plants and animals. Furthermore, because mRNA is the intermediate molecular species for protein biosynthesis, mRNA levels are indicative of gene expression. For this reason, mRNA sequences are used for the production of expressed sequence tags (EST) libraries. However, cellular levels of mRNA are not necessarily reliable markers for protein levels. It is, therefore, of paramount importance to establish the protein profile of a cell, which not only gives the relative number of proteins, but also the form in which they exist and post-translational modification such as glycosylation, acylation, ubiquitination, phosphorylation or proteolytic processing involved in protein activation. All these processes are involved in controlling the activity and location of a protein in the cell.

PROTEIN COMPOSITON OF A CELL

To make matters more complex, the protein composition of a cell and the post-translational modifications of proteins vary at different stages of the cell cycle, in metabolic and environmental stress, in cell-to-cell signalling and in individuals with diseases. Tumours, for example, often show altered expression and activity patterns of key proteins as compared to healthy tissue. Since these proteins are related to growth control, carcinogenesis can generally be viewed as some lack of control in growth or the unhindered multiplication of cells which should no longer divide or are programmed to die (ageing, apoptosis).

Because all somatic cells contain the full genome, but use only part of it for regular activity, up and down regulation of genes is especially important during the development of these cells, where a single cell multiplies and differentiates into specialised cell types, tissues and organs. The imprinting of gene activity patterns is a process where the cells control the levels of gene products and behave as recessive or dominant genes. This is known as gene dose effect and is well studied for X-chromosome-related genes that contain one copy in males and two copies in females. The level of proteins often affects metabolic and second messenger pathways and is used as a fine-tuning control mechanism. The cellular mechanisms of such gene dose effects are often not understood Fig. 8.1.

MACROMOLES AND CELLULAR STRUCTURE

Furthermore, not all macromolecules and cellular structures are synthesised off a linear template. In fact, RNA and protein synthesis are the only molecular species directly encoded for by DNA. Everything else—and this includes the protein modifications mentioned earlier—is guided by molecular interactions, sequential synthesis and spatial separation known as compartmentalisation. Good examples of biological macro-molecules lacking a gene template are polysaccharides and protein and lipid glycosylation. Polysaccharides (carbohydrates) exist as linear, as well as branched, multimers and although polymer sequences are consistently reproduced by the cellular machinery (proteins catalyse carbohydrate synthesis), these sequences are not encoded by other linear, molecular templates as DNA codes for protein synthesis. Instead, polysaccharide synthesis is a sequential catalytic activity performed by the spatial arrangement of enzymes within the cell. Its own gene encodes each enzyme of such a pathway. Groups of enzymes that synthesise polysaccharides are therefore not independent, since the lack of a single protein in the pathway makes it defective.

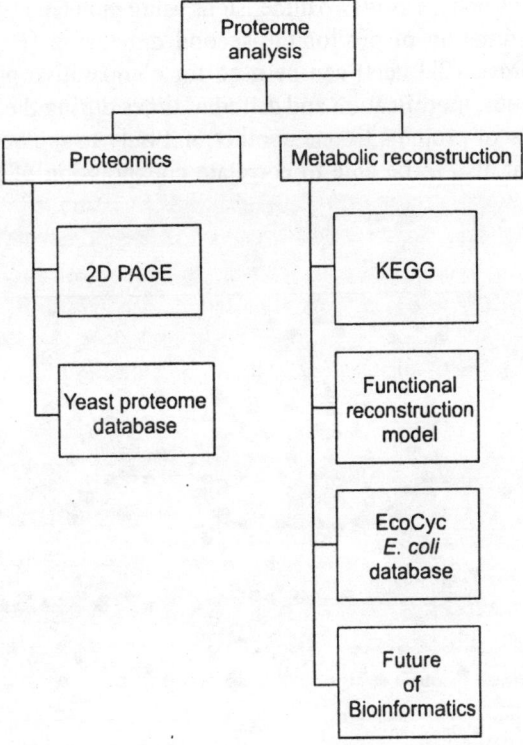

Fig. 8.1. Proteome analysis.

It is, therefore, important to understand the structure of enzymatic pathways. Comparing not only individual genes across species, but entire pathways yields additional information about newly discovered DNA sequences. Are pathways identical across species? Are all enzymes of the same pathway homologs expressing similar degrees of identity? Are certain enzymes in pathways more important or more conserved than others? Do some species have alternative pathways to generic ones, while others do not? Finding the answers to such questions is the true challenge of biology in the twenty-first century. The Internet (or any equivalent form of public communication) will be instrumental in this discovery process. It will provide the databases necessary for comparing the protein composition of a cell or an organism as a function of metabolic activity and disease from the period of conception to the moment of death.

Collection of Protein of a Given Cell

The task of organising the collection of proteins of any given cell type or organism has recently given rise to a new science called proteomics, which attempts to look at the combination and expression patterns of a cell's or an organism's proteins at any given moment. It basically tries to understand the organisational complexity of the enzymatic machinery of cells.

The word proteomics refers to the idea that all proteins of any given organism are necessarily linked in their fate with each other. Understanding this inter-relationship is important in understanding their biology, including their evolutionary traits.

Biochemical Techniques of Proteomics

Proteomics makes use of a biochemical technique invented in the early 1970s where proteins are analytically separated on polymer gel electrophoresis in two dimensions using molecular weight for the first dimension and electrical charge as a function of pH for the second dimension (Fig. 8.2). The so-called two-dimensional gel electrophoresis (2D gels) can be used for comparative purposes to identify proteins that exist in different quantities, modification and different times during the life cycle of an organism. It is important to compare sets of proteins to one another, not only to replace the more tedious work of studying single proteins, but also to be able to correlate coexpression of proteins and to relate these patterns to cellular activity.

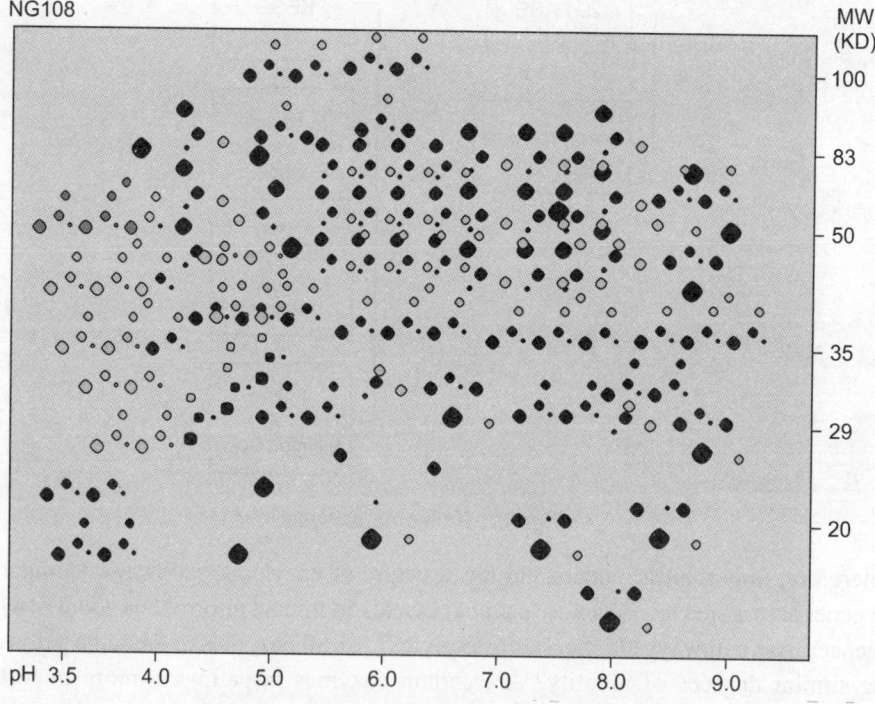

Fig. 8.2. 2D polyacrylamide gel showing protein contents of eukaryotic cell type: proteins extracted from the mammalian cell line NG108 are separated according to molecular weight [MW in kilodalton (KD)] on Y-axis and according to charge in a pH gradient ranging from 3.5 to 10 (X-axis). Each spot represents an individual protein type. Intensities reflect protein concentrations. Proteins can be extracted from gel matrix for biochemical analysis (sequencing, mass spectrometry).

Proteomics is a formidable approach because many proteins have never been characterised on 2D gels (or characterised at all) and a biochemist's most time-consuming work is to unambiguously identify the spot on an analytical gel as a specific protein, modified protein or fragment thereof. As previously mentioned, 2D gels give two pieces of information: size and charge. Both physical parametres depend on the cellular condition at the time the protein was isolated and purified. The calculated molecular weight of a protein based on its DNA sequence often does not exactly match the experimentally determined value from gel electrophoresis, because the latter reflects the overall solubility and mobility of a protein within the gel matrix. The mobility in the direction of molecular weight not only depends on the true molecular weight of the protein, but more accurately reflects the charge/unit weight of the protein. Therefore, changing the pH of the system changes the mobility because the number of charges-per-unit weight is changed and not every protein with the same molecular weight has the same charge/unit weight ratio. The precise determination of the actual molecular weight and sequence of a protein spot on a gel is crucial for such interpretation.

Identification of Protein Spots

Modern analytical and automated systems assist in the large-scale identification of these protein spots (Fig. 8.3). Proteins of interest can be digested within the gel matrix and the resulting peptides are extracted and subjected to high mass accuracy MALDI-MS (matrix-assisted desorption ionisation mass spectrometry) analysis. Here, peptide fragments are ionised and their charge/mass ratio is determined. The mass-charge ratio is matched to all possible amino acid sequence combinations. If the matching is ambiguous, the peptide fragment must be micro-sequenced and the sequence subjected to a database search using BLAST algorithms. If many fragments from a single 2D gel spot match the same sequence in the database (e.g. GenBank), the protein corresponding to this spot has been successfully identified.

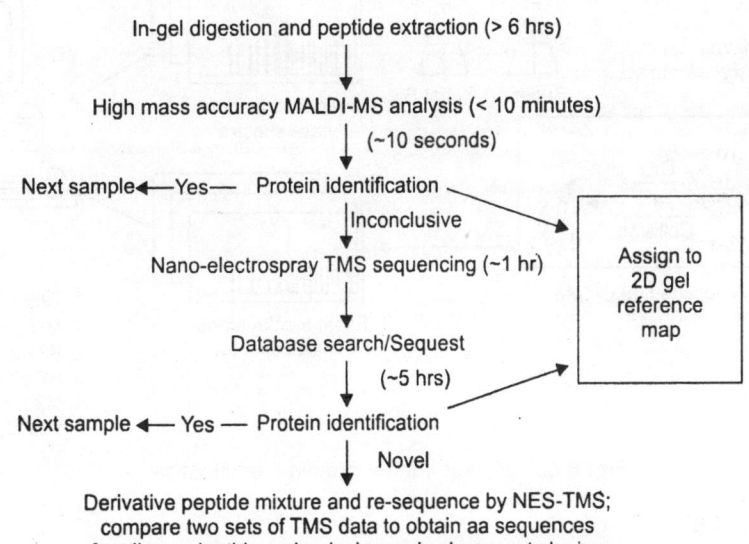

Fig. 8.3. Strategies for the identification of proteins from 2D gels.

The matching is often not straightforward because of the potential chemical modification of the peptide fragments. These post-translational modifications come from cellular processes used to control protein activities. These modifications affect net charge, reactivity and solubility of proteins. Modifications such as phosphorylation add negative charges to the protein, thus influencing its mobility during electrophoresis. A single negative charge has the equivalent effect of decreasing the molecular weight of a protein by 2 kDa or roughly 15 to 18 (noncharged) amino acids. Glycosylation also affects the molecular weight of a protein, but not necessarily its pH dependence. Because of the existence of multiple modifications that affect the apparent mobility of a protein on a gel in a similar way, the interpretation of small differences in mobility of proteins on 2D gels is not always easy and requires careful biochemical analysis.

The entire process of peptide fragment identification has been automated over the last several years (Fig. 8.4). Automated processes require special robotic equipment, as well as customised software. Again, computers play a central role in controlling and analysing the process. An autosampler collects peptide fractions from a HPLC column chromatography which separates peptides according to size. Very small volumes are used in capillary columns and subjected to nano-electrospray ionisation for mass spectrum analysis. Experimental and predicted mass spectra are used to generate cross-correlation data to identify the sequence of the extracted peptide fragments. If several fragments from a single 2D gel spot match a single amino acid sequence entry in the database, a protein is identified.

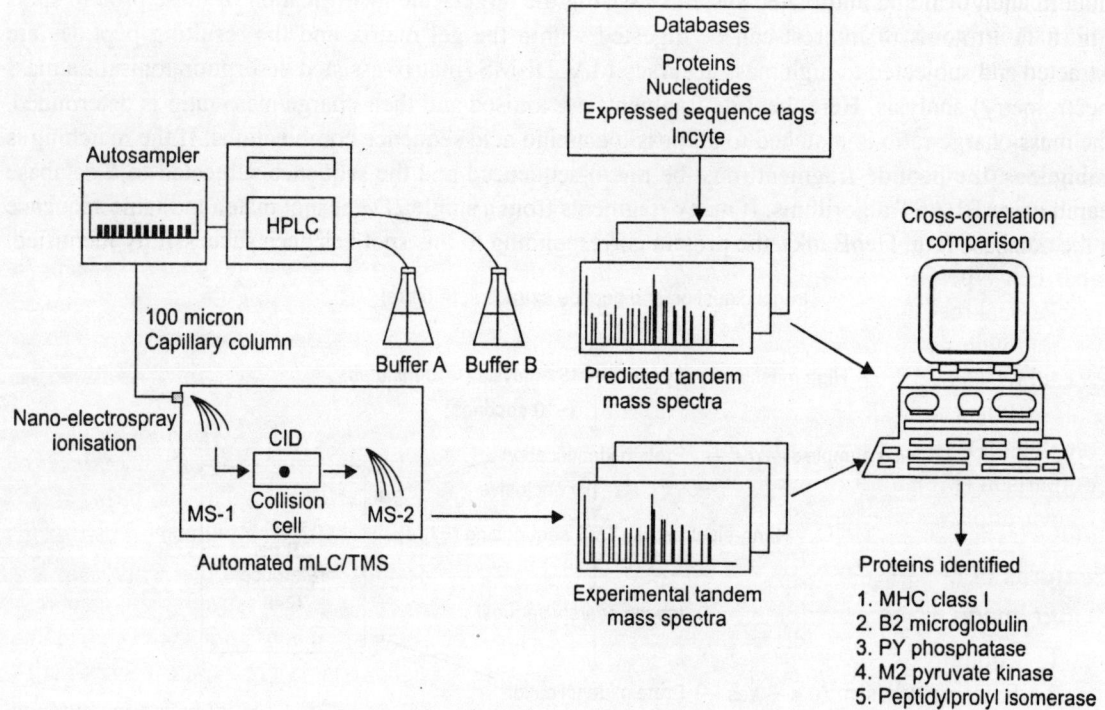

Fig. 8.4. Fully automated protein identification.

2D-PAGE AT EXPASY

The first step in proteomic analysis of cellular mechanisms is to compare 2D gels of cellular extracts obtained after stimulating a cell with an activator (such as insulin on liver cells) with those obtained under metabolic resting conditions. Many public databases include a growing number of such reference gels for preliminary identification of the charge and molecular weights of a novel protein. A public proteome database (SWISS-2D-PAGE) has been established at the Geneva University Hospital,

Switzerland (http://www.expasy.ch). This database is one of eight intended to help scientists understand organisms at the functional level by directly studying gene products (proteins) and their corresponding post-translational modifications. The site is organised to access the 2D database interactively, to provide online help, technical manuals for 2D gel electrophoresis and services such as running gels upon submission of samples, training courses (not online courses, you have to travel to Geneva) and software packages for the analysis of 2D gels.

The 2D database at Expasy contains electrophoretic information on 16 tissues and organisms, including yeast, *E. coli*, Dictyostelium and human cell types (platelet, red blood cell, macrophage, plasma protein, lymphoma, liver, kidney, two leukemia cell lines, cerebrospinal fluid and intestinal epithelial cells). Known proteins can be found by searching for an accession number (SWISS-PROT) or clicking on 2D gels with marked spots. The putative locations of new proteins can be identified if the amino acid sequence is known. The hypothetical molecular weight and charge are used to place the protein on the gel. However, and this is an important caveat for 2D gel electrophoresis, theoretical values often differ from experimental values due to solubility behaviours of proteins in gels and actual post-translational modification of the amino acids. Many proteins yield multiple spots on 2D gels for this reason, so this information is valuable to the biochemist in understanding the function of a protein within a cellular environment.

A look at those gels shows that the majority of spots are not linked to any known protein. New technology is being developed to more quickly identify proteins on 2D gels. Biochemical analysis using micro sequencing of peptide fragments and mass spectrometry of these fragments is the analog approach in sequencing nucleic acid libraries.

Once a protein is identified in one cell type or organism, its expression level can be compared in other cell types or tissues, potentially revealing different levels of expression and modes of post-translational modifications. This task of comparing protein expression levels is hardly a trivial one. The way a protein runs on a gel greatly depends on the purification procedure, source and electrophoresis procedure. Comparison, therefore, requires cautious interpretation regarding relative positioning of spots and their intensities. SWISS-2D-PAGE offers an analysis package for rapid image manipulation, complete 2D analysis, worldwide comparison for referencing and automated gel matching and comparison (Melanie II 2D Analysis Software, developed by Denis Hochstrasser at Melanie Group in Geneva, http://www.expasy.ch/melanie/MelanieII/description.html). The features of Melanie II include:

Features of Melanie II

Rapid image manipulation

1. Zooming.
2. Filtering (smoothing, contrast enhancement, background subtraction).
3. Gel flipping.
4. Gel stacking for better visualisation.
5. Image stretching.

Complete 2D analysis

1. Automatic spot identification and analysis.
2. Gaussian spot modelling.
3. Gel overlay display.
4. Point-and-click interface.

5. Embedded landmarks.
6. pI/MW setting.
7. Extended reports.
8. Histograms.
9. Statistical data analysis.

Worldwide comparisons

1. Multiple gel display.
2. Fast, automatic gel comparison and matching.
3. Reference gels for comparison to all other gels.
4. Creation of synthetic gels by merging a set of gels.
5. SWISS-2D-PAGE master gels.
6. Network and online links to biological databases, including SWISS-2D-PAGE and SWISS-PROT through Expasy.
7. World Wide Web server.

Data import/export

1. Gel printing.
2. Image import/export from and to TIFF and PPM.
3. Data export to Excel and other applications.
4. Data export as Melanie I format to public statistical and heuristic clustering programs.

SPECIALISED 2D-PAGE DATABASES

There are two specialised proteomic databases that compare expression profiles associated with toxins and xenobiotics: the Rodent Molecular Effects Database at Oxford's Glycosciences and a keratinocyte database at the Danish Centre for Human Genome Research at http://biobase.dk/cgi-bin/celis. The latter provides a database for knockout and transgenic animals, meaning that specific genes have been inactivated or added to the germ lines of the animals. The absence or addition of genes should be observable at the protein level by a missing or additional spot on a 2D gel. ESA, Inc.'s neurological disease database specialises in Alzheimer's, Parkinson's and Huntington's diseases through protein differential display.

The yeast proteome database™ (YPD) from proteome, Inc. (www.proteome.com) is an example of how entrepreneurial efforts tap into a vast amount of existing data in the current literature and combine it into a specific new form; in this case, the collective knowledge of all proteins of the micro-organism *Saccharomyces cerevisiae*, baker's yeast.

YPD is an encyclopaedia of all yeast proteins known and predicted from the yeast genome project connecting basic biophysical and functional data like molecular weight from mass spectrometry, amino acid sequences (from genome sequences) and function (from published literature). Currently, about 30 new yeast proteins are being characterised at different levels of information and 3000 proteins are known to some degree (how many ORFs and URFs). In addition, homology-based information that cross-references yeast with human, for example, is valuable to researchers who may use yeast as a model organism to perform initial studies on proteins that are used similarly in human metabolism and physiology. The data going into YPD and 2D gel maps in general include molecular weight information gained from mass spectrometry, the charge and chemical modification information gained from the amino acid sequence and functional information largely gained from published data.

METABOLIC RECONSTRUCTION

Kyoto Encyclopaedia of Genes and Genomes—KEGG

The kyoto encyclopaedia of genes and genomes (KEGG) is an effort to provide a means to compute pathways of molecular and cellular processes. KEGG is part of the Japanese human genome program at the Institute for chemical research, Kyoto University (http://www.genome.ad.jp:80/kegg/). Although the technical challenges and underpinnings of KEGG are the same as those of NCBI, KEGG addresses the complex interaction of proteins in cells from the perspective of metabolic interaction. Their philosophy includes finding answers to some of the common questions of modern molecular biology such as: what do we know about the relationship between the sequence of a gene and the function of the protein? What is the protein-folding problem in the cellular context? What are the challenges and problems facing the functional reconstruction problems or how can we understand the relationship between the genome and the organism—its development and morphology? The goal of KEGG, therefore, is to build a functional map starting with available components within various molecular catalogs. The functional maps represent metabolic and regulatory pathways. The molecular catalogs include genome maps, base sequences, gene allocations (physical map, inheritance map) and LIGAND databases (enzymes, compounds and elements).

Functional Reconstruction Model

Other databases and organisations have information similar to KEGG's, but with a notable exception: KEGG also has a deductive database. Here, the user can compute pathways and binary relations with the goal of computing wiring diagrams of genes and molecules. This should lead to an understanding of cells as being a complex, self-assembling system whose components and the relationship between them are fully understood. This is known as the functional reconstruction model. In KEGG's words, the genome is simply a 'warehouse of parts...and all the regulatory signals in the genome are simply bar codes to retrieve them. In this view the blueprint of life is written in the entire cell as a network of molecular interactions'. To gain an understanding of this network of molecular interactions, KEGG uses prediction tools for the computation of novel relationships based solely on the contents of its individual catalogs (the warehouse). These tools can be found through the 'Search and compute with KEGG' link.

How can we reconstruct a biological organism? KEGG's approach uses a hierarchical view of an organism, most easily viewed as atomic levels, molecular levels and network levels (pathways). KEGG uses a system for data representation that structures a database according to the number of links between its components.

Elements of the catalog database include molecules (protein structures, metabolites), genes (sequences) and genomes (Fig. 8.5). Pathway maps connect elements from the catalog database through binary relations, which are molecular interactions (structure) and genetic interactions (function). Interactions of more than two units are called networks and include metabolic pathways (molecular and genetic), genomes (linear and circular), hierarchies (classification, taxonomy) and neighbours (sequence similarities, structural similarities). KEGG introduces the integration of genomic information with pathways to reflect the biological reality within a cell. This allows the individual scientist to search for proteins or genes of new or related pathways in model organisms other than the one being investigated. Missing structural information can quickly be obtained by finding homologs in 'neighbours' whose structure has been solved. Novel pathways may be predicted by entering starting and end points of substrate and product and selecting an appropriate organism.

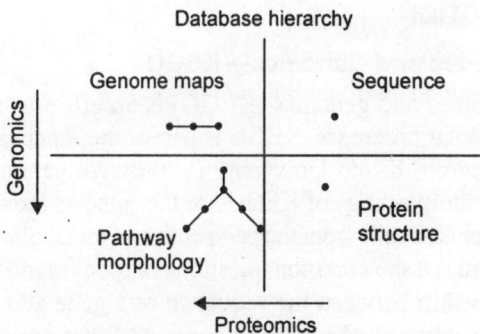

Fig. 8.5. Database hierarchy.

E. coli Metabolic Database: EcoCyc

The bacterium *E. coli* is the ultimate laboratory test subject for geneticists, molecular biologists, microbiologists and biochemists. It is also extremely important to human health and physiology, as it is part of our gastrointestinal system. Unfortunately, *E. coli* is also an opportunistic pathogen, i.e. it can cause lethal infections if it enters our bloodstream. It is recognised by most people for its role in food poisoning caused by meat contamination, most often in undercooked hamburger meat. Its close genetic relationship to the bacteria *Salmonella typhimurium* (a problem found mostly in poultry) makes the integrative knowledge of its metabolism, genetics and health problems a pressing yet fascinating issue.

EcoCyc from Pangea systems, Inc. (http://www.pangeasystems.com) addresses the integration of the classic biochemical pathways (metabolism) of *E. coli* with its complete genome sequence information. For example, the metabolic pathways for amino acid synthesis in *E. coli* involve several enzymes that are often coregulated at gene expression levels. Thus, sensitive proteomics techniques should be able to see shifts in spot density, not only for one protein, but for several different ones. New pathways or homologous pathways in recently studied organisms with limited sequence information may be detected by proteomic means. Similar to KEGG, EcoCyc uses chemical compound libraries that list the molecules involved in each biological reaction, the molecular weight of the compound and in many cases, its chemical structure. The EcoCyc KB has a number of uses. It is an electronic reference source for *E. coli* biologists and for biologists who work with related micro-organisms. Scientists can visualise the layout of genes within the *E. coli* chromosome or of an individual biochemical reaction or of a complete biochemical pathway (with compound structures displayed). The navigation capabilities allow the user to move from a display of an enzyme to a display of a reaction that the enzyme catalyses or of the gene that encodes the enzyme. The interface also supports a variety of queries, such as generating a display of the map positions of all genes that code for enzymes within a given biochemical pathway. In addition to being a reference source for individual facts, the EcoCyc KB allows complex computations related to the metabolism, such as design of novel biochemical pathways for biotechnology, studies of the evolution of metabolic pathways and simulation of metabolic pathways. The EcoCyc KB is also being used for computer-based education in biochemistry. (From: http://ecocyc.PangeaSystems.com/ecocyc/ecocyc.html).

The *E. coli* metabolic database nevertheless provides us with a considerable body of knowledge that is easily accessible from a PC terminal. As of January 2002, the following numbers of objects were contained in the latest version of EcoCyc:

1. 4909 *E. coli* genes.
2. 804 enzymes encoded by these genes.

3. 829 metabolic reactions occurring in *E. coli*.
4. 124 metabolic pathways occurring in *E. coli*.
5. 1303 chemical compounds involved in *E. coli* metabolism.
6. 79 tRNAs.
7. 45 2-component signal transduction proteins.

What keeps the bacterium alive? This question looms in the minds of life scientists and the answer seems frighteningly close. The creators of EcoCyc talk about 'an *in silicio* model of *E. coli* metabolism that can be probed and analysed through computational means'. This suggests that experimenting on the model of metabolic pathways instead of the biochemical (wet bench) model will someday be as possible as a computer simulating nuclear tests thus replacing the actual tests which are detectable seismographically by the enemy. Further, it suggests that the encyclopaedia will someday be transformed into a workbench—an electronic laboratory rather than an electronic library.

Where Should We Be in the Future?

At the current level of database integration and the combination of general information, the Internet is an open-ended, badly annotated and unedited 'database'. There are infinite numbers of existing hyperlinks and the task of searching for correct and complete information is often difficult and sometimes impossible. Small companies are often founded on the realisation that editorial work, annotation and human intervention are needed to enable the life science community to make full use of the existing information. Annotation is costly, but can sell well if it is customised to the needs of the end user. For entrepreneurs, selling compounded information to the industry can be very lucrative, since the time and expertise required for scientists to work together with computer engineers can be financially prohibitive. Selling information over the internet—information that is already available in unprocessed form—is vulnerable to exploitation. The interface between proprietary and academic information and the struggle for new patents on life forms feeds companies such as proteome and Pangea systems.

Spatial organisation of cellular components is central to the function of a cell, yet this aspect of supramolecular structures is poorly understood. It boils down to how cells build the necessary building blocks at the right place and the right time. Self-assembly systems are part of a new interdisciplinary branch of biology and chemistry that addresses such problems—chemistry beyond the molecule.

ANALYSING DATA FROM 2D-PAGE GELS

Raw Data from 2D-PAGE gels

Two-dimensional polyacrylamide gel electrophoresis (2D-PAGE) is a method used to separate proteins according to charge and mass. The resolution of the technique is such that thousands of proteins can be distinguished, providing a diagnostic protein fingerprint of any particular sample. After the gel has been run, it is stained to reveal the position of individual proteins. These appear as spots of varying size, shape and intensity. The role of bioinformatics in protein gel analysis is the extraction of useful information from the positions and intensities of the protein spots. 2D-PAGE data can be used to derive general information on protein expression profiles without any knowledge of which specific proteins are actually present on the gel. However, the most powerful approach to 2D-PAGE experiments is to couple the expression analysis with protein annotation by mass spectrometry.

Data Processing

Data are extracted from 2D-PAGE gels in several stages. First, the stained protein gel is scanned to obtain a digital image. Individual protein spots are then detected and quantified and the intensity of the signal for each spot is corrected for local background.

The quality of the digital image is important since its spatial resolution determines how accurately protein spot sizes are recorded and its densitometric resolution determines how accurately the intensity of each spot is recorded. Protein spot measurement involves a special set of problems that are not found with microarray data. The features on a microarray are arranged in a precise grid and the signals tend to be regular, discrete and nonoverlapping. Conversely, the signals in a protein gel are irregularly distributed, the spots vary widely in morphology and it is often the case that spots join together in clumps or lines that are difficult to resolve. Several algorithms are available which address these issues and generally these are based on either Gaussian fitting or laplacian of gaussian (LOG) spot detection. Spots whose morphology deviates from a single Gaussian shape can thus be interpreted using a model of overlapping shapes. A simpler approach is line and chain analysis, in which columns of pixels from the digital image are scanned for peaks in signal density. This process is repeated for adjacent pixel columns allowing the algorithm to identify the centres of spots and their overall signal intensity (signal volume). A further approach is known as watershed transformation (WST). In this method, pixel intensities are viewed as a topographical map so that hills and valleys can be identified. This is useful for separating clusters, chains and shouldered spots (small spots overlapping with larger ones) and also for merging regions of a single spot. The output of each method is a spot list, in which each individual protein spot is identified by the x and y coordinates of its centre.

Gel Matching

An important application of 2D-PAGE is the analysis of differential protein expression. This can be used, for example, to look for proteins that are induced or repressed by particular treatments or drugs, to look for proteins associated with disease states or to look at changes in protein expression during development. Differential protein expression can only be studied by running a series of 2D-PAGE gels with alternative samples and searching for novel spots or spots whose intensity changes significantly in different gels. Note that any observed changes, for example the presence of a novel protein spot, may not reflect the synthesis of a new protein. Instead, the new spot may reflect the post-translational modification of an existing protein, for example phosphorylation or glycosylation. Such modifications can radically alter the mass or charge of a protein, leading to different migration behaviour during electrophoresis.

Due to minute variations and inconsistencies in the chemical and physical properties of electrophoretic gels, it is impossible to exactly reproduce the conditions of anyone electrophoresis experiment. This means that, even in a series of gels using exactly the same sample and electrophoresis parametres, the positions of individual protein spots are never the same. In order to compare serial gels and identify novel protein spots or spots that vary in intensity, it is necessary to use gel matching. Generally this involves establishing the positions of several unambiguous landmark spots and then using algorithms to match the positions of the remaining spots (Fig. 8.6). To bring the spots from two gels into register, simple image manipulations such as stretching and rotating can be carried out. This may be assisted by incorporating spot intensities and the (physical) distances between neighbouring spots as variables in the algorithm. For example, an approach known as propagation involves determining the distance between a given landmark spot and all neighbours. If matches are found on other gels, the neighbouring spots can be used as new landmarks and the process reiterated. An implementation of such algorithms is available as the program MELANIE II. This is available to download for use on Windows-based computers (www.expasy.ch/ch2d/melanie) but cannot be used on-line.

Image analysis of two-dimensional gels

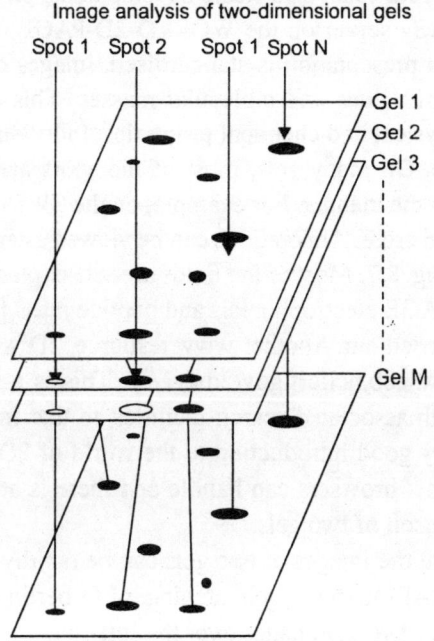

Fig. 8.6. Principle of gel matching. Individual spots are compared and matched across a series of 2D-PAGE gels.

Protein Expression Matrices

Once protein expression data have been recorded they are built into a protein expression matrix. This is similar in principle to the gene expression matrix. Spots, representing proteins, are arranged in rows, while experimental treatments are listed in columns. The data points in the matrix represent signal intensities for each spot. Comparison of values along a given row can identify proteins whose expression levels change according to different treatments. As with gene expression data, multivariate statistical analysis can group data by similar expression profiles, which can be used both for classification purposes or clustering.

2D-PAGE Databases

The results from 2D-PAGE experiments are generally stored in 2D-PAGE databases, which use gel images as a basis for protein annotation. Digital images from 2D-PAGE gels are presented and each protein spot acts as a link to further information such as protein name, molecular mass, pI value, annotations from the SWISS-PROT database, bibliographic references and if appropriate, graphs showing how spot intensities vary over a series of gels. Some 2D-PAGE databases are free standing and may come packaged with gel analysis software. For example, the analysis suite PDQUEST incorporates its own database, which may be installed locally and used to store the 2D-PAGE experimental data from a single laboratory. There are also free software packages available that can be used to set up 2D-PAGE databases, such as Make2ddb.

The construction of 2D-PAGE databases on the world wide web (www) allows 2D-PAGE data to be shared and compared over the Internet. There are over 30 such databases currently available, many showing 2D-PAGE data either for specific organisms or specific systems. For example, the HEART-2D-PAGE contains 2D-PAGE data related to heart development, physiology and disease. All these pages are indexed by the ExPASy server on the WORLD-2D-PAGE (http://www.expasy.ch/ch2d/2d-index.html). The format of data presentation is standardised. Images of 2D-PAGE gels are presented overlain with a grid showing pI values and molecular masses. This allows each protein spot to be identified on the basis of its physical and chemical properties. Individual spots can be clicked, linking the user to an annotation page. On many gels, most of the spots are not annotated and those with annotations are highlighted in some manner. For example, on the SWISS-2DE database each annotated protein spot is marked with a red cross. Annotations can be viewed as an original SWISS-PROT file, an example of which is shown in Fig. 8.7. Most of the fields are self-explanatory, but note that the 2D field may include data on both 2D-PAGE electrophoresis and peptide mass fingerprinting (Topic K2) where such experiments have been carried out. Another www resource, 2D web gel (2DWG) can be found at the following URL: http://www.lecb.ncifcrf.gov/2dwgDB/. This is a catalog of some of the 2D gel images found on the www, with associated search facilities so that images can be abstracted by key words. 2DWG represents a very good introduction to the world of 2D gels. The images are stored in formats such as GIF that Internet browsers can handle and there is an associated Java applet, called Flicker, to facilitate the comparison of two gels.

The basis of flickering is that the images of two gels can be rapidly alternated to identify matching spots. Another useful applet is CAROL (http://gelmatching.inf.fu-berlin.de/Carol.html) which uses point pattern matching to compare any two gel images over the Internet.

Raw Data from Mass Spectrometry

Mass spectrometry (MS) is a method for accurately determining the mass/charge ratio (m/z) of ions in a vacuum, thus allowing the precise determination of molecular masses. These raw data can be used in three different approaches for the identification of proteins. In peptide-mass fingerprinting, a protein is digested with a specific cleavage agent (usually the enzyme trypsin) and the masses of each of the resulting peptides are determined. These masses are then used in correlative database searching to identify the protein. In fragment ion searching, peptide fragments are generated as above and then fragmented in a collision cell between two quadrupole mass analysers (this is called tandem MS, often abbreviated to MS/MS) or by a process known as post-source decay, which occurs when matrix-assisted laser desorption/ionisation (MALDI) MS is used at a higher acceleration voltage than usual. The resulting fragment ions are short peptide fragments.

The molecular masses of such fragments can be used to search not only protein databases, but also other sequence repositories including dbEST. Both these approaches require that the protein in question has been identified and its sequence deposited. Where this is not the case, *de novo* sequencing can be carried out. In this method, peptide ladders are generated either by sequential chemical degradation of terminal amino acid residues or by separating the fragment ions generated as above into nested sets. Mass differences between sequential fragments correspond to the known masses of individual amino acids, thus allowing protein sequences to be deduced without any correlative information from sequence databases.

```
ID    ACTB_HUMAN; STANDARD; 2DG.
AC    P02570;
DT    01–AUG–1993 (Rel. 00, Created)
DT    01–DEC–2000 (Rel. 13, Last update)
DE    Actin, cytoplasmic 1 (Beta-actin):
GN    ACTB.
OS    Homo sapiens (Human).
OC    Eukaryota; Metazoa; Chordata; Craniata; Vertebrata; Euteleostomi;
OC    Mammalia; Eutheria; Primates; Catarrhini; Hominidae; Homo.
OX    NCBI_TaxID = 9606;
MT    CSF_HUMAN, ELC_HUMAN, HEPG2_HUMAN, HEPG2SP_HUMAN, LIVER_HUMAN,
MT    LYMPHOMA_HUMAN, PLASMA_HUMAN, PLATELET_HUMAN, RBC_HUMAN, U937_HUMAN,
MT    KIDNEY_HUMAN, HL60_HUMAN, CEC_HUMAN, DLD1_HUMAN.
IM    CSF_HUMAN, ELC_HUMAN, HEPG2_HUMAN, HEPG2SP_HUMAN, LIVER_HUMAN,
IM    LYMPHOMA_HUMAN, PLASMA_HUMAN, PLATELET_HUMAN, RBC_HUMAN, U937_HUMAN,
IM    KIDNEY_HUMAN, HL60_HUMAN, CEC_HUMAN, DLD1_HUMAN.
RN    [1]
RP    MAPPING ON GEL.
RX    MEDLINE=93162045; PubMed=1286669; [NCBI, ExPASy, EBI, Israel, Japan]
RA    Hochstrasser D.F., Frutiger S., Paquet N., Bairoch A., Ravier F.,
RA    Pasquali C., Sanchez J.-C., Tissot J.-D., Bjellqvist B., Vargas R.,
RA    Appel R.D., Hughes G.J.;
RT    'Human liver protein map: a reference database established by
RT    microsequencing and gel comparison.';
RL    Electrophoresis 13:992–1001(1992).
RN    [2]
```

... Several more literature references follow...

```
CC    –!– SUBUNIT: SINGLE CHAIN WHICH CAN BIND UP TO 4 OTHER CHAINS.
2D    –!– MASTER: CSF_HUMAN;
2D    –!–   PI/MW: SPOT 2D–000C1S=5.24/44747;
2D    –!–   MAPPING: MATCHING WITH THE PLASMA MASTER GEL [2].
2D    –!– MASTER: ELC_HUMAN;
2D    –!–   PI/MW: SPOT 2D–000ED0=5.21/41208;
2D    –!–   PI/MW: SPOT 2D–000ED7=5.12/41300;
2D    –!–   MAPPING: MATCHING WITH THE LIVER MASTER GEL [2].
2D    –!– MASTER: HEPG2_HUMAN;
2D    –!–   PI/MW: SPOT 2D–00030B=5.15/41700;
2D    –!–   PI/MW: SPOT 2D–00030Z=5.09/41700;
2D    –!–   PI/MW: SPOT 2D–00031Z=5.23/41272;
2D    –!–   MAPPING: MATCHING WITH THE LIVER MASTER GEL [2].
2D    –!– MASTER: HEPG2SP_HUMAN;
2D    –!–   PI/MW: SPOT 2D–000952=5.27/38525;
2D    –!–   PI/MW: SPOT 2D–000954=5.16/38400;
2D    –!–   PI/MW: SPOT 2D–000955=5.22/38223;
2D    –!–   PI/MW: SPOT 2D–000959=5.11/38223;
2D    –!–   MAPPING: MATCHING WITH THE PLASMA MASTER GEL [2].
2D    –!– MASTER: LIVER_HUMAN;
2D    –!–   PI/MW: SPOT 2D–0000WF=5.26/41839;
2D    –!–   PI/MW: SPOT 2D–0000WN=5.19/41722;
2D    –!–   PI/MW: SPOT 2D–0000WO=5.22/41605;
2D    –!–   MAPPING: MATCHING WITH A PLASMA GEL [1].
```

Fig. 8.7. (Contd ...)

```
2D   -!- MASTER: LYMPHOMA_HUMAN;
2D   -!-   PI/MW: SPOT 2D-0007PE=5.26/41898;
2D   -!-   PI/MW: SPOT 2D-0007PQ=5.15/42194;
2D   -!-   MAPPING: MATCHING WITH THE LIVER MASTER GEL [2].
2D   -!- MASTER: PLASMA_HUMAN;
2D   -!-   PI/MW: SPOT 2D-00050N=5.28/43590;
2D   -!-   PI/MW: SPOT 2D-00050Q=5.24/43244;
2D   -!-   MAPPING: IMMUNOBLOTTING [3].
2D   -!-   NORMAL LEVEL: PLATELET CONTAMINATION.
2D   -!- MASTER: PLATELET_HUMAN;
2D   -!-   PI/MW: SPOT 2D-000FWX=5.27/41946;
2D   -!-   PI/MW: SPOT 2D-000FZ5=5.18/41400;
2D   -!-   PI/MW: SPOT 2D-000FZM=5.06/41400;
2D   -!-   PI/MW: SPOT 2D-000FZN=5.30/41400;
2D   -!-   MAPPING: MATCHING WITH RBC AND LIVER MASTERS [5].
2D   -!- MASTER: RBC_HUMAN;
2D   -!-   PI/MW: SPOT 2D-00064D=5.20/42104;
2D   -!-   PI/MW: SPOT 2D-00064O=5.14/42209;
2D   -!-   PI/MW: SPOT 2D-00064W=5.27/42104;
2D   -!-   MAPPING: IMMUNOBLOTTING [3] AND MATCHING [4].
2D   -!- MASTER: 0937_HUMAN;
2D   -!-   PI/MW: SPOT 2D-000CXH=5.23/41807;
2D   -!-   MAPPING: MATCHING WITH THE LIVER MASTER GEL [2].
2D   -!- MASTER: KIDNEY_HUMAN;
2D   -!-   PI/MW: SPOT 2D-000N5T=5.18/41212;
2D   -!-   PI/MW: SPOT 2D-000N5U=5.25/41503;
2D   -!-   PI/MW: SPOT 2D-000N67=5.14/41406;
2D   -!-   PI/MW: SPOT 2D-000N6J=5.12/41309;
2D   -!-   MAPPING: MATCHING WITH THE LIVER MASTER GEL AND IMMUNODETECTION [6].
2D   -!- MASTER: HL60_HUMAN;
2D   -!-   PI/MW: SPOT 2D-000YZK=5.25/41925;
2D   -!-   PI/MW: SPOT 2D-000Z0A=5.15/41390;
2D   -!-   PI/MW: SPOT 2D-000ZOG=5.08/41497;
2D   -!-   MAPPING: MATCHING WITH THE LIVER MASTER GEL  [7] [8].
2D   -!- MASTER: CEC_HUMAN;
2D   -!-   PI/MW: SPOT 2D-000TWW=5.05/41396;
2D   -!-   PI/MW: SPOT 2D-000TWX=5.11/41497;
2D   -!-   MAPPING: MATCHING WITH THE LIVER MASTER GEL  [9].
2D   -!- MASTER: DLD1_HUMAN;
2D   -!-   PI/MW: SPOT 2D-001E5J=5.15/41545;
2D   -!-   PI/MW: SPOT 2D-001E5O=5.19/41545;
2D   -!-   PI/MW: SPOT 2D-001E6E=5.10/41391;
2D   -!-   PEPTIDE MASSES: SPOT 2D-001E5J: 976.504; 1132.57; 1198.7; 1516.72; 1790.89; 1954.05;
2D         2231.02; TRYPSIN.
2D   -!-   PEPTIDE MASSES: SPOT 2D-001E5O: 976.464; 1132.53; 1198.7; 1516.7; 1790.87; 1954.05;
2D         2231.07; TRYPSIN.
2D   -!-   PEPTIDE MASSES: SPOT 2D-0J1E6E: 976.513; 1132.57; 1516.73; 1790.89; 1954.04;
2D         2231.05; TRYPSIN.
2D   -!-   MAPPING: MASS FINGERPRINTING  [10].
CC   ------------------------------------------------------------------------------
CC   This SWISS-2D-PAGE entry is copyright the Swiss Institute of Bioinformatics.
CC   There are no restrictions on its use by non-profit institutions as long as
CC   its content is in no way modified and this statement is not removed. Usage
CC   by and for commercial entities requires a license agreement (See
CC   http://www.isb-sib.ch/announcer/ or send an email to license@isb-sib.ch).
CC   ------------------------------------------------------------------------------
DR   SWISS-PROT; P02570; ACTB_HUMAN.
DR   Siena-2D-PAGE; P02570; ACTB_HUMAN.
//
```

Fig. 8.7. Example SWISS-2D-PAGE entry (for human actin B). Some material has been deleted for brevity as shown. Note the extensive 2D data, which includes information from 2D-PAGE experiments and mass spectrometry.

Virtual Digests

It would be impossible to link peptide mass data to proteins in sequence databases such as SWISS-PROT without first knowing the expected peptides from such proteins. This information can be obtained by carrying out virtual digests that is, theoretical digests based on the known protein sequence and the known specificity of the cleavage agent used.

Cleavage agents with high specificity are most suitable and the endoproteinase trypsin, which cleaves a polypeptide chain after each basic amino acid (lysine or arginine) providing the next residue is not a proline, is the most widely used. Given a protein of known sequence, the tryptic peptides can be predicted. For example, a protein with the sequence shown below:

MCLTAKGAATCSATFRYLIFALSLATKPACALLASALLARACATTAVA

would generate the following tryptic peptides:

MCLTAK GAATCSATFR YLIFALSLATKPACALLASALLAR ACATTAVA

The four peptides provide four theoretical molecular masses. Correlation between these theoretical masses and the actual masses obtained in a mass spectrometry experiment would provide very convincing evidence for a database match.

Of course the same molecular masses could be obtained in many other ways. Each of the four peptides has a potentially very large number of anagrams (same amino acids in a different order), which would all have the same molecular mass.

Theoretically, this places limitations on the usefulness of the technique but in practical terms the chances of a series of peptides from the same protein generating spurious matches to the same deposited protein sequence because of permutations in the order of amino acids are very small indeed. Generally, correlation between two or more peptides is taken to be unambiguous confirmation of a database match. Another theoretical limitation is that the amino acids leucine and isoleucine have the same molecular masses. This provides a small technical problem in *de novo* sequencing, but for peptide mass fingerprinting and fragment ion fingerprinting it does not have a practical impact.

Dual Digests

Peptide mass fingerprinting allows the rapid identification of proteins if they are already represented in databases such as SWISS-PROT. Where this is not the case, both peptide mass fingerprinting and fragment ion searching can be used to match mass spectrometry data to other sequence databases, including the expressed sequence tag (EST) database dbEST.

The problem with this approach is that the databases contain a large amount of irrelevant data (e.g. noncoding sequence and other 'noise'), which can reduce the efficiency of the search. More confidence can be placed in any results if dual digests are carried out (i.e. combining the information from two protease digests using enzymes with different specificities, such as trypsin and endoproteinase LysC). Another approach is to carry out a single digest with the protein in the native state and then carry out the same digest after modifying the protein, for example by methylation.

Furthermore, since lysine (K) and arginine (R) are two of the most common amino acids in proteins, there is a relatively large number of doublets and triplets (e.g. RR, KKR, KRK). Trypsin cleaves randomly at such sites generating peptide fragments with ragged termini. More confidence can be placed in database hits that are compatible with such peptides because this is effectively the same as searching with a larger number of peptides.

Database Search Tools

A number of algorithms have been developed for sequence database searching using MS data. Among these, the most commonly used is SEQUEST, which works by searching for all peptides in the specified database(s) with the same mass as a given peptide ion.

Then, a virtual digest is performed on the matched protein and a theoretical mass spectrum generated. The data from the theoretical mass spectrum are then compared to the experimental data and the best matches are scored.

In a different approach, peptide mass data are used to generate a collection of possible sequences and this profile is used as a query in a modified BLAST or FASTA search. A program called Lutkefisk has been developed for this purpose. Many software resources for the analysis of MS data are available over the Internet and some are listed in Table 8.1.

Table 8.1. Internet resources for MS-based protein identification.

Resource	URL	Features and comments
CBRG, ETH-Zurich	cbrg.inf.ethz.ch/Masssearchtml	Peptide mass search
European molecular biology Laboratory (EMBL), Heidelberg	www.mann.embl-heidelbergde/Services/ PeptideSearch/PeptideSearchIntro.html	Peptide-mass and fragment ion search
ExPASy	www.expasy.ch/tools/#proteome	Peptide-mass and fragment ion search
Mascot	www.matrix-science.com/cgi/index.pl? page/home.html	Peptide-mass and fragment ion search
Rockefeller University, New York	prowl.rockefeller.edu/	Peptide-mass and fragment ion search
SEQNET, Daresbury, UK	www.seqnet.dl.ac.uk/Bioinformatics/ welapp/mowse	Peptide-mass and fragment ion search
University of California	prospector.ucsf.edu	Peptide mass (MS-Fit) and fragment ion (MS-Tag) search
	donatello.ucsf.edu	As above, on-line access
University of Washington	Thompson.mbt.washington.edu/sequest/	Instruction on how to get the SEQUEST fragmention search program

Limitations of MS Analysis

Although a powerful technique for protein annotation and sequencing, there are some limitations to MS, which need to be taken into account when interpreting and analysing experimental data. One of the most important factors to take into account is that MS data may not match any database entry due to the presence of an unknown post-translational modification.

Where such modifications are known, exact mass differences between unmodified and modified amino acids can be predicted. Indeed several algorithms, including SEQUEST, have built-in parametres for detecting such modifications.

However, the presence of a modified residue should always be confirmed experimentally. Another potential problem is the occurrence of nonspecific proteolysis. This depends on the purity of the cleavage agent used. Many algorithms will carry out peptide mass searches without a specified cleavage agent to take nonspecific proteolysis into consideration.

A common problem is that protein spots isolated from 2D-PAGE gels often contain a mixture of proteins and these contaminants may be difficult to identify. Finally, imperfect matches may result because the actual protein does not exist in the database, but a close homolog from the same species or a different species, which may have a related sequence, does exist. This is often the case if a protein contains a single nucleotide polymorphism leading to two or more variants. Programs such as MS-BLAST and CID entify use sequence candidates from tandem mass spectrometry data as the input for a homology search.

SECTION IV

COMPUTERS AND THEIR APPLICATIONS IN BIOINFORMATICS

## Chapter 9

Installing Bioinformatics Software in a Server-Based Computing Environment

INTRODUCTION

To support a diverse institutional program of genomics projects, it is often necessary to have an equally diverse and comprehensive software base. Although programs may come from many sources, it is important to make them easily accessible to the user community on a single computing platform. This chapter will outline the strategies for installing programs for a server-based molecular biology software resource, accessed by a large user base.

It is assumed that the reader is familiar with basic UNIX commands and concepts. The approaches discussed here are implemented in the BIRCH system (Website: http://home.cc.umanitoba.ca/~psgendb), but are generally applicable to any centralised multiuser software installation. The important parts of the process are described in either program documentation or UNIX documentation. The tricks and conventions that help to simplify the installation process will also be highlighted. This should give the novice an idea of what to expect before wading through the documentation.

RUNNING COMPUTER SOFTWARE

Software Frameworks for Bioinformatics

Software is a collective term for the various different programs that can run on computers. Software is distinguished from hardware, which refers to physical devices such as the processor, disk drives and monitor. On a stand-alone computer, software is divided into two categories: system software and application software. System software essentially comprises the computer's operating system and any other programs required to run applications, while application software is installed by the user for specific purposes (e.g. word processing, image analysis, etc.). On networked computers programs can also be run remotely. The same applies to computers attached to the internet.

Programs and Programming Languages

Computer programs can be written in a variety of programming languages, which are conventionally described in terms of three levels. The first level is machine code, which is the binary code used by the computer's own processor. The second level includes a number of languages known as assembly languages. The third and subsequent levels are grouped as higher-level languages and include widely used programming languages such as Pascal and C. Programs written in assembly or higher-level programming languages must be converted into machine code before they will run. For assembly languages, this process is known as assembly and for higher-level languages it is known as compilation. In Windows,

199

files in machine code are known as executable files and have the extension .exe. There are no rules or conventions for naming such files in UNIX systems and they are known as executable images. These files can be created and stored in the computer's memory until the operating system is told to run them. Alternatively, assembly or compilation can be carried out 'on the fly' if programs are executed remotely, for example over the internet.

Scripts and Scripting Languages

Executable files (Windows) and executable images (UNIX systems) are written in machine code and are run by the computer's processor. Other program files are designed to be executed by another program, and such files are known as scripts. There are a variety of scripting languages that can be used, including Microsoft Visual Basic, JavaScript and PERL. Script languages are easier work with than compiled languages, but take longer to process, so they are ideal for short programs.

Popular Languages in Bioinformatics

A number of programming, scripting and markup languages are popular with bioinformaticists because they are versatile and can integrate a wide variety of types of data either in a stand-alone environment or over the Internet. Some of these languages are discussed below:

HTML and JavaScript

HTML

HTML is hypertext markup language, a language used to specify the appearance of a hypertext document, including the positions of hyperlinks. Since HTML is not a programming language, basic hypertext documents are static. JavaScript is a popular scripting language that adds to the functionality of hypertext documents, allowing web pages to include such features as pop-up windows, animations and objects that change in appearance when the mouse cursor moves over them.

Java

Java is a versatile and portable programming language that is designed to generate applications that can run on all hardware platforms, from large servers to individual PCs, without modification. The Java source code is based on C++ and can be run in a stand-alone fashion or from within a hypertext document, in which case it is called an applet (small application). When executed, a Java program is converted into an intermediate language called bytecode, which is compiled into machine code as the program runs. Browsers must incorporate a Java plug-in interpreter called Java Virtual Machine for this purpose. Java applets may take a long time to download but the performance of the applet is not dictated by activities of the server. Java is a full programming language and is not the same as JavaScript, which is a scripting language. The names are similar because both languages use a similar syntax. As discussed above, JavaScript is used primarily to enhance world wide web (www) pages, while Java has a much broader scope.

PERL

Practical extraction and reporting language (PERL) is a versatile scripting language, which is widely used in bioinformatics for applications such as the analysis of sequence data. PERL is a free product, providing compatibility with Windows, UNIX or other operating systems. It has excellent facilities for file handling and uploading and downloading files over the www.

XML

XML stands for extensible markup language. This is a new standard markup language that allows files to be described in terms of the types of data they contain. As a replacement for HTML, XML has the advantage of controlling not only how data are displayed on a www page, but also how the data is processed by another program or by a database management system.

Running Programs Over the Internet

Software does not have to be downloaded and installed on local computers but can be run over the Internet. This can be achieved in two ways. If the programs are client-side, they are supplied for example as JavaScript or Java applets that are embedded in HTML within a hypertext document. The utility of these programs might be limited by the capacity of the local machine. Furthermore, although both Internet Explorer and Netscape Navigator support JavaScript, the script is interpreted in slightly different ways by the two browsers. There is currently no clean solution to this problem. The alternative is to use common gateway interface (CGI) programs or Java servlets, in which case the software is run on the server itself (the programs are server side). Server side programs can be written in machine code or in a scripting language such as PERL or Java. It is easy to detect whether the software is running on a server because the URL will typically end with the extension. cgi. The performance of CGI programs is dependent on the number of current users (the server load). Some servers avoid bottlenecks by carrying out client instructions (e.g. homology searches) in their own time and then E-mailing the results to the client.

COMPUTER OPERATING SYSTEMS

Operating Systems

On modern computers, the operating system is a master program that manages all peripheral hardware (e.g. monitor, keyboard, disk drives) and allows other software applications to run. There is a low-level operating system, sometimes called the basic input-output system (BIOS), which is largely or entirely in firmware (i.e. software stored in read-only memory). The BIOS handles activities such as deciding what to do when the computer is switched on after a cold start, reading and writing to disks, responding to input, displaying readable characters on the monitor and producing diagnostics. The higher-level operating system then takes over and the computer acquires a typical graphical user interface (GUI) such as Windows. Files that contain instructions for the operating system are called batch files in Windows and shell scripts in UNIX systems. For example, the Windows batch file AUTOEXEC.BA T is required to initialise the disk operating system when you switch on your PC (see below).

Windows

Windows is the most familiar operating system on home and office PCs and is wholly owned by Microsoft Corporation. Most stand-alone PCs currently run on Windows 95 or Windows 98 (often grouped as Windows 9x) or Windows Me. These operating systems are derived from the earlier Microsoft Disk Operating System (MS-DOS) and a GUI simply called Windows. From the launch of Windows 95, the GUI was integrated into the operating system and opens automatically when the operating system is loaded. Plain text files can be viewed without the benefit of the GUI using the DOS shell (a shell is an interactive interface between the user and an operating system, i.e. the part of the program that interprets and executes user commands). The DOS shell can be accessed from Windows by selecting Start,

Programs, MS-DOS Prompt. MS-DOS and early versions of Windows were designed to run on stand-alone PCs. Now networks of computers are commonplace, Windows has been developed as a multi-user operating system. In Windows NT and Windows 2000, different users can have access to both personal and common files, which may all be located on a central server. The latest version of Windows, Windows XP, is available tailored for either home (stand-alone) or business (network compatible) use.

UNIX

Although Windows is the most popular operating system on PCs, most commercial workstations and servers run under variations of an operating system called UNIX. Unlike Windows, UNIX is not owned by any of the large computer companies and since it is written in the standard programming language C, it has been modified and improved by many individuals, academic instructions and commercial companies for specific applications. There have been several public domain releases of operating systems that conform to the UNIX standard, such as GNU and LINUX. In particular, LINUX has become very popular in the scientific community. LINUX can be downloaded from the Internet or purchased at a nominal charge from one of several distributors. There are numerous GUIs for UNIX-like systems, which can be made to look like the familiar Windows or MacOS desktops. These include GNOME (GNU network object model environment), KDE (K desktop environment) and CDE (common desktop environment).

Other Operating Systems

Some older servers use the VMS operating system from the Digital Equipment Corporation (DEC). Apple Macintosh computers have their own operating system called MacOS, which has its own GUI. There is no simple way to view files on an Apple Macintosh without using the GUI. Other operating systems include OS/390, OS/400 and z/OS, which are used on some IBM computers.

SOFTWARE DOWNLOADING AND INSTALLATION

Downloading Methods

Computer software is often obtained on media such as floppy disks or CDs. CDs are the most versatile, not just because of their capacity (650 MB for a standard 72 minute disk and even more with data compression), but also because the standard file system, known as ISO 9660, is interpreted by all major computer platforms including Windows, MacOS and UNIX. However, it is often more convenient to download programs and other files from a local computer network or from the Internet. A file is downloaded when it is copied from a remote source onto a local computer. Conversely, a file is uploaded when it is copied from a computer's hard drive to a remote source. Downloading from the Internet can be achieved in three ways:

1. Files can be downloaded directly from a hypertext document.
2. Files can be obtained from an FTP server.
3. Files can be received by E-mail.

Downloading from a Hypertext Document

This is the simplest method and is usually a case of clicking the appropriate hypertext link. In many cases, the browser will automatically detect the embedded file type and initiate a download procedure. The user on the local computer is allowed to specify the destination of the downloaded file and its name, if the default name (from the server) is not appropriate or will overwrite an existing file. In other cases, clicking may attempt to open the file remotely, so it may be necessary to right click (on PCs) or hold (on Apple Macs) the link with the mouse and choose 'save as' to download the file. It is strongly recommended to have virus-checking software installed and running if you are performing regular downloads!

Downloading from an FTP Server

FTP stands for file transfer protocol and is a standard system for exchanging files over the internet. FTP servers may restrict access to authorised individuals, who have to enter a username and password to gain access to the files. However, in many cases access is free, and users can log in anonymously and download whatever they like. This is known as anonymous FTP. FTP servers host sites that contain lists of files arranged in a hierarchical directory. Files for public access are often located in a directory called 'public' or 'pub'. Some dedicated search tools, such as Archei, are available to locate specific files by searching directories of FTP sites. Otherwise, standard world wide web (www) search engines can be used to locate files. Note that for FTP sites running on UNIX servers, the file names are case sensitive. This is not the case for sites based on a Windows operating system or MacOS.

Nowadays, anonymous access to FTP sites is usually achieved by typing the name of the FTP server in an Internet browser address window or clicking on an appropriate link. Both Internet Explorer and Netscape Navigator support anonymous FTP. Such sites have addresses with the configuration ftp.name.org or similar, although the user may be required to type ftp:/ftp.name.org in the address bar of the browser rather than using the standard hypertext transfer protocol (http://......). Alternatively, a dedicated FTP program may be used to access the files. Such programs may have either a text or graphical user interface. Once the FTP site has been accessed, the anonymous user may be asked to log in and give a password, which should be 'anonymous' and an e-mail address respectively. The following UNIX-style commands are then used to access and download files:

ls	List directory of files on remote server
cd pub	Change directory to public files
cd pub/sequence	Change directory to public files in the directory 'sequences'
get sequence.gz	Download a file called sequence.gz (the suffix is explained below)
bye	Log off

FTP has some limited help facilities which can be accessed using the commands 'help' or '?'. The following commands are useful if large files are being downloaded:

prompt	Do not prompt for multiple access
verbose	Do not display output on the screen
mget*.gz	Multiple get all files with the specified name (* is used as a wildcard)
bg	Put the job in the background

Receiving Programs by E-mail

Programs and other files can also be received by e-mail. This is achieved by appending the file to the e-mail message as an attachment, which can be downloaded (saved) by the recipient. In many cases, the format of the attached file will be recognised automatically. However, with some local mail clients, the original format of the file may not be recognised and will be interpreted by default as a text file, in which case a program such as Microsoft Word is opened automatically and tries to read and present the data as text. This is generally successful for text documents but for other files, for example executable programs, images and other multimedia objects, the result is a random mix of letters, numbers and other characters.

Archiving and Compression

Most FTP sites store files in a compressed format, which reduces the file sizes (and therefore speeds up downloading) and also allows many files to be compressed together in a single entity called an archive. Different computer platforms have different compression systems, which are revealed by the file suffix. For Windows systems, files are usually compressed using PkZip or WinZip and have the extension .zip. For Apple Macintosh systems, the programs Stuffit and DropStuff are widely used. The compression formats include BinHex (suffix .hqx), Stuffit (suffix .sit) and self-extracting archive (suffix .sea). UNIX systems support UNIX compress and gzip (suffix .Z or .gz) for compression and tar (suffix .tar) for archiving.

Installation Methods

Once a program has been downloaded it must be installed and run on the local computer. If the file or file archive was compressed, it must first be uncompressed (expanded, unzipped, uncrunched, etc.) using utilities such as PkUnzip or Stuffit Expander. There are some very useful programs that allow cross-platform archiving and compression/uncompression. For example, UUencode will convert binary files from Windows, MacOS or UNIX platforms into ASCII format and allow their expansion on any of these machine types.

Once a program file is uncompressed it can be installed. In a Windows or MacOS environment, this can be achieved using the operating system utilities for installation or the expanded archive may include a file with the name install.exe or start.exe, which must be run from the desktop.

UNIX programs are usually distributed as source code because the C compiler and other programming utilities are part of the UNIX standard. If the downloaded file is called 'package.tar.gz' or 'package.tar.Z', the first job is to uncompress it using the instructions 'gunzip package.tar.gz' or 'uncompress package.tar.Z' and then to unpack the archive with 'tar xf package.tar'. This will recreate the file system. In a fairly simple case the new file system might contain a file called Makefile and the package should then be compiled with instructions such as: (i) make all, (ii) make test, (iii) make clean, and (iv) make install. With very simple cases, 'make' alone should suffice.

More complex packages may not have a Makefile and the authors may have written a script conventionally called configure. In this the user types './configure' to run the script and it will produce some diagnostics. The purpose of configure is to explore the local operating system, find out what utilities are available and already installed and (assuming there is no problem) to create Makefile.

DATABASE MANAGEMENTS

Flat Files and Markup Languages

On a computer system, a file is a discrete collection of bytes that can be manipulated (moved, copied, deleted, etc.) as a single entity. A file may either constitute a program or a data file that is processed by a program (e.g. a document that can be read by Microsoft Word). In the context of bioinformatics, files are used to store structured biological data. Most raw biological data can be stored in the form of text, for example nucleotide and protein sequences, protein structural co-ordinates and matrices of gene expression profiles. Text files can be handled by various software applications such as text editors (e.g. SimpleText), Internet browsers (e.g. Internet Explorer, Netscape Navigator) and word processor applications (e.g. Microsoft Word, Corel WordPerfect). Other types of biological data are stored as images, for example gene expression patterns and pictures of two-dimensional-protein gels. In some cases, the raw data in the images are converted into numbers that can be stored in text files. For example, this is the case for microarray image data.

Most software applications that handle text include a markup language that specifies how the text should be displayed on screen or in a printed document. These instructions comprise hidden character sets, known as tags. In Microsoft Word, for example, the markup language controls the font, size, colour, paragraph structure, etc. of the text. Other familiar markup languages include HTML (hypertext markup language), which controls the display of text on www pages and enables hyperlinks to be inserted and XML (extensible markup language), which allows the integral description of data objects. Such tags are often transparent, however, if the text is used by another software application, such as a sequence analysis program. Therefore, it is best to save biological data files in a simple format with no markup language. These text-only files are known as flat files. Text editor programs such as SimpleText and NotePad are suitable for handling flat files and flat files can be generated in word processor programs such as Microsoft Word by saving as text only.

Databases

A database is a collection of structured information, often stored in the form of flat files in the case of bioinformatics data. Individual database entries are known as records and each record comprises the same set of fields (categories of data). For example, in a sequence database such as GenBank, each record represents a deposited sequence and fields include accession number, sequence name, taxonomy of source species, literature references and the sequence itself. Computer databases are usually associated with software that allows the information to be accessed, amended and searched. This software is known as a database management system (DBMS) and also controls the security and integrity of the data. Searches are made possible by indexing the records, which in the case of flat files is achieved by looking for text strings in particular fields. In the case of a sequence database, the accession number could be used for index purposes. Several different types of database are used in bioinformatics.

A relational database is organised as tables, each table comprising a group of records (also known as tuples) with the same fields (known as attributes). This allows related data to be linked (reassembled) as required without reorganising the original tables. For example, a sequence table might contain records with the attributes accession number and protein sequence, while a function table might contain records with the attributes accession number and protein function. Matching attributes in different tables can be joined to bring together related records, in this case linking protein sequence and protein function. The industry-standard language used to interrogate and process data in a relational databases is SQL (symbolic query language). This is incorporated into familiar and widely used relational database management systems such as Microsoft Access and Oracle.

An object-oriented database has a more flexible organisation, that is, it does not depend on the formal 'table; row and column' format of relational databases. Data are defined as objects, which have a class hierarchy, that is, they can be grouped into classes and subclasses, etc. in a hierarchical manner. Properties attributable to classes of objects are inherited through the hierarchy; these may be general in the upper levels of the hierarchy but may become more specialised in the lower levels. Properties or procedures attributable to data objects are known as methods. The flexibility of the data organisation in object-orientated databases allows more complex relationships between datasets to be modeled than is possible with relational databases. Object-oriented database management systems are also capable of handling multimedia objects (pictures, videos and audio files) while relational DBMSs are often restricted to numbers, alphanumeric text and dates. Pure object-oriented DBMSs include Object Store and ONTOS DB. ACeDB (A *C. elegans* database) is an example of a customised object-oriented database. It is more common to see bioinformatics databases incorporating relational DBMS features in an object-oriented programming environment. Such object-relational DBMSs are generally accessed using a language based on SQL.

Developments in object-oriented programming have led to attempts to have object definitions that are common across different computer systems. This is useful for the integration of distributed databases, that is, databases that are physically stored on two or more separate computer systems. An interface definition called common object request brokering architecture (CORBA) has been developed which can be used to integrate large distributed bioinformatics databases. Software such as CORBA that functions as a conversion or translation layer in distributed systems is sometimes called middleware.

GUIDING PRINCIPLES FOR INSTALLATION

There are five guiding principles for installation and use that should be applied to help ensure a smooth operation:

1. Any user should be able to run any program from any directory simply by typing the name of the program and arguments. It should not be necessary to go to a specific directory to run a program.
2. System administration should be kept as simple as possible. This saves work for the Bioadmin[1], as well as increasing the likelihood that things will function properly ([1] Since bioinformatics software may be installed by a specialist other than UNIX system staff, the term bioadmin will refer to the person installing and maintaining bioinformatics software, distinct from system administrators).
3. Avoid interruption of service during installation and testing.
4. The Bioadmin should never have to modify individual user accounts.
5. Even if you have root access, do most of your work on a regular user account. Log in as root only when necessary.

NETWORKED COMPUTING ENVIRONMENT

The casual computer user learns only a narrow computing model: the PC mode. PCs are based on the idea that each person has their own computer that is completely self-contained, with all hardware, software and data residing physically on the desktop. Provisions for multiple users on a single machine (e.g. separate home directories, user accounts, file permissions) may exist, but are seldom taken into account by PC software developers. Each PC becomes a special case with special problems. The work of administration grows with the number of computers. Software has to be purchased and independently installed for each machine. Security and backup are often not practised.

UNIX greatly simplifies the problem of computing with a network-centric approach, in which any user can do any task from anywhere. Figure 9.1 illustrates computing in a network-centric environment. All data and software reside on a file server which is remotely mounted to one or more identically configured compute servers. Programs are executed on a compute server, but displayed at the user's terminal or PC. Regardless of whether one logs in from an X11 terminal, a PC running an X11 server, a PC using the VNC viewer or an internet appliance the user's desktop screen looks the same and opens to the user's HOME directory. Consequently, any user can do any task from any device, anywhere on the internet.

LEVERAGING THE MULTI-WINDOW DESKTOP

The installation process involves moving back and forth among several directories, which is most effectively accomplished by viewing each directory in a separate window. One of the issues that makes the typical PC desktop awkward to use is the one window owns the screen model. In MS-Windows, most applications default to take up the entire screen. One moves between applications using the task bar. Although it is possible to resize windows so that many can fit on one screen, this is seldom done, in MS-Windows. On Macintosh, even when multiple windows are present, they depend on the menu at the top of the screen. This requires the user to first select a window by clicking on it and then to choose an item from the menu at the top of the screen. Even worse, the menus often look almost identical from program to program, so that it is not obvious when the focus has shifted to a new application.

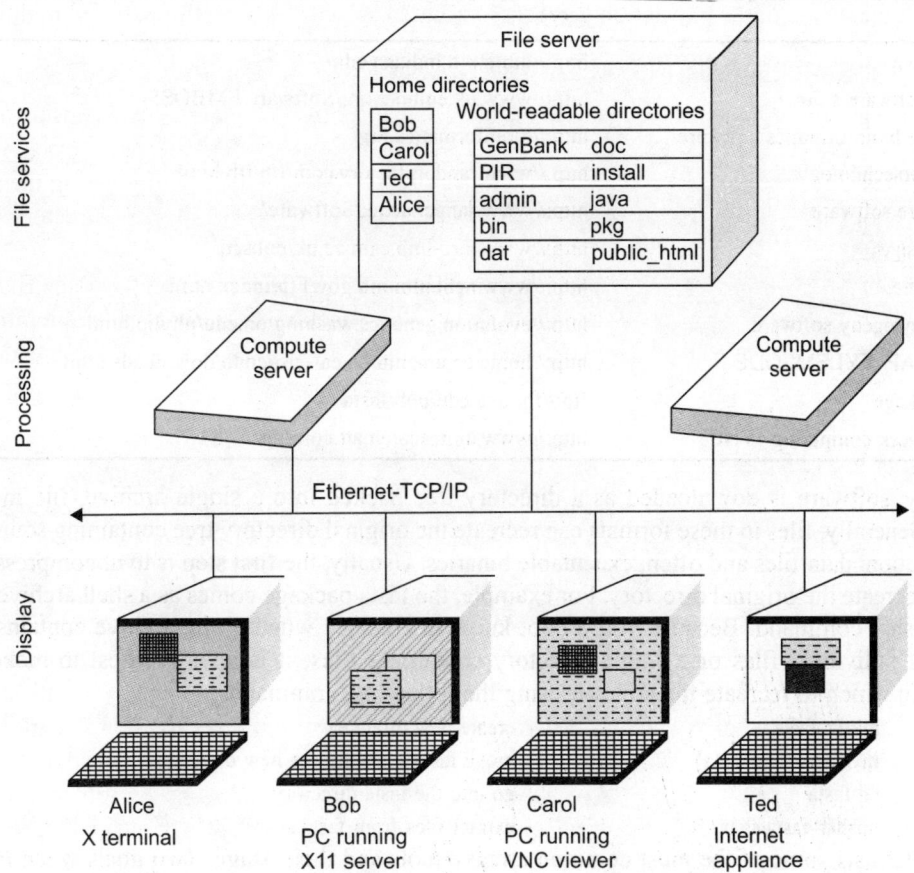

Fig. 9.1. Network-centric computing.

On UNIX desktops, menus are found within the windows themselves. This decreases the amount of distance the eye has to cover. Focus moves with the mouse and does not need to be switched with the taskbar. The user simply moves from one window to another to work. Because UNIX tends to be oriented towards multiple windows, UNIX users tend to favour larger monitors. More screen real estate means more space for windows. The screen is crowded because it was generated at 1024 × 768 resolution. Although this is a common resolution for PCs, the UNIX community tends to work with larger monitors, at 19″ diagonal or larger, running at 1280×1000 or higher resolution. To provide further real estate, UNIX desktops such as CDE, KDE and GNOME support switching between several desktops at the push of a button.

FINDING AND DOWNLOADING SOFTWARE

Table 9.1 has a short and by no means exhaustive list of sites where freely available sequence analysis software can be downloaded. USENET newsgroups such as bionet.software contain announcements of new software and updates, as well as discussion on molecular biology software.

Table 9.1. Sources of free downloadable software.

Source	URL
IUBio archive	http://iubio.bio.indiana.edu/
EMBOSS software suite	http://www.uk.embnet.org/Software/EMBOSS/
Open source bioinformatics software	http://bioinformatics.org/
Linux for biotechnology	http://www.randomfactory.com/lfb/lfb.html
Sanger centre software	http://www.sanger.ac.uk/Software/
Staden package	http://www.mrc-lmb.cam.ac.uk/pubseq/
NCBI FIP site	http://www.ncbi.nlm.nih.gov/Ftp/index.html
PHYLIP Phylogeny software	http://evolution.genetics.washington.edu/phylip.html
BIRCH, FSAP, XYLEM, GDE	http://home.cc.umanitoba.ca/~psgendb/downloads.html
FASTA package	ftp://ftp.uva.edu/pub/fasta/
Virtual network computing (VNC)	http://www.uk.research.att.com/vnc/

Usually, software is downloaded as a directory tree packed into a single archive, file in various formats. Generally, files in these formats can recreate the original directory tree containing source code, documentation, data files and often, executable binaries. Usually, the first step is to uncompress the file and then recreate the original directory. For example, the fasta package comes as a shell archive created using the shar command. Because you do not know in advance whether the archive contains a large number of individual files or a single directory containing files, it is always safest to make a new directory in which to recreate the archive, using the following, commands:

mkdir fasta	create new directory
mv fasta.shar fasta	move fasta.shar into the new directory
cd fasta	go into the fasta directory
unshar fasta.shar	extract files from fasta.shar

Table 9.2 lists some of the most common archive tools and their usage. Two goals when installing software are to: (i) avoid interruption of service for users during installation and testing, and (ii) having the option of deleting programs after evaluation. For example, a separate directory called install could hold separate directories for each package during the installation.

UNDERSTAND THE PROBLEM BEFORE YOU BEGIN

For many standard office tasks, it is possible to get by without ever reading the documentation. In molecular biology, the task itself often has enough complexity that it may not be possible to simply launch, point and click. In practice, it is almost always faster to read the documentation before trying to install. Each program will have installation instructions.

Table 9.2. Archive commands.

File extension	Utility	Archive command	Unarchive command
.tar	UNIX tar	To create a tar file from a directory called source: tar cvf source.tar source	To recreate the directory: tar xvf source.tar
.zip	ZIP	To create a compressed archive file called source.zip: zip source source	To recreate the directory: unzip source
.shar	UNIX shar	To create a shar file from a directory named source: shar source > source.shar	To recreate the directory: unshar source.shar or chmod $u + x$ source.shar or shar source.shar[a]
.gz	GNU zip	To compress a file with: gzip source > source.gz	To recreate the directory: gunzip source
.Z	compress	To compress source. tar: compress source.tar	To uncompress source.tar.Z: uncompress source.tar.Z
.uue	uuencode	To encode source.tar.Z using ASCII characters: uuencode source.tar.Z source.uue	To recreate the original binary file: uudecode source.uue

[a] .shar files are actually shell scripts that can be executed to recreate the original directory.

These will let you know about important options like where the final program files will reside and which environment variables must be set. Reading the documentation at this stage gives you a chance to learn more about what the program does and to decide if it is really what you need. This weeding out phase can save a lot of unnecessary compiling, organising and testing.

COMPILATION

Program distributed as source code, for which no binaries are available, will require compilation and linking steps. Although these procedures vary somewhat with the language in which they are written, most of the common packages use protocols of the C and C++ family of languages. In addition to source files (.c), code items such as type definitions, which need to be shared, are found in header files (.h). When you compile, the code from the header files is inserted into C code and the .c file translated to machine code, which is written as object modules (.o). Next, the compiler calls a linked, which links object modules into a final executable file. In most programs, object modules from standard libraries (e.g. Tcl/Tk) are also linked. These are typically linked dynamically, meaning that only a reference to the libraries is made and the actual library modules are loaded each time the program is run. Consequently, dynamic linking saves disk space. However, when a program depends on libraries that may not be found on all systems, static linking can be accomplished, in which object modules are written to the final executable code file. Static linking favours portability at the expense of disk space. A short list of the types of files frequently encountered during installation appears in Table 9.3.

Virtually all scientific program packages automate these procedures using the make program. The *make* program reads a Makefile, containing compilation, linking and installation options. For cross-platform compatibility, it is common to include separate Makefiles for each platform (e.g. SGI, Linux, Windows, Solaris). For example, the fasta package has a file called Makefile.sun for Solaris systems. Copy Makefile.sun to Makefile and edit Makefile as needed for your system. At the beginning of the

Makefile, variables are often set to specify the final destinations for files. On our system, fasta's Makefile would be edited to change the line reading XDIR = /seqprog/sbin/bin to XDIR = /home/psgendb/bin. Because this directory is in the $PATH for all BIRCH users, the new programs become available to all users as soon as the files are copied to this location.

Table 9.3. Common file types and file extensions.

File extension	File type
.c	C source code
.h	C header
.o	Compiled object file
no extension	Executable binary file
.1, .l	UNIX manual page
.makefile, .mak	Makefile

Typing make executes the commands in Makefile, compiling and linking the programs. It is best to run make in a terminal window that supports scrolling, so that all warning and error messages can be examined. This is particularly important because one can then copy error messages to a file to provide the author of the program with a precise description of the problem. If the authors do not receive this feedback, the problems do not get fixed. However, feedback must be precise and detailed.

If make is successful, executable binary files, usually with no extension, are written to the target directory. This may or may not be the current working directory. Many Makefiles require you to explicitly ask for files to be copied to the destination directory by typing make install.

In some cases, testing can be carried out at this point, particularly if a test script is included with the package. In the fasta package several test scripts are found. For example, ./test.sh will run most of the fasta programs with test datafiles.

Note: './' forces the shell to look for test.sh in the current working directory. Unless '.' was in your $PATH, it would not be found. However, it is generally considered insecure to include '.' in your $PATH.

It is important to check test scripts to see where they look for executable files. For example, if the script sets $PATH to '.' (the current directory) or if programs are executed with a statement such as ./fasta33, then the shell will look for an executable file in the current directory. If the directory for the executable file is not explicitly set, the shell will search all directories in your $PATH to find an executable file. This could either result in a *command not found* message or if earlier copies of the programs were already installed, older programs will execute, not the newly compiled programs.

INSTALLATION

In the BIRCH system, all files and directories are found in a world-readable directory specified by the $DB environment variable.

Thus, $DB/bin, $DB/doc and $DB/dat refer to directories containing executable binaries, documentation and datafiles used by programs, respectively, as summarised below.

$DB/bin

Although $DB/bin could in principle be set to refer to /usr/local/bin, it is probably best to keep the entire $DB structure separate from the rest of the system. This approach has the advantage that the Bioadmin need not have root privileges. All files in $DB/bin should be world-executable.

One practice for managing program upgrades is to create a symbolic link to point to the current production version of the program. For example, a link with the name fasta might point to fasta3:

lrwxrwxrwx 1 psgendb psgendb 6 Jul 18 09:45/home/psgendb/bin/fasta3 -> fasta*

To upgrade to fasta33:

rm fasta

ln -s fasta33 fasta

lrwxrwxrwx 1 psgendb psgendb 6 Jul 18 09:45/home/psgendb/bin/fasta33 -> fasta*

Aside from giving users a consistent name for the current most recent version of the program, this type of stable link eliminates the need to modify other programs that call the upgraded program.

$DB/doc

Documentation files for software should be moved to this directory. Ideally, the complete contents of this directory should be Web-accessible. Where a program or package has more than one documentation file, create a separate subdirectory for each program. All files should be world-readable.

$DB/dat

A program should never require that ancillary files such as fonts or scoring matrices be in a user's directory. These should always be centrally installed and administered, transparently to the user. Datafiles required for programs, such as scoring matrices, lists of restriction enzymes and so forth should be moved to this directory. Generally, each program should have its own subdirectory. All files should be world-readable.

$DB/admin

This directory contains scripts and other files related to software administration. First time BIRCH users run the *newuser* script, to append a line to the user's login file:

> source/home/psgendb/admin/login.source

And to the .cshrc file:

> source/home/psgendb/admin/cshrc.source

These files respectively contain commands that are executed when the user first logs in and each time a program is started. All environment variables, aliases and other settings required to run these programs are set in these files. Having run *newuser* once, a user should never have to do any setup tasks to be able to run new or updated programs. When a new program is added, the environment variables and aliases needed are specified in cshrc.source and therefore become immediately available to the user community. The net effect is that the bioadmin should never have to go to each user's account when a new program is installed.

Where programs require first-time setup, such as a configuration file being written to the user's $HOME directory, the program should be run from a wrapper script that checks for the presence of that file. If the file is not present, the script writes a default copy of the file to $HOME. The user should never have to explicitly run a setup script before using a program.

All directories that are to be accessible to users must be world searchable (world executable), as well as world-readable. For example, to allow users to read files in $DB/doc/fasta, both $DB/doc and $DB/doc/fasta must be world executable.

Use:

Chmod a+rx $DB/doc/fasta

Special Considerations for Complex Packages

Some packages come as integrated units whose components cannot be moved out of their directory structure to $DB/bin, $DB/dat and $DB/doc. Packages of this type are installed in $DB/pkg. A good case in point is the Staden Package (Table 9.1). The BIRCH login.source file contains the following lines:

Initialise Staden Package Settings
Setenv STADENROOT $DB/pkg/staden
Source $STADENROOT/staden.login

that cause the commands in staden.login to be executed when the user logs in. This script in turn sets several environment variables referencing files in the $STADENROOT directory. As well, login.source adds $DB/pkg/staden/solaris-bin to the $PATH. This illustrates that there are sometimes no simple solutions. On one hand, it would be desirable to simply copy all Staden binaries into $DB/bin. However this has the effect of making it difficult to identify the origin of specific programs in $DB/bin as being part of the Staden Package. On the other hand, symbolic links from $DB/bin to each of the programs in $DB/pkg/staden/solaris-bin would provide a compromise. This would require that links be individually maintained.

Documentation and data can be linked more easily in $DB/doc. The following command:

In -s $STADENROOT/doc staden

creates a link to the Staden documentation directory, while in $DB/dat and

In -s $STADENROOT staden

creates a link to the main Staden directory, from which the user can find several directories with sample datafiles. In this fashion, the $DOC and $DAT directories appear to contain staden subdirectories.

On Linux systems, complex packages are maintained using programs such as Red Hat Package Manager (RPM). RPM automates package installation, often requiring no user input. As files are copied to their destinations, their locations are recorded in the RPM database (/usr/lib/rpm). In addition to installation, RPM automates package updating, verification and deinstallation. Tools such as RPM make it possible to install software in system directories such as /usr/local/bin or /usr/bin without making these directories unmanageable. The one disadvantage is that installation in system directories can only be accomplished with root permissions.

Special Considerations for Java Applications

Java applications should be installed in a central location, such as $DB/java. Ideally, all that should be required is the inclusion of $DB/java in the $CLASSPATH environment variable. The java virtual machine (JVM) would search this location at runtime. However, the precise commands needed to launch an application vary, so that no single solution exists. For example, some applications are completely contained in a single .jar file, while others require a complex directory structure containing large numbers of objects and datafiles. Consequently, Java applications should be launched from wrappers: short scripts that reside in $DB/bin and call the application. For example, a script called $DB/bin/readseq runs the Java implementation of readseq (available from IUBio, see Table 9.1).

CALLING PROGRAMS FROM A GRAPHIC FRONT-END

Several options exist for unifying a large software base with a graphic front end. Programs such as GDE (Table 9.1), SeqLab from the GCG package (see Website: http://www.accelrys.com) or SeqPup (see Table 9.1, IUBio) allow the Bioadmin to add external programs to their menus, as specified in easy-to-edit configuration files. In general, the user selects one or more sequences to work with and then chooses a program from the main menu. A window pops up, allowing parametres to be set. The front end then generates a UNIX command to run the program with these parametres, using the selected sequences.

In many cases, it is best for the front end to call a wrapper that verifies and checks the parametres and sequences, then executes the program. This is especially important for programs from packages such as FSAP or PHYLIP (Table 9.1), which operate through text-based interactive menus. If a prompt does not receive a valid response, programs of this type may go into an infinite loop that prompts for a response.

LAUNCHING PROGRAM FROM THE WORKSPACE MENU

The workspace menu is yet another avenue through which users can find programs. Figure 9.2 shows a CDE workspace menu organised categorically.

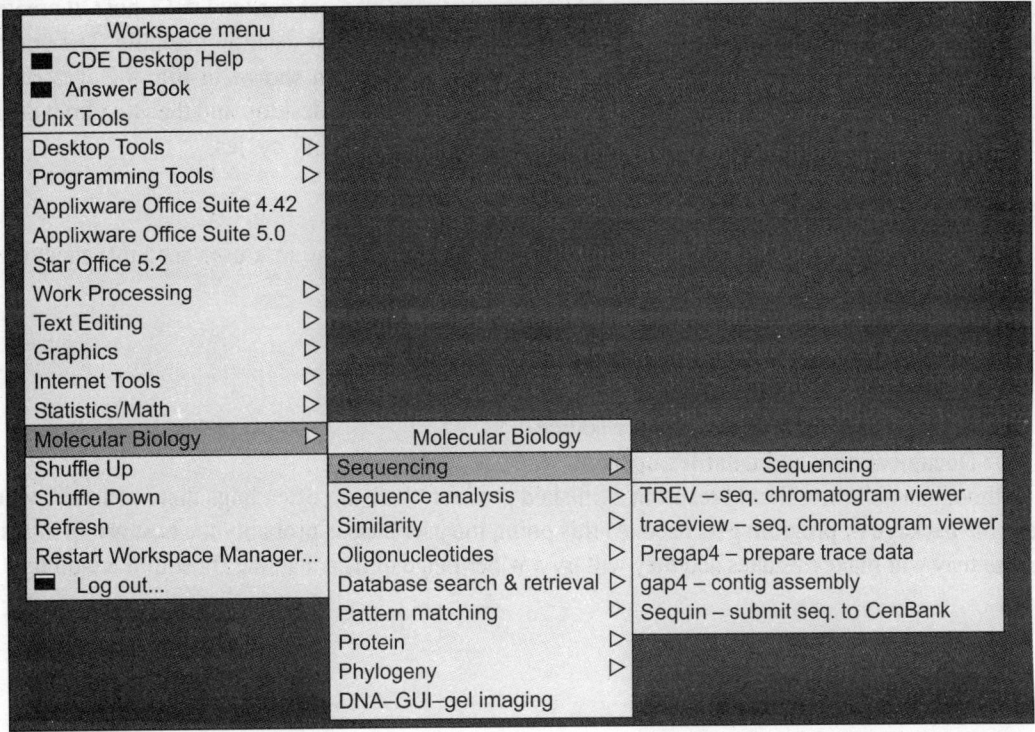

Fig. 9.2. The CDE workspace menu.

At the highest level are the main categories of programs, including standalone items for office packages. The molecular biology menu is further divided into submenus. For example, the Sequencing submenu contains programs that together cover all steps in the sequencing process, including reading the raw chromatograms, vector removal, contig assembly and submission to GenBank. The downside of the workspace menu is that it is incomplete, as command line applications, cannot be launched from the workspace menu.

One should be able to launch GUI applications from the workspace menu, defaulting to the user's $HOME directory. In the CDE desktop, this is specified in the .dt directory. Most recent UNIX desktops, such as CDE 1.4 and GNOME use tree-structured directories to define the structure of the workspace menu. Again, it is important to avoid having to update individual user accounts. The easiest way is to create a directory for molecular biology programs on the Bioadmin's account and have new users run a script creating a symbolic link from their workspace menu directory (e.g. .dt/Desktop) to the Bioadmin's directory. Subsequently, all updates to the Bioadmin's menu will become available to all users.

TESTING

Testing should not be carried out using the account that owns the programs (e.g. root). Testing should always be done in a regular user account. One reason is that testing on a user account will uncover incorrect permissions. This is likely the single most common installation error. At the same time, it is probably also best to test in a subdirectory, rather than in the $HOME directory, to fully demonstrate that the program can be run from anywhere.

Using VNC (Table 9.1), one can easily eliminate login/logout cycles between your Bioadmin account and your user account. The vncserver is an X11 server that runs on a networked UNIX host. It creates an X11 screen in memory. To display that screen, run vncviewer on your desktop machine. The complete UNIX desktop appears in a window. For example, the entire screen shown in Fig. 9.2 was run in a vncviewer window. Thus, switching back and forth between the user desktop and the Bioadmin desktop is as easy as switching between windows, facilitating rapid test-modify cycles.

INSTALLATION CHECKLIST

Before announcing updates or new programs, go through the package in a user account, checking the following:
1. All files world-readable (chmod a+r filename).
2. All binaries world-executable (chmod a+x filename).
3. All directories world-searchable (chmod a+x directoryname).
4. Environment variable set in cshrc.source.
5. Documentation and datafiles updated.

Although installation should result in a finished product, there are often bugs that need to be worked out as the package or program gets used. At this point, the user base is probably the best group of testers, because they will make mistakes and they will try a wider range of data than the Bioadmin would try.

## Chapter 10

Management of a Server-Based Bioinformatics Resources

INTRODUCTION

The strategies for managing a server-based molecular biology software resource, accessed by a diverse user community has been discussed in the previous chapters. It assumes that the reader is familiar with basic UNIX commands and concepts. The approaches discussed here are implemented in the BIRCH system (see website: http://home.cc.umanitoba.ca/~psgendb) but are generally applicable to any centralised multiuser software installation.

Most major UNIX distributions now come with graphic tools that simplify many administration tasks. It is, therefore, realistic to act as your own *sysadmin*. In fact many of the principles discussed are valid in the larger context of a general purpose multiuser system. Although general system administration is a broad field, particular attention should be paid to: daily and weekly backups, both onsite and offsite; security, including rapid installation of security patches; management of user accounts; and disk space to minimise the work and know-how needed on the part of the user. These topics are beyond the scope of this chapter and are covered extensively in books on system administration, on USENET newsgroups in the compo section and at various HOWTO websites.

KEY FACTORS AND CONSIDERATIONS

The key factors and considerations when implementing the system are:
1. A user base with a diverse set of needs and usually minimal informatics training.
2. A diverse software base, comprised of programs from many authors, in many languages and in many styles.
3. Documentation written in many formats and styles.
4. A complex networked server system.
5. Limitations of disk space and computing resources.

This chapter builds on the organisational scheme and to summarise, the resource is located in a world-readable directory tree referenced by the $DB environment variable. Program binaries, documentation and ancillary datafiles are located in $DB/bin, $DB/doc and $DB/dat, respectively. To use the resource, user accounts are set up by running the newuser script. This appends a set of configuration commands from $DB/admin/login.source and $DB/admin/cshrc.source to their .login and .cshrc files. The commands in these files are executed when a user logs in or starts a new shell. Thus, as the central configuration is updated, all users have immediate access to the updates.

MANAGING DOCUMENTATION

Documentation is the user's entry point into the system. Keeping documentation organised, accessible and updated accomplishes several tasks. First, it helps to bring out difficulties that users may face when running programs. Second, it forces the Bioadmin to see the software base from the user's perspective. Third, well-organised documentation works to the Bioadmin's advantage, making it easy to refer users to the appropriate documentation, rather than having to answer the same question over and over. While installation of documentation should be straightforward, there are a few considerations for providing a consistent web-accessible documentation library.

HTML

HTML is rapidly becoming the most common format for documentation because of its dynamic capabilities and universal availability. However, it is probably best to keep a local copy of the program documentation on your website, rather than simply linking to the author's website. An author's website will probably describe the most recent version of the software, which may not be installed on your system. If the author stops supporting a software package, he or she may no longer keep documentation on a website. Thus, installation of a local copy of the documentation that was obtained at the time the package was installed is guaranteed to accurately describe the version of the software currently installed.

UNIX Manual Pages

BIRCH has a directory for manual pages called $DB/manl. All files in this directory should be in the form name.l (where l stands for local). In login.source, the line:

setenv MANPATH $MANPATH\:$DB

tells UNIX to look for the manual pages in this directory, as well as in any other directory specified in the system's $MANPATH. For example, to read the documentation for align, the user types man align and the file $DB/manl/align.l will be displayed. To display on the web, UNIX manual pages can be converted to ASCII text by redirecting the output from the man command to an ASCII file, e.g.

man fasta > fasta.txt

Postscript and PDF

Although PostScript viewers are usually available on most UNIX workstations, acroread, the Adobe Acrobat Reader, has been universally adopted. Therefore, it is probably safest to convert postscript files to PDF for web accessibility using ps2pdf, e.g. ps2pdf primer3.ps, will create a file called primer3.pdf. ps2pdf is included with most UNIX distributions.

ASCII Text

All web browsers can display ASCII text. It should be noted that file extensions such as .txt or .asc are probably best to use, because these are not commonly used by application software. ASCII files with .doc extensions should be changed to some other extension to avoid confusion with Microsoft WORD files.

Word Processor Documents

Import filters are often less than satisfactory. Therefore, when documentation is in a format specific to a word processor such as WordPerfect, StarOffice Writer, Applix Words or Microsoft Word, it is best to convert it to the PDF format. Some programs can directly save or print to PDF, while others can only print to PostScript. For the latter, convert to PDF using ps2pdf as noted earlier.

COMMUNICATING WITH THE USER BASE

Login Messages

Brief announcements can be printed at the user's terminal by including a statement such as cat ~psgendb/admin/Login_Message the in login.source, where Login_Message contains a few lines of text with the current announcements. This message is printed in each terminal window.

Web Site Organisation

The BIRCH website provides a number of views to the system (Fig. 10.1). The New User section provides documents that describe BIRCH, how to set up accounts, and how to learn the system. The Documentation section provides tutorials and other resources for users to develop their informatics skills while getting useful work done. Finally, the complete online documentation is available in the Software and Database sections, describing the full functionality of the system. All login messages are archived in the file WHATSNEW.html, which can be viewed in a scrolling window entitled BIRCH ANNOUNCEMENTS. This file provides links to more detailed information than appears in login messages, so that even users who have been away from the system for a while won't miss important changes.

Discussion Groups

Although online discussions can be conducted through a mailing list, these often become an annoyance as the number of users increase and the number of lists one subscribes to increases. Most web browsers such as Netscape and Internet Explorer/Outlook Express, as well as third-party applications, can be used to read and participate in discussions on USENET newsgroups. Many users are familiar with worldwide groups, including the bionet groups (e.g. bionet.software, bionet.molbio.genearrays). However, it is also possible to have local newsgroups on any system that operates a newsserver, as do most campus UNIX systems.

The local news Bioadmin can easily create a group such as local.bioinformatics or local.genomics that will be accessible to the local user community.

Remote Consultation Using VNC

Remote consultation on UNIX platforms is now greatly enhanced by Virtual Network Computing (VNC). VNC is a package of programs freely distributed by AT&T (Website: http://www.uk.research.att.com/vnc/). In essence, vncserver creates an XII desktop session on a remote login host, which keeps an image of the screen in memory. A copy of vncviewer, running on a PC or workstation anywhere in the world with a high-speed internet connection, can display and control the screen as if it were running locally. VNC is available for MS-Windows, Macintosh and UNIX. The vncviewer can also run as a Java applet in a web browser, so that vncviewer does not have to be installed on the local machine: Thus, regardless of where you are, your UNIX desktop looks and acts the same.

For remote consultation, assume that a user has phoned the Bioadmin with a problem. If it cannot be easily described over the phone, the user changes their VNC password using vncpw and tells the Bioadmin the new password. Next the user starts up a copy of vncserver:

```
vncserver -alwaysshared
New 'X' desktop is mira:8
```

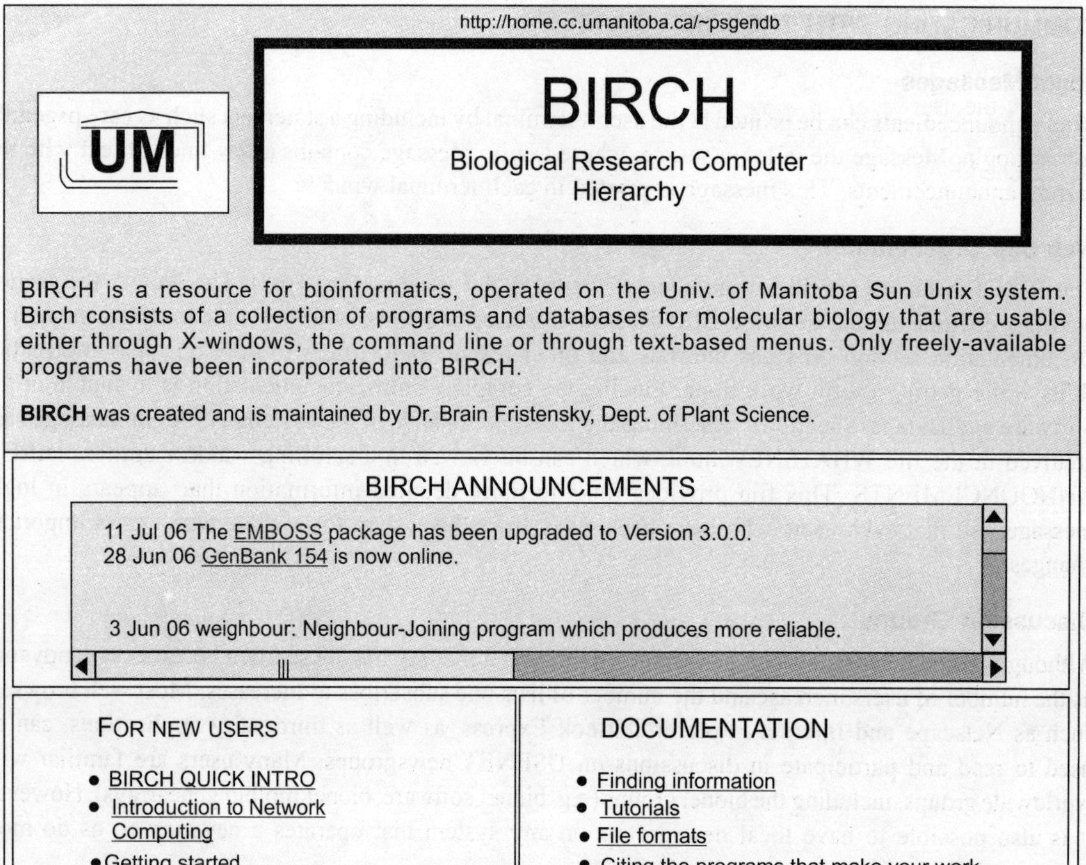

http://home.cc.umanitoba.ca/~psgendb

BIRCH

Biological Research Computer
Hierarchy

[UM]

BIRCH is a resource for bioinformatics, operated on the Univ. of Manitoba Sun Unix system. Birch consists of a collection of programs and databases for molecular biology that are usable either through X-windows, the command line or through text-based menus. Only freely-available programs have been incorporated into BIRCH.

BIRCH was created and is maintained by Dr. Brain Fristensky, Dept. of Plant Science.

BIRCH ANNOUNCEMENTS

11 Jul 06 The EMBOSS package has been upgraded to Version 3.0.0.
28 Jun 06 GenBank 154 is now online.

3 Jun 06 weighbour: Neighbour-Joining program which produces more reliable.

FOR NEW USERS

- BIRCH QUICK INTRO
- Introduction to Network Computing
- Getting started
- Using CDE
- Using Unix

DOCUMENTATION

- Finding information
- Tutorials
- File formats
- Citing the programs that make your work possible

SOFTWARE

Hightlights of selected software applications

- Molecular Biology Software
- Genetics Software
- Gene Array Software
- ACN Software List
- X-windows Software summary
- Downloadable Software

DATABASES

- GenBank (DNA/RNA): /home/psgendb/GenBank
- PIR (protein): /home/psgendb/PIR
- GenPept – translation of GenBank CDS (protein) features: /home/psgendb/GenPept
- ACeDB – Laboratory Database Management

LINKS

- Molecular Biology etc.
- Bioinformatics

Fig. 10.1. Organisation of web-based documentation on the BIRCH home page (see Website: http:// home.cc.umanitoba.ca/~psgendb).

The alwaysshared option makes it possible for more than one user to simultaneously display the same desktop. The message tells the user that vncserver has created desktop 8 on host mira.

Next, the user and Bioadmin each type: vncviewer mira:8 followed by the password, and the same vncviewer window will appear on both of their screens. If connecting via a browser, vncviewer would be launched by setting the URL to http://mira.cc.umanitoba.ca:5808, where the last two digits in 5808 indicate the screen number.

Now, both the user and Bioadmin can see and control the same desktop while discussing the various operations over the phone. The user can run a-program that is causing difficulty and the Bioadmin can see everything that happens. The Bioadmin can demonstrate in real time what the user should be doing and if necessary, datafiles or configuration files such as .cshrc can be examined.

At the end of the session, the Bioadmin reminds the user to kill the VNC session by typing vncserver. -kill :8 and to change their VNC password.

The real value of VNC becomes apparent when travelling. For example, applications such as Powerpoint produce static presentations and most people travel with their own lap top to ensure that it will work. As long as a fast Internet connection is available, the full functionality of the desktop can be demonstrated anywhere there is a computer and a data projector.

DETECTING, HANDLING AND PREVENTING PROBLEMS

A multiuser system poses challenges in terms of managing shared resources, such as CPU time, memory, disk space and network bandwidth. Usually it is possible to design a system that will minimise user errors and in most cases UNIX is intrinsically protected from most catastrophes. For example, so that the permissions are explicitly set otherwise, a user can only read or modify files belonging to him and usually these can only reside in the $HOME directory.

Disk Space

$HOME directories should always reside in a separate file system and user quotas should be set, regardless of how much disk space exists. The one filesystem that is potentially troublesome is /tmp, which is writeable by all users. In the event that /tmp becomes full, programs that need to write temporary files may hang, resulting in a filesystem full error. The best way to avoid this problem is to have applications write temporary files to the current working directory, so that in the worst case, only the user is affected.

CPU Time

Monitoring CPU usage

Keeping track of CPU usage is critically important. The top command gives you a real-time picture of the most CPU intensive jobs currently running on the host you are logged into.

If you type top at the command line, your system will generate similar information to the following:

last pid: 13912; load averages: 2.61, 1.64, 1.31 13:48:41

504 processes: 488 sleeping, 1 running, 6 zombie, 7 stopped, 2 on cpu

CPU states: 16.4% idle, 65.7% user, 17.9% kernel, 0.0% iowait, 0.0% swap

Memory: 640M real, 17M free, 846M swap in use, 3407M swap free

PID	Username	THR	PRI	NICE	SIZE	RES	STATE	TIME	CPU	COMMAND
11371	umamyks	13	10	0	77M	71M	CPU/0	23: 19	64.27%	matlab
27668	frist	10	58	0	97M	56M	sleep	3:06	3.49%	soffice.bin

13894	frist	1	33	0	3344K	1672K	cpu/1	0:01	1.65%	top
13898	umnorthv	1	58	0	6424K	4352K	sleep	0:00	0.82%	pine.exe
1629	mills	7	0	0	9992K	7840K	sleep	0:24	0.42%	dtwn
13704	mhbasri	1	38	0	1464K	1360K	sleep	0:01	0.31%	elm.exe
9797	syeung	1	58	0	1000K	816K	sleep	267:53	0.28%	newmail
6914	umtirzit	8	58	0	13M	3992K	sleep	26:38	0.23%	dtmail
26524	mgarlich	1	58	0	9376K	6960K	sleep	0:10	0.23%	dtterm
29993	simosko	1	58	0	6824K	4528K	sleep	0:21	0.23%	pine.exe
7937	jayasin	1	58	0	6112K	3816K	sleep	6:55	0.22%	Xvnc
4483	francey	7	48	0	9904K	7920K	sleep	0:24	0.21%	dtwm
206	root	6	58	0	76M	8024K	sleep	458:13	0.20%	automountd
27272	frist	7	58	0	11M	8376K	sleep	0:35	0.20%	dtwm
580	syeung	1	48	0	2376K	1976K	sleep	2:56	0.19%	irc-2.6

This display is updated every few seconds in the terminal window. To quit, type q. The top command has many options. For example, you can sort jobs by memory used or list only jobs under a given userid. The owner of a job can also kill that job using top. Type man top for full documentation.

The ps command with no arguments tells which jobs are running in the current shell (the current window):

```
ps
```

PID	TTY	Time	CMD
2122	pts/l04	0:00	dsdm
27401	pts/l04	2:18	mozilla-
27376	pts/l04	0:00	netscape
2082	pts/104	0:00	zwgc
27384	pts/l04	0:00	netscape
27396	pts/l04	0:00	run-mozi
2024	pts/l04	0:18	Xvnc
2041	pts/l04	0:00	Xsession
27305	pts/l04	0:01	csh
27381	pts/l04	0:00	netscape
27457	pts/l04	0:14	java_vm

while

```
ps -u userid
```

tells which jobs are running under a given userid on the host you are logged into.

The following list summarises the types of tasks that tend to require a lot of processing time:

Jobs that tend to be CPU-intensive

1. Phylogenetic analysis:
   (a) Distance matrix methods (e.g. neighbour joining, FITCH): Very fast, the amount of time increases in a linear fashion with the number of sequences.
   (b) Parsimony (e.g. DNAPARS, PROTPARS): Moderately efficient, the amount of time increases exponentially with the number of sequences.

    (c) Maximum likelihood (e.g. DNAML, PROTML, fastDNAML): Very slow, the amount of time increases according to a FACTORIAL function of the number of sequences.

2. Sequence database searches: The amount of time that is required is proportional to product of sequence length and database size; use high k values to speed up a search; protein searches are faster than DNA.

3. Multiple sequence alignments (e.g. CLUSTALX): Cluster type alignments scale linearly in proportion to the number of sequences.

4. Retrievals of large numbers of sequences: The time required is linear, related to number of sequences.

5. The efficiency of any sorting operation with a large number of items depends on the sort algorithm used.

6. Statistical and mathematical packages (e.g. SAS, MATLAB).

Jobs that should never be CPU intensive

If the following applications are using significant percentages of CPU time, they are not functioning normally and are probably runaway jobs:

1. Graphic front ends: Programs such as GDE, SeqLab or SeqPup by themselves do almost nothing. If you see one using a substantial amount of CPU time, it is probably a runaway job. One exception is when reading large sequence files, e.g. large numbers of sequences or very long sequences that are placed in memory for analysis.

2. Most user apps (e.g. word processors, mailers, spread sheets, drawing programs).

3. Desktop tools (e.g. text editors, filemanagers).

4. Most UNIX commands.

5. Web browsers: For short bursts browsers can be very CPU-intensive, but this should not persist for more than a minute or two.

Managing long-running jobs

On any multitasking system, all jobs are assigned priorities that govern the amount of CPU time allocated to them. In UNIX, the nice command determines the priority. Most user commands default to a nice value of 0. This is especially important for applications run through a graphic interface, which need to work in real time. The higher the nice value, the less CPU time a job will be allocated, and the less of a load it puts on the system. Programs known to be CPU intensive can, therefore, be set to run at low priority. A higher nice value prevents the program from taking large amounts of time at high loads, but does not prevent it from utilising CPU resources when the load on the system is light.

    CPU-intensive tasks such as database searches or phylogenetic analysis should be run from wrappers, i.e. scripts that set parametres before running the program. The name of the program is preceded by the nice command. For example, to run fastDNAml at the default priority, a wrapper might contain the line:

nice fastDNAml arguments... &

    The default priority for nice varies from system to system. In the BIRCH system, most sequence programs are launched from the GDE interface by calling wrappers that run programs using nice. As well, termination of the command line with an ampersand (&) tells the shell to run the task in the background. Thus, a user can launch a long-running job, quit GDE and logout without terminating the job. When the program is completed, the output is written to the file, which the user can access when logged in during the next session.

In some cases, programs that use a graphic interface will perform analyses that require very long execution times. The problem with this design is that the user must remain logged in to the terminal from which the program was launched, because quitting the program would terminate the analysis. One can circumvent this problem by running jobs of this type from a vncviewer window. Killing a vncviewer window has no effect on the applications currently running and the user can open up the same screen at any time from anywhere. This has the added benefit of making it easy to remotely monitor the progress of long-running jobs.

Killing runaway jobs

Sometimes a program will not correctly handle an error and will begin using up large amounts of CPU time. Unless the Bioadmin has root permissions, it is necessary to ask either the owner of the job or a sysadmin to kill it. For example, a runaway netscape job might show up thus when running the top command:

PID	USERNAME	THR	PRI	NICE	SIZE	RES	STATE	TIME	CPU	COMMAND
25779	frist	13	22	0	24M	11M	cpu/0	23:19	64.27%	netscape

To kill the job, root or the owner would type: kill -925779.

Applications that do not normally use a lot of CPU time, but may be prone to runaway execution, could be contained by running them from a wrapper, in which the ulimit command is issued prior to running the program, e.g. ulimit -t 900, limiting CPU time in the current shell to 900 seconds (15 min).

## Chapter 11

Databases

INTRODUCTION

Computers serve four interdependent functions in bioinformatics: communications, computation, control and storage. Embedded computer controllers, in sequencing machines, fermentation tanks and bioreactors direct the programmable robotic arms that automate intricate processes and markedly decrease the need for human operators. When time is of the essence, computer-controlled devices are superior to manual operations, in part because they can operate virtually unattended around the clock.

As a communications device, not only has the computer helped researchers craft more journal articles in less time than at any other point in history, but an increasingly large proportion of academic research information appears online. Up until the mid-1990s, newly discovered nucleotide sequences from human and other species of DNA were published in printed journals, requiring that researchers interested in using computer techniques to explore the sequence either key in the sequences by hand or use optical character recognition (OCR) systems to automatically capture the printed sequences and translate them into in machine-readable form. Today, no researcher would think of consulting a printed journal for a nucleotide sequence, but would immediately turn to either one of the numerous public databases on the Web or one of the value-added commercial databases. Furthermore, if a printed journal article isn't referenced by one of the electronic databases, such as PubMed, then the chances of the article ever being read in any form are low.

As computational devices in bioinformatics, computers are used for tasks that range from searching for nucleotide sequences and visualising protein folding patterns to simulating complex 3D protein-protein interactions, for applications ranging from drug discovery to biomaterials research and development. As an example of computer processing power focused on numeric computation in bioinformatics, consider that Celera Genomics' network of 800 Compaq AlphaServers has the capacity to compare up to 250 billion genomic sequences per hour generated by its hundreds of robotic gene sequencing machines. Even lesser-endowed companies and academic centres are creating high-performance Beowulf clusters for bioinformatics work. These massively parallel systems that are constructed from dedicated PC hardware are generally affordable and available to anyone.

Researchers at another pharmacological powerhouse. GlaxoSmithKline (GSK), are studying how individual variations in the genetic code cause adverse drug reactions in some patients. To pursue this research, GSK partners with biotech research firms who store clinical data from drug trials and correlate it with the patient's genetic information to create a genetic profile of patients at risk. Similarly, clinicians with the Mayo Clinic in Minnesota are working with researchers to identify gene markers that indicate which patients should respond to specific anticancer therapy. Elsewhere, pharmaceutical research firms are using genetic traits to predict whether a patient will respond to therapy as well as the likelihood of serious side effects. Several biotech startups are developing panels of DNA tests that will allow clinicians to quickly determine how patients metabolise drugs so that dosage regimens can be tailored to their individual metabolism.

All of these activities revolve around database technology. For example, both communications and computation operations in bioinformatics depend on data that have to be maintained. Electronic databases maintain data in a persistent, nonvolatile form that allows operations to be repeated and compared with other operations, with the results communicated to other researchers and developers. The electronic database—a file composed of records, each containing fields together with a set of operations for searching, sorting, recombining and other functions—is the silicon, plastic and iron-oxide equivalent of the experimenter's private notebook and the basis for electronic publishing to the scientific community.

As an illustration of how central databases are to the molecular biology research and development, consider a sampling of the public bioinformatics databases listed in Table 11.1. Perhaps the best-known of the hundreds of DNA sequence databases accessible through the Internet are the international nucleotide sequence database collaborators GENBANK, supported by the National Centre for Biological Information (NCBI), the DNA DataBank of Japan (DDBJ) and the European Molecular Biology Laboratory (EMBL). Another major database, PubMed, which is maintained by the U.S. National Library of Medicine, is a key resource for biomedical literature.

Table 11.1. Public bioinformatics databases accessible via the internet.

Database type	Example	Note
Nucleotide	GenBank	One of the largest public sequence databases
Sequence	DDBJ	DNA DataBank of Japan
	EMBL	European Molecular Biology Laboratory
	MGDB	Mouse Genome Database
	GSX	Mouse Gene Expression Database
	NDB	Nucleotide Acid Database
Protein sequence	SWISS-PROT	Swiss Institute for Bioinformatics and European Bioinformatics Institute
	TrEMBL	Annotated supplement to SWISS-PROT
	TrEMBLnew	Weekly, preprocessed update to TrEMBL
	PIR	Protein Information Resource
3D structures	PDB	Protein DataBank
	MMDB	Molecular Modelling Database
	Cambridge Structural database	For small molecules
Enzymes and compounds	LIGAND	Chemical compounds and reactions
Sequence	PROSITE	Sequence motifs
Motifs	BLOCKS	Derived from PROSITE
(Alignment)	PRINTS	A superset of BLOCKS
	Pfam	Protein families database of alignments and hidden Markov models
	ProDOM	Protein Domains

(Contd...)

Database type	Example	Note
Pathways and complexes	Pathway	Metabolic and regulatory pathway maps
Molecular disease	OMIM	Online Mendelian Inheritance in Man
Biomedical	PubMed	Contains Medline
Literature	Medline	Medical Literature
Vectors	UniVec	Used to identify vector contamination
Protein mutations	PMD	Protein Mutant Database
Gene expressions	GEO	Gene Expression Omnibus
Amino acid indices	Aaindex	Amino Acid Index Database
Protein/peptide literature	LITDB	Literature database for proteins and peptides
Gene catalog	GENES	KEGG Genes Database

The nucleotide sequence databases and PubMed represent the extremes of the spectrum from sequences of base pairs to their relevance in disease and the practice of medicine. Other online databases, such as the protein sequence database SWISS-PROT and the online mendelian inheritance in man (OMIM) database—a molecular disease database that links human genes and genetic disease—provide data that is somewhere between the two ends of the spectrum. For example, SWISS-PROT contains sequence motifs (where a motif is a small structural element that is recognisable in several proteins, such as the alpha helix) that are often associated with particular functions, linking structure and function. Popular representatives of so-called alignment databases are PROSITE and BLOCKS, for sequence motif and motif alignment data, respectively.

Public structural databases are represented by the cambridge structural database for small molecules and the protein data bank (PDB) for macromolecules. The PDB, which is maintained by the research collaboratory for structural bioinformatics (RCSB), includes publicly available 3D structures of proteins, nucleic acids and carbohydrates, as determined by X-ray crystallography and NMR spectroscopy. The PDB serves as the source data for other databases, such as the molecular modelling database (MMDB), which is used to construct 3D images of the molecules involved.

In addition to the public databases, there are a rapidly increasing number of private databases created and maintained by for-profit companies and laboratories associated with academic institutions. For example, the LifeSeq database from Incyte Genomics, Inc, contains gene sequences from humans, rats and mice. Regardless of whether databases are public or private, most have particular functions and uses in bioinformatics and entire books could easily be devoted to their construction, maintenance and use. However, because of volatility in the commercial database space and evolving associations among academic laboratories, the specifics of particular databases will change markedly over time. As such, it's more important for the reader to understand the general concepts and issues that apply to all biological databases, whether they're custom, in-house systems or public databases administered by the various government agencies.

For example, one characteristic of biological databases that is virtually universal is the enormity of their contents. To the delight of the sagging post-eCommerce information technology industry, the data-handling requirements associated with even modest biological databases often necessitate considerable investment in hardware, software and personnel. Consider that as of mid-2002, GenBank, the repository of nucleotide sequences for a variety of species that forms the basis for much bioinformatics research, contained data on over 17 billion base pairs stored in over 15 million sequence records. Similarly, Incyte Genomics' LifeSeq commercial database contained over a terabyte (1000 gigabytes) of data, with a system capacity of 70 terabytes. Many companies in the bioinformatics space have database system capacities in excess of 200 terabytes (2,00,000 gigabytes, equivalent to about 3,10,000 CD-ROMs), in the form of multiple, refrigerator-sized racks of hard drives. Creating archives is an inherent challenge in any database system. So is integrating information in different formats from multiple databases. The difficulty of these tasks is accentuated by the sheer enormity of the volume of data involved.

Given the central role databases and database technology plays in bioinformatics, at a minimum, researchers, managers and scientists in the field should not only become fluent in the language of database technology, but should also understand how biomedical databases form the basis of all bioinformatics research and development efforts. In addition, readers should appreciate that database technology is most valuable in the biotech industry when it enables the integration of research, development, clinical activity, manufacturing and selling and marketing. Data take on added value when they leave the confines of a workstation and become incorporated into shared public and private databases, applications and products.

To this end, this chapter gives all overview of database technology and its uses in bioinformatics, with a focus on shared or multi-user database systems. Topics range from the database management process, database models, interfacing databases to the Internet for collaboration, archiving, to the practical challenges associated with establishing a local database. The likely future of bioinformatics database technology is also discussed. The first section, 'definitions', provides a review of key definitions that readers should be familiar with to understand the following discussions. The 'data management' section provides a functional overview of the typical data-management challenges faced by researchers in the biotechnology field. These researchers typically work with locally generated data, the public genomic databases and data from collaborators in associated areas, such as clinical medicine. The 'data life cycle' section continues the functional overview by exploring the normal life cycle of data, from creation to disposal and how this cycle can be managed. 'Database technology' reviews the more technical issues associated with biomedical databases, from the architecture of databases and database management systems to database models and data capture. The 'implementation' section illustrates how an understanding of these technical issues translates to practical database installations. Finally, 'Endnote' looks to the near horizon and suggests impending developments in biomedical databases and the challenges of moving forward to a fully integrated biomedical database system.

DEFINITIONS

Databases, which provide the long-term memory of computer operations, take on a variety of names, depending on their structure, contents, use and amount of data they contain. Two technologies often confused with databases are disk servers and file servers. A disk server is a node in a local area network that acts as a remote disk drive. A disk server can be divided into multiple volumes, some of which are shared by all users on the server and others of which can be accessed only by a specific user, as defined by username and password login. At the next level in sophistication is the file server, which can be thought of as a disk server with intelligence. A file server not only stores files, but manages the network requests for them and maintains order as users request and modify files.

The file server, like the disk server, supports movement and cataloging of files, but, unlike a true database, the contents of a file server are unavailable without the use of some other application. With both disk servers and file servers, separate applications must be used to open documents for reviewing and editing. In this regard, most disk and file servers work like extensions to the computer operating system. Files can be identified, copied, deleted and otherwise managed at a very high level. For our purposes, file servers and disk servers can be considered as extensions to the internal workstation hard drive that may be configured is a shared volume so that collaborators on the same network can share data stored on the server.

At the simplest level of a true database is the data repository, a database used as an information storage facility, with minimal analysis or querying functionality. A data repository is a structured, systematically collected storehouse of data distilled or mirrored from a single application, such as a sequencing machine, microarray analyser or clinical system (Fig. 11.1).

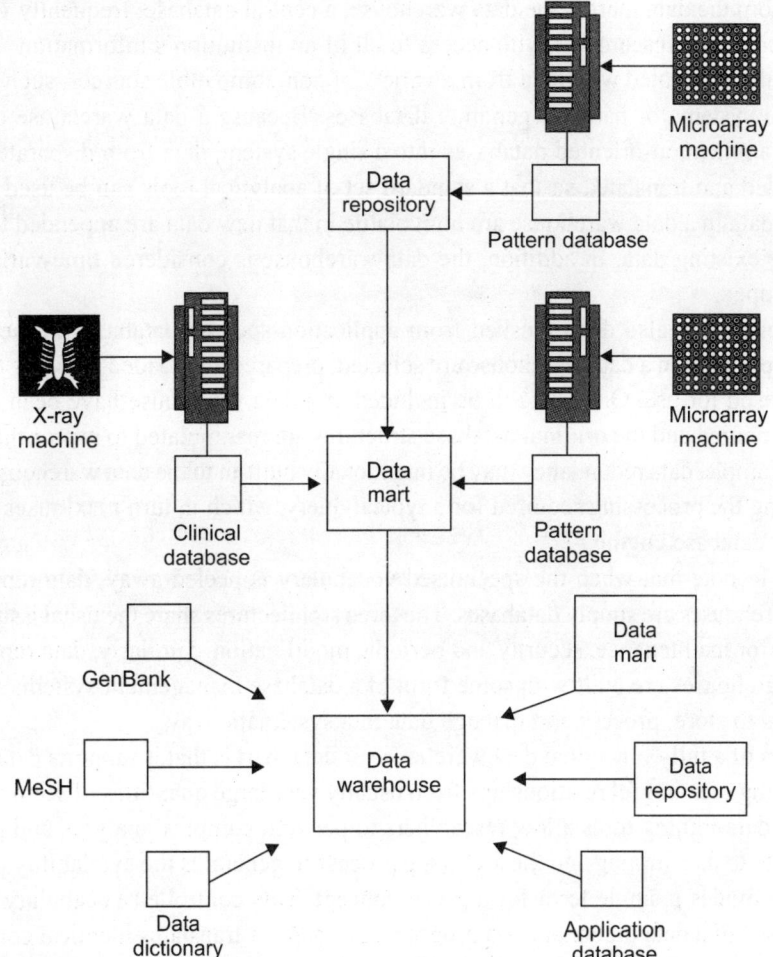

Fig. 11.1. Database nomenclature. Data repositories, data marts and data warehouses differ primarily in the diversity of data sources that contribute to their contents.

One advantage of using a data repository instead of the original database in the host application or device is that longitudinal studies are possible because all data in the host application are mirrored and stored in the repository. For example, because of storage limitations or because the local database is always in use, it may be virtually impossible for a researcher to compare data from multiple runs of a sequencing machine. Another advantage of using a data repository instead of the original database is that it offloads the query functions that are available through native applications to the database management system that enables efficient control and management of the data repository.

Next up the hierarchy of complexity and capability is the data mart, a searchable database system, organised according to the user's likely needs. Like a data repository, a data mart has a narrow focus on data that is specific to a particular research project or task. That is, a data mart contains a subset of the data contained in other databases as opposed to all indiscriminate mass copying of all the data from another database. The major difference between a data mart and a data repository is that a data mart contains data extracted or mirrored—copied in real time—from multiple application databases.

One step up from the data mart is the data warehouse, a central database, frequently very large, that can provide authenticated researchers with access to all of an institution's information. That is, a data warehouse is usually populated with data from a variety of non-compatible sources, such as sequencing machines, clinical systems or national genomic databases. Because a data warehouse combines data from a variety of application-oriented databases into a single system, data from disparate sources must be cleaned, encoded and translated so that a standard set of analytical tools can be used with the data. Furthermore, the data in a data warehouse are nonvolatile in that new data are appended to the database and never replace existing data. In addition, the data warehouse is considered time-variant in that the data are time-stamped.

The data warehouse is also distinguished from application-specific databases in the way the data destined for incorporation in a data warehouse are selected, prepared and loaded and how the underlying database is optimised for use. Once data to be included in a data warehouse have been identified, the data are cleaned, merged and the original database structures are manipulated to mirror those of the data warehouse. For example, data redundancy may be intentionally built-in to the data warehouse architecture, thereby minimising the processing required for a typical query, which in turn maximises the efficiency of the underlying database engine.

It's important to note that when the specialised vocabulary is peeled away, data repositories, data marts and data warehouses are simply databases. The three architectures share the usual issues of database design, provision for maintenance, security and periodic modification. Similarly, data repositories, data marts and data warehouses are built with some form of a database management system, a program that allows researchers to store, process and manage data in a systematic way.

One of the uses of a fully functional data warehouse or data mart is that it supports data mining—the process of extracting meaningful relationships from usually very large quantities of seemingly unrelated data. Specialised data-mining tools allow researchers to perform complex analyses and predictions on data. A prerequisite to data mining and the archiving process in general is the availability of a controlled vocabulary that provides a single term for a given concept. This controlled vocabulary is most often implemented as part of a data dictionary—a program that maps or translates identical concepts that are expressed in different words, phrases or units into a single vocabulary.

Related to the concept of databases is the data archive—a nonvolatile holder for data that are infrequently accessed—that is optimised for data recovery and data longevity. Strictly speaking, an archive needn't be a database. Archives are commonly made on multi-gigabyte tape cartridges that are stored offsite in environmentally controlled conditions to minimise the chances of data loss.

Armed with these core definitions, the reader can proceed with this chapter, which considers databases from a functional, data-management perspective before exploring the core technologies.

DATA MANAGEMENT

A central tenet in applied information technology is that process should drive technology. If there is an obvious need that is only partially or inefficiently addressed, it's much easier to introduce a technology to address the need than it is to eradicate the need through technology alone. There are exceptions, of course, in that some individuals will adopt a new technology simply because it's new. Marketing professionals refer to these prospects as innovators and early adopters—technophiles who take joy in owning the first model of a new technology before it's available to the public or their peers. However, for most of the population—the early and late majority—technology is a means to an end. For most researchers in bioinformatics, database technology is the means to handling the enormity of data and information that is created, manipulated and communicated every day. Consider the various components in the biological data-management scenario in the pharmacogenomic laboratory depicted in Fig. 11.2.

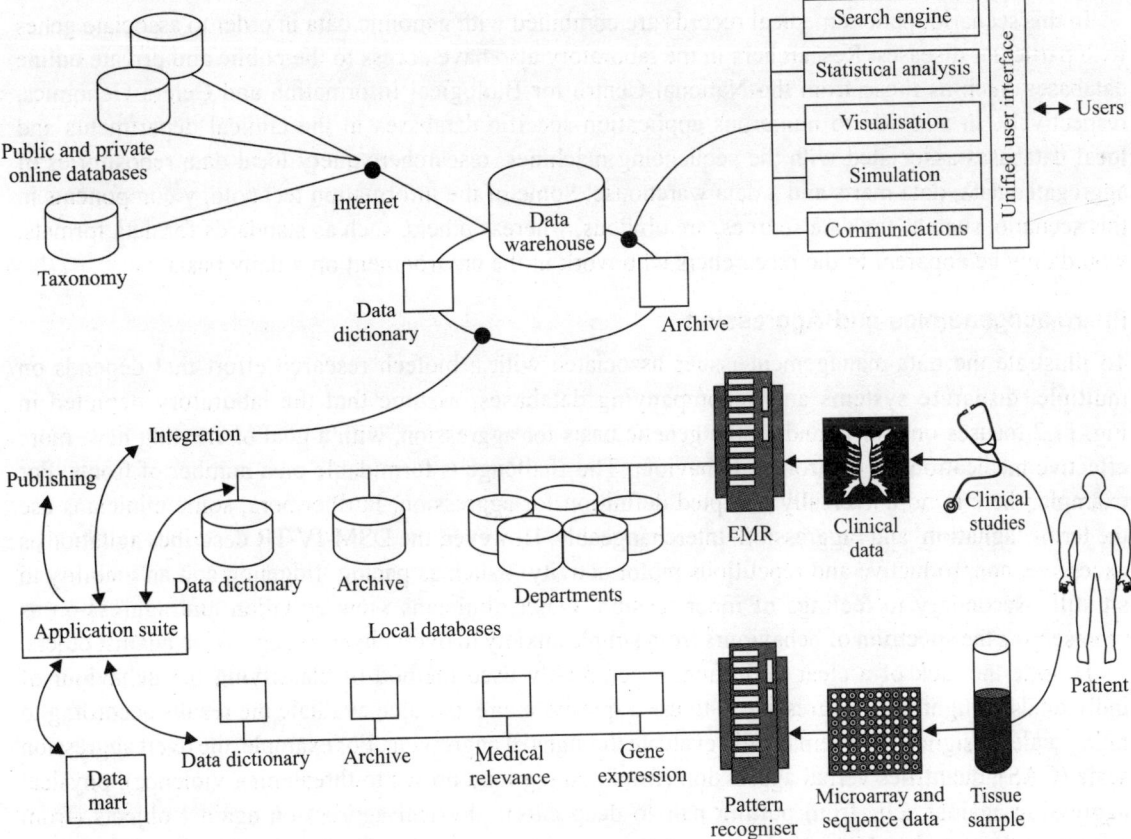

Fig. 11.2. Data management. In this data-management scenario for a pharmacogenomic laboratory, data of various types are acquired from a variety of sources, incorpated into the data warehouse, used by a variety of applications and archived for future use. Data created locally may be published electronically, serve as the basis for a paper publication and may be used in a variety of applications from drug discovery to genetic engineering.

This data-management scenario is similar to that followed by several commercial biotech ventures, such as deCODE Genetics, the commercial venture in Iceland that is headed by a former Harvard Medical School professor who recognised the advantage of having access to a genetically homogeneous population for pharmacogenomic R&D. Because the majority of Iceland's population dates back only to the time of the original Viking settlers around 800 AD and there are meticulous records of family history, every native's genetic heritage is available online through a government-run database. In addition, the researchers at deCODE, through a hotly debated arrangement with the Icelandic government, purchased the exclusive rights to access every citizen's medical records, most of which are in electronic form.

Because of the similarity of the genetic code in the closed population, DNA samples from families that suffer from particular diseases can be compared to those of closely related families who are disease-free. Through data mining, researchers at deCODE hope to identify the genes responsible for a variety of diseases, such as osteoarthritis. The competitive advantage of the company isn't the latest sequencing or microarray machines; it's their ability to integrate data from Iceland's family tree and medical record databases with deCODE's own patient DNA database and to manage that data in a way that supports the company's research objectives.

In this scenario, patient medical records are combined with genomic data in order to associate genes with particular diseases. Researchers in the laboratory also have access to the public and private online databases, such as those from the National Centre for Biological Information and Celera Genomics, respectively. In addition to numerous application-specific databases in the clinical departments and local databases associated with the sequencing machines, researchers query local data repositories of aggregated data, data marts and a data warehouse. Some of the information technology components in this scenario, such as the data sources, are obvious, whereas others, such as standards for data formats, would only be apparent to the researchers who work in the environment on a daily basis.

Pharmacogenomics and Aggression

To illustrate the data-management issues associated with a biotech research effort that depends on multiple, disparate systems and accompanying databases, assume that the laboratory depicted in Fig. 11.2 focuses on understanding the genetic basis for aggression, with a goal of creating new, more effective medications to control the behaviour. The challenge is formidable on a number of fronts. For example, there is no universally accepted definition for aggression. Furthermore, some clinicians use the terms 'agitation' and 'aggression' interchangeably. However, the DSM-IV-TR describes agitation as excessive, nonproductive and repetitive motor activity—such as pacing, fidgeting and an inability to sit still—secondary to feelings of inner tension. Other clinicians view agitation and aggression as representing the spectrum of behaviours from simple anxiety to overt physical aggression against others.

Despite the lack of a clear definition, a commonly used method of classifying the behaviour of individuals thought to be aggressive is to use a questionnaire and then evaluate the results according to rating scales designed to systematically evaluate the signs of aggression. For example, the overt aggression scale (OAS), quantifies verbal aggression (from making loud noises to threatening violence), physical aggression against self (from pulling hair to deep cuts), physical aggression against objects (from slamming doors to breaking windows) and physical aggression against other people (from threatening gestures to breaking bones). However, even this widely recognised scale isn't all-inclusive. For example, it doesn't distinguish between acute and chronic aggression. Although there is no universally accepted boundary between acute and chronic aggression, a one-month timeframe is often used as the break point. The distinction between acute and chronic aggression has practical significance because patients diagnosed with chronic aggression are eligible for insurance coverage for behavioural modification and pharmacological treatment, including the use of antipsychotic drugs, while drugs for patients diagnosed with acute aggression are not covered by insurance.

Researchers in the lab might use an online literature reference database, such as PubMed, to identify prior research in academia and perhaps published reports from other companies working on the genetic basis of aggression. A reasonable place to start in the search for prior research would be the National Library of Medicine's online MeSH browser, shown in Fig. 11.3. The browser offers a definition for the term 'aggression' and provides two MeSH trees to indicate there are two applicable contexts—behavioural symptoms and social behaviour.

In addition, the browser lists the allowable qualifiers for aggression that can be used to restrict or limit search results. As defined on the MeSH site (www.nlm.nih.gov/MBrowser. html), these qualifiers are:

1. CL (classification): Used for taxonomic or other systematic or hierarchical classification systems.
2. DE (drug effects): Used with organs, regions, tissues or organisms and physiological and psychological processes for the effects of drugs and chemicals.
3. PH (physiology): Used with organs, tissues and cells of uni- and multi-cellular organisms for normal function. It is also used with biochemical substances, endogenously produced, for their physiologic role.
4. PX (psychology): Used with nonpsychiatric diseases, techniques and named groups for psychologic, psychiatric, psychosomatic, psychosocial, behavioural and emotional aspects and with psychiatric disease for psychologic aspects; used also with animal terms for animal behaviour and psychology.
5. RE (radiation effects): Used for effects of ionising and nonionising radiation upon living organisms, organs and tissues and their constituents and upon physiologic processes. It includes the effect of irradiation on drugs and chemicals.

The most relevant of these qualifiers for the researcher's work is probably drug effects (DE), to identify articles that deal with the physical and psychological aspects of drugs and chemicals dealing with aggression. In addition, articles dealing with radiation effects (RE) may also be relevant, especially if the articles describe radiation-induced genetic mutations associated with aggression in rats or primates.

With the relevant MeSH search terms and contexts defined, the next step would be to conduct an online search of the biomedical literature dealing with aggression using the online bibliographic database PubMed. The search on PubMed would likely return citations such as Antonio Moniz's surgical removal of the frontal lobes of the brain to control aggressive behaviour. The search would also reveal work on twin studies in Denmark in the late 1980s that suggests aggressiveness is a personality trait with a genetic component because twins raised apart have similar aggressiveness scores.

The PubMed search would also reveal work on attempting to identify the genetic basis for aggression in other animals, including lobsters, rats and fruit flies. For example, researchers at Harvard and the University of Basel in Switzerland experimented with fruit flies to quantify aggressive behaviour as a function of genetic makeup. Pairs of fruit flies were allowed to fight over females and the genetic profiles of the winners were studied for systematic differences among those of more submissive losers. One difference noted in the study is that there are significant variations in levels of certain neurotransmitters, including serotonin and dopamine, in the brains of the more aggressive combatants. However, these studies leave many questions unanswered, such as the contribution of physical strength or experience to winning a bout. As in human conflicts, the better fighter, not necessarily the more aggressive fighter, may be victorious.

MeSH Heading	Aggression
Tree Number	F01.145.126.125
Tree Number	F01.145.813.045
Annotation	Human and animal; 'aggression' in French is translated 'stress' and indexed under a STRESS heading; 'agressologie' = STRESS
Scope Note	A form of behaviour which leads to self-assertion; it may arise from innate drives and/or a response to frustration; may be manifested by destructive and attacking behaviour, by covert attitudes of hostility and obstructionism or by healthy self-expressive drive to mastery. (Dorland 27th ed)
Allowable Qualifiers	CL DE PH PX RE
Unique ID	D000374

Behaviour and behaviour mechanisms [F01]
    Behaviour [F01.145]
        Behavioural symptoms [F01.145.126]
            Affective symptoms [F01.145126.100]
        † Aggression [F01.145.126.125]
                Agonistic behaviour [F01.145.126.125.100]
        Catatonia [F01.145.126.156]
        Child reactive disorders [F01.145.1261.59]
        Coprophagia [F01.145.126.175]
        Delusions [F01.145.126.200]
        Depersonalisation [F01.145.126.300]
        Depression [F01.145.126.350]
        Encopresis [F01.145.126.837]
        Enuresis [F01.145.126.856]
        Hearing loss, functional [F01.145.126.875]
        Malingering [F01.145.126.925]
        Mental fatigue [F01.145.126.937]
        Obsessive behaviour [F01.145.126.950]
        Paranoid behaviour [F01.145.126.962]
        Schizophrenic language [F01.145.126.975]
        Self-injurious behaviour [F01.145.126.980]
        Stress, psychological [F01.145.126.990]

Fig. 11.3. National library of medicine medical subject heading descriptor data and tree structure for 'Aggression'. The tree structure puts the term in the context of a behavioural symptom. A second tree that defines a social behaviour context for the term is not shown here.

Armed with information on aggression from the medical literature, the researchers might hypothesise that a new drug that moderates the production of serotonin in the brain may be useful in controlling aggressive behaviour. They establish a study using volunteers who have been screened according to the overt aggression scale and they use a battery of clinical studies to rule out nongenetic causes for aggressive behaviour. The clinical examination includes a general history and physical, with a neurological examination, medication history and mental status examination, as well as chest X-ray, EEG, MRI and lumbar puncture. The objective of this testing is to identify patients in which abnormal behaviour might be due to causes such as head trauma, infection or brain tumors. For example, meningitis, an infection of the spinal fluid, can result in behaviour consistent with aggression and apprehension. Volunteers for the study would also be subject to standard laboratory tests, including urine drug screening, blood-alcohol concentration, serum drug concentrations and a thyroid profile to screen for patients who are taking illicit drugs or who have metabolic diseases that could contribute to abnormal behaviour. These and similar clinical data are stored in an electronic medical record (EMR) in the format described in Table 11.2.

Table 11.2. Typical electronic medical record (EMR) contents. The EMR contains both objective signs, such as physical examination findings, as well as subjective patient symptoms, including chief complaint and review of systems.

Data category	Description
Chief complaint	Patient's primary reason for the medical visit
History of present illness	History of onset of clinical signs and symptoms
Medications	Current list of medications the patient is using
Past medical history	Relevant past medical history, including hospital admissions, surgeries and diagnoses
Family history	History of family diseases, such as diabetes, cancer, heart disease and mental illness
Social history	Use of drugs, smoking, job stability, housing, living conditions, incarceration
Review of systems	Patient's recollection of symptoms and current medical problems, such as trouble sleeping at night or panic episodes and results of tests
Physical examination	The clinician's hands-on examination of the patient, including head, eyes, ears, nose, throat, chest and extremities
Laboratories	Includes blood glucose, cholesterol and drug levels
Studies	X-ray, MRI, CT and EKG
Progress notes	Record of temporal progression of signs and symptoms, laboratories and studies for the length of the study or admission

The components of the EMR report rarely exist in a single, unified database, but reside in the separate, domain specific databases that may exist within a single hospital or clinic or be dispersed geographically across a region or country. Regardless of their relative proximity to each other, laboratory, radiology, cardiology, hematology, internal medicine and other clinical departments typically maintain their own medical-record systems. What's more, each application may be supported by a different operating system, use a different underlying database—some of which may be outdated—and execute on a completely different hardware platform. For example, the pharmacy system might run under UNIX on a Sun Server using a Sybase database, whereas the clinical radiology system might run under VMS on a VAX server with an Oracle database. Within each department or clinic, these differences are usually irrelevant unless data have to be shared with other departments. The traditional method of creating a composite view of a patient's clinical status is to generate custom reports, which is time-consuming and expensive. The modern approach to the EMR is to create one or more central databases derived from and yet completely independent of, each of the application databases and to optimise these databases for research and analysis. In order to create a comprehensive record that can be queried, the data from the various clinical systems have to be integrated, usually with the assistance of a data dictionary that translates various clinical databases to common formats so that the data can be more easily combined. The data dictionary is, in simplest terms, a collection of information about naming, classification, structure, usage and administration of data that originates from a variety of sources. The data dictionary is perhaps most useful in addressing the problem of data element ambiguity. For example, within a biotech enterprise composed of variety of commercial and in-house applications, a given data element may be defined differently within different applications.

Patient age might be defined in months within a clinical pathology system, whereas patient age within the microarray database and the data dictionary might be represented in years. The data dictionary can be used to reconcile the two systems, providing an appropriate data transform between the two representations. For example, the appropriate transforms to move between the representations used by the pathology and microarray systems for patient age might be:

Patient age (data dictionary) = Patient age (microarray) = Patient age (pathology)/12

The data dictionary can also impose a standard vocabulary on the system so that clinical findings can be identified unambiguously. For example, one clinical system might refer to heart attack as 'M.I.', another as 'Myocardial Infarction' and yet another as 'Heart Attack'. By imposing a standard vocabulary, the data dictionary allows data from the various systems to be combined into a unified view of the patient that can be more easily mined for patterns. This view is typically maintained in a data mart, as illustrated in Fig. 11.4. The data mart contains a subset of the data that resides in the individual databases combined with contents from these databases translated into a standard format that can be efficiently mined for data.

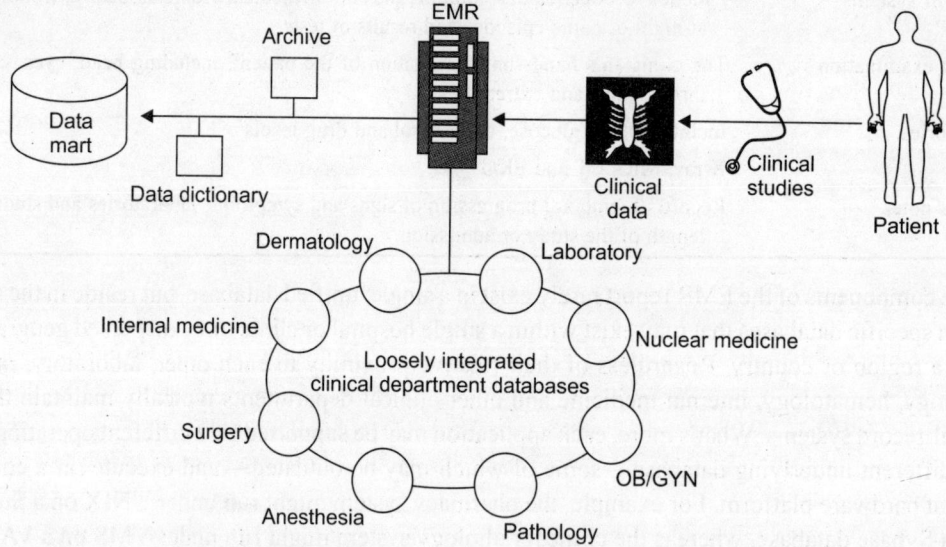

Fig. 11.4. Integration of clinical data. To create an EMR capable of supporting efficient data mining, a data dictionary is used to impose a standard format and vocabulary on data stored in the clinical data mart.

A parallel situation exists in the bioinformatics component of the patient data management. As depicted in Fig. 11.5, patients provide DNA source material for analysis in the form of tissue samples, which are processed for microarray analysis, generating thousands of data points. These data are then processed by a pattern-recogniser program to identify significant patterns. Researchers rely on local databases of gene expression, medical relevance and a data dictionary to provide a common language and format for the data. Links to the large public genomic databases provide, additional reference material. As with the clinical data, the composite genomic data are stored in a data mart for efficient manipulation and analysis through a suite of applications. Ideally, relevant data from clinical applications are combined in the data mart as well.

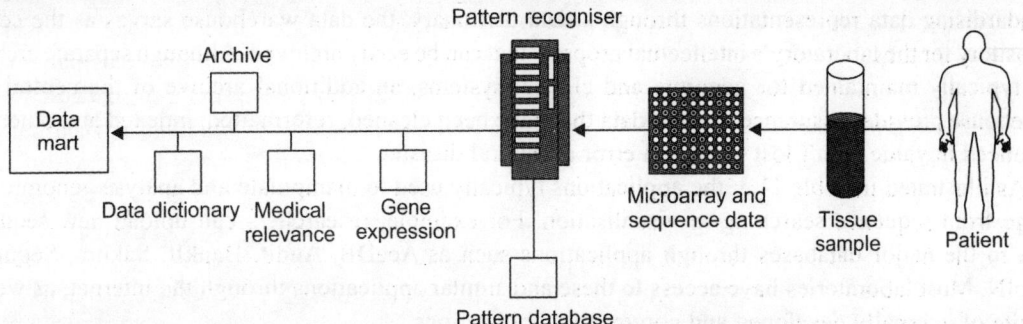

Fig. 11.5. Integration of bioinformatics data. Like clinical data, bioinformatics data from a variety of sources and in numerous formats are combined in a data mart to enhance data management.

One advantage of building and maintaining a data mart that combines data from genomic and clinical sources is that data can be manipulated and visualised by applications that offer a single, combined view of the data that may provide a unique insight into their correlation and relevance. As shown in Fig. 11.6, when clinical laboratory (Serotonin), psychological (overt aggression scale or OAS) and genetic (Gene) data are readily available in a common format, they can be combined to provide a quick qualitative and quantitative view of how behaviour, gross biology and genomic information relate to each other and how they correlate with aggressive behaviour.

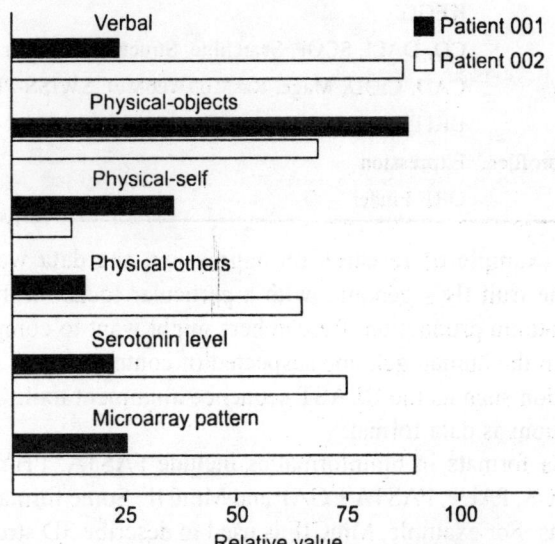

Fig. 11.6. Aggressive behaviour versus microarray data. A view of aggressive behaviour in two closely related patients as a function of clinical laboratory (Serotonin), psychological (overt aggression scale or OAS) and genetic (gene) data. Compared to patient 002, patient 001 has a relatively high score on the physical aggressiveness against the objects component of the OAS and low scores on serum serotonin and microarray patterns.

In addition to locally generated clinical and genetic data, the typical pharmacogenomic laboratory has access to data in private and public online databases. Ideally, subsets of often-used data are integrated with local data in the laboratory's data warehouse, making the data readily available for searching, statistical analysis, visualisation, simulation and communications. In addition to homogenising and standardising data representations through a data dictionary, the data warehouse serves as the central repository for the laboratory's intellectual property that can be easily archived. Although separate archives are typically maintained for genomic and clinical systems, an additional archive of the central data warehouse provides assurance that the data that have been cleaned, reformatted, indexed and otherwise enhanced in value aren't lost to human error or natural disaster.

As illustrated in Table 11.3, the applications typically used to manipulate and analyse genomic data range from sequence searching to visualisation. For example, researchers can upload new sequence data to the major databases through applications such as AceDB, Audit, BankIt, Sakura, Sequin or WebIN. Most laboratories have access to these and similar applications through the internet, as well as a suite of internally developed and commercial applications.

Table 11.3. Genomic applications. A variety of public and private applications are available for analysis of genomic data, many of which are designed to work on the large public databases. Listed here are publicly funded applications.

Application	Examples
Sequence search	BLAST, BLASTN, CLUSTALW, FASTA, MOTIF, PBLAST, TBLASTIN
Submission	AceDB, Audit, BankIt, Sakura, Sequin, WebIN
Information retrieval	Entrez, DBGET, IDEAS
Linkage	LocusLink
Portal	KEGG
Structure match	CD, DALI, SCOP, Searchlite, Structure Explorer, VAST
Visualisation	CAD, Cn3D, Mage, RasMol/WebMol, SWISS-PDBViewer, VRML, WebMol
Protein-protein interactions	BRITE
Microarray gene expression profiles	Expression
Open-reading frame locator	ORF Finder

Continuing with the example of research on aggression, the data warehouse might contain a compilation of data on the fruit fly's genome, with a particular focus on the sequence that relates to genes responsible for serotonin production. Researchers might want to compare sequences in the fruit fly's genome with those in the human genome suspected of contributing to serotonin neurotransmitter control, using an application such as the BLAST sequence alignment tool. One consideration in using one of the online applications is data format.

The most popular data formats in bioinformatics include FASTA, PHYLIP, MAML (Microarray Markup Language), NEXUS, PAUP, FASTA + GAP and MmCIF. Some formats are specific to particular data types and applications. For example, MmCIF is used to describe 3D structures, whereas FASTA is used to describe sequence data. As shown in Fig. 11.7, the FASTA format begins with a single-line description, followed by lines of sequence data. The description line is distinguished from the sequence data by a greater-than (>) symbol in the first column. Sequences, which should be shorter than 80 characters in length, are represented in the standard International Union of Biochemistry International Union of Pure and Applied Chemistry (IUB/IUPAC) amino acid and nucleic acid codes. Exceptions are that lowercase letters are accepted and are mapped into upper-case; a single hyphen or dash can be used to represent a gap of indeterminate length; and in amino acid sequences, U and * are acceptable letters.

FASTA format

A sequence in FASTA format begins with a single-line description, followed by lines of sequence data. The description line is distinguished from the sequence data by a greater than (>) symbol in the first column. An example sequence in FASTA format is:

>g i½532319½pir½TVFV2E½TVFV2E envelope protein
ELRLRYCAPAGFALLKCNDADYDGFKTNCSNVSVVHCTNLMNTTVTTGLLLNGSYSENRT
QIWQKHRTSNDSALILLNKHYNLTVTCKRPGNKTVLPVTIMAGLVFHSQKYNLRLRQAWC
HFPSNWKGAWKEVKEEIVNLPKERYRGTNDPKRIFFQRQWGDPETANLWFNCHGEFFYCK
MDWFLNYLNNLTVDADHNECKNTSGTKSGNKRAPGPCVQRTYVACHIRSVIIWLETISKK
TYAPPREGHLECTSTVTGMTVELNYIPKNRTNVTLSPQIESIWAAELDRYKLVEITPIGF
APTEVRRYTGGHERQKRVPFVXXXXXXXXXXXXXXXXXXXXXXXXXVQSQHLLAGILQQQKNL
LAAVEAQQQMLKLTIWGVK

Sequences, which should be shorter than 80 characters in length, are expected to be represented in the standard International Union of Biochemistry-International union of pure and applied chemistry (IUB/IUPAC) amino acid and nucleic acid codes, with these exceptions: lower-case letters are accepted and are mapped into upper-case; a single hyphen or dash can be used to represent a gap of indeterminate length; and in amino acid sequences, U and * are acceptable letters. Before submitting a request, any numerical digits in the query sequence should either be removed or replaced by appropriate letter codes (e.g. N for unknown nucleic acid residue or X for unknown amino acid residue). The nucleic acid codes supported are:

A	→	adenosine	M	→	A C (amino)
C	→	cytidine	S	→	G C (strong)
G	→	guanine	W	→	A T (weak)
T	→	thymidine	B	→	G T C
U	→	uridine	D	→	G A T
R	→	G A (purine)	H	→	A C T
Y	→	T C (pyrimidine)	V	→	G C A
K	→	G T (keto)	N	→	A G C T (any)
			–		gap of indeterminate length

For programs that use amino acid query sequences, such as BLASTP and TBLASTN, the accepted amino acid codes are:

A	alanine	P	proline
B	aspartate or aspargine	Q	glutamine
C	cystine	R	arginine
D	aspartate	S	serine
E	glutamate	T	threonine
F	phenylalanine	U	selenocysteine
G	glycine	V	valine
H	histidine	W	tryptophan
I	isoleucine	Y	tyrosine
K	lysine	Z	glutamate or glutamine
L	leucine	X	any
M	methionine	*	translation stop
N	asparagine		gap of indeterminate length

Fig. 11.7. The FASTA format. This is a standard data format for use with online sequencing databases.

Complexity

The pharmacogenomic laboratory exploring the genetic basis for aggression illustrates several key characteristics of data management in the biotech industry. Foremost is the complexity of data management, as summarised in Table 11.4. There are numerous data sources, including the volunteer patients, clinical studies, genomic studies and public and private online databases. Similarly, there are a variety of applications that can be. brought to bear on genomic and clinical data and the biomedical literature, including search engines, statistical analysis applications, visualisation tools, simulations, communication applications, database management systems, electronic medical record (EMR) systems and genomic analysis recognition and manipulation, including sequence recognition.

Table 11.4. Complexity and data management. The typical R&D environment in a biotech firm encompasses an array of data sources, applications, formats, interfaces and integration tools.

Data category	Examples
Data sources	Patient, clinical studies, genomic studies, public databases, private databases
Applications	Search engines, statistical analysis, visualisation, simulation, communications, database management system, electronic medical record, genomic
Databases	Public, private, taxonomy, clinical, genetic, local, external, archives
Data Formats	FASTA, PHYLIP, MAML, NEXUS, PAUP, FASTA + GAP and MmCIF, proprietary clinical formats, local application formats
Interfaces	Local databases, online databases, data warehouse, application
Integration tools	Data dictionary, network, standards

Furthermore, many of the dozens of databases involved in pharmacogenomic research and development use proprietary formats. This is especially true of clinical systems, many of which are speciality-specific. For example, standard image formats for radiology databases include digital imaging and communications in medicine (DICOM) and the American college of radiology/national electrical manufacturers association (ACR/NEMA) standards. These standards were developed primarily to facilitate multi-vendor connectivity to promote the development of picture archiving and communications systems (PACS), but they have no provision for linking images with genomic systems, such as gene expression databases.

The typical research laboratory must develop and maintain numerous interfaces between applications and databases to provide the logical connectivity for data communications through the network infrastructure. The simple network illustrated in Fig. 11.2 glosses over the inner complexity of the dozens of standards used through a typical information system, a problem at least partially addressed by data dictionaries and conversion utilities. For example, few laboratories or medical facilities provide the degree of connectivity suggested by this discussion. The vast majority of hospitals in the U.S. use paper charts to record patient history and physical findings, for example.

Perhaps 5 per cent of hospitals have a functional EMR and most of these are partial implementations that provide only summary information. Furthermore, these systems typically require researchers and clinicians to learn several arcane languages and procedures to access all data that may be relevant to a given patient. For example, clinicians may have to log in to a pathology system to check urinalysis results, a radiology system to read the report on a patient's latest image studies and an admission, discharge, transfer (ADT) system to verify the patient's insurance provider. Similarly, although many clinical studies are multimedia-rich, most radiology and pathology images, EKG tracings, pulmonary function test curves and other graphical materials are maintained in separate databases that aren't connected to the main hospital or clinic network.

One approach to minimising or hiding the complexity of the data-management process is to create a single, integrated user interface. Just as the Windows or Macintosh operating systems hide the complexity of computer operations from users, a unified user interface to a network of disparate applications can hide the complexity of the data sources and various applications used to manipulate the data. This unified user interface may take the form of a web portal or the workstation's operating system. For example, the flavours of UNIX for the PC, Macintosh and dedicated UNIX workstations each provide various views of local and networked applications. The challenge with hiding complexity this way is that the constant changes in how data are actually managed in the background requires parallel updating of the user interface that provides a front end to the system.

The data-management process is much more involved than simply sending data to a database and retrieving it later. As discussed in the following sections, the databases used in bioinformatics research presents a variety of challenges, many of which pertain to all phases of the data life cycle, issues such as security, standards, interoperability, longevity of data, access and version control, the use of encryption and minimising access time. The data life cycle and the relevant issues that arise at each stage in the life of data are discussed in the rest of this chapter. Finally, issues that pertain to data repositories are discussed: database technology, database architecture and database management systems.

DATA LIFE CYCLE

In the data-management process, data are authored by clinicians and researchers and generated directly by research and test equipment, used by a variety of applications, repurposed or modified for other uses and archived for future study. Eventually, the data are disposed of, freeing the data warehouses and other hardware from the overhead of maintaining low-value data. The overall process, from data creation to disposal, is normally referred to as the data life cycle, as depicted in Fig. 11.8. The highlights of each stage are described there.

Data Creation and Acquisition

The process of data creation and acquisition is a function of the source and type of data. For example, in the scenario depicted in Fig. 11.8, data are generated by sequencing machines and microarrays in the molecular biology laboratory and by clinicians and clinical studies in the clinic or hospital. Depending on the difficulty in creating the data and the intended use, the creation process may be trivial and inexpensive or extremely complicated and costly. For example, recruiting test subjects to donate tissue biopsies is generally more expensive and difficult than identifying patients who are willing to provide less-invasive (and painful) tissue samples. In addition to cost, the major issues in the data-creation phase of the data life cycle include tool selection, data format, standards, version control, error rate, precision and accuracy. These metrics apply equally to clinical and genomic studies. In particular, metrics such as error rate, precision and accuracy are more easily ascribed to machine-generated data, whether from clinical laboratory studies or microarray analysis. For example, optical character recognition (OCR), which was once used extensively as a means of acquiring sequence information from print publications, has an error rate of about two characters per hundred, which is generally unacceptable.

Subjective information created by hands-on clinical analysis and entered into the computer system through the use of manual transcription, voice recognition data-input systems or desktop or hand held computers, is much more difficult to validate. What's more, there is significant variation in subjective interpretation of clinical studies.

For example, five seasoned radiologists will typically provide five different interpretations of the same chest film or other radiographic study. In addition to the quality of the initial clinical observation, there are errors introduced by the hardware, software and processes involved in capturing data, from keyboard and mouse to optical character recognition and voice recognition.

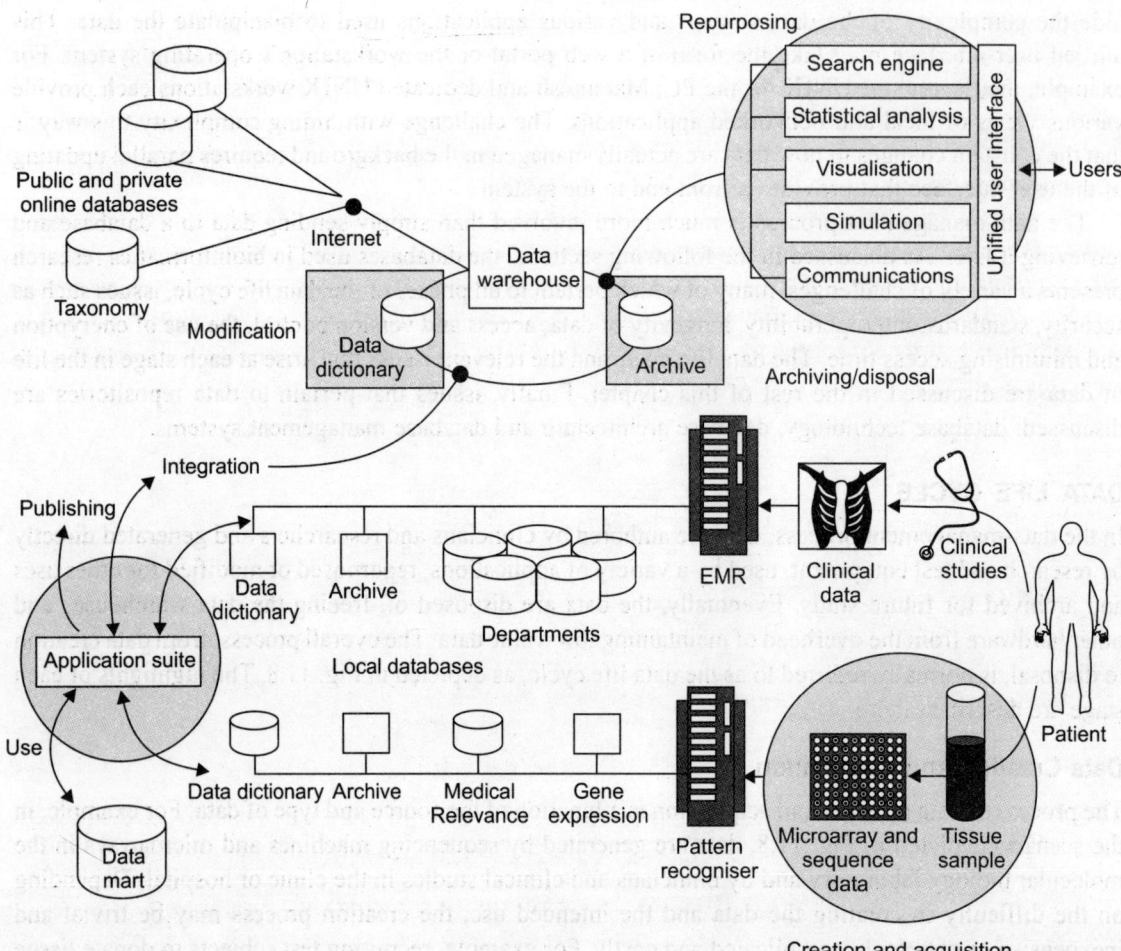

Fig. 11.8. Data life cycle. Key steps in the process include data creation and acquisition, use, modification, repurposing and the end game—archiving and disposal. The same process applies to data in a desktop workstation or, as in this illustration, to a large pharmacogenomic operation with multiple, disparate systems.

The creation and acquisition or patient data raises several ownership and privacy concerns. One of the greatest challenges regarding acquisition of clinical data is the health insurance portability and accountability act (HIPAA), which mandates security and privacy of patient data. The act requires all health plans, clearinghouses and providers of healthcare services to adopt national standards for electronic transactions and information security by mid-2004. Technologies that support user authentication, from password-protection schemes to biometric security technologies and data encryption are key to ensuring compliance with the act. Although there is not yet a parallel guideline for genomic data, it is likely that legislation in this area will materialise as soon as public awareness of the privacy issues becomes widely apparent.

Use

Once clinical and genomic data are captured, they can be put to a variety of immediate uses, from simulation, statistical analysis and visualisation to communications. Issues at this stage of the data life cycle include intellectual property rights, privacy and distribution. For example, unless patients have expressly given permission to have their names used, microarray data should be identified by ID number through a system that maintains the anonymity of the donor.

Data Modification

Data are rarely used in their raw form, without some amount of formatting or editing. In addition, data are seldom used only for their originally intended purpose, in part because future uses are difficult to predict. For example, microarray data may not be captured expressly for comparison with clinical pathology data, but it may serve that purpose well. The data dictionary is one means of modifying data in a controlled way that ensures standards are followed. A data dictionary can be used to tag all microarray data with time and date information in a standard format so that they can be automatically correlated with clinical findings (Fig. 11.9).

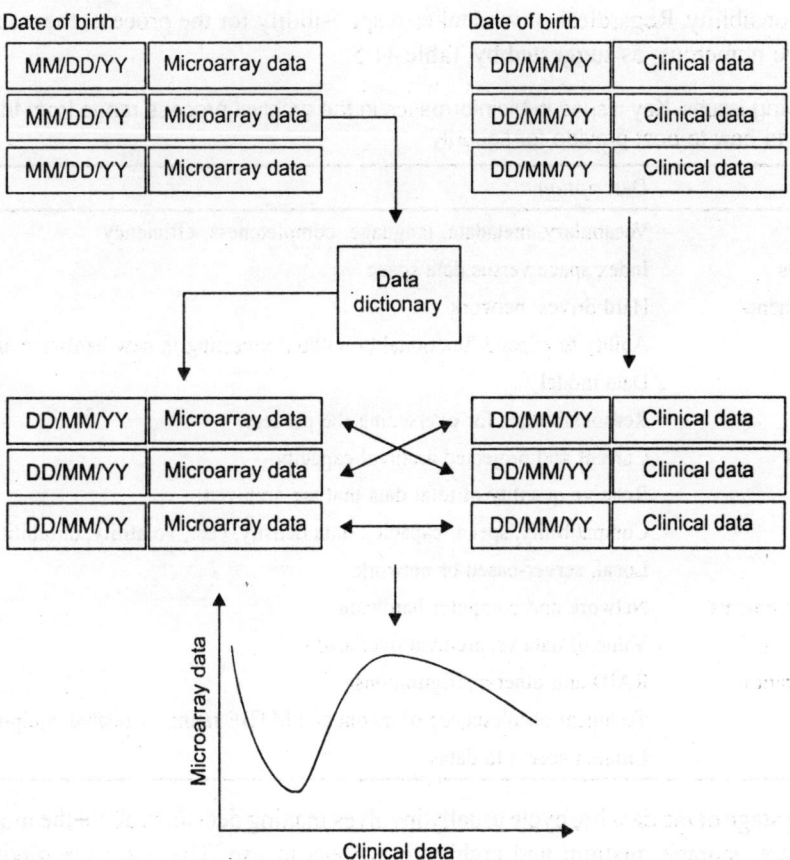

Fig. 11.9. Data dictionary-directed data modification. The time and date header for microarray data can be automatically modified so that it can be easily correlated with clinical findings.

Data that are modified or transformed by the data dictionary are normally stored in a data mart or data warehouse so that the transformed data are readily available for subsequent analysis without investing time and diverting computational resources by repeatedly reformatting the data. In the example in Fig. 11.9, the relationship between microarray data and clinical data, such as activity at a particular gene locus and overt aggression score, can be more easily computed because the data can be sorted and compared by date of birth. That is, the more likely transformed data will be used in analysis in the future, the more valuable the data warehouse and the data dictionary.

Archiving

Archiving, the central focus of the data life cycle, is concerned with making data available for future use. Unlike a data repository, data mart or data warehouse, which hold data that are frequently accessed, an archive is a container for data that is infrequently accessed, with the focus more on longevity than on access speed. In the archiving process—which can range from making a backup of a local database on a CD-ROM or Zip® disk to creating a backup of an entire EMR system in a large hospital—data are named, indexed and filed in a way that facilitates identification later. While university or government personnel archive the large online public databases, the archiving of locally generated data is a personal or corporate responsibility. Regardless of who takes responsibility for the process, the issues associated with archiving are numerous, as suggested by Table 11.5.

Table 11.5. Archiving issues. Key issues in bioinformatics in the archival process range from the scalability of the initial solution to how to best provide for security.

Issue	Description
Indexing	Vocabulary, metadata, language, completeness, efficiency
Space Requirements	Index space versus data space
Hardware Requirements	Hard drives, network
Scalability	Ability to expand functionality without investing in new hardware and software
Database design	Data model
Archival process	Responsibilities for overseeing the process
Space requirements	Current and projected archival capacity
Completeness	Relative quantity of total data that are archived
Media selection	Compatibility, speed, capacity, data density, cost, volatility, durability and stability
Location	Local, server-based or network
Infrastructure-requirements	Network and computer hardware
Relative value	Value of data vs. archival overhead
Hardware Configuration	RAID and other configurations
Longevity	Technical obsolescence of media and MTBF rating of related equipment
Security	Limited access to data

The archiving stage of the data life cycle usually involves making decisions about the most appropriate software, hardware, storage medium and archiving process to use. There are the obvious issues of media cost and longevity, security standards, the type of hardware to use to store the data and the software that will facilitate storage and later retrieval. For example, selecting the optimal storage medium for the archiving process is a function of the frequency with which archived data are accessed, the budget and the volume of data involved.

The hardware involved in the archiving process may include a PC-based CD-ROM burner, a large database server that's networked to a number of workstations and routinely backed up onto magnetic tape or a network-based storage that may be located offsite. As discussed later in this chapter, each option has security, cost and performance issues. The software tools selected for archiving data also define the usability and performance of the data archive, especially regarding data indexing and retrieval functions.

After data have been created and, if necessary, modified for use and before it can be archived, it's typically named, indexed and filed to facilitate locating it in the future. As such, the filing system, naming conventions and accuracy and specificity of indexing limit die efficiency with which the data can be located later. For example, each document can be assigned one or more keywords, but if the keywords aren't appropriate, the keyword vocabulary is undefined or not enforced or too few keywords are used, then a document may be effectively lost in the system. Not only the choice and number of keywords, but the indexing hierarchy can make data hard to find.

The process of data archiving is far more important than the associated technology, in that the best software and hardware are useless if they aren't used. Of the technical issues involved in archiving gene sequences, microarray analysis and other bioinformatics data, scalability is typically the most important. Even relatively small laboratories generate megabytes of data every week, which is fuelling demand for very-large-capacity archival storage devices.

One of the primary determinants of archive capacity is the storage media—the physical material used to form a tape, disk or cartridge. In addition to capacity, media can be characterised in terms of compatibility, speed, data density, cost, volatility, durability and stability. Compatibility is the ability of media to function within a particular software and hardware environment. Speed is a multi-faceted performance characteristic that encompasses both the time to locate data (seek time) and the time to write it to or download it from the media (data transfer rate), all of which are functions of the construction of the supporting hardware and electronics. Seek time may be several hundred milliseconds for a CD-ROM, a few milliseconds for a hard drive and a few microseconds for a flash memory card. Capacity—the maximum amount of data the media can store—is a function of the media construction, the tolerance of the casing or cartridge for tape- and disk-based media and the technology used to read and write the data. Capacity is also a function of data density, which is in turn a function of the media, the drive mechanism and the error coding and compression technologies. Error-control and compression schemes in hard drives and other media allow higher data densities than the raw media would support otherwise.

Cost is a function of the raw materials involved in the creation of media, but has more to do with what the market will bear and what the competition has to offer. Volatility, a characteristic normally ascribed to solid-state memory, refers to the status of the data when external power is removed. Flash memory, like magnetic disk or tape, is considered relatively nonvolatile and can hold data for years without loss.

Durability refers to the physical properties of the media that contribute to the longevity of the surface, mechanisms and housing, if any, during normal use. For example, the bearings and other components in the rotational system of a hard drive undergo wear and tear over time. Stability reflects the physical properties of the media in a given environment that contribute to the longevity of the media and therefore the data, in a dormant state. For example, the bearings, metal and plastic parts are subject to the same problems that beset every complex electro-mechanical device. Lubrication dries out, leaving bearing dry and without protection, rubber becomes brittle, plastic parts deform and dust and lint accumulate in the cooling system. Furthermore, the magnetic patterns induced in the iron-oxide coating on the disk platters fade over the years, especially in the heat. Similarly, the plastic-based optical media of a CD-ROM is susceptible to damage from high humidity, rapid and extreme temperature fluctuations and contamination from airborne pollution. Over time, oil from our fingers can also damage the plastic surface of a CD-ROM. Fluctuations in temperature and humidity can also cause shrinking and expansion of magnetic tape, distorting the position of data tracks, resulting in data loss.

The longevity or life expectancy of the devices in an archive system is usually expressed in the mean time between failure (MTBF) rating. The MTBF, an estimate of the failure rate of a device during its expected lifetime, is one metric that can be used to estimate the life span of an archive. Typical MTBF fatings for tape drives and commercial-grade hard drives are over 20 years. However, this figure assumes ideal conditions of constant low temperature and humidity, freedom from biological agents, statio-electricity discharges and mechanical abuse. Another consideration is that even if a tape survives a decade or more in fireproof safe, it's likely that the data it contains will be inaccessible because of changes in tape-drive standards. Most of the disk packs, tapes and magnetic cartridges that were standard archival media a decade ago are incompatible with current computer hardware.

Archives vary considerably in configuration and in proximity to the source data. For example, servers typically employ several independent hard drives configured as a redundant array of independent disks (RAID system) that function in part as an integrated archival system. The idea behind a RAID system is to provide real-time backup of data by increasing the odds that data written to a server will survive the crash of any given hard drive in the array. RAID was originally introduced in the late 1980s as a means of turning relatively slow and inexpensive hard disks into fast, large-capacity, more reliable storage systems. RAID systems derive their speed from reading and writing to multiple disks in parallel. The increased reliability is achieved through mirroring or replicating data across the array and by using error-detection and correction schemes. Although there are seven levels of RAID, level 3 is most applicable to bioinformatics computing. In RAID–3, a disk is dedicated to storing a parity bit—an extra bit used to determine the accuracy of data transfer—for error detection and correction. If analysis of the parity bit indicates an error, the faulty disk can be identified and replaced. The data can be reconstructed by using the remaining disks and the parity disk.

For example, in Fig. 11.10, disks A–D are dedicated to data and disk P is used to store the parity bit. In this case, an odd number of '1' bits corresponds to a high ('1') parity bit. When data are written in parallel to the data disks, the corresponding parity bit is stored on the parity disk. Immediately after the data are written to the data disks, the data are read and the parity bits are compared. The discrepancy noted in Fig. 11.10 is typical of a case when there is an error on one disk. The error on disk 'C' can be repaired or if groups of errors are suddenly becoming apparent indicating imminent disk failure, then the entire disk can be replaced. Another approach is to create archives on separate media on a regular basis and transport the media offsite to a safe location that would survive natural or man-made disaster at the main computing facility. A related tactic is to use network-based storage from a third-party vendor and export data to the offsite storage electronically. However, third-party archives have greater security risks than archives that can be controlled and maintained locally.

Repurposing

One of the major benefits of having data readily available in an archive is the ability to repurpose it for a variety of uses. For example, linear sequence data originally captured to discover new genes are commonly repurposed to support the 3D visualisation of protein structures.

One of the major issues in repurposing data is the ability to efficiently locate data in archives. The difficulty in locating data once it's been incorporated into a storage system depends on the volume of data involved. Efficient retrieval is a function of the hardware and database management software, the effectiveness of the user interface and the granularity of the index. For example, nucleotide sequence data indexed by chromosome number would be virtually impossible to locate if the database contains thousands of sequences indexed to each chromosome.

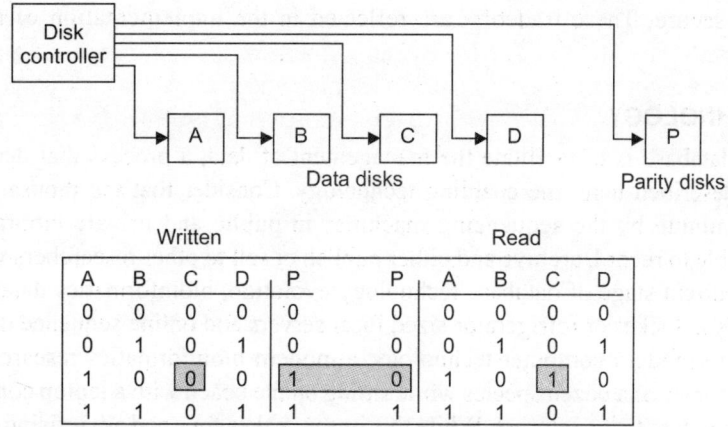

Fig. 11.10. RAID–3. Data disks are read and written to in parallel, providing speed, while a dedicated parity disk provides increased reliability through error detection and correction. In this example an error in disk C is detected by a different parity bit (P), indicating that the data read from disks A–D don't agree with what was written to the disks. Although the parity bit is usually based on a comparison of bytes on the data disks, bits (0 or 1) are used here for clarity.

Issues in the repurposing phase of the data life cycle include the sensitivity, specificity, false positives and false negatives associated with searches. The usability of the user interface is also a factor, whether free-text natural language, search by example or simple keyword searching is supported. In addition, the provisions for security can affect the ease with which data can be located and repurposed. An overly complex security procedure that requires revalidation of user identity every five minutes could deter even the most well-intentioned researcher.

Disposal

The duration of the data life cycle is a function of the perceived value of the data, the effectiveness of the underlying process and the limitations imposed by the hardware, software and environmental infrastructure. Eventually, all data die, either because they are intentionally disposed of when their value has decreased to the point that it is less than the cost of maintaining it or because of accidental loss. Often, data have to be archived because of legal reasons, even though the data is of no intrinsic value to the institution or researcher. For example, most official hospital or clinic patient records must be maintained for the life of the patient. As such, earmarking data for disposal is normally based on the quality and relevance of the data, as opposed to the age of the data. Researchers in a laboratory working with sequence data might be investigating single genes in turn, moving from one gene to the next. When sequence data from one gene is no longer necessary, it can be discarded from the local data warehouse leaving room for the next gene's sequence data—whether the data are stored on an internal disk in a Linux workstation or a central data warehouse.

Managing the Life Cycle

Managing the data life cycle is an engineering exercise that's a compromise between speed, completeness, longevity, cost, usability and security. For example, the media selected for archiving will not only affect the cost, but the speed of storage and longevity of the data. Similarly, using an in-house tape backup facility may be more costly than outsourcing the task to networked vendor, but the in-house approach is likely to be more secure. These tradeoffs are reflected in the implementation of the overall data-management process.

DATABASE TECHNOLOGY

The purpose of a database is to facilitate the management of data, a process that depends on people, processes and as described here, the enabling technology. Consider that the thousands of base pairs discovered every minute by the sequencing machines in public and private laboratories would be practically impossible to record, archive and either publish or sell to other researchers without computer databases. At the current stage of database technology evolution, bioinformatics databases are housed on large hard drives in locker or refrigerator sized local servers and online sequence data bases such as GenBank. Thanks to modern computer technology, a modern bioinformatics researcher can compare and contrast the genomes of a dozen species while sitting on the beach with a laptop computer connected through a wireless modem to the Internet. While this image makes for good advertising copy, in practice, most researchers are tied to wet laboratories that generate, manipulate and store vast quantities of experiment-specific data. In this context, the database technology empowers researchers to store their data in a way that it can be quickly and easily accessed, manipulated, compared to other data and shared with other researchers.

The concept of a database is necessarily coloured by the current state of the technology, just as a state-of-the-art bioinformatics workstation, operating at Gigahertz clock speeds with a gigabyte or more of RAM and banks of hundred-gigabyte hard drives, would easily outperform one of the early supercomputers, database technology is constantly evolving. Within our lifetimes, the contents of GenBank will easily fit into the working memory of a handheld computer and our concept of what constitutes a 'large' database will have to be adjusted accordingly. Even so, there is more to the concept of a database—whether it's referred to as a repository, data warehouse, data mart or local database—than raw capacity.

The volatility of the data, the concept of working memory and the interrelatedness of data, regardless of the volume of data involved, are distinguishing features of the various forms of memory systems or databases. For example, from the perspective of working memory, the function of a data warehouse is to move data from a variety of sources and prepare the data for incorporation into working memory. Similarly, a data warehouse or other database is distinguished from an archive in that the data in an archive are much further removed from working memory. An archive might be stored on optical platters, magnetic tapes or other media that is held in an offsite fireproof safe or underground building. Furthermore, the archive is typically engineered for longevity and the ability to be reconstituted and not for speed of access. A database, in contrast, is a live, working system that forms the centerpiece for biotech R&D activities.

Functionally, the relationship between various database technologies can be compared to the information stored in the body, as depicted in Fig. 11.11. Just as it's inefficient to have papers strewn about an office, out of order, difficult to identify and distracting the user's attention from the documents that should be addressed, our genetic information is stored in the genome, tightly packed, out of harm's way and yet accessible. The data are there, as in an archive, but not immediately available. Focusing on the individual chromosomes, data are more readily available, but still packed away so that they don't interfere with cellular processes. As subsets of data are moved out of the chromosome to the work environment, through the process of transcription, data are more readily available for use. Finally, at the translation stage, the data serve as the basis for the current work (as data do for computer applications), whether creating proteins according to the Central Dogma or attempting to locate a matching gene in a pattern-matching application.

The analogy depicted in Fig. 11.11 highlights the concept of working memory. Data are pulled from archives, whether they reside in the double helix of a chromosome or on a tape cartridge and are put in position where they can either be acted upon or direct other activities. In the cell, the activity is protein synthesis. In the workstation, this activity can be identifying a nucleotide sequence, predicting the 3D structure of a protein or modelling how multiple proteins interact at the molecular level.

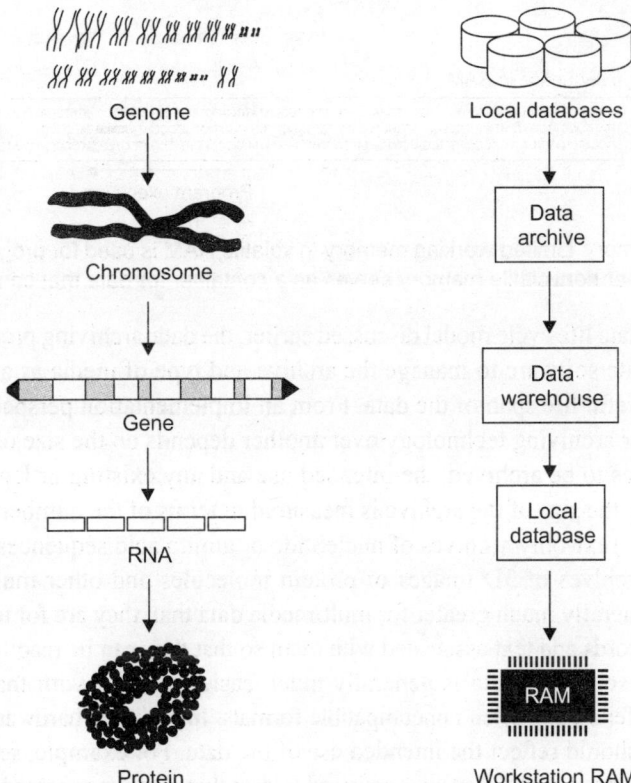

Fig. 11.11. Organic analog of database hierarchy. The database hierarchy has many parallels to the hierarchy in the human genome. Data stored in chromosomes, like a data archive, must be unpacked and transferred to a more immediately useful form before the data can be put to use.

For example, as illustrated in Fig. 11.12, a pattern-matching program that is searching for a match in a long nucleotide sequence works on the sequence in local, high-speed, active (and volatile) memory—the computer's RAM. As soon as the length of nucleotide sequence that can fit in RAM is searched, it is discarded and replaced by a new sequence that is copied (akin to transcription) from the hard disk, flash memory or other nonvolatile storage media. Just as RNA is discarded after it has been involved in the translation process to make room for the next set of instructions from the DNA, the data in RAM are constantly refreshed and updated under the direction of the computer's CPU.

Volatility, working memory and the volume of data that can be handled are key variables in memory systems such as databases. In addition, there is the quality of interrelatedness; just as the genes in the chromosomes are associated with each other by virtue of their physical proximity, the data in a database are interrelated in a way that facilitates use for specific applications. For example, nucleotide sequences that will be used in pattern-matching operations in the online sequence databases will be formatted according to the same standard—such as the FASTA standard.

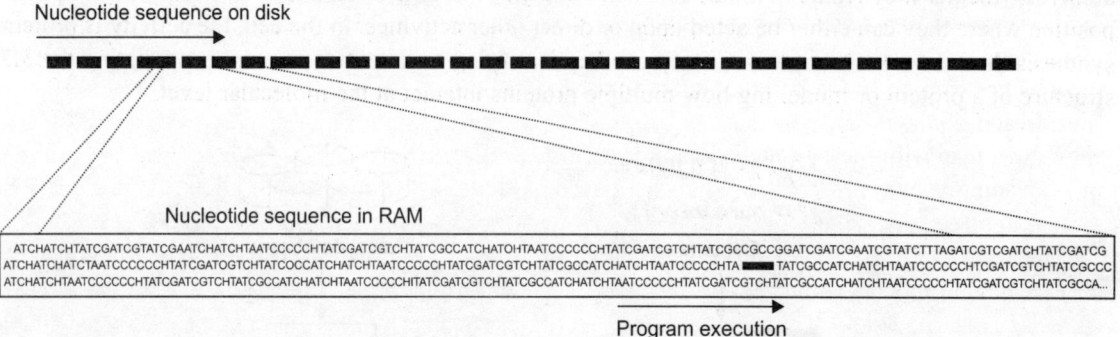

Fig. 11.12. Working memory. Limited working memory in volatile RAM is used for program execution, whereas an expansive disk or other nonvolatile memory serves as a container for data that can't fit in working memory.

As reflected in the data life cycle model discussed earlier, the data-archiving process involves indexing, selecting the appropriate software to manage the archive and type of media as a function of frequency of use and expected useful life span of the data. From an implementation perspective, the key issues in selecting one particular archiving technology over another depends on the size of the archive, the types of data and data sources to be archived, the intended use and any existing or legacy archiving systems involved. For example, the size of the archive is measured in terms of the number of items and the space requirements per item. Text-only archives of nucleotide or amino acid sequences generally require less space per item than archives of 3D images of protein molecules and other multimedia. Not only are space requirements generally much greater for multimedia data than they are for text, but images usually require additional keywords and text associated with them so that they can be readily located in an archive.

Similarly, a single source of data is generally much easier to work with than data from multiple, disparate sources in different and often noncompatible formats. In addition, hardware and software used in the archiving process should reflect the intended use of the data. For example, seldom-used data can be archived using a much less powerful system, compared to data that must be accessed frequently. Finally, it's rare to have the opportunity to initiate a digital archiving program from scratch. Normally, there is some form of existing (legacy) system in place whose data has to be converted to be suitable for archiving.

The simplest approach to managing bioinformatics data in a small laboratory is to establish a file server that is regularly backed up to a secure archive. To use the hardware most effectively, everyone connected to the server copies their files from their local hard drive to specific areas on the server's hard drive on a daily basis. The data on the server are in turn archived to magnetic tape or other high-capacity media by someone assigned to the task. In this way, researchers can copy the file from the server to their local hard drive as needed. Similarly, if the server hardware fails for some reason, then the archive can be used to reconstitute the data on a second server.

As noted earlier, from a database perspective, file servers used as archives have several limitations. For example, because the data may be created using different applications, perhaps using different formats and operating systems, searching through the data may be difficult, especially from a single interface other than with the search function that is part of the computer's operating system. Even then, there is no way of knowing what particular files hold. For example, the files in a library of 3D protein-folding images created in a graphics modelling package may be labelled according to one researcher's experiment and not for general use. That is, there is typically no automated way of instituting a controlled vocabulary for all users to abide by.

There are other practical limitations as well. For example, in a small work group of perhaps a dozen researchers, it's tempting to make an open file-sharing system without security procedures. However, this practice can result in accidental loss of information through inadvertent deletion or modification of files. In addition, without a database, it's difficult to control for versions or updated copies of particular files, other than with file-naming conventions. Furthermore, combining data from different applications in a meaningful way to assist in analysis may be arduous and time-consuming without a database system in place.

The need for greater control over the intellectual capital of a biotech R&D laboratory usually necessitates the understanding and use of database technology. Just as particular wet-laboratory equipment provides a mix of features that supports some experiments and yet hinders others, databases are available in a wide spectrum of designs that are optimised for specific types of operations at the expense of others. The overall architecture, the underlying models supporting the database and database management system that supports the model provided by one database system may be ideal for managing nucleotide sequence data, but unwieldy for managing 3D protein structures, for example. Furthermore, a homegrown database that is developed without knowledge of outside standards may be unusable or inefficient when used with public-domain software, such as the locally executable BLAST application.

Database Architecture

One of the greatest challenges in bioinformatics is the complete, seamless integration of databases from a variety of sources. This is not the case now, primarily because when databases such as GenBank and SWISS-PROT were designed, their architectures were designed primarily to support their particular function. Working with other systems was a secondary concern. However, with the proliferation of data and the standardisation on the Web as the main means of access to these data, integration has become a major concern. Without some form of database integration, the researcher who seeks to correlate a symptom such as aggression with a genetic abnormalities must query several databases to compare clinical behaviour with genetic abnormalities. Furthermore, because the amount of data in many of the molecular biology databases is growing at an exponential rate, there usually aren't sufficient resources to modify the basic architecture of these databases.

There are exceptions, such as PubMed Central, where data from disparate databases, each with their own data formats and underlying architectures, have been combined into one common structure. However, because of the time and cost involved in converting database architectures, a better approach, when the option is available, is to use an architecture that not only supports immediate needs, but that also makes provision for future integration with other database systems. For this reason, knowledge of database architecture is key to anyone practising bioinformatics. In addition, an understanding of database architectures can facilitate working with existing or legacy systems.

From a structural or architectural perspective, database technology can be considered either centralised or distributed. In the centralised approach, typified by the data warehouse, data are processed in order to fit into a central database. In a distributed architecture, data are dispersed geographically, even though they may appear to be in one location because of the database management system software. In each case, the goal is the same—providing researchers with some means of rapidly accessing and keeping track of data in a way that supports reuse. This is especially critical in large biotech laboratories, where large, comprehensive patient and genomic databases support data mining and other methods that extract meaningful patterns from potentially millions of records.

A centralised architecture, such as that illustrated in Fig. 11.13, concentrates all organisational activity in one location. This can be a formidable task, as it requires cleaning, encoding and translation of data before they can be included in the central database. For example, once data to be included in a data warehouse have been identified, the data from each application are cleaned (typos and other errors are identified and removed or corrected) and merged with data from other applications. In addition, there are the usual issues of database design, provision for maintenance, security and periodic modification.

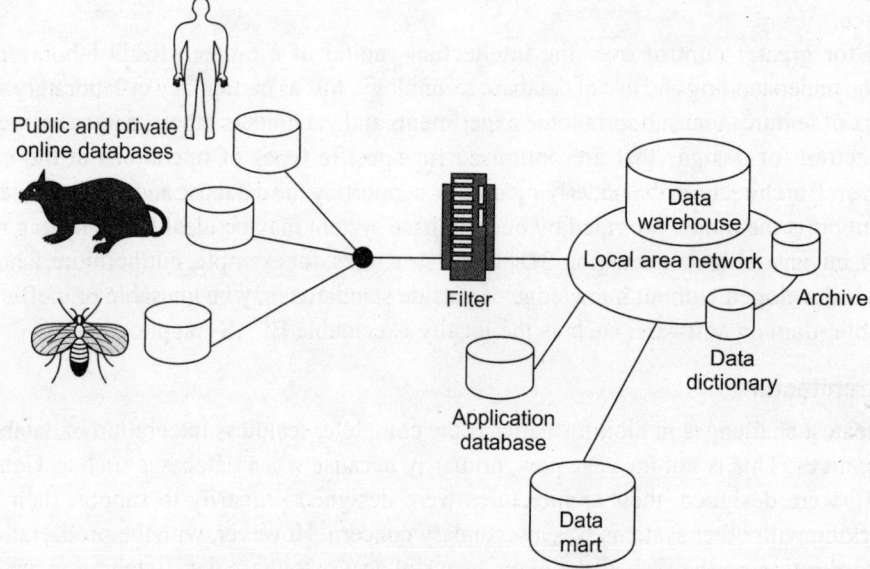

Fig. 11.13. Centralised database architecture. A centralised database; such as a data warehouse, combines data from a variety of databases in one physical location.

A data warehouse isn't simply a large hard disk, but a database system implemented on a tiered storage system that reflects access time, cost and data longevity constraints. For example, some data may reside on fast magnetic media, such as hard disks and other data may reside on slower optical media. The goal is to keep the right information flowing to the right people in the most intelligent form as quickly and efficiently as possible, which includes making provision for the storage of both frequently and seldom-accessed data.

In contrast to a centralised architecture, distributed database architecture is characterised by physically disparate storage media. One advantage of using a distributed architecture is that it supports the ability to use a variety of hardware and software in a laboratory, allowing a group to use the software that makes their lives easiest, while still allowing a subset of data in each application to be shared throughout the organisation. Separate applications, often running on separate machines and using proprietary data formats and storage facilities, share a subset of information with other applications. A limitation of this common interface approach, compared to a central database, is that the amount of data that can be shared among applications is typically limited. In addition, there is the computational overhead of communicating data between applications.

A challenge of using an integrated approach is developing the interfaces between the databases associated with each application. When there are only a few different applications and operating systems to contend with, developing custom interfaces between different databases may be tenable. However, with multiple applications and their associated databases, the number of custom interfaces that must be developed to allow sharing of data becomes prohibitive. For example, with 5 different databases, 9 different custom interfaces would have to be developed. For 6 different databases, 11 interfaces would be needed. Because of the work involved, a typical scenario is incomplete integration, as shown in Fig. 11.14.

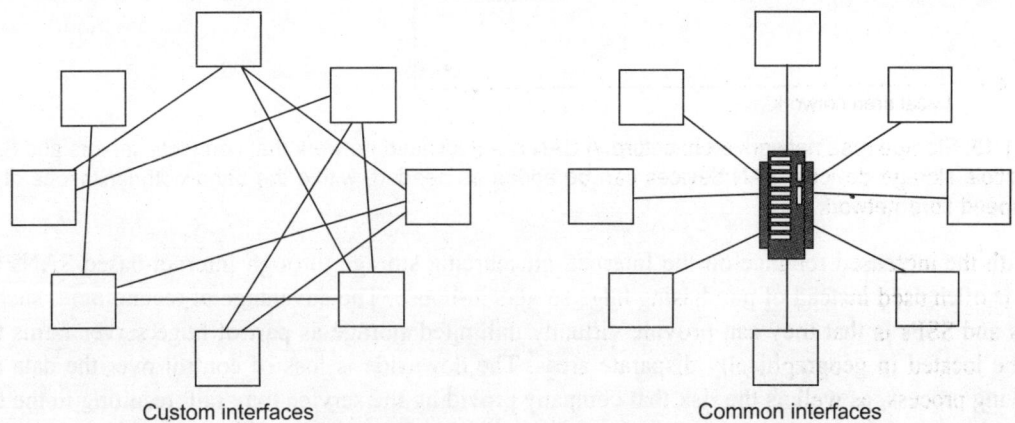

Custom interfaces   Common interfaces

Fig. 11.14. Distributed database integration. Distributed databases can be configured to share data through dedicated, one-to-one custom interfaces (left) or by writing to a common interface standard (right). Custom interfaces incur a work penalty on the order of two times the number of databases that are integrated.

A better solution to integrating incompatible databases is to write interfaces to a common standard. For example, in clinical medicine, most application vendors are compatible with the health level 7 (HL 7) interface protocol, which allows radiology, laboratory and pathology systems to exchange a subset of their data, such as patient demographics, diagnosis, drug allergies and current medications.

Full database integration is much more than simply moving data to a single hard disk. A file server can store data from dozens of various applications and yet have no integration between applications. Similarly, just as a single hard disk can be formatted so that it appears as several logical volumes or drives, a distributed physical architecture can function like a logical centralised database. Taking this analogy one step further, there are hybrid database architectures that combine aspects of centralised and distributed architectures to provide enhanced functionality or reduced cost. For example, the storage area network (SAN) architecture is based on a separate, dedicated, high-speed network that provides storage under one interface (Fig. 11.15). With the appropriate software, a SAN can be configured to provide the functionality of a central data warehouse, including provision for making available an unlimited subset of the data from each application database.

In addition to SANs, there is a variety of other network-dependent database architectures. For example, network attached storage (NAS) is one method of adding storage to a networked system of workstations. To users on the network, the NAS acts like a second hard drive on their workstations. However, a NAS device, like a file server, must be managed and archived separately. A similar approach is to use a storage service provider (SSP), which functions as an application service provider (ASP) with a database as the application.

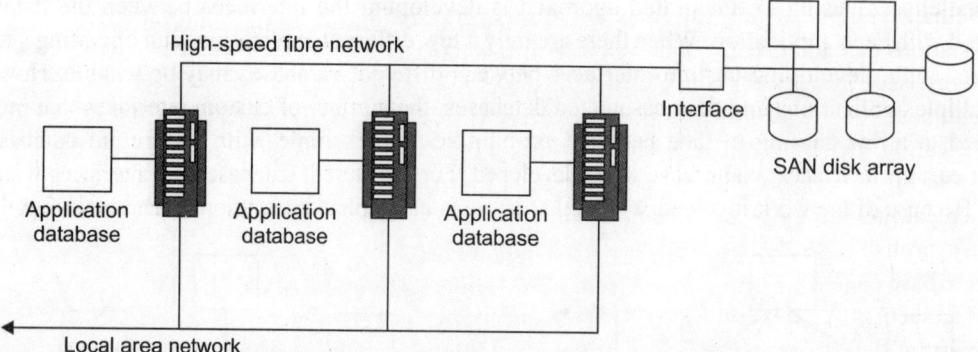

Fig. 11.15. Storage area network architecture. A SAN is a dedicated network that connects servers and SAN-compatible storage devices. SAN devices can be added as needed, within the bandwidth limitations of the high-speed fibre network.

With the increased reliance on the Internet, outsourcing storage through Internet-based SANs and SSPs is often used instead of purchasing huge servers in-house. The advantage of technologies such as SANs and SSPs is that they can provide virtually unlimited storage as part of huge server farms that may be located in geographically disparate areas. The downside is loss of control over the data and archiving process, as well as the risk that company providing the service may fail, resulting in the loss of valuable research and production data. In addition, like NAS, SANs and SSPs only address additional storage space, not integration.

Database Management Systems

The database management system (DBMS) is the set of software tools that works with a given architecture to create a practical database application. The DBMS is the interface between the low-level hardware commands and the user, allowing the user to think of data management in abstract, high-level terms using a variety of data models, instead of the bits and bytes on magnetic media. The DBMS also provides views or high-level abstract models of portions of the conceptual database that are optimised for particular users. In this way, the DBMS, like the user interface of a typical application, shields the user from the details of the underlying algorithms and data representation schemes.

In addition to providing a degree of abstraction, the DBMS facilitates use by maximising the efficiency of managing data with techniques such as dynamically configuring operations to make use of a given hardware platform. For example, a DBMS should recognise a server with large amounts of free RAM and make use of that RAM to speed serving the data. A DBMS also ensures data integrity by imposing data consistency constraints, such as requiring numeric data in certain fields, free text in others and image data elsewhere. A researcher isn't allowed to insert a numerical sequence in the space assigned for a nucleotide sequence, for example.

The DBMS also guards against data loss. For example, a DBMS should support quick recovery from hardware or software failures. A DBMS can guard against data corruption that might result from two simultaneous operations on a given data item. The most common example is prohibiting two users from simultaneously manipulating the same data. In addition, a DBMS adds security to a database, in that a properly constructed DBMS allows only users with permission to have access to specific data, normally down to the level of individual files. Multi-level user password-protection schemes can be used to allow only graphic designers to view intermediate graphic data and those in marketing to view only final versions. Using intranets that limit data communications within a predefined group of workstations can add greatly to the security of a database.

A key issue in working with a DBMS is the use of metadata or information about data contained in the database. Views are one application of metadata—a collection of information about naming, classification, structure and use of data that reduces inconsistency and ambiguity. For example, as shown in Fig. 11.16, one way to think about the application of metadata is to consider the high-level biomedical literature a means of simplifying and synthesising the underlying complexity of molecular disease, protein structure, protein alignment and protein and DNA sequence data. From this perspective, data are base pair identifiers derived from observation, experiment or calculation, information is data in context, such as the relationship of DNA sequences to protein structure and metadata is a descriptive summary of disease presentations that provides additional context to the underlying information. The use of metadata as an organisational theme makes the centralised data-management approach easier to maintain and control. For example, a simple file-server system typically lacks the contextual framework and interrelatedness of information and data provided by a database management system. As a result, there is no automated way to manage the contents of individual files and folders that may be included on the file server.

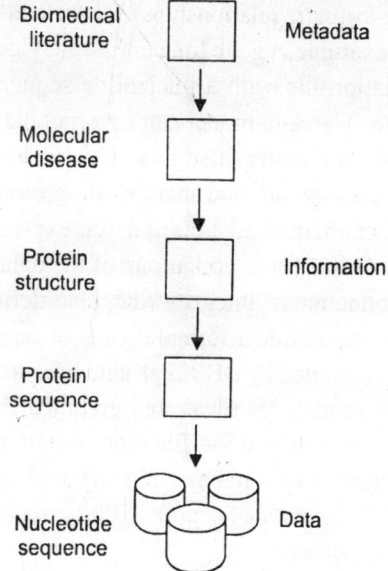

Fig. 11.16. Metadata, information and data in bioinformatics. Metadata labels, simplifies and provides context for underlying information and data.

Commonly used commercial DBMS packages in bioinformatics include products from Microsoft, Oracle, Sybase, IBM, MySQL AB and InterSystems. In addition, there are dozens of proprietary and academic systems developed for particular niche applications that many bioinformatics researchers employ as well. Regardless of whether the technology is rooted in academia or business, virtually every DBMS can be described using three levels of abstraction: the physical database, the conceptual database and the views. The point of using these abstractions is that they allow researchers to manipulate huge amounts of data that may be associated in very complex ways by shielding database designers and users from the underlying complexity of computer hardware. The physical database is the low-level data and framework that is defined in terms of media, bits and bytes. This low-level abstraction is most useful for anyone who has to deal directly with data and files.

The conceptual database, at a somewhat higher level of abstraction than the physical database, is concerned with the most appropriate way to represent the data. This level of abstraction more closely approximates the needs of database designers who deal with DBMS data representation and efficiency issues such as the data-dictionary design. The conceptual database is defined in terms of data structures (an organisational scheme, such as a record) and the properties of the data to be stored and manipulated. The most common methods of representing the conceptual database are the entity-relationship model and the data model.

The entity-relationship model focuses on entities and their interrelationships in a way that parallels how we categorise the world. For example, common database entities in bioinformatics are the human being, protein sequences, nucleotide sequences and disease processes about which data are recorded. Similarly, every entity has some basic attribute, such as name, size, weight (a particular protein may have a known weight) or charge. Relationships within the model are classified according to how data are associated with each other, such as one-to-one, one-to-many or many-to-many. For example, a length of DNA may be translated to one mRNA sequence (a one-to-one relationship) and a gene may give rise to several proteins (a one-to-many relationships). These and other relationships can be used to maintain the integrity of data. For example, a gene (one entity) may generate more than one protein, but the gene, having a one-to-one relationship with a nucleotide sequence, shouldn't be associated with more than one nucleotide sequence. The data model can enforce this one-to-one relationship.

The conceptual database can also be represented as a data model. Like entity-relationship models, data models provide a means of representing and manipulating large amounts of data. A data model consists of two components—a mathematical notation for expressing data and relationships and operations on the data that serve to express manipulations of the data. Like entity-relationship models, data models may also contain a collection of integrity rules that define valid data relationships. These various components work together to provide a formal means of representing and manipulating data.

The most common data models supported by DBMS products are flat, network, hierarchical, relational, object-oriented and deductive data models, as illustrated graphically in Fig. 11.17. Even though long strings of sequencing data lend themselves to a flat file representation, the relational database model is by far the most popular in the commercial database industry and is found in virtually every biotech R&D laboratory. However, virtually every data model illustrated in Fig. 11.17 has applications in bioinformatics, from flat to semi-structured.

The flat data model is simply a table without any embedded structure information to govern the relationships between records. As a result, a flat file database can only work with one table or file at a time. Strictly speaking, a flat file doesn't really fit the criteria for a data model because it lacks an embedded structure. However, the lack of an embedded structure is one reason for the popularity of the flat file database in bioinformatics, especially in capturing sequence data. A sequence of a few dozen characters may be followed by a sequence of thousands of characters, with no known relationship between the sequences, other than perhaps the tissue sample or sequence run. As such, a separate flat file can be used to efficiently store the sequence data from each sample or run. In order to make the management of large amounts of sequence or other data more tenable, a model with an embedded structure is required.

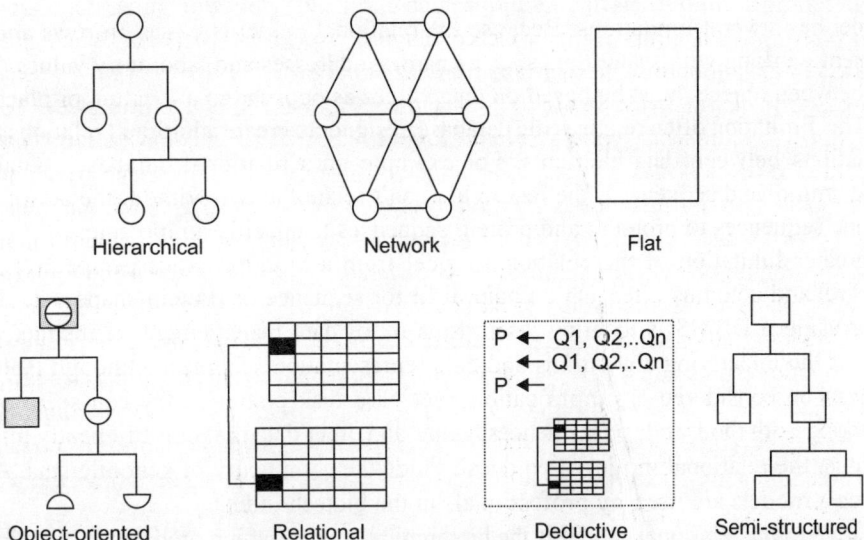

Fig. 11.17. Data models. The most common data models in bioinformatics are relational, flat and object-oriented.

The relational model, is based on the concept of a data table in which every row is unique. The records or rows in the table are called tuples; the fields or columns are variably referred to attributes, predicates or classes. Database queries are performed with the select operation, which asks for all tuples in a certain relation that meet a certain criterion—for example, a query such as 'Which authors write about neurofibromatosis?' To connect the data of two or more relations, an operation called a join is performed. A record is retrieved from the database by means of a key or label, that may consist of a field, part of a field or a combination of several fields. Supporting this data model so that it's easy for someone to direct a search for the record that contains the particular value of the key is the purpose of a relational DBMS. Consider querying a bibliographic database with an 'author_subject_table', using the Structured Query Language (SQL) statement:

SELECT *.* FROM author_subject_table
WHERE subject = 'Neurofibromatosis'

A useful feature of the relational model is that records or rows from different files can be combined as long as the different files have one field in common. Theoretically, records with a common field can be combined or joined with an unlimited number of files. The price paid for this flexibility is extended access time. That is, in a database design that doesn't take likely use patterns into account, performance suffers. A large amount of processor time will be spent extracting information from the system as the database program performs joins and other operations. This performance penalty is a reason for not simply polling application databases for data. It's far better, from a performance perspective, to move the data into a separate data repository, a second database that is optimised for the desired searching and analysis.

The attraction of the ubiquitous relational model is that it is mature, stable, reliable, well understood and well suited for a number of different applications in bioinformatics. The basic concepts involved with the relational model are easily grasped; data are populated into rows and columns in a table and tables are associated with one another by joining fields that match in the two tables. However, the relational model has several limitations. Because the relational model is based on rows and columns, it's most efficient working with scalar data such as names, addresses and laboratory values. That is, all relationships between objects must be based on data values as opposed to a location or place-holder in the database. This limitation often requires the database designer to create additional relations to describe logical associations between data elements. For example, in a relational database containing both nucleotide and amino acid sequences, the researcher can't relate the two without the aid of tables that relate nucleotide sequences to proteins and protein sequences to specific amino acids.

An even greater limitation of the relational model from a bioinformatics perspective is that the metaphor of rows and columns often isn't a natural fit for sequence or protein shape data. Recall that one reason for using a DBMS is to allow users to think of data management in abstract, high-level terms, instead of the underlying algorithms and data representation schemes. Although tables of rows and columns can be considered a simplification over hard disk platters, they can seem obtuse to a researcher working with thousands of sequences, genes and other data that don't fit neatly into a tabular metaphor. That is, the relational model often doesn't hide the complexity of genomic data. As a result, various other data models are used by professionals in the biotech industry.

One alternative to the relational model is the hierarchical model, which predates the relational model by a decade. Unlike the flexible relational model, permanent hierarchical connections are defined when the database is created. Within the hierarchical database model, the smallest data entity is the record. That is, unlike records in a relational model, records within a hierarchical database are not necessarily broken up into fields. In addition, connections within the hierarchical model don't depend on the data. The hierarchical links, sometimes called the structure of the data, can best be thought of as forming an inverted tree, with the parent file at the top and children files below. The relationship between parent and children is a one-to-many connection, in that one parent may produce multiple children.

The basic operation on the hierarchical database is the tree walk, proceeding from parent to child. Data can be retrieved only by traversing the levels of the hierarchy according to the path defined by the succession of parent fields. This unidirectional convention causes certain relationships to be difficult to extract from the database, even though they may be explicit in the data. For example, one characteristic of the hierarchical model is that information must often be repeated. Returning to the author-subject database example, under the topic of neurofibromatosis, if an author wrote more than one paper on the subject, the author's name and contact information would be repeated throughout the database.

The hierarchical model was once very popular in medicine, in the form of the massachusetts general hospital utility multi-programming system (MUMPS) database language, which was used to develop one of the first electronic medical record (EMR) systems. A reason for the initial popularity of MUMPS in the early 1960s was that the data model is a good fit for clinical data, which tends to follow a standard topic outline, which is hierarchical. For example, patients at the top of the hierarchy have child nodes containing the elements of the EMR, including chief complaint, diagnosis and laboratory results, as defined in Table 11.2. The limitation, noted earlier, is that for every patient admission, certain data must be repeated, such as the patient's address, billing information and other demographic information.

The hierarchical model remains significant in bioinformatics if only because a library of clinical information resides in databases following this model. For example, a descendent of MUMPS called simply M is the standard for EMRs in the Veterans Administration hospitals throughout the U.S.

Because of the storage inefficiency of the hierarchical model for some types of data, the network model was developed in the late 1960s. For example, the network model is more flexible than the hierarchical one because multiple connections can be established between files. These multiple connections enable the user to gain access to a particular file more effectively, without traversing the entire hierarchy above that file. Unlike the one-to-many relationship supported by the hierarchical model, the network model is based on a many-to-one relationship. The network model is significant in bioinformatics in that it may play a significant role in the architecture of the great global grid and other web-based computing initiatives.

One of the most significant alternatives to the relational database model is the object-oriented model in which complex data structures are represented by composite objects, which are objects that contain other objects. These objects may contain other objects in turn, allowing structures to be nested to any degree. This metaphor is especially appealing to those who work with bioinformatics data because this nesting of complexity complements the natural structure of genomic data (Fig. 11.18).

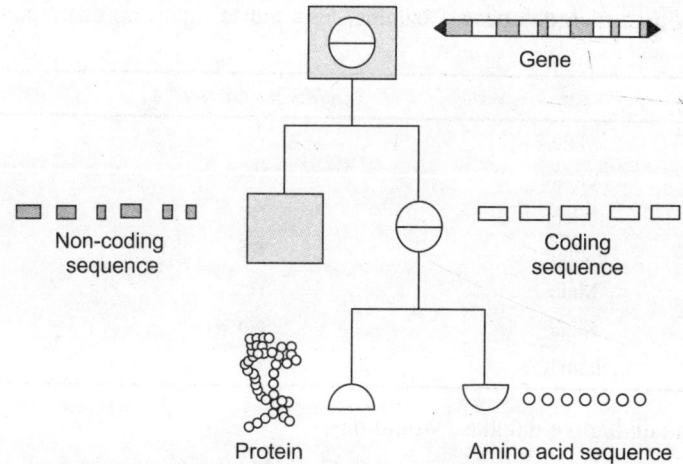

Fig. 11.18. Object-oriented data representation. The object-oriented data model is natural for hiding the complexity of genomic data.

The object-oriented model combines the natural structure of the hierarchical model with the flexibility of the relational model. As such, the major advantage of the object-oriented model is that it can be used, to represent complex genomic, information, including nonrecord-oriented data, such as textual sequence data and images, in a way that doesn't compromise flexibility. Furthermore, with an object-oriented DBMS, it's possible to use arbitrary data types and complex relationships can be queried without having to create resource-intensive joins between tables. The object-oriented model is considered optimum for, handling genomic data, because it allows combinations of data to be treated as single entities. Instead of thinking about a gene with exons, introns, mRNA, nucleotide sequences, associated proteins and their 3D shapes as a separate sound file, a separate video file and a separate text document, researchers can simply work with the gene object. Although the object-oriented approach holds great promise in bioinformatics, it still lags far behind relational technology in the global database market. In addition, because of the flexibility and power of the relational design, many of the object-oriented DBMS products on the market are based on extensions of commercial relational database packages. Because of the added overhead, the performance of these hybrid object-oriented systems is necessarily less than that of either a pure relational or an object-oriented system.

In addition to object-oriented models built on relational model technology, a variety of other models that are optimum for bioinformatics work can be constructed from relational technology. For example, the deductive model is an extension of the relational database with a logic programming interface based on the principles of logic programming. The logic programming interface is composed of rules, facts and queries, using the relational database infrastructure to contain the facts.

The database is termed deductive because from the set of rules and the facts it is possible to derive new facts not contained in the original set of facts. Unlike logic programming languages such as PROLOG, which search for a single answer to a query using a top-down search, deductive databases search from bottom-up, starting from the facts to find all answers to a query.

For example, using the format 'patient (Patient ID, Sex, Mother Carrier, Father Trait),' data in the deductive database describing a sex-linked recessive gene such as red-green colour blindness could be represented in a relational table as in Table 11.6.

Table 11.6. Data for a deductive database. Columns, from left to right, represent patient ID, sex, mother carrier and father trait.

Patient ID	Sex	Mother carrier	Father trait
001	Male	Yes	Yes
002	Female	Yes	No
003	Male	No	Yes
004	Female	No	Yes
005	Male	Yes	No
006	Male	No	No
007	Female	Yes	Yes

A relevant rule in a deductive database would be:

Potential Carrier ← (Sex = Female) AND (Mother Carrier = Yes)

That is, the patient is a potential carrier if the sex of the patient is female and the patient's mother is a known carrier. Males with the gene exhibit the disease or red-green colour blindness. However, because the gene involved in colour blindness is maternal, then the state of the father's colour acuity is irrelevant. The query:

← Patient ID (X, potential carrier)

would return the list of patients that should be tested for the genetic anomaly, in this case Patient 002 and Patient 007 from Table 11.6. Despite the obvious uses of deductive databases in bioinformatics, most deductive databases are either academic projects or internally developed and have yet to enter the ranks of commercial relational database products.

One more model worth mentioning is loosely defined as the semi-structured model. This model is a hybrid between a flat file and a hierarchical model, typically written as a text document in eXtensible markup language (XML). The major advantage of the semi-structured model (which, like a flat file, isn't really a model *per se*) includes the ability to revise the structure to match new requirements on-the-fly. Like the hybrid model, however, there is a likely repetition of data.

Regardless of the model, at the highest level of abstraction of the DBMS is the view. That is, views are abstract models of portions of the conceptual database. Each view describes some of the database entities, attributes and relationships between entities in a format convenient for a specific class of user or application. For example, researchers in a pharmacogenomic firm working with an application to report sequencing results do not need to know about patient findings. Similarly, clinicians in the pharmacology department may not need access to sequence results, but may require access to patient files. Thus, there may be one view of the database for the sequencing department and one for the proteomics department. As described in the following section, the view abstraction has application in user interface design.

INTERFACES

Databases don't stand alone, but communicate with devices and users through external and user interfaces, respectively. Getting data into a database can come about programmatically as in the creation of a data warehouse or data mart through processing an existing database. More often, the data are derived from external sources, such as user input through keyboard activity or devices connected to a computer or network. Common sources of input data include mouse and keyboard activity, voice recognition, barcode readers, wireless devices and RF-ID tags. Electronic Data recorders, sequencing machines and a variety of test equipment can also provide data for inclusion in the database, according to device communications standards. A variety of standards, such as the IEEE 1073 Point of Care Medical Device Communications standard, define the format, speed and protocol of communications between workstations and external devices (Fig. 11.19).

Getting data into a database is of little value unless the data can also be retrieved. As illustrated in Fig. 11.19, the most common methods for extracting data from a database are based on the Internet or an intranet and languages such as the Common Gateway Interface (CGI), the PHP: Hypertext Processor (PHP) and Java. In each case, the user issues a command from the workstation that is interpreted in the server. Results of the database query are then processed by language system and HTML is sent to the user's browser. In this scenario, the computational overhead is borne by the server.

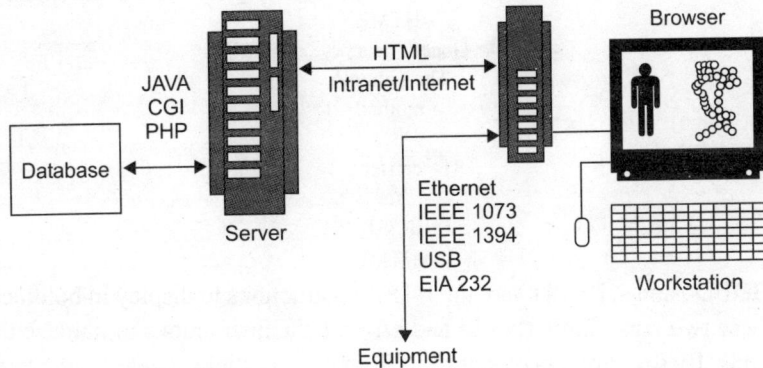

Fig. 11.19. External Interfaces. Databases communicate with equipment and users through a variety of external interfaces.

Each system handles high-lever database queries differently: For example, to perform a query using CGI, the user submits a query through a Web browser and the server executes a program, a CGI script and the user's query is passed to the database via CGI. The program then returns information to the server via CGI and this information is formatted into an HTML Web page that is displayed through the user's browser.

Similarly, the PHP interface offloads database query functions to the server, which handles the query, formats results and conveys these to the user via standard HTML. Although PHP, which was originally referred to as personal home page/forms interpreter (PHP/FI), is less established than CGI, it is considerably more powerful as a database interface. For example, unlike other scripting languages for Web page development, PHP offers excellent connectivity to most of the common databases, including Oracle, Sybase, MySQL, ODBC and many others. Java is also a server-side language that shares many of the database interface features of CGI and PHP. In addition, like PHP, Java uses a language that loosely resembles C.

CGI, PHP and Java are all dependent on the server hardware for performance and don't make additional demands for space or execution time on the workstations that are accessing data. This is in contrast with JavaScript, which has little to do with Java. JavaScript runs on the client side of the interface and, as such, can be malicious because of JavaScript viruses, JavaScript, while providing interactivity to Web pages, is much less useful as a database query tool compared to CGI, PHP or Java.

Regardless of the language used to extract data from a database, the data have to be displayed on the user's monitor in an appropriate, understandable and attractive way. This component of the user interface is most easily handled with a separate style sheet that defines the characteristics for the display device. In this paradigm, data to be displayed are first extracted from the database and coded in XML, a markup language for the Web that classifies content, but doesn't define how it should be displayed. A separate style sheet, in the form of an extensible stylesheet language (XSL) document, specifies how the data are to be displayed in the user's browser.

Using the XML/XSL approach, modifying the manner in which data are displayed can be done without changing the XML Document and involves simply modifying the relevant style sheet. Similarly, if the data change, only the XML document need be changed, not the style sheet. For example, consider the differences in how wireless content appears in HTML, XML and XSL for the following database report.

Genetic History: The patient's mother is carrier for BCG1.

In standard HTML, which combines data and formatting instructions, the source code could appear as:

```
<HTML>
<BOLD> Genetic History: </BOLD>
The patient's
<I> mother </I>
is a
<I> carrier </I>
for
<I> BCG1 </I>.
</HTML>
```

Notice that <BOLD> and </BOLD> are the HTML instructions to display in boldface type whatever comes between these two tags. Similarly <I> and </I> are the instructions to italicize the type between these two commands. By decoupling content from format instructions, changes in content can be made without the need to modify the formatting instructions given in the style sheets. Here's an example (formatted for clarity), using XML to categorise the data and XSL source code to describe formatting:

```
<PHRASE>
<GENETIC_CATEGORY> Genetic History: </GENETIC_CATEGORY>
The
<SUBJECT> patient's </SUBJECT>
<PARENT> mother </PARENT>
is
<GENOTYPE> recessive </GENOTYPE>
for
<GENE> BCG1 </GENE>
</PHRASE>
```

Assuming that the data are destined to be displayed on a wireless PDA with a monochrome display, one that supports bold and italic text formatting, the associated XSL source code could take the form:

FORHAT 'GENETIC_CATEGORY' = BOLD
FORMAT 'PARENT' = ITALICS
FORMAT 'GENOTYPE' = ITALICS
FORMAT 'GENE' = ITALICS

Furthermore, because the data in XML is decoupled from the display information in XSL, the symptom can be displayed in italics on the PDA and, for example, in red bold text on a laptop with a colour display.

IMPLEMENTATION

Even with all of the public-domain databases accessible through the Internet, there will be research tasks that necessitate using a local database. The reasons vary from a need to collect, analyse and publish sequence information inside a small laboratory to establishing a massive data warehouse as part of a pharmacogenomic R&D effort. In either case, the general issues and challenges are the same, albeit in different degrees of severity. As shown in Table 11.7, the major database implementation issues range from the storage capacity requirements and cost to scalability and security.

Table 11.7. Bioinformatics database implementation issues.

Issue	Description
Accessibility	Ease of use, support for multiple mental models and database abstractions
Archiving	Support for the archival process, including software and hardware and offsite storage facilities
Capacity	Local and remote data storage capacity, including space for expansion of the database
Connectivity	Connectivity through local and wide area networks, intranets and the internet
Control	Internal vs. third-party control of data, which may be an issue with storage service providers and other internet-based commercial storage options
Cost	Initial, operating and indirect (need to upgrade current network hardware and software, purchase additional peripherals) costs
Data dictionary	Design, implementation and maintenance of the data dictionary
Data Formats	Data formats supported by the database
Data Input	Hardware, software and processes involved in feeding data into the database, from keyboard and voice recognition to direct instrument feed and the internet
Data Model	Flat files, relational, hierarchical, network, object-oriented or semi-structured
DBMS software	Robustness, scalability, performance, cost, vendor reputation (if commercial), support available (if open source)
Dependencies frequency	Dependence on primary databases for populating the database, especially regarding update provision for validating data to minimise propagation of errors
Disaster recovery	Procedural, hardware and software provisions for disaster recovery, including error recovery mechanisms
Export/import capabilities	Provisions for importing and exporting data to and from different file formats

(Contd...)

Issue	*Description*
Hardware requirements	Hard disks, controllers, backup hardware, production and staging servers for large database projects
Indexing	Indexing methodology, including selection and use of the most appropriate controlled vocabulary
Integration	Integration with other databases
Intellectual property	Ownership of sequence data, images and other data stored in and communicated through the database
Interfaces	Connectivity with other databases and applications
Legacy systems	How to deal with legacy data and databases
Licensing	For vendor-supplied database systems, the most appropriate licensing arrangement
Life span	The MTBF for the hardware as well as the likely useful life of the data
Load testing	The maximum number of simultaneous users that can be supported by the DBMS
Maintenance	Cost and resource requirements
Media	The most appropriate disk, tape cartridges and CD-ROM media
Normalisation	Avoiding errors by representing data one way, one time and in one place
Operating environment	Ensuring proper power and operating temperature and humidity
Operating system	UNIX, Linux, Windows, MacOS or mini/mainframe OS
Output	Format of database output
Privacy	Provision for preserving confidentiality of data
Performance	Access time and data throughput
Query language	Proprietary or standard query language
Redundancy	Hot backups, shadowing and RAID systems
Resource requirements	Hardware, software and operating and development personnel
Scalability	Ability to handle greater data volume with added hardware and/or software upgrades
Security	Limits on user access, from username-password combinations to biometrics, as well as encryption of sessions
Stand-Alone vs. Network	And multi- vs. single user
Standards	From media format to operating system, query language and data models
Utilities	Availability of software tools for data recovery
Vendor viability	Commercial viability of the hardware and software vendors supplying database tools and platform

For example, a milestone in designing and implementing a database is defining the type of data to be stored. This decision will then imply the most appropriate data model and type of DBMS to employ. If the data are nucleotide sequences, then a reasonable choice would be a semi-structured database based on XML-tagged text files. However, if the data are images of 3D protein structures and key words, then either an object-oriented or a relational database would likely be more appropriate. Even though the representation of rows and columns may not be optimum for mapping protein structures onto a database, factors such as support from a commercial relational database vendor and support might dictate use of a relational product.

Consider the process involved in creating a central data warehouse of a scale appropriate for the pharmacogenomic laboratory discussed at the beginning of this chapter. The six-stage process usually involves these phases: planning; data consolidation; data transformation; selective archiving; data distribution; and ongoing maintenance.

In the planning stage, arguably the most important phase of data warehouse development, representatives from administration, R&D and information technology departments decide exactly what to include in the data warehouse. Ideally, the data warehouse content should reflect the questions likely to be asked. For example, researchers might want to correlate microarray values with specific clinical diagnoses and administrators might want to compile summaries of average sequence run costs. Because of practical cost, resource and performance limitations, it's normally impossible to store every data element from every application in a data warehouse. The planning phase directly impacts the eventual cost and functionality of the data warehouse.

In the consolidation phase, the selected data from each application database are restructured. This typically involves adding fields and relations to reflect how the data will be used in the data warehouse. The goal in the consolidation phase is to provide an efficient framework that supports queries likely to be asked, as determined in the planning stage.

The data transformation stage of data warehouse development involves transforming the consolidated data into a more useful form through summarisation and packaging. In summarisation; the data are selected, aggregated and grouped into views more convenient and useful to users. Packaging involves using the summarised data as the basis of graphical presentations, animations and charts.

Selective archiving involves moving older or infrequently accessed data to tape, optical or other long-term storage media. Archiving saves money by sparing expensive magnetic, high-speed storage and minimises the performance hit imposed by locally storing data that is no longer necessary for outcomes analysis.

The distribution phase makes data contained in the data warehouse available to users. Providing for distribution encompasses front-end development so that users can easily and intuitively request and receive data, whether in real-time or in the form of routine reports. Push technologies, including e-mail alerts, can be used to distribute data to specific users. The Web is also a major portal for accessing the data.

Maintenance is the final, ongoing stage of data warehouse development. However, creating a data warehouse involves much more than simply designing and implementing a database. Even if there is a process in place for extracting, cleaning, transporting and loading data from sequence machines, bibliographic reference databases and other molecular biology applications and distribution tools are both powerful and intuitive, the data warehouse may not be sustainable in the long-term. For example, the process of extracting, cleaning and reloading data can be prohibitively expensive and time-consuming. A sustainable data warehouse provides a real benefit to users to the degree that not only is the return worth the original development, but that it is valuable enough to warrant continual redesigning and evaluation to meet changing demands.

Infrastructure

From a hardware perspective, implementing a database requires more than servers, large hard drives, perhaps a network and the associated cables and electronics. Power conditioners and uninterruptible power supplies are needed to protect sensitive equipment and the data they contain from power surges and sudden, unplanned power outages. Providing a secure environment for data includes the usual use of username and passwords to protect accounts. However, for higher levels of assurance against data theft or manipulation, secure ID cards, dongles and biometrics (such as voice, fingerprint and retinal recognition) may be appropriate.

Secure ID cards are credit card-sized pseudorandom number generators that are synchronised with a similar generator on the server. Users enter the 16-digit number displayed on the secure ID card for their password to gain access to the system. Biometric security systems use personal biological characteristics such as a fingerprint, voice or the pattern of capillaries on the retinae to verify the identity of a user. Dongles are hardware keys that applications look for on either the serial or USB port of a workstation before users can access their data and applications. Dongles can be considered as a form of hardware-based encryption. Dedicated, high-speed hardware capable of high-speed encryption and decryption are available options as well.

Encryption is the use of a key or code to scramble a message so that it can only be deciphered by someone with knowledge of the key and the algorithm used to encrypt the original message. From a practical perspective, encryption is the processing of data so that it's at least challenging for casual eavesdroppers to read, even if the data are intercepted.

For web-based databases, secure socket layer (SSL) is the dominant security protocol. Information transmitted over the web using SSL is automatically encrypted and only when the user's web browser and the computer serving: content have the same key can they communicate. Both Netscape and Internet Explorer support the optional use of SSL.

One of the limitations of SSL is that it's wedded to the client/server architecture, where a secure session is established, through which any amount of data may be securely transmitted for the duration of the session. A complimentary communications protocol that makes use of encryption is secure hypertext transfer protocol (S-HTTP), a protocol that is designed to transmit individual messages securely over the web. That is, SSL provides a secure communications channel for the length of the connection between the client and the server, regardless of whether or not data is flowing from one to the other. In contrast, S-HTTP is more appropriate for short communications that only uses the channel when data are moving from sender to receiver.

Regardless of whether SSL or S-HTTP is used, at the core of communications over the Internet is an encryption technology called public key encryption (PKE), which is based on a pair of keys or data strings: One key is public, known or at least knowable to everyone and one key is private, known only to the sender. The private key, which is not shared with anyone, is used to decrypt information that's been encrypted by someone using the public key. In other words, encoding uses a generally available public key and decoding is performed using a private key available only to the intended recipient. PKE is like a physical padlock, where one key is used to lock a padlock and another key to open it.

Thus, looking to the immediate future, the database technologies that will most likely have a significant impact on bioinformatics are the ones that deal with systems integration, the process in which disparate computer applications and systems can share data. Because the applications in a typical biotech laboratory are often cobbled together from different vendors and custom, in-house development and may be running on multiple generations of hardware, system integration is still a custom-programming task. As a result, integrating every database in an organisation can take months of effort, considerable expense and have only mixed results. Part of the challenge is that, due to the relative youth of the bioinformatics arena, the market has yet to respond to the need for commercial integration tools that address the specific needs of the community. Two areas in which rapid innovation is required for database integration and overall improved interoperability of bioinformatics tools are vocabulary standards and DBMSs.

Although organisations such as NCBI and the national library of medicine are actively involved in developing tools for the molecular biologist working in the field of bioinformatics, a vocabulary of bioinformatics has yet to be defined. As a result, most data warehouses and data dictionaries are based on ad-hoc compilations of existing vocabularies with additions made on an as-needed basis. Part of the challenge of creating a standard bioinformatics vocabulary is determining the appropriate level of granularity needed to adequately describe everything from nucleotide sequences and protein structure to species data. This challenge is intensified as the focus of bioinformatics research shifts from nucleotide sequencing to proteomics, which necessarily includes phenotypic expression data stored in clinical systems. As a result, an all-encompassing vocabulary must increasingly incorporate data in the medical record and public health as well.

In the area of DBMSs, although the relational model currently dominates the market, the complexity of clinical and laboratory data is driving many researchers to seriously consider other DBMS technologies, such as object-oriented DBMSs. While there is a great deal of interest in object-oriented approaches to supporting bioinformatics computing, the information technology community is still expressing caution toward the technology. This is partly because many object-oriented database systems are incomplete, in that they lack backup and recovery functions. In addition, data models often conflict, the languages supported by vendors are proprietary, scalability is unproven and the systems require huge amounts of memory and computational resources. In the recent past, vendors have partially addressed these and other limitations of ODBMs, but performance and scalability concerns remain.

Several vendors are building what they consider the next generation of bioinformatics database systems, but it's uncertain which of these systems will establish a standard. As such, the most promising technologies in the systems integration arena are aimed at the general computing market, such as web services, storage area networks, storage service providers or application service providers.

Time will tell which of these models, if any, can be shown to be economically—as opposed to simply technologically—viable. In most cases, this translates to technologies that are transparent to the research workflow, thereby augmenting current processes and contributing to effectiveness of R&D.

By far the most significant challenges surrounding the effective use of database technology in bioinformatics relate to issues of security, privacy and bioethics and how these issues will eventually affect legislation that will either support or hamper advances in the field. Consider the privacy and security issues, associated with having an individual's medical records and DNA analysis available online and instantly available to teachers, employers, the courts, police, the FBI and, inevitably, hackers. For now, the challenge is achieving the level of database integration that would make these issues a reality. At best, integration is limited to what internet and intranet technology can support, through both fixed or hard-wired links and, more commonly, through dynamic links provided by online search engines.

Chapter 12

Statistics

INTRODUCTION

This chapter explores the practical considerations involved in applying statistical techniques to modern bioinformatics challenges. It illustrates the range and complexity of issues that arise in controlling for the variability (which, in this discussion, encompasses errors) associated with microarray experiments and other bioinformatics work. 'Statistical concepts' introduces the underlying concepts of randomness and variability, while the 'microarrays' section provides an overview of the microarray experimental process. The 'imperfect data' section reveals the numerous potential sources of variability in microarray experiments.

The 'basics' section relates microarray experiments to fundamental statistical concepts, while 'quantifying randomness' discusses how randomness and variability are assigned to devices and processes. 'Data analysis' discusses how experimental output data are evaluated and 'Tool selection' examines the criteria for statistical analysis tool selection. The 'statistics of alignment' and 'clustering and classification' sections illustrate the practical application of statistical concepts. 'On the horizon' introduces the technological innovations that bioinformatics is pushing forward, often ahead of the theoretical statistical underpinnings. 'Endnote' addresses the implication of succumbing to the pressure to treat statistics as a black box solution to modern research challenges.

This chapter, like any book on statistical methods, should be considered a roadmap to potential issues to consider in discussing the selection of statistical methods with an expert statistician familiar with bioinformatics issues.

STATISTICAL CONCEPTS

Given the breadth of bioinformatics, the statistical concepts relevant to the field could easily fill a bookcase, much less a single chapter. As listed in Table 12.1, typical applications of statistics in bioinformatics range from clinical diagnosis and descriptive summaries to gene hunting and nucleotide alignment. Many of these applications are far removed from the traditional definition of a statistic, which is simply a value calculated from a sample. For example, consider that clinicians dealing with the efficacy of specific therapy in treating a genetic disease typically focus on disease prevalence (the number of cases of an illness or condition that exists at a particular time in a defined population). They also assess clinical and genetic tests for the probability of a negative result, given that the condition under consideration is absent (their sensitivity) and for the probability of a positive result, given that the condition under consideration is present (their sensitivity) and for the predictive value (the probability that a condition is present, based on the results of a test). The process of diagnosing patients potentially suffering from genetic disorders typically encompasses quantifying uncertainty and using statistical methods to predict long-term outcomes.

Table 12.1. Applications of statistics in bioinformatics.

Clinical diagnosis
Descriptive summaries
Equipment calibration
Experimental data analysis
Gene expression prediction
Gene hunting
Gene prediction
Genetic linkage analysis
Laboratory automation
Nucleotide alignment
Population studies
Protein function prediction
Protein structure prediction
Quantifying uncertainty
Quality control
Sequence similarity

In most cases, statistics are gathered in order to estimate population characteristics or parametres. Furthermore, these parametres are typically unknown and unknowable. Further still, because a statistic is an estimate of a parametre, it is likely in error and much of statistical work is devoted to quantifying the magnitude of this error.

At this point in the discussion of statistics, it's important to consider the basic concepts of randomness and probability as they relate to bioinformatics. Biological systems are inherently random, meaning that they involve variables that have undetermined value but definite probability. The first fruit fly to escape from a container of 50,000 flies when the container lid is opened may be male or female, for example. Even though the sex is a random event, the probability is 0.5 that the sex of the fly is male—assuming no external forces have been at work to affect the natural balance of fruit fly sex. Probability, the likelihood that an event will occur, is expressed as the ratio of the number of favourable outcomes in the set of outcomes divided by the total number of possible outcomes. Similarly, a stochastic system involves or shows random behaviour.

Despite the apparent randomness at the organism level, when the same events are viewed at the population and ecosystem levels, they often appear as deterministic behaviours. That is, they have an outcome that can be predicted because all of its causes are either known or are the same as those of previous events. The concepts of evolution and chaos theory describe patterns in apparently random events that appear systematic and predictable over several generations. Chaos theory describes the unpredictability inherent in every system, in which apparently random changes occur because of a system's extreme sensitivity to small differences in initial conditions. A small increase in the earth's average temperature may drastically alter life on earth over several centuries, for example.

Mutations, chance mating, random environmental pressures and the relative contribution of parents to the genotype of their offspring all lend themselves to statistical interpretation. An important distinction in biological systems is that some processes or measurements are either present or absent (discrete), while others are variable within some range (continuous). For example, a particular nucleotide is either at a location within a sequence or it isn't, just as a pea from one of Mendel's sweet pea plants either was round or wrinkled. In contrast, the expression of a gene, as measured by the fluorescence of a spot on a microarray slide, may range from absent to weak or pronounced. For example, consider a patient genetically predisposed to adult onset or Type II Diabetes. In many cases, by altering their behaviour to include a low-calorie diet and regular exercise, a patient can control the symptoms of the disease—and presumably the expression of some genes. As such, bioinformatics methods encompass not only traditional statistics, but probability and stochastic processes, with both continuous and discrete variables.

Progress

Many advances in statistics were rooted in anecdotal observations that predated the development of formal mathematical proofs or models. For example, the first model of Mendel's work, Punnet squares (Fig. 12.1), was developed about 50 years after Mendel's original observations. R.C. Punnet developed the model to illustrate the range of possible allele pairings and to calculate the probability of each pairing. Using Mendel's mating of pea plants with round and wrinkled peas, Punnet's model predicts that the offspring will have four genotypes and a probability ratio of:

$$1\,RR : 2\,Rr : 1\,rr$$

with a phenotype of:

$$3\ \text{round} : 1\ \text{wrinkled}$$

Punnet's model was soon extended by others, including his associate G.H. Hardy, to a more generalisable form. For example, the Hardy-Weinberg Principle, proposed in 1908, states that, in the absence of forces that change generations in populations, when random mating is permitted, the frequencies of each allele will tend to remain constant throughout the following generations. Work by subsequent scientists, such as the British statistician Ronald Fisher, further quantified the observations of Mendel, Punnet, Hardy and others.

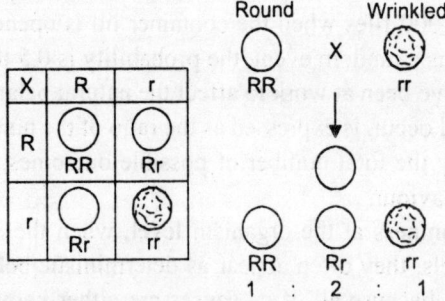

Fig. 12.1. Probability and Punnet squares. The model illustrates how the relative probability of a genotype relates to a given genotype mating.

When Fisher applied his statistical methods to Mendel's work in the 1930s, he showed that Mendel's figures were too perfect. With the small sample size used by Mendel, his findings, which agree with the ratios predicted by Punnet's squares, would be unlikely to be observed. Whether this apparently intentional error was the result of Mendel's manipulation of the data or as some historians assert, due to incorrect reporting by his support staff, is unknown.

In terms of complexity, Mendelian genetics, while a milestone in the development of our understanding of genetics, pales in comparison to many of the statistical challenges of modern molecular biology. Even though many researchers work with statistics through the special function keys on their calculators or a dedicated statistical analysis program, the application of statistics is much more than simple data analysis. For example, statistical methods provide the basis for modern genomic and proteomic laboratory automation. Automating manual operations like pipetting not only saves time but, properly implemented, automation can eliminate or minimise many sources of variability and provide for a more robust experimental procedure. The rapid advances in bioinformatics, such as sequencing most of the human genome, have been possible because of the availability of statistical methods that compare and manipulate data representative of nucleotide sequences and computer-enabled laboratory automation. Machines— perhaps more appropriately referred to as robots—have been used to automate error-prone, manual procedures such as micro-pipetting to the point that computer-based tools can quickly analyse the data they produce in the time that it would have taken to simply set up a manual experiment.

Moving to the wet lab, sequencing machines generate data on thousands of base pairs per hour and microarray experiments can collect data on the expression of tens of thousands of genes in a few hours. There are numerous potential sources of variability in the microarray experimental process and consequently a concomitant need for statistical processing. For these reasons, an examination of microarray technology represents a reasonable avenue to introducing many of the practical statistical concepts relevant to bioinformatics.

MICROARRAYS

Microarrays offer an efficient method of gathering data that can be used to determine the expression patterns of tens of thousands of genes in only a few hours. Microarray methods allow researchers to examine the mRNA from different tissues in normal and disease states to determine which genes and environmental conditions can lead to disease. Similarly, microarray methods can be used to determine which genes are expressed in which tissues and at which times during embryonic development. Spotting, the first widely used method of gene expression analysis using microarrays, is described by the process flow diagram in Fig. 12.2 and depicted graphically in Fig. 12.3. In preparation for a traditional spotting microarray experiment, several microarrays are created on a membrane, in a gel matrix or most often, on a scrupulously clean microscope slide made of low-fluorescence glass. When glass slides are used as a substrate, they are coated with a nonfluorescing compound to which known DNA sequences can easily adhere. Next, a solution containing expressed genes is applied to (spotted on) the treated face of each slide. This spotting is performed by mechanical robot controlled by micro pens or sprayers at a density of tens of thousands of spots per square inch. After the spotting process, the slides are heated and dried. Because loosely attached DNA can migrate from one spot to another during an experiment, the next step in processing involves removing loosely attached DNA from the microarrays by washing each slide in alcohol and then immersing them in boiling water for several minutes. A control is then run on one microarray with a known cDNA probe to verify that the reagents are active and on the microarrays in sufficient density to run additional experiments. With the prepared microarrays in hand, the next step is to create an experimental sample or probe.

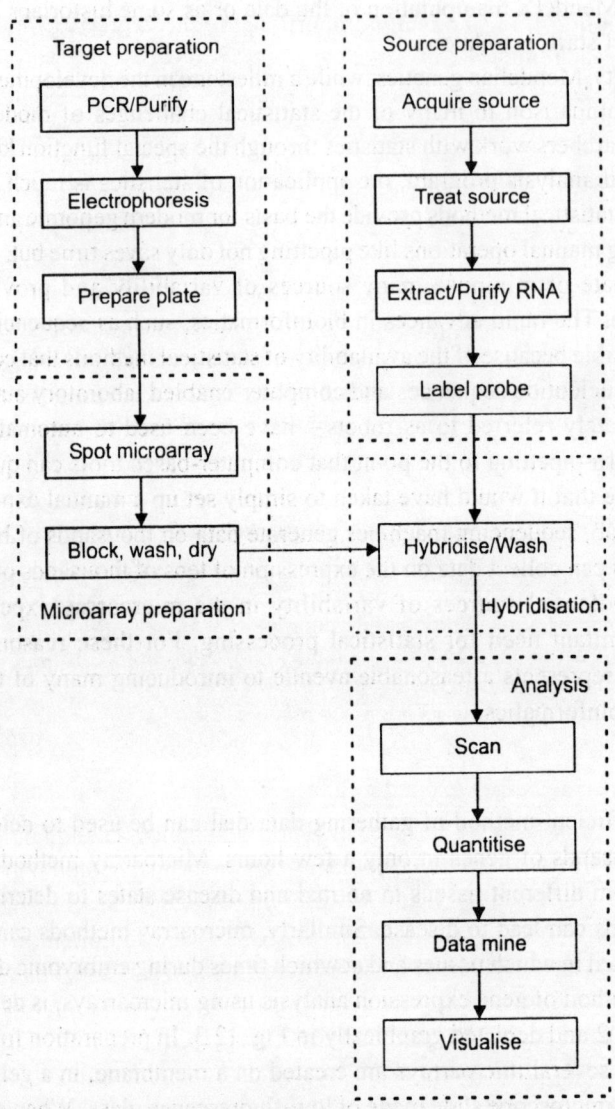

Fig. 12.2. Microarray spotting process flow.

To create a probe, a tissue sample is harvested by laser capture microdissection or other comparable method. Next, the mRNA from a few cells is isolated, purified, amplified, processed and labelled with fluorescent nucleotides, eventually yielding fluorescent (typically red) cDNA. The sample is then incubated with a similarly processed cDNA reference (typically green). The labelled probe and reference are then mixed and applied to the surface of one of the prepared DNA microarrays, allowing fluorescent sequences in the probe-reference mix to attach to the cDNA adherent to the glass slide.

The attraction of labelled cDNA from the probe and reference for a particular spot on the microarray depends on the extent to which the sequences in the mix complement the DNA affixed to the slide. A perfect complement, in which a nucleotide sequence in a strand of cDNA exactly complements a DNA sequence affixed to the slide, will attach more strongly (hybridise) to the DNA sequence than will a strand of cDNA in which alignment isn't perfect. The strength of adherence, as well as the success in competing for a spot on the slide, is directly proportional to the degree to which the cDNA and DNA sequences complement each other.

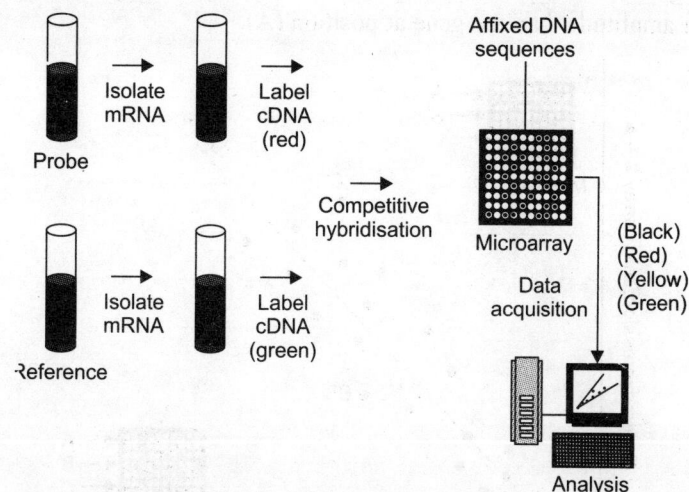

Fig. 12.3. Microarray spotting. Labelled probe and reference cDNA is competitively hybridised on a microarray prepared with known DNA sequences. Hybridisation may not occur (no fluorescence or black), may be solely from the reference (green fluorescence), solely from the probe (red fluorescence) or a mixture of reference and probe (yellow). Other ratios of probe-to-reference mixtures result in colours between green and red in the spectrum.

The populated microarray is then excited by a laser and the resultant fluorescence at each spot in the microarray is measured. If neither the experimental nor the reference samples hybridise with the genes at a given spot on the slide—indicating that there are no sequences in either the probe or the reference that are complementary to the DNA on the slide—the spot won't fluoresce. However, if hybridisation is predominantly with the probe, the spot will be red. Conversely, if hybridisation is primarily between the reference and the DNA affixed to the slide, the spot will fluoresce green. If cDNA from the probe and reference samples hybridise equally at a given spot—indicating that they share the same number of complementary nucleotides in the appropriate sequence—the spot will be yellow. Similarly, various ratios of probe-to-reference hybridisation with the slide-mounted DNA result in colours somewhere in the spectrum between red and green. An analysis of the location, extent and exact proportions of red-to-green fluorescence provides a semi-quantitative measure of gene expression in the tissue sample. That is, even though the fluorescence is digitised and read by computer, the relative value of the ratios is more exactly determined than is the absolute fluorescence value, in part because of the variability in the quantity and quality of DNA that is affixed to the slide during microarray preparation.

An obvious point for the application of statistical methods is at the final stage of the experiment, where tens of thousands of data points, each indicating relative gene activity, may need to be analysed. However, the random variability associated with every stage of the process has to be considered before the final data can be analysed in a meaningful way.

A quick check for data validity is to create a scatter plot of fluorescence data from two identically treated microarrays. As shown in Fig. 12.4, the ideal condition is when gene expressions as measured by the microarrays are identical, as indicated by data on the 4S-degree ID line, as in (A). If the amplitude of gene expression on one microarray is greater than the other, data fall off the ID line, as in (B) and (C). The scatter plot also provides a measure of gene expression amplitude, in that the greater the distance from the origin, the greater the expression amplitude. For example, the gene plotted at position (C) has a greater expression amplitude than the gene at position (A).

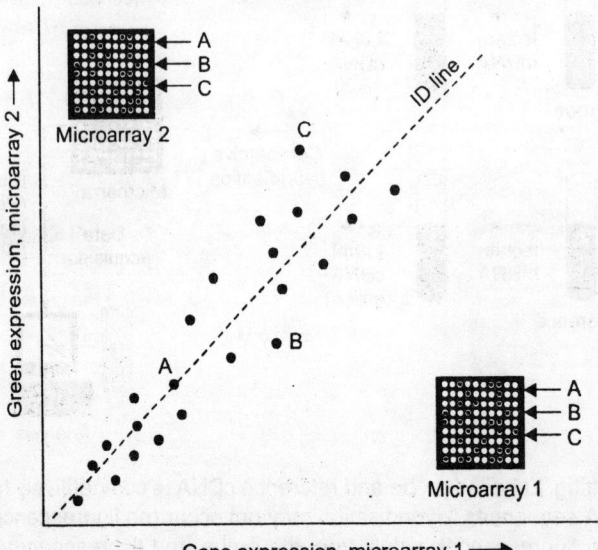

Fig. 12.4. Microarray results analysis. Scatter plot illustrating inter-microarray variability in two identically treated microarrays, microarray 1 and microarray 2 ideally, all data points fall on the ID line, as illustrated by data point (A).

The common reasons for variability in spotting, as reflected by deviation from the ID line, are listed in Table 12.2. Reasons for variability in spotting results include variability in the microarray surface chemistry, inaccuracies in the various instruments used to prepare the reagents and monitor the environment and fluctuations in the temperature, humidity and other hybridisation conditions. Variations in the degree of DNA attachment to the slide, in the volume of cDNA applied during the spotting process and in the location of spots on the microarray slide are often caused by the robot and other mechanical equipment.

Table 12.2. Sources of variability in spotting.

Binding of cDNA to microarray
cDNA volume deposited
Digitisation of spot intensities
Environmental conditions
Experimental design
Hybridisation of RNA to DNA
Instrument error
Locating spotted areas
Microarray surface chemistry
Quality of spotted genes on array
Reagent preparation
Spot placement (Robot Arm Accuracy)

Assuming a microarray passes scatter plot analysis, the microarray data are typically arranged in the form of an expression matrix. Whereas data on the microarray don't necessarily follow a particular pattern, the standard expression matrix is arranged by gene and experimental condition, as illustrated in Fig. 12.5. Conditions may indicate elapsed time since some event, such as the activation of another gene or local environmental changes, such as an increase in temperature or the start of drug therapy. Although four experimental conditions are shown for each gene in this illustration, there is no inherent limitation in the relative number of conditions or genes that can be represented in the expression matrix, within the total capacity of the microarray. For example, there may be seven experimental conditions applied to one gene and three to another.

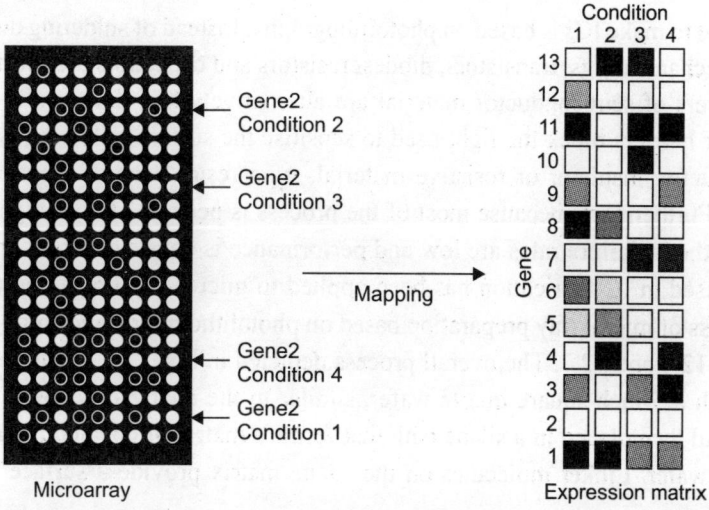

Fig. 12.5. Mapping microarray data to an expression matrix. Note the lack of correlation between physical experimental position on the microarray and the mapping of data in the expression matrix. Although shown here in grayscale, the individual squares in the gene expression matrix are normally represented by the fluorescence colour of the corresponding microarray spot.

The expression matrix format is a more human-readable form than a reproduction of arbitrarily arranged microarray data. A colour version of an expression matrix is more useful in publications and for quick visual inspection of experimental results than is a table of relative red and green fluorescence amplitude values. The standard expression matrix format also means that it's possible to spot a microarray with an arbitrary pattern of genes-condition cDNA without regard to how the data will eventually be displayed. Note that the data used for analysis is actually based on the digitised (numerical) value of the relative red and green fluorescence of the spots on the microarray.

In many respects, the spotting process, which was developed at Stanford University, has many parallels with the early digital electronic computers. The first commercially successful digital computers, such as the UNIVAC line, used discrete components and mechanical means—including punched paper cards—to work with the system. Individual components were soldered by hand to create the thousands of circuits. Because of variability in the tubes and components, the circuits had to be tuned by hand. There were often failures of individual components because of device failure or because the solder joints of components and cables eventually failed. Because construction was done by hand and because every computer was built with thousands of components—each of which varied somewhat from their ideal values and performance—it took a month or more to produce a computer system. This investment in time was well worth it. Compared to earlier computational methods, the early digital electronic computers shaved countless hours off the time required to compile a census or compute the trajectory of a projectile.

Even though the first discrete-component electronic digital computers worked well, because of the time required to create and test each computer, customers were limited to large corporations, the military and the government. The situation changed with the introduction of the integrated circuit (IC). Not only did the development of the IC allow for much smaller computers, but component count and variability dropped precipitously. As a result, reliability increased, prices dropped and computers became affordable to a mass market.

The process used to make ICs is based on photolithography. Instead of soldering discrete components by hand or with mechanical jigs, transistors, diodes, resistors and capacitors are formed by a process in which multiple layers of semiconductor material are alternatively laid down on a ceramic or silicon substrate. Masks or barriers block the light used to sensitise the surface, allowing it to accept the next layer of semiconductor, insulator or resistive material. As a result, tens of thousands of ICs can be produced in days. Furthermore, because most of the process is performed with high-tolerance, mostly nonmechanical methods, failure rates are low and performance is consistent from one IC to the next.

The approach used in IC fabrication has been applied to microarray preparation and analysis. For example, the process of microarray preparation based on photolithography and solid-phase chemistry is illustrated in Figs. 12.6 and 12.7. The overall process depicted in Fig. 12.6 illustrates how commercial process begins with a 5-inch square quartz wafer, similar to the quartz discs used to create ICs. The wafer is washed and then placed in a silane bath that forms a matrix of covalently linked molecules on the surface of the wafer. Linker molecules on the silane matrix provide a surface that may be light-activated.

In the photolithography process, illustrated in Fig. 12.7, fenestrated masks are placed over the coated wafer and exposed to UV light. The UV light exposes linkers, which are then available for nucleotide coupling. A solution containing a single type of deoxynucleotide (A, T, C or G) is flushed over the surface, where the nucleotide attaches to the exposed linkers. The process is repeated with additional masks until the oligonucleotides on the surface of the wafer are 20–25 nucleotides in length.

Each wafer can produce between about 50 to 400 individual microarrays, each of which can hold up to 5,00,000 probes, depending on the yield of the process. In comparison, each glass slide in the spotting process can hold perhaps 30,000 spots. The quartz wafer is diced and each of the individual arrays is packaged for use, just as the semiconductor wafers are diced and the individual components are mounted in a plastic or ceramic housing. A sample of the packaged microarrays is tested by running control hybridisations. A quantitative test of hybridisation is run using standardised control probes before the microarrays are available for use in competitive hybridisation experiments. The hybridisation process is essentially identical to that used in the spotting process outlined in Fig. 12.3.

A comparison of spotting and the Affymetrix process, summarised in Table 12.3, reveals that spotting is associated with quicker setup and modification times. What's more, the spotting process results in more variability and lower density because it relies on mainly mechanical means. The Affymetrix process excels at providing absolute, quantitative results instead of qualitative results, in part because the oligonucleotides are of a fixed length and known quantity.

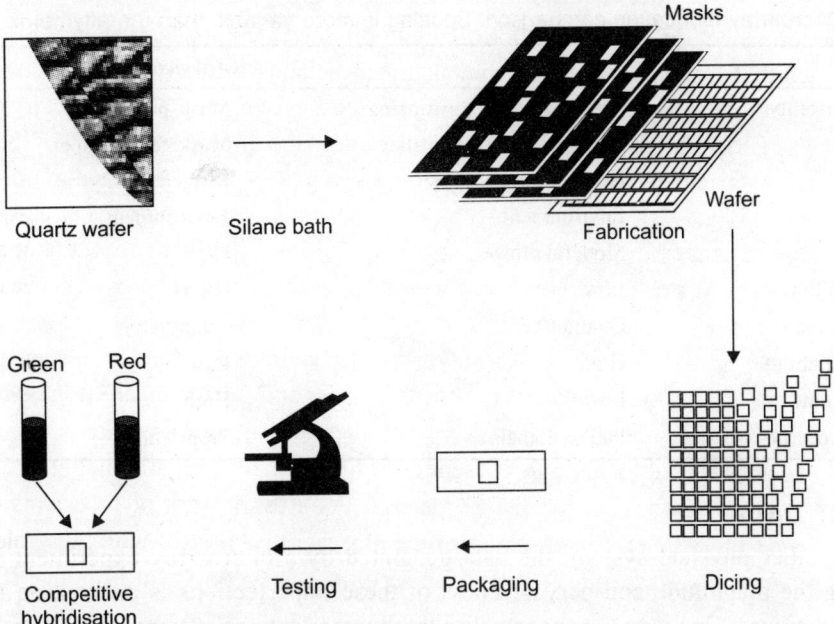

Fig. 12.6. Affymetrix microarray preparation process. The process parallels that used in the microcomputer industry used to create ICs. The technology offers much higher capacity and more quantitative results compared to microarray spotting.

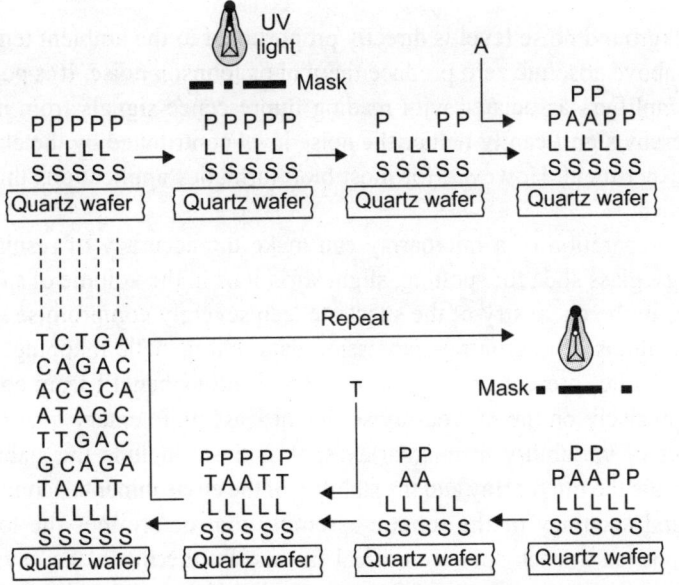

Fig. 12.7. Details of the affymetrix microarray fabrication. L—Linker molecules. S—Silane matrix. P—Protective layer. The process is repeated until the oligonucleotides are around 20 nucleotides long.

Table 12.3. Microarray fabrication comparison. Spotting is more variable than the affymetrix process.

Factor	Spotting	Affymetrix
Source of variability	Mechanical pin positioning	Mask positioning
	Bonding of cDNA to slide	Mask fenestrations
	Reagent purity	Reagent purity
	Environment	Environment
Repeatability	Moderate/low	High
Layout design time	Low	High
Analysis possible	Qualitative	Quantitative
Inter-array variability	High	Low
Modification time	Low	High
Intellectual property	Public domain	Proprietary

IMPERFECT DATA

As in every other physical system, the data generated by a microarray experiment are imperfect. Determining the magnitude and pervasiveness of these imperfections is one reason for employing statistical techniques. One way to conceptualise these imperfections is as noise in the communications channel. This noise is due to limitations of the equipment, reagents, tissue samples and deficiencies in the overall process. Some of this noise is unavoidable and can at best only be reduced. For example, microarrays are commonly created on glass slides. However, the glass, like the coating that allows DNA to adhere to the slides, fluoresces slightly when it is excited by the laser light used to read spots on the microarray.

Similarly, the background noise level is directly proportional to the ambient temperature, in that all conductors operated above absolute zero produce thermal or Johnson noise. It is possible to operate the image sensors and amplifiers associated with reading fluorescence signals from microarrays close to absolute zero and thereby significantly reduce the noise level contributed by the electronics equipment associated with the experiment. However, for most bioinformatics applications this approach to noise reduction is not practical.

Variations in the preparation of a microarray can make the accuracy of results questionable. For example, in preparing a glass slide for spotting, slight variations in the volume of substrate deposited on the slide or variations in the chemistry of the substrate, can severely compromise subsequent analysis. Although some applications of microarray expression data, like genetic mapping, are associated with binary measurements (either present or absent), most applications benefit from consistent volumes of materials deposited precisely on the microarray so that at least rudimentary qualitative measurements can be made. Sources of variability in microarray spot analysis include the stability of the spotting technology used to create the microarray and the stability of the environmental conditions. For example, the reproducibility and accuracy of the robotic assembly that determines the location and volume of DNA material deposited at each spot are critical factors. Furthermore, the environment, including humidity, temperature and amount of particulate matter in the air, can add additional variables that must be considered. For example, if the relative humidity is too high, then the samples in the microarray may not evaporate as fast as expected. Because of unavoidable variability in the spotting process, active areas on microarrays are commonly printed in triplicate to provide an internal control.

Variability in microarray experimental results is also a function of the methods used in the data acquisition phase of a microarray experiment. For example, the two most popular methods of capturing data from a microarray are scanning and spotting. In scanning, a laser illuminates each point in the microarray separately. Variability in the data is commonly due to inaccuracies in positioning the laser over each area where a spot is expected, as illustrated in Fig. 12.8. In addition, there is a trade-off between the diametre of the excitatory laser beam and the relevance of the fluorescence data. A beam that is only slightly larger than the expected spot size (high specificity) theoretically provides the least amount of extraneous fluorescence noise, assuming that the spot in the microarray is in the expected location, with the reading laser superimposed over the spot. A wider excitatory beam will control for variability in spot location, at a cost of more chances of fluoresce from contamination, slide coating and the underlying glass contributing to the fluorescence signal.

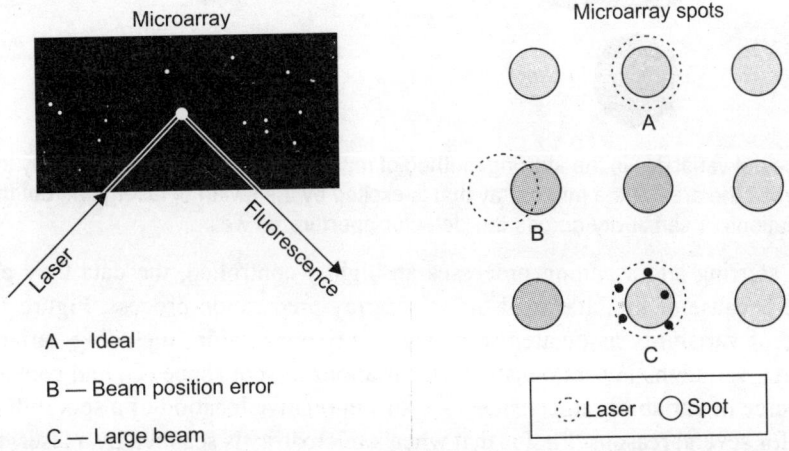

Fig. 12.8. Sources of variability in reading microarray spots through spotting. The ideal situation (A) is when the excitatory laser beam is tightly focused on a single microarray spot. However, achieving this level of perfection requires accurate positioning of both the spot and the reading equipment. If beam position is off the mark (B), gene expression data will be underrepresented. Using a larger beam than absolutely necessary; and (C) incorporates a full spot in the analysis, even if the spot placement isn't ideal.

In the starring approach to gene expression analysis, a large swath of laser light excites many spots in the microarray at a time (see Fig. 12.9), producing a fluorescence pattern resembling a field of stars—hence the name. The fluorescence pattern is captured by a photo detector; processed and analysed. In starring, the major sources of variability are nonuniformity in illumination intensity and differences in the sensitivity of the image-detection circuitry over the area of the microarray being read. For example, because the intensity of the fluorescence signal is a function of the power of the reading laser, if the power of the laser beam falls off significantly near the edges of a field, then the level of gene expression represented by those spots will be underrepresented. Similarly, the expression of genes represented by spots excited by the centre of the beam will be overrepresented. Even if the excitation intensity is uniform across the area of the microarray being read, the characteristics of the image capture optics and associated circuitry can introduce artifacts in the fluorescence signal strength because of nonuniform sensitivity to light across the area being measured. For example, the sensitivity of the detector may vary from one edge of the detector to the next. As a result, unless these effects are addressed in the final analysis, the gene expression figures will be invalid.

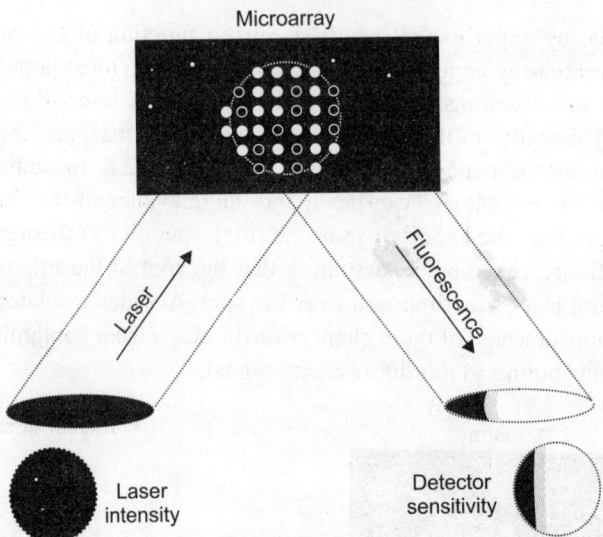

Fig. 12.9. Sources of variability in the starring method of reading a microarray. Not only may the laser intensity be nonlinear across the area of the microarray that is excited by the swath of laser light, but the photodetector may exhibit variations in sensitivity across the detector aperture as well.

Even if the starring and scanning processes are tightly controlled, the data they produce may be highly variable because of limitations of the microarray preparation process. Figure 12.10 illustrates several sources of variability associated with microarray preparation, including variations in relative spot location (A), variations in spot density (B), variations in spot shape (C) and contamination (D).

The first source of variability to consider—a shift in relative location of a spot in the microarray—is problematic for several reasons. First is that when a microarray is scanned by a laser, a displaced spot won't read as strongly as it would otherwise because part of the spot may be outside of the field of the exciting laser beam. This type of variability can be addressed somewhat if starring is used to read the microarray because image-recognition technology can be used to identify spot location on the captured image. Image-recognition software can search the immediate vicinity where a spot is expected and appropriately adjust the location of the image pixels that are read.

Variations in spot density due to uneven adherence of cDNA to the slide during the spotting process may result in erroneous output signal interpretation, depending on the statistical method used to analyse spot intensity. Variations in spot shape and deviations from expected spot location result in errors in intensity reading of spot fluorescence. Starring and scanning are both susceptible to variations in spot shape. In starring, a mask is used to limit the extent of the area read on the captured image, even though the excitatory laser beam covers many spots at once. The opposite is true of scanning, in that the image capture device is receptive to fluorescence signals from anywhere on the microarray. However, only a small area of the array is excited at a time. As a result, a misshapen spot may not contribute fully to its expected fluorescence intensity. Contamination of the microarray, whether from dust or extraneous organic material in the slide coating, is another source of variability that is difficult to counteract. Contamination can interfere with automated spot-locating technologies used with starring and partially obscure spots in the microarray so that they can't be properly scanned. Contamination can also give false positive indications of the level of gene expression when it is highly fluorescent and falls on spots that would otherwise not fluoresce.

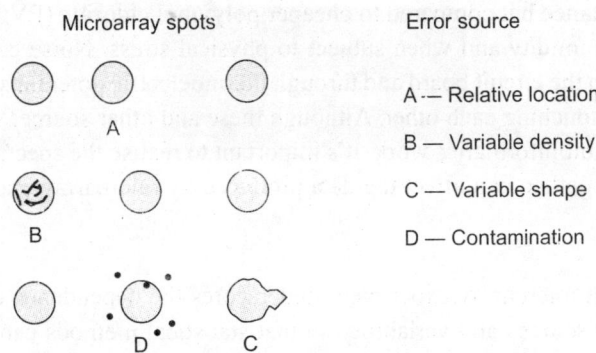

Fig. 12.10. Common sources of variability associated with microarray preparation. These sources of error affect both the spotting and starring methods of microarray reading.

At a higher level is variability due to the overall system operation and processes. Sources of process variability include photobleaching, in which the exciting laser or other light bleaches the fluorescing dye, rendering the scanned spots useless for subsequent analysis. Photobleaching, which is a function of laser intensity and the time the laser dwells on each spot, is problematic when the microarray reading process is interrupted mid-way through a reading cycle and restarted. The previously excited area on the microarray may be faded relative to the unread in the microarray. This may be problematic when gene activity corresponding to dual or multiple excitations is compared with areas of single excitation.

In addition to process variation, there is also variability due to the particular equipment used in the microarray system. Some of this variability or noise may be due to improper design or because of overwhelming noise level in the environment. For example, data acquisition devices are subject to noise from magnetic fields from nearby wiring and devices. There are also short-term errors due to equipment warm-up and long-term drift with time because of ageing of the electronic components.

Variation can be introduced by instrument loading and perturbation of the system under study or by crosstalk. Crosstalk occurs when, for example, light from one channel or flourescent colour bleeds over to a detector intended for another signal. Using emission filters that block potential interfering light signals can minimise it. Variability can be introduced by noise in the power supply, by memory effects (image persistence) on the image sensors due to previous exposures and by drift of sensor sensitivity and amplifier gain with time. Simply using the measuring equipment as it's intended to be used can demonstrate susceptibility to errors. For example, there is the issue of instrument loading, in that following Heisenberg's uncertainty principle, it's generally impossible to measure something with absolute accuracy without changing its value to some degree. For example, because of photobleaching by the laser, the process of reading a microarray also erases data from the microarray, making subsequent readings less accurate. Imperfections in measuring equipment can introduce variation in the data. For example, because insulation used on wires is imperfect, there is current leakage and equipment noise. In addition, spurious signals can be induced by mechanical stress on wires and electronic components (the Piezoelectric effect), by friction, such as when materials rub together (the triboelectric effect) or when insulation quality changes due to high humidity or because of surface contamination. Noise can also be induced by current-carrying cables and wires located near the measuring equipment.

Deciding on components to use in constructing a microarray system or other complex measuring system is a compromise between price, performance and the intended use. For example, ceramic insulators have a high volume resistance but compared to cheaper polyvinyl chloride (PVC) insulators, they are a source of noise at high humidity and when subject to physical stress. Noise can also be produced by electrochemical effects on the circuit board and through thermoelectric potentials induced by conductors of different composition touching each other. Although these and other sources of low-level noise may not be relevant in typical bioinformatics work, it's important to realise the spectrum of possible sources of variation that, taken together, can affect the data produced by microarray experiments.

BASICS

The overview of a typical microarray experiment underscores the dependence of bioinformatics work on an awareness of error sources and variability so that statistical methods can be used to control for their effects on experimental results.

Randomness

One of the key statistical concepts highlighted by the microarray experiment is that data are inherently noisy and that randomness is inherent in any sampling process. Furthermore, randomness is inherent in and a necessary component of, biological systems. Whereas the randomness in mechanical systems and electronic circuitry is often minimised as much as is economically possible, randomness is an integral component of the workings of biological systems. Mutations and the distribution of maternal and paternal genetic material during meiosis are biological processes that reflect the dependence of biodiversity on the randomness of biological processes.

Every measurement system introduces noise—random variability—into the desired signal. This noise can be minimised by controlling the external environment (for example, by reducing the ambient temperature in a system designed to make very low-level measurements) or more often, by reducing the bandwidth of the system, using statistical techniques. For example, by reducing the bandwidth of acceptable (good) data, it can be more readily differentiated from bad data and made more apparent and available. Even though statistical techniques can be used to filter data during the final analysis of a gene expression experiment, reliance on statistical analysis of the final results alone isn't optimal. For example, although analysis of intra-array spot fluorescence intensity can be used to control for contamination and other sources of variability, a better approach is to minimise variability in the overall process. As a result, there will be more experimental data and less need to run controls that add to the experimental overhead without contributing directly to gene expression discovery.

The microarray experiment also illustrates how conventional mechanical systems are more variable than their electronic counterparts. Compared to computers and other so-called finite-state machines defined in silicon and software, conventional mechanical systems such as robotic arms and micro-pipettes are much more variable in their operation. One of the greatest potential sources of variability in the placement of cDNA solution on a prepared glass slide microarray is the robotic assembly that performs the spotting of the microarray. What's more, the amount of cDNA that actually adheres to the slide can vary widely as well, as a function of the slide coating, the ambient environmental conditions and the presence of contaminants. Estimating the variability contributed by the mechanical and biochemical systems—through computer modelling or direct measurement—provides an indication of the expected value of the data. Nanotechnology may eventually reduce the variability of computer-enabled mechanical systems to the point that it is comparable to that of digital electronic circuitry.

Variability is Cumulative

Regardless of whether the source is mechanical, biological or electronic, variability is cumulative, in that noise introduced in the early stages of a system propagates and is amplified by later activity in the system. For example, extraneous genetic material commingled with the cDNA used to create a microarray will add to the fluoresce activity measured from each spot. This not only adds to the noise level of the system and decreases the effective dynamic range of the experiment, but the fluoresce activity at otherwise quiescent locations in the microarray will be amplified by the PMT or CCD-based system and digitised. Unless the variability can be quantified through control experiments, the gene expression conclusions suggested by the data analysis will be incorrect.

Controlling variability is a key component of process management. Managing the chain of processes in the microarray experiment involves controlling variability through computer-enabled statistical controls. For example, correlating gene expression of microarray runs in a timely manner is impractical without computer-based statistical analysis and visualisation tools. One reason is that noise and variability are dynamic; most complex systems get noisier and accumulate variability with time—hence the need for timely recalibration.

Approximation

The microarray experiment also illustrates that statistical summaries, probability-based predictions and estimates of variability introduced by various processes are at best approximations. For example, Punnet's square allows a researcher to predict, with some degree of certainty, the outcome of mating pea plants with specific characteristics. The degree to which the predictions hold is based on sample size and the extent to which the explicit and implicit assumptions of the model are upheld. That is, sample size, external variables that may affect pea plant phenotype, the method of recording and analysing data and the basic design of the model all affect the accuracy of results.

Interface Noise

Much of bioinformatics work involves interfacing mechanical, biological and electronic systems, each of which has its own nonlinearities, variability and noise sources. Furthermore, each interface introduces noise and variability in the overall process. For example, translating analog fluorescence intensity to a digital signal introduces noise, decreases overall system dynamic range and adds nonlinearities and variability to the gene expression data. Similarly, the mechanical and optical-to-digital interfaces in a nucleotide sequencing machine contribute noise, errors and random variability to sequence data.

Assumptions

Most statistical methods assume basic premises that hold regardless of the specific application in bioinformatics. For example, one of the most popular statistical pattern classification methods is Bayes' Theorem, developed by the clergyman Thomas Bayes in the 18th century. His theorem, applied to such problems as determining the probability that disease is present given that a gene is shown to be expressed in a microarray experiment, combines the prior probabilities of outcomes together with the conditional probabilities of various input features in order to reach a conclusion.

Using the odds-likelihood form of Bayes' Theorem, the probability that a patient has a particular disease can be calculated from three parametres: the pretest probability of the patient having the disease, the probability that the test is positive in diseased people and the probability that the test is positive in nondiseased people.

For example, given that probability (p) and odds are related as follows:

$$odds = \frac{p}{1-p}$$

$$p = \frac{odds}{1+odds}$$

In addition, the relationship between pretest and post-test odds is:

Post-test odds = pretest odds × likelihood ratio

Expressed in the odds-likelihood form of Bayes' Theorem, this relationship appears as:

$$\frac{p[D|R]}{p[-D|R]} = \frac{p[D]}{p[-D]} \times \frac{p[R|D]}{p[R|-D]}$$

Using this equation, assume that the pretest odds of a patient having a particular genetic disease is 0.50 and that it's known that the probability that a gene expression test is positive in people with the genetic disease is 0.65 and that the probability that the same gene expression test is positive in people without the disease is 0.20. The post-test odds that the patient has the disease given a positive gene expression test result is calculated as:

Post-test odds = pretest odds × likelihood ratio

$$\text{Pretest odds} = \frac{0.50}{1-0.50} = \frac{0.50}{0.50} = 1$$

$$\text{Likelihood ratio} = \frac{0.65}{0.20} = 3.25$$

Post-test odds = $1 \times 3.25 = 3.25{:}1$

Converting odds to probability:

$$p = \frac{odds}{1+odds} = \frac{3.25}{1+3.25} = 0.77$$

That is, the post-test odds that the patient is suffering from the disease is 0.77, up from even odds prior to the gene expression test results. A better test—one with a greater likelihood ratio—would have provided a greater increase in post-test odds that the patient has the disease.

The most significant limitation of Bayes' Theorem is that the input features must not only be independent of each other, but they must be either present or absent. Furthermore, the possible outcomes must be mutually exclusive and there can be only one outcome.

A basic assumption in many statistical analyses is that the sample mean tends to approach the population mean, given a large enough sample size or enough smaller samples. Descriptive statistics such as mean, mode, median and variance—a measure of how dispersed the values are around the distribution mean—are measures of this central tendency. For example, the Punnet's Square accurately predicts the expected probability of genotypes and phenotypes, but only for sufficiently large sample sizes. A single, random sample of only four plants might reveal all wrinkled peas, despite the expected result of one wrinkled to three smooth offspring.

Sampling and Distributions

Much of statistics deals with obtaining as much information as possible from small samples. The question is how large a sample is large enough considering it's usually unrealistic to measure every data element, even if they are generated by a sequence machine or other automatic device. We estimate population mean and variance by sampling population data and drawing inferences from the sample data, based in part on assumptions of how the data are distributed in the population.

Popular distributions used in statistical analysis of discrete random variables include the binomial, hypergeometric and poisson distributions. The more well-known Normal distribution is used for analysis of continuous random variables. A special case of the Normal distribution is the z-distribution, which is normally distributed data with a mean of zero and a standard deviation of one (Fig. 12.11). The distinction between distributions of continuous and discrete variables is important because many statistical methods are valid only when used with data drawn from populations with specific distributions. For example, the analysis of discrete random variables, such as the position of a nucleotide on a given sequence, may use techniques based on a binomial distribution, but may not use techniques that assume a normal distribution. If assumptions of distribution aren't valid, then the relevance of the analysis should be downplayed accordingly.

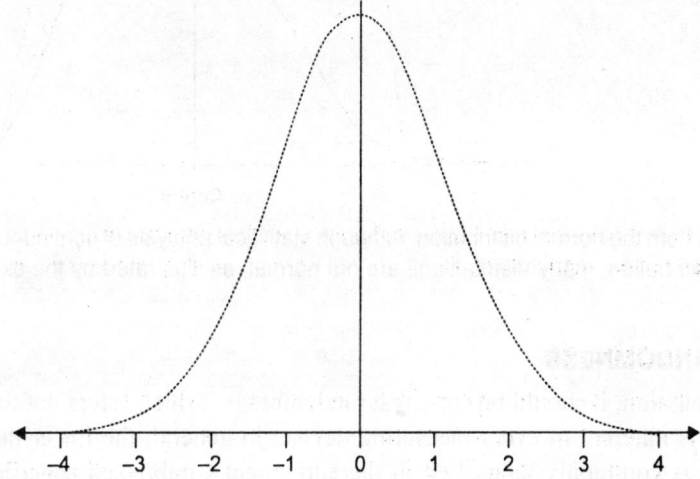

Fig. 12.11. The z-distribution. This distribution is a special case of the normal distribution, with mean of zero and a standard deviation of one.

Returning to the starring method of capturing fluorescence intensity data, the response characteristics of the image-capture electronics results in a skewed distribution (Fig. 12.12). Aberrations in the exciting laser and fluorescence intensity detector in a microarray experiment result in a peaked and skewed distribution, compared to the ideal (dotted line) distribution that is flat across the area excited by the laser.

Hypothesis Testing

Hypothesis testing, in which a hypothesis (often termed the 'null hypothesis' because it is a negatively stated hypothesis that a researcher suspects is incorrect) is assumed to hold unless there is enough evidence to reject it, is another basic statistical method. In microarray work, a typical hypothesis is that two microarrays that have been subjected to the same spotting and hybridisation process will produce identical gene expression fluorescence results. The degree to which this hypothesis is true can be estimated by examining the gene expression scatter plots created from data gleaned from each microarray and correlating the values mathematically.

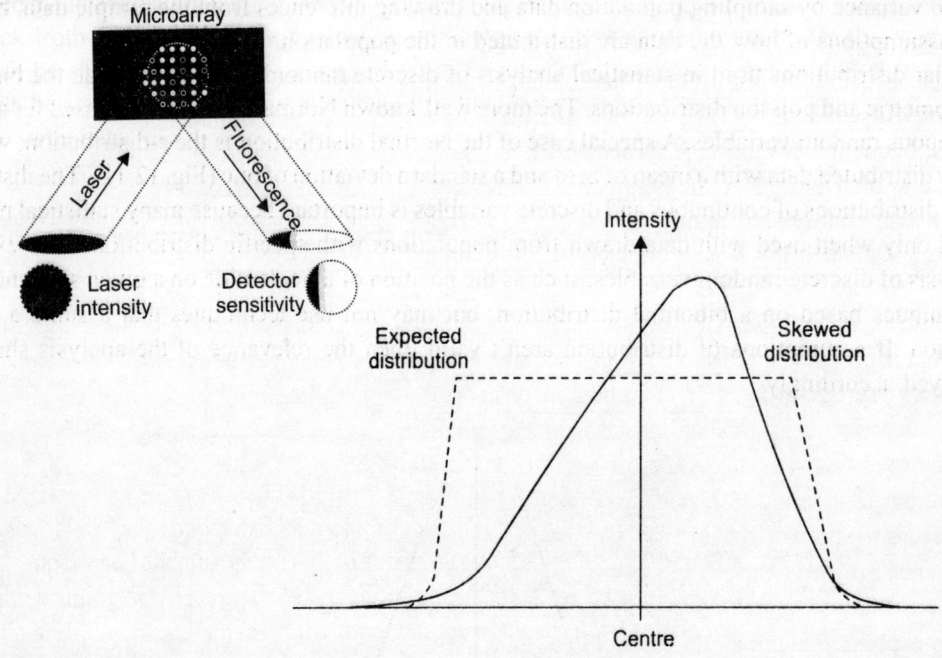

Fig. 12.12. Deviations from the normal distribution. Although statistical analysis of continuous, random variables assumes a normal distribution, many distributions are not normal, as illustrated by the skewed and expected distributions.

QUANTIFYING RANDOMNESS

From the earlier discussion, it should be clear that randomness—which refers not to the data, but how they are obtained—is inherent in every measuring device. In general, the lower the randomness, the better. Randomness is commonly quantified in the equipment's published specifications document, which characterises the equipment's performance in terms of accuracy, resolution (precision), repeatability, stability and sensitivity.

Accuracy—the degree to which a data value being measured is correct—is usually expressed as plus or minus a percentage of the reading, as '± (0.2 per cent)'. The accuracy of digital systems is further defined in terms of the number of counts of the least significant digit, such as '± (0.2 per cent + 1 count)'. Resolution, sometimes referred to as precision, is the ability of an instrument to resolve small differences. In a digital system, resolution is often expressed in terms of the number of bits available to represent signal. For example, in a 4-bit digital device, there are 2^4 or 16 discrete steps.

Consider an analog-to-digital (A-to-D) converter, a device that converts continuously variable analog signals, such as the intensity of fluorescence emitted by a spot in a microarray, to digital values. If a 4-bit A-to-D converter has full-scale capacity of 16 volts, then the resolution is one volt. Signals are rounded to the nearest integer, so that 0.5, 1.2 and 3.6 volts are represented as 1, 1 and 4 volts, respectively. In general, the higher the resolution, the greater the accuracy of a device.

Sensitivity—the ability of a device to detect low-level signals—is a function of the resolution and the amount of noise in the system. For example, continuing with the example of the 4-bit A-to-D converter with a 16-volt full-scale capacity, the maximum sensitivity would be 0.5 volts, assuming a perfect, noiseless system. However, as noise is added to the system, the sensitivity decreases as a function of the amplitude and time distribution of the noise. That is, the higher the signal-to-noise ratio, the higher the effective sensitivity of the device.

Repeatability is the ability of an instrument or system to provide consistent result. For example, the initial intensity of a spot's fluorescence, as measured with a photomultiplier tube, should ideally agree with a subsequent measurement. Repeatability is related to stability, which is the ability of an instrument or device to provide repeatable results over time, assuming certain environmental conditions, such as ambient temperature, are maintained within a certain range and the process of photo bleaching is consistent. Repeatability is also affected by any changes in the data source caused by the measurement process.

An instrument may provide highly repeatable results, but the results may be inaccurate unless the instrument is properly calibrated. All instruments are subject to changes in accuracy over time, whether or not they are operating. For example, an ordinary mercury thermometre is subject to a change in accuracy because of changes in the glass housing, which crystallises and contracts over several years. Accuracy specifications are, therefore, stated in terms of time, such as within one year of calibration. The accuracy of a calibration standard limits the maximum accuracy of the equipment being calibrated.

In assessing the capabilities of a microarray experiment system, one measure of overall system performance is the dynamic range of the system—the ratio of the maximum signal level to the minimum signal level that can be measured or represented. The dynamic range of a microarray system, which is typically expressed in terms of orders of magnitude, is a function of the scanner electronics, the chemical dynamic range of the chemicals used and the biological dynamic range of the system under investigation. All else being equal, a system with a greater dynamic range is capable of greater precision and accuracy in quantifying the relative gene expression. Furthermore, the dynamic range of the system is limited by the element in the signal chain with the smallest dynamic range.

Although the biological dynamic range is usually an unchangeable, parametre, there is some latitude in selecting reagents with the greatest dynamic range and even more choice in the microarray electronics. Consider that the detector used in the image-acquisition component of a microarray system is commonly either a solid-state charge-coupled-device (CCD) or a glass and vacuum photomultiplier tube (PMT). The choice of one device over the other involves a tradeoff between cost, sensitivity, complexity and dynamic range. A PMT is larger and much more fragile than a solid-state CCD and requires a more complex power supply because of the PMT's much higher operating voltage. In addition, a PMT is also more easily damaged than a CCD. However, a PMT provides superior sensitivity and dynamic range compared to a CCD.

Both CCD and PMT components exhibit nonlinearities outside of their optimal operating ranges. For example, both devices saturate at some input level, so that increases in signal strength aren't matched with corresponding increases in output, as illustrated in Fig. 12.13. In general, there is a tradeoff between the amplification possible and the extent of the linear region. For example, operating a PMT at the highest voltage and gain that the device will tolerate may produce phenomenal signal gain, but at the expense of a severely compressed linear operating region. This nonlinearity has the effect of compressing the dynamic range of the device.

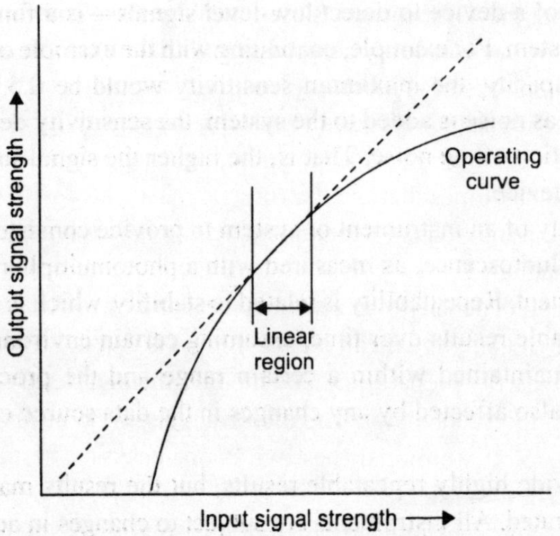

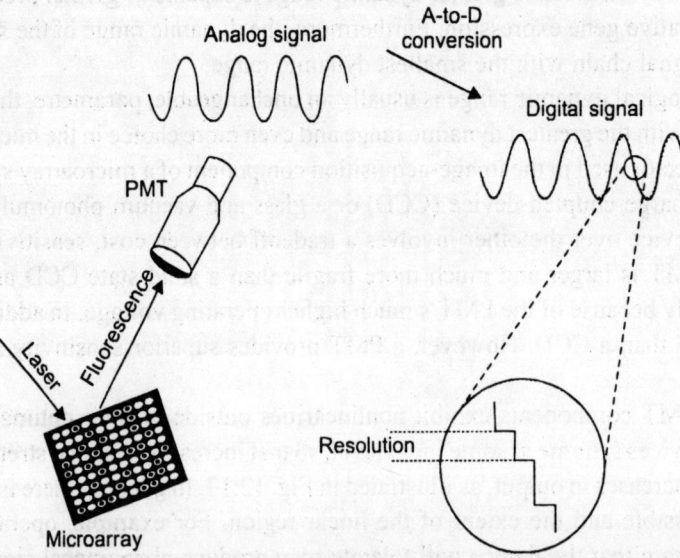

Fig. 12.13. Detector operating curve. Although only one curve is shown here, most signal detectors are associated with a family of operating curves.

DATA ANALYSIS

Once a fluorescence signal is detected, it has to be quantitised or digitised before it can be manipulated statistically. The digitisation or A-to-D conversion is performed at a fixed sampling frequency, with a converter rated at a certain dynamic range, as measured in bit depth (Fig. 12.14). For example, a 16-bit A-to-D converter can process a signal into one of (2^{16}) or 65,636 levels, a dynamic range of over 4 orders of magnitude—which is generally considered the minimum for gene expression applications.

Fig. 12.14. Analog-to-Digital conversion. The dynamic range of the microarray experiment is limited by the resolution or bit depth of the A-to-D conversion process, as illustrated by the magnified view of the digital signal.

The output of the digitiser, typically a 16-bit TIFF (.tif) file, is fed to the workstation for analysis and visualisation. One reason that the TIFF format is used over the more common and space-efficient JPEG (.jpg) format, is that JPEG format uses lossy compression. If data from the image digitiser are discarded in the compression process, the result is a compressed dynamic range of the overall system.

Analysis of the fluorescence data includes a check for microarray-to-microarray variability using a scatter plot, as illustrated earlier in Fig. 12.4. However, assuring microarray-to-microarray agreement in gene expression levels first assumes that the fluorescence associated with each spot can be adequately quantified. The most common methods of accomplishing this is to rely on simple descriptive statistics, such as mean, mode and median.

The mean is the average pixel density over a spot, corresponding to the average fluorescence intensity (Fig. 12.15). The advantage of using the mean intensity level is that it decreases error due to variance in DNA deposition during microarray preparation. The mode is the most likely intensity value, represented by the highest peak in the fluorescence plot. The mode is resistant to outlier values, but the measure is unstable when the intensity plot is bimodal (has two major peaks). The median, the mid-point in the intensity plot, is also resistant to outliers.

Other measures of assessing spot intensity include the total pixel intensity—the sum of all pixels corresponding to fluorescence in an area. However, the total intensity value is sensitive to the amount of DNA deposited on a spot in the microarray. The volume measure is the sum of signal intensity above background noise for each pixel. Although there are several additional means of quantifying spot fluorescence, the most common measure is the mean, followed by the mode and median descriptive statistics.

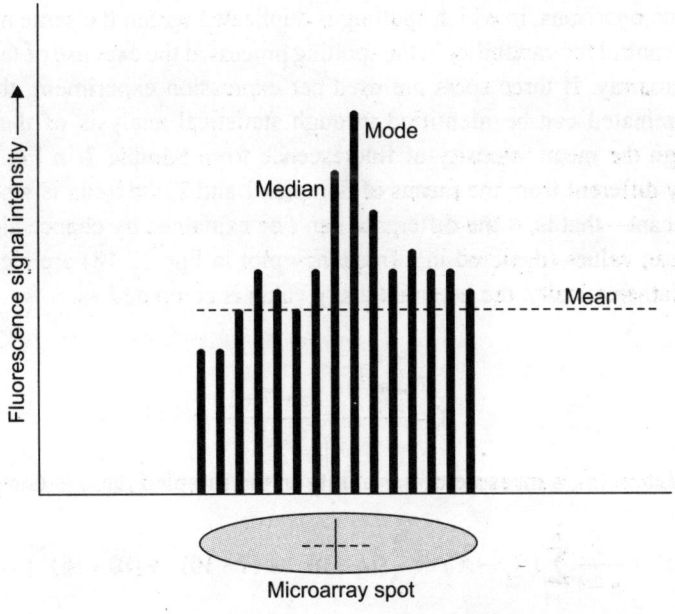

Fig. 12.15. Microarray fluorescence statistical analysis.

Possible fluorescence intensity distributions associated with common spotting errors are illustrated in Fig. 12.16. Notice that each distribution results in a different mean and median intensity reading, even though the gene expression in each case is identical. The role of statistical analysis in reading the intensity value associated with each spot is to control for variability—a challenge that isn't always possible. For example, when a microarray is contaminated, simple statistical analysis on individual spots offers little in the way of reducing variability or noise. However, inter- and intra-microarray comparisons can be used to identify contamination and other sources of variability.

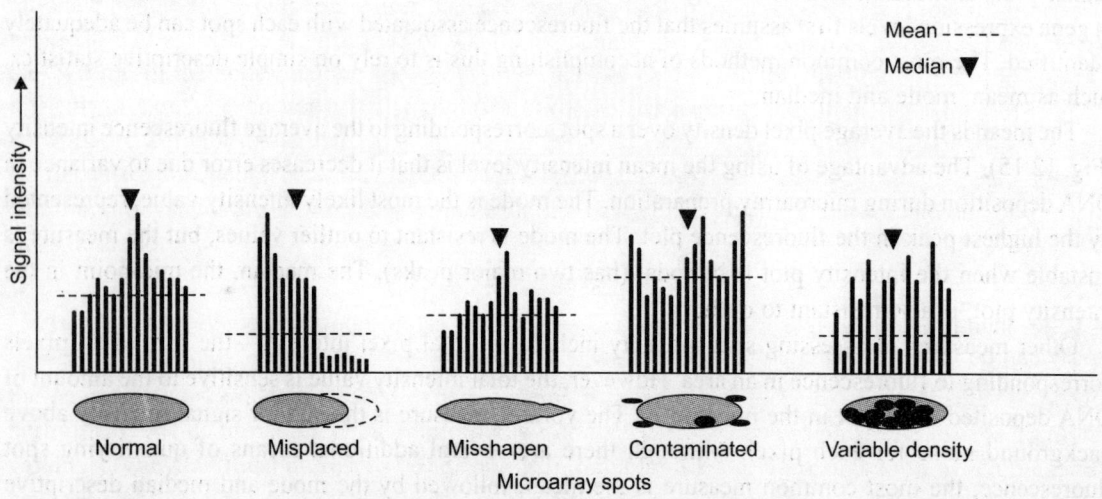

Mean -----
Median ▼

Normal   Misplaced   Misshapen   Contaminated   Variable density

Microarray spots

Fig. 12.16. Microarray spot intensity distributions.

Intra-microarray comparisons, in which spotting is duplicated within the same microarray, allow the statistical analysis to control for variability in the spotting process at the expense of fewer gene expression experiments per microarray. If three spots are used per expression experiment, then one of the three spots that are contaminated can be identified through statistical analysis of the relative intensities (Fig. 12.17). Although the mean intensity of fluorescence from Sample 3 in Fig. 12.17 is, by visual inspection, obviously different from the means of Samples 1 and 2, the issue is whether this difference is statistically significant—that is, if the difference can't be explained by chance alone. Whether or not the differences in mean values (depicted in a frequency plot in Fig. 12.18) are significant depends on the cutoff criteria. Mathematically, the mean intensity value is computed as:

$$\overline{X} = \frac{\sum_{i=1}^{n} X_i}{i} = \frac{6 + 7 + 10}{3} = 7.67$$

The standard deviation (s), a measure of variability in the sampled data, is computed as:

$$s^2 = \frac{1}{n-1} \sum_{i=1}^{n} (X_i - \overline{X})^2 = \frac{1}{2}[(6-10)^2 + (7-10)^2 + (10-10)^2]$$

$$s^2 = \frac{1}{2}[(-4)^2 + (-3)^2 + (0)^2] = \frac{1}{2}(16 + 9) = 12.5$$

$$s = \sqrt{12.5} = 3.54$$

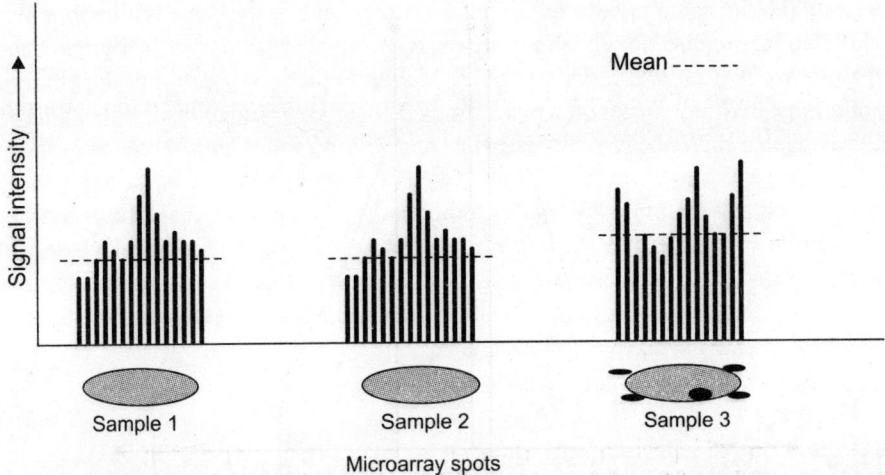

Fig. 12.17. Intra-microarray intensity comparisons. Statistical analysis of the means of relative fluorescence intensity can be used to programmatically identify a contaminated sample (far right) that can be discarded from the final gene expression analysis, thereby reducing variability in the experiment.

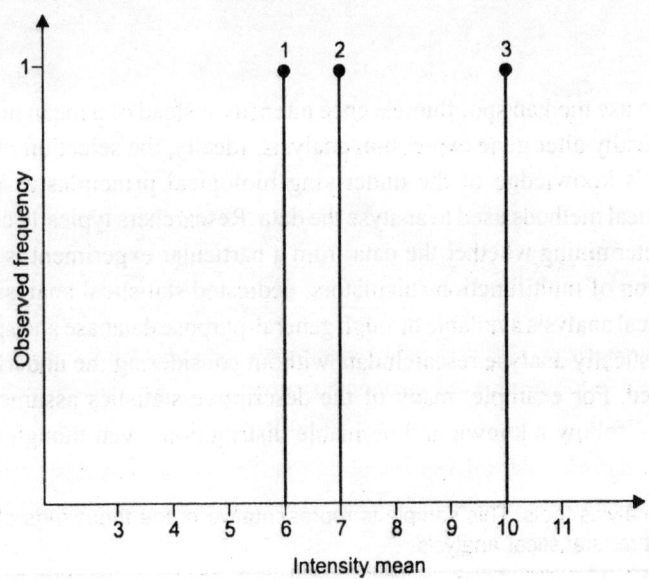

Fig. 12.18. Observed frequency of differences between means. The intensity values associated with sample 3 appears to be different from the values derived from samples 1 and 2. The scale of intensity mean values is arbitrary.

The standard deviation is useful in defining the distribution of data in terms of z-scores, which are measures that represent the deviation of a specific observation from the mean divided by the standard deviation. Given a standard deviation(s) of 3.54, the mean intensity levels of the three samples are all within about one standard deviation of the mean—much better than the typical criterion for inclusion of within the typical four z-scores (four standard deviations from the mean), as illustrated in Fig. 12.19.

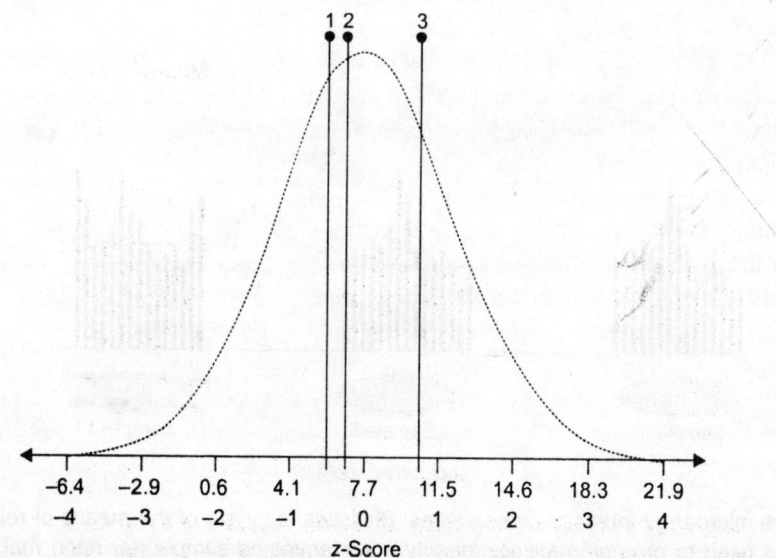

Fig. 12.19. z-scores of mean intensity values. All values are within one z-score (one standard deviation from the mean).

TOOL SELECTION

An arbitrary decision to use median spot fluorescence intensity instead of a mean or mode measurement, for example, can drastically alter gene expression analysis. Ideally, the selection of a statistical method reflects the researcher's knowledge of the underlying biological principles as well as the inherent limitations of the statistical methods used to analyse the data. Researchers typically consider the statistical methods used when determining whether the data from a particular experiment is valuable to them.

With the proliferation of multifunction calculators, dedicated statistical analysis software packages (Table 12.4) and statistical analysis available through general-purpose database and spreadsheet programs, it's all too easy to statistically analyse research data without considering the underlying assumptions of the statistical tools used. For example, many of the descriptive statistics assume that the population data—the parametres—follow a known and definable distribution, even though the distribution may be unknown.

Table 12.4. Statistical analysis tools. This sample is representative of the thousands of tools available on the market for statistical analysis.

Type of tool	Examples
Dedicated,	SAS, Minitab, Matlab, Decision Pro, MVSP, SimStat,
General-purpose	NCSS, PASS, SISA, Statistica, S-Plus, R, Splus, SPSS,
	Perl, SigmaStat, Statview, Prism, Mathematica, ProStat
Ancillary:	Microsoft excel
General-Purpose	
Bioinformatics-specific	BLAST, VAST, BioConductor
Excel add-ons	Analyse-it, XLStat, XLStatistics

Similarly, even though Bayes' Theorem assumes independence of variables, it's often used to estimate probabilities of co-occurring events that may be linked in some way. In addition, it's possible to spend months on an experimental design and end up with worthless data because the sample size or composition of the experimental groups is insufficient to address the question at hand. In the vernacular of statisticians, the experimental design has insufficient power to reject the null hypothesis.

Selecting the statistical methods and tools most appropriate for a problem requires an understanding of the assumptions of the available statistical methods, the underlying biology, the data requirements, the validity of the overall experimental design and computational requirements. One way of assessing the performance of a set of statistical tools is to determine its sensitivity and specificity. Given a criterion for when to call a test abnormal, sensitivity is the percentage of actual positives that are counted as positive, whereas specificity is the percentage of actual negatives that are rejected. Expressed another way, sensitivity is the number of true positives divided by the sum of true positives and false negatives, as illustrated in Fig. 12.20. Similarly, specificity is the number of true negatives divided by the sum of false positives and true negatives.

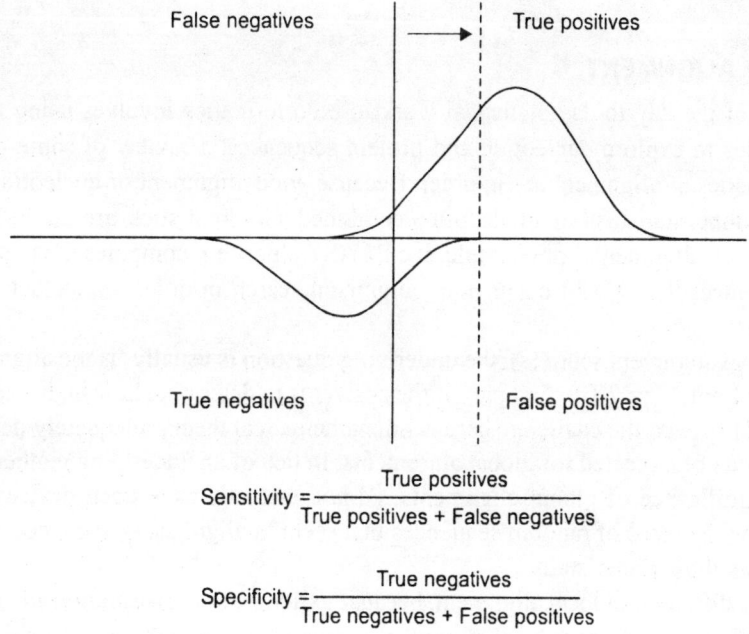

$$\text{Sensitivity} = \frac{\text{True positives}}{\text{True positives} + \text{False negatives}}$$

$$\text{Specificity} = \frac{\text{True negatives}}{\text{True negatives} + \text{False positives}}$$

Fig. 12.20. Sensitivity and Specificity. Both are a function of the number of true and false positives and negatives. Moving the cutoff value (vertical bar) to the right (dotted line) results in almost no false positives at the expense of fewer true positives.

Another way to evaluate the sensitivity and specificity of a statistical test is to determine its receiver operating characteristic (ROC) curve, as shown in Fig. 12.21. The ROC curve is a plot of a test's sensitivity versus 1—specificity or true-positive rate versus false-positive rate. The higher the curve of a test, the greater its discriminative ability. Every point along an ROC curve corresponds to test sensitivity and specificity at a given threshold of abnormal. All else being equal, a test with the greatest discriminative ability (Test A) is superior to a test with lower discriminative ability (Test B).

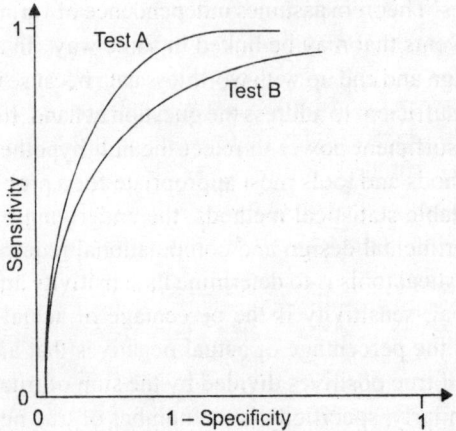

Fig. 12.21. Receiver Operating Characteristic (ROC) curves for the two tests shown here, Test A provides superior discrimination over Test B.

STATISTICS OF ALIGNMENT

Given that much of the day-to-day statistical work in bioinformatics involves using tools that utilise statistical principles to explore nucleotide and protein sequences, a review of some of the principles related to the statistics of alignment are in order. Because good alignment of nucleotide sequences can occur by chance alone, statistical methods, often combined with heuristics, are used to help determine the significance of an alignment. For example, the BLAST algorithm computes the expected frequency of matching sequences that should occur in an alignment search in order to conduct a more efficient search.

In calculating an alignment score (s), the underlying question is usually 'is the alignment score high enough to suggest homology'? The first part of the answer is to determine how high a score could occur by chance alone. However, the challenge here is no mathematical theory adequately describes statistics of the scores that can be expected for global alignments. In lieu of an underlying mathematical basis for computing the significance of global alignments, ad-hoc methods have been devised for comparing alignment scores with scores of random sequences that seem to align, using sequences the same length and composition as those under study.

The situation is different for local alignment, because extreme value distribution adequately describes the expected distribution of random local alignment scores. By relating the observed direct score to the expected distribution, the statistical significance of alignment can be assessed.

A statistic commonly used in alignment searches is the z-score, which is a measure of the distance from the mean, measured in standard deviation units. If each sequence to be aligned is randomised and an optimal alignment is made, the result is a series of scores (s) for the alignment of two sequences, with a mean (μ) and standard deviation (δ). In this scenario, the z-score (z) is computed as:

$$z = \frac{S - \mu}{\delta}$$

The advantage of a z-score over a simple percentage score is that it corrects for compositional biases in the sequence and accounts for the varying length of sequences. The problem with using a z-score to assess whether an alignment occurred by chance is that a ż-score assumes a normal distribution. However, alignment data don't follow a normal distribution. As a result, a higher z-score should be taken as a threshold of significance.

Distributions have different uses in bioinformatics statistical works. Binomial distributions are used for spotting stretches of DNA with unusual nucleotide sequences and pairwise sequence comparisons. Normal distributions are used for modelling continuous random variables, with applications such as the statistical significance of pairwise sequence comparison. Multinomial distributions are used for spotting stretches of DNA with unusual content, distinguishing tests for introns by composition and quantifying relative codon frequency.

Relying solely on purely mathematical methods for statistical analysis without incorporating heuristics or knowledge of the underlying biology can often lead to incorrect conclusions. For example, a run of pure C-G sequences in a sequence to be aligned will likely match many C-G-rich regions in a sequence database. Based on this knowledge, masks can be used to hide these regions from the database search, allowing the search algorithm to ignore these regions during the search process.

CLUSTERING AND CLASSIFICATION

Two statistical operations commonly applied to microarray data are clustering and classification. Clustering is a purely data-driven activity that uses only data from the study or experiment to group together measurements. Classification, in contrast, uses additional data, including heuristics, to assign measurements to groups. Two of the most common methods of clustering gene expression data are hierarchical clustering (Fig. 12.22) and k-means clustering (Fig. 12.23). Mathematically, hierarchical clustering involves computing a matrix of all distances for each expression measurement in the study, merging and averaging the values of the closest nodes and repeating the process until all nodes are merged into a single node. One of the many options of computing the matrix of distances involves evaluating the relative ranking of the measures of red and green fluorescence intensities taken from the expression matrix associated with a given microarray study.

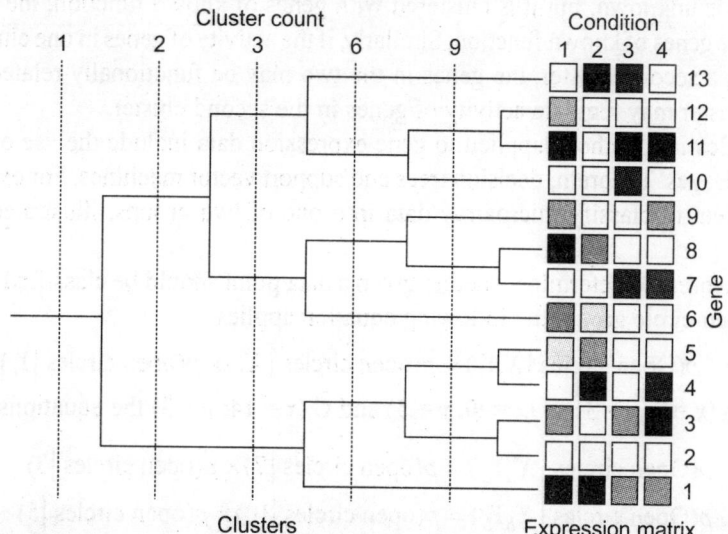

Fig. 12.22. Hierarchical clustering. Data in the expression matrix can be clustered to an arbitrary depth.

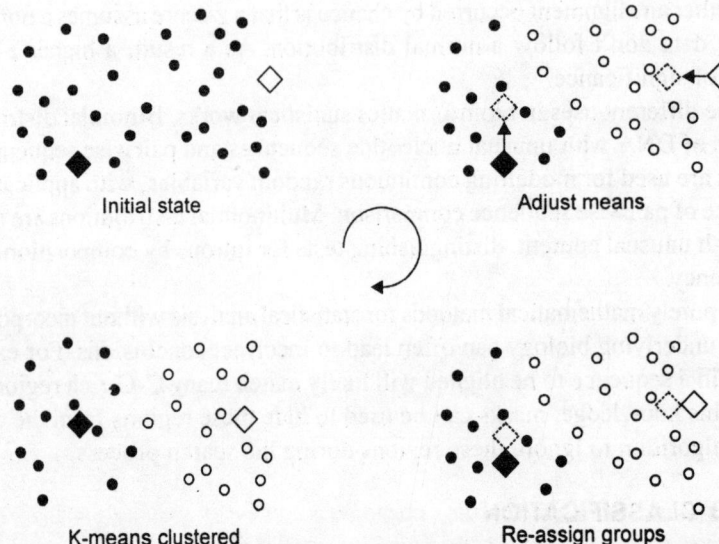

Initial state   Adjust means

K-means clustered   Re-assign groups

Fig. 12.23. K-means clustering, Items are assigned to the nearest cluster and the cluster centres (squares) are recalculated. This process is repeated until the cluster centres don't change significantly. In the end, there are two clusters, one with filled circles and one with empty circles.

K-means clustering involves generating cluster centres (squares in Fig. 12.23) in *n*-dimensions and computing the distance of each data point to each of the cluster centres. Data points are assigned to the closest cluster centre. A new cluster position is then computed by averaging the data points assigned to cluster centre. The process is repeated until the positions of the cluster centres stabilise.

Clustering microarray gene expression data is useful because it may provide insight into gene function. For example, if two genes are expressed in the same way, they may be functionally related. In addition, if a gene's function is unknown, but it is clustered with genes of known function, the gene may share functionality with the genes of known function. Similarly, if the activity of genes in one cluster consistently precedes activity in a second cluster, the genes in the two may be functionally related. For example, genes in the first cluster may regulate activity of genes in the second cluster.

Common classification methods applied to gene expression data include the use of linear models, logistic regression, Bayes' Theorem, decision trees and support vector machines. For example, consider using Bayes' Theorem to classify microarray data into one of two groups, illustrated graphically in Fig. 12.24.

Using Bayes' Theorem to determine whether given a data point should be classified as a member of, for example, the open-circle group, the following equation applies:

$$p(\text{Open circles} \mid X_i Y_i) = p(\text{open circles} \mid X_i) \times p(\text{open circles} \mid Y_i)$$

For the data point A ($x = 7, y = 3$), B ($x = 10, y = 5$) and C ($x = 14, y = 3$) the equations take the form:

$$p(\text{Open circles} \mid X_a Y_a) = p(\text{open circles} \mid 7) \times p(\text{open circles} \mid 3)$$

$$p(\text{Open circles} \mid X_b Y_b) = p(\text{open circles} \mid 10) \times p(\text{open circles} \mid 5)$$

$$p(\text{Open circles} \mid X_c Y_c) = p(\text{open circles} \mid 14) \times p(\text{open circles} \mid 3)$$

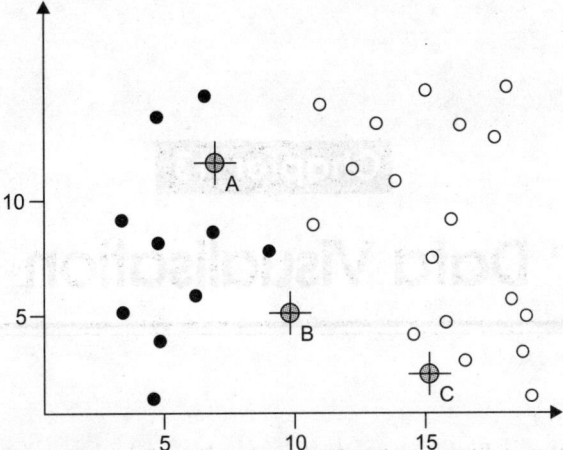

Fig. 12.24. Bayes' theorem example. The data points A, B and C can be classified using Bayes' theorem.

Visually, the data point C in Fig. 12.24 can reasonably be classified as a member of the open-circle group. Conversely, the probability that data point A is a member of the open-circle group is high. The main issue surrounds the cutoff probability for evaluating the equations. If the probability must be high in order to accept the hypothesis that a given data point is a member of the open-circle group, then data point B may not be able to be classified in the open-circle group and may best be assigned to another group.

## Chapter 13

Data Visualisation

INTRODUCTION

We evolved as visual creatures, highly dependent for our survival on our virtually instantaneous, visual pattern-recognition skills. When faced with predator or prey, our ancestors who were able to assess the situation quickly and take the appropriate action survived. Day-to-day survival favoured the quickest pattern recognisers.

In the modern, digital society, when it comes to communicating or understanding complex concepts and vast amounts of data quickly, the optical cortex is still the best processor going. The rise of TV as a universal portal for disseminating image-intensive news and entertainment, joined recently by the multimedia-rich Web, is a testament to our ability to immediately evaluate graphical content without conscious, focused mental processing.

Although there are exceptions, it's often difficult for even highly trained professionals to intuitively evaluate strings of text or tables of data so that they can act on them quickly. This is especially true when we are inundated throughout the day with data from a variety of sources, each source competing for attention. Everyone from aircraft pilots, drivers, anesthesiologists and nuclear power plant operators to molecular biologists rely on graphical displays to operate equipment and communicate findings to others.

Consider that the typical physician understands or is at least familiar with the concepts of statistical sensitivity and specificity as applied to the interpretation of routine laboratory test results. However, when asked to apply these concepts to their everyday practice of reviewing tables of numerical laboratory test values, most cannot calculate when a test result is far enough from normal to warrant further investigation. For this reason, many laboratories report laboratory results to physicians in a tabular, numeric form in which each value is accompanied by a normal range and a simple graphic to show how it relates to what is generally accepted as the normal range.

The list of blood values for a male patient shown in Fig. 13.1 is representative of how simple graphics are used at many hospitals and clinics to allow physicians to quickly visualise significantly abnormal results. In this example, the fasting blood glucose and hematocrit levels are outside of their normal ranges. The degree of abnormality can be calculated by looking at the range of normal values. However, because of the difference in ranges, it isn't immediately clear that the fasting blood glucose level is significantly out of normal range and that the hematocrit is just outside of normal. The advantage of the graphic is that the data ranges are normalised so that the distance outside of the normal range brackets has the same relative significance across all laboratory results.

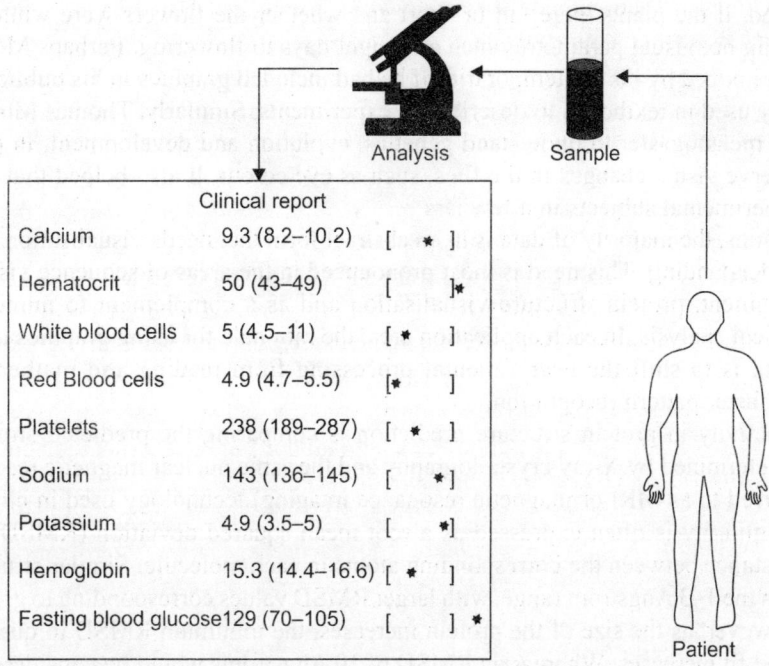

Fig. 13.1. Visualisation aids to tabular clinical laboratory data.

Although the hemoglobin level is outside of its normal range, it may be acceptable clinically. It may be temporarily elevated if the patient is dehydrated, for example. Making this clinical decision is the physician's responsibility, based on her experience. However, before the physician can make this assessment, she must be able to quickly identify values that are significantly out of normal range—which is where visualisation aids are most valuable.

The value of using graphical representations of data to provide added meaning and context is also evident in the field of neuroscience, where 3D visualisation technologies such as functional magnetic resonance imaging (fMRI) have supplanted the squiggly lines of the electroencephalograph (EEG). Functional MRI, which is based on the nuclear magnetic resonance of protons to produce proton density maps, empowers researchers to observe activity in the brain—as a 3D colour image of the gross brain—when the patient is asked to perform different mental tasks. Particular patterns of activity are also associated with personality traits, from aggression and risk-aversion to depression.

Although these and other data have been available in the form of EEGs, before such advanced visualisation technologies as fMRI, these patterns were not readily discernable, evert to researchers who spent most of their time interpreting EEGs. Thanks to fMRI, researchers and clinicians with only minimal knowledge of neuroanatomy and neurophysiology can see changes in patterns of colour on the brain surface and correlate the patterns with a patient's mental activity.

A major challenge in molecular biology has long been making sense of an abundance of potentially confusing data—even prior to the start of automated nucleotide sequencing of the human genome. Perhaps for this reason, some of the most influential advances in the field have been based on highly visual research. For example, in performing the basic research that formed the basis for his laws of inheritance, Mendel focused on readily visible, obvious traits of pea plants that he could definitively recognise and categorise. He and his attendants could unequivocally determine whether the peas were round or wrinkled, if the plants were tall or short and whether the flowers were white or purple. He avoided measuring nonvisual parametres such as weight days to flowering. Perhaps Mendel's findings would have been noticed by his contemporaries if he had included graphics in his publication similar to the type currently used in textbooks to describe his experiments. Similarly, Thomas Morgan decided to use Drosophilae melanogaster to understand genetics, evolution and development, in part because he could easily observe visual changes in the flies, such as eye colour. It also helped that he could house thousands of experimental subjects in a few jars.

In bioinformatics, the majority of data is in an abstract form that needs visualisation technologies to enhance user understanding. This need is most pronounced in the areas of sequence visualisation, user interface development, protein structure visualisation and as a complement to numerical analyses, especially statistical analysis. In each application area, the rationale for using graphics instead of tables or strings of data is to shift the user's mental processing from reading and mathematical, logical interpretation to faster pattern recognition.

A common activity in protein structure prediction is comparing the predicted structure with one experimentally determined by X-ray crystallography and the same nuclear magnetic resonance imaging (NMR, also referred to as MRI or magnetic resonance imaging) technology used in clinical medicine. The degree of similarity is often expressed as a root mean squared deviation (RMSD) figure, which represents the distance between the corresponding atoms in each molecule. Similar structures typically have an RMSD in the 1–3 Angstrom range, with larger RMSD values corresponding to greater deviations in similarity. However, as the size of the protein increases, the minimum RMSD to qualify for what is considered a good fit increases. Whereas an RMSD of 10 Angstroms would be considered a poor fit for a small protein, it might be considered excellent for a longer protein with several hundred amino acids.

Consider the challenge of comparing the protein structures depicted in Fig. 13.2. Although the RMSD value provides a quantitative measure of closeness of fit, visualising the overlap of structure pairs is more intuitive. In addition to being more intuitive than simple RMSD values, the visualisation provides additional information—just as the graphics in Fig. 13.1 add value to a simple tabular listing of clinical data. Even though the RMSD values for the four pairs of structures is identical, there is clearly a difference in what the value represents in each case. The difference between the experimental and predicted structures in (a) is uniformly distributed. However, in (b) most of the molecules match exactly. The single point of deviation is responsible for the majority of the RMSD score. In (c) there is considerable mismatch in structure, but because of the small number of atoms involved in the calculation, the RMSD score seems to indicate a good match. For example, even though the larger molecules in (d) have the same RMSD score, the overlap is much tighter along the entire length of the proteins.

Regardless of the visualisation technologies used, the underlying assumption is that, for most researchers, the perceptual clues in graphical displays can enhance immediate understanding of the data being presented. Visualisation technologies can provide an intuitive representation of the relationships among large groups of objects or data points that could otherwise be incomprehensible, while providing context and indications of relative importance.

This chapter explores data visualisation techniques applicable to bioinformatics, from methods of generating 3D renderings of protein structures to creating maps of the physical location of genes on the chromosomes. The 'sequence visualisation' and 'structure visualisation' sections explore the technologies available to help researchers visualise nucleotide sequence data and protein structure data, respectively. The remainder of the chapter deals with the underlying technologies. For example, the 'user interface' section looks at how visualisation techniques can make bioinformatics applications more easily understood and learned. 'Animation versus simulation' explores difference between the two technologies, as applied to visualisation. The 'general purpose' section explores the use of general-purpose software and hardware technologies that can be applied to bioinformatics. The 'on the Horizon' and 'Endnote' sections consider the prospects of practical virtual reality and other near-future visualisation technologies.

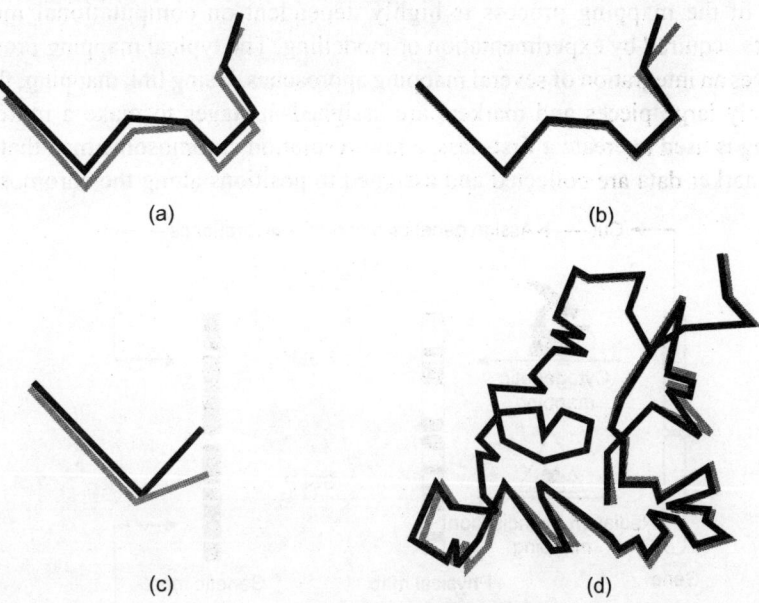

Fig. 13.2. The challenge of structure comparison. Each pair of protein backbones has the same RMSD value, but different relative amounts of structure similarity. Visualisation, together with the RMSD value, provides the best indicator of structure similarity. (a) Uniformly distributed difference; (b) localised difference; (c) significant difference with few atoms; (d) small difference with many atoms.

SEQUENCE VISUALISATION

Working with strings that represent nucleotide sequences is like programming in machine code. Although it's humanly possible to program a computer with strings of 0s and 1s, it's an arduous, error-prone, time-consuming process that doesn't lend itself to efficiency or easy maintenance and one that requires extensive program documentation. A step up from machine code is Assembly language, which allows programmers to use mnemonics such as 'CLR' to clear a buffer and 'ADD' to add two values. However, the programmer is still forced to think in terms of low-level CPU instructions. As a result, the programmer is constantly switching between a high-level problem such as how to best rotate a molecule in 3D space and a low-level problem, such as whether to use integer or floating-point math in the rotation algorithm.

Further up the programming hierarchy are languages such as C++, BASIC and HTML that insulate programmers from the underlying computational hardware infrastructure and allow them to work at a level nearer the application purpose. Higher still are the flow diagrams or storyboards—maps of sorts— that provide a graphic overview of the application that can be understood and critiqued by nonprogrammers. Returning to nucleotide sequence work, the parallel to these storyboards are gene maps-high-level graphic representations where specific sequences reside on a chromosome.

Sequence Maps

When it comes to visualising nucleotide sequences, the obvious organisational metaphors are the amino acids, proteins, chromosome segments and genes. Just as flow diagrams can be used to provide content and a high-level description of how the various components of a program are organised and function, gene maps provide a high-level view of relative and absolute gene and nucleotide sequence location.

The accuracy of the mapping process is highly dependent on computational methods used to manipulate the data acquired by experimentation or modelling. The typical mapping process, illustrated in Fig. 13.3, involves an integration of several mapping approaches. Using link mapping, the chromosome is cut into relatively large pieces and markers are assigned in stages to make a more detailed map. Cytogenic mapping is used to create a first-pass, a low-resolution chromosome map that becomes more detailed as more marker data are collected and assigned to positions along the chromosome.

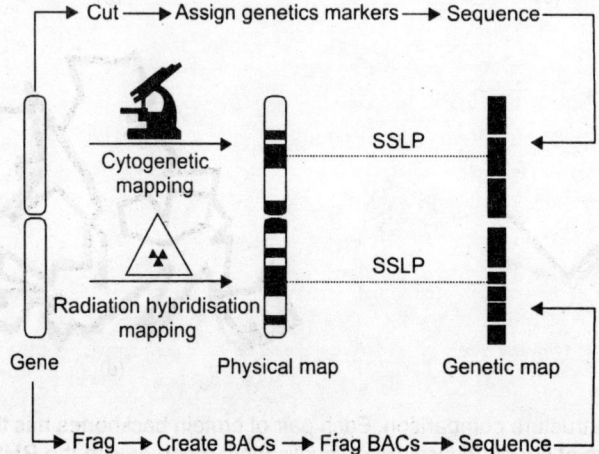

Fig. 13.3. Gene mapping processes. A variety of techniques are available for creating physical and genetic maps.

Sequence mapping involves first breaking up the chromosome at random into large fragments, which are then cloned with bacteria to make a bacterial artificial chromosome (BAC). These BACs are ordered in such a way as to maximise the contiguous regions while using the minimum number of BACs. Because BACs are too long to sequence, each one is broken at random into fragments that can be handled by a sequencing machine—less than around 500 nucleotides—and each fragment is sequenced. In this way the sequence of each BAC and eventually of each contiguous region, are defined. The result is a physical map that may have a few gaps between contiguous regions.

STRUCTURE VISUALISATION

One of the primary activities in proteomics R&D is determining and visualising the 3D structure of proteins in order to find where drugs might modulate their activity. Other activities include identifying all of the proteins produced by a given cell or tissue and determining how these proteins interact. The current methods available for realising these later activities include time-consuming protein purification and X-ray crystallography—both activities that take significant time, even with robotic automation. As such, it's generally understood by the molecular biology research community that the sequencing of the human genome, which will likely take several more years to complete, is relatively trivial compared to definitively characterising the proteome.

Barring the introduction of some new technology, cataloging, interpreting and dissecting the proteome will take many years. Unlike a nucleotide sequence, which is a relatively static structure, proteins are dynamic entities that change their shape and association with other molecules as a function of temperature, chemical interactions, pH and other changes in the environment. Grasping the static structure of the approximately 30000 proteins of the human proteome is difficult enough for many researchers, much less their potentially unlimited variation.

In contrast to visualising the sequence of nucleotides on a strand of DNA, visualising the primary structure of a protein adds little to the knowledge of protein function. More interesting and relevant are the higher-order structures.

For example, understanding the docking of two proteins is greatly facilitated by visualising the two 3D structures interacting in 3D space. Visualising a protein's tertiary structure is valuable in comparing protein structure predictions.

Visualisation Tools

The list of technologies in Table 13.1 only hints at the hundreds of available visualisation tools that are either available or underdevelopment in bioinformatics. The vast majority of bioinformatics-specific tools are shareware utilities developed with government funding, supplemented with a few dozen commercial offerings.

Many tools are hardware-or process-specific. For example, there are dozens of graphical interfaces or visualisation tools made expressly for microarray devices and the data they generate. Some of these tools are written in low-level computer languages such as C++ and others are adaptations of high-level tools, such as the graphical user interface editors that ship with commercial database engines. In addition to these bioinformatics-centric tools, there are general-purpose visualisation technologies that can be used in bioinformatics applications.

Table 13.1. Visualisation technologies. Visualisation tools leverage the pattern-recognition capabilities of the viewer's visual apparatus as opposed to the logical, intellectual capabilities that can be more easily saturated.

Visualisation Tool	Examples
Nucleotide location	Map viewer
Protein structure	SWISS-PDBViewer, WebMol, RasMol, Protein Explorer, Cn3D, VMD, MolMol, MidasPlus, Pymol, Chime, Chimera
User interface	Third-Party Browsers, VRML, Java Applets, C++
General-purpose software	Microsoft Excel, Strata Vision 3D, Max3D, 3D-Studio, Ray Dream Studio, StatView, SAS/Insight, Minitab, Matlab
General-purpose hardware	Stereo Goggles, Data gloves, 3D (Stereo) Displays, Haptic Devices

Rendering Tools

Most of the imaging work in bioinformatics involves data from the protein data bank (PDB) or the Molecular Modelling Database (MMDB). Searching for a structure is typically through protein name or ID. For example, data in the PDB is accessible by name or four-letter identifier. Note from the summary information in PDB that the Glutamine Synthetase molecule is represented by almost 46,000 atoms, which explains in part why rendering the data is so computationally expensive. The resolution listed for the data the RMSD is 2.89 Angstroms.

Representative protein structure rendering programs available as free downloads from the Internet include RasMol, Cn3D, PyMol, SWISS-PDBViewer and Chimera. A summary of the features of these programs are shown in Table 13.2.

Table 13.2. Application feature summary. Some of the more popular protein structure rendering programs are summarised here. All of these programs are available from the Internet at no cost for noncommercial users.

Feature	RasMol	Cn3D	PyMol	SWISS-PDBViewer	Chimera
Architecture	Stand-alone	Plug-in	Web-enabled	Web-enabled	Web-enabled
Manipulation power	Low	High	High	High	High
Hardware requirements	Low/Moderate	High	High	Moderate	High
Ease of Use	High; command-line language	Moderate	Moderate	High	Moderate; command-line language and GUI
Special features	Small size; very easy to install and use; established user base; highly portable	Powerful; GUI	Powerful; GUI; ray-tracing option	Powerful; GUI	Powerful; GUI; built-in extensions for collaboration
Output quality	Moderate	Very high	High	High	Very high
Documentation	Good	Good	Limited	Good	Very good
Support	Online and users groups	Online and users groups	Online and users groups	Online and users groups	Online and users groups
Speed	High	Moderate	Moderate	Moderate	Moderate/Slow
OpenGL support	Yes	Yes	Yes	Yes	Yes
Extensibility	No	No	Yes; supports Python	No	Highly extensible; supports Python
Operating systems	Universal	Universal	Universal	Universal	Universal

USER INTERFACE

The user interface is the veneer that hides the intricacies of the computer hardware and software and presents users with images, sounds and graphics that they can interact with on a cognitive level. Properly constructed, the user interface focuses the computer user's attention on what's being presented—a protein structure, for example—not on the image-rendering software or the display hardware. Every computer application and every workstation has a user interface defined by hardware and software. Whether the workstation is running a computer operating system such as Microsoft Windows, a Web browser extension designed to draw 3D protein structures, such as WebMol or a Web-based nucleotide sequence viewer, such as Map Viewer, it's the user interface that defines the usability and usefulness of the underlying application and accessibility of the associated data.

The user interface determines the density of information that can be presented to the user, as defined by Information Theory, for which the user interface is the medium through which the data flow. As shown in Fig. 13.4, the application—a 3D protein visualisation tool, for example—is the information source and the data created by the application is the message. The computer interface hardware, including the video card and monitor, is the transmitter. The user interface, including the buttons and other graphics rendered on the computer monitor, serves as the medium. In this model, the irrelevant data includes components of the system that interfere with the message generated by the application, such as superfluous graphics, distracting colours and other irrelevant data that appear on the computer monitor, which only serves to confuse the user.

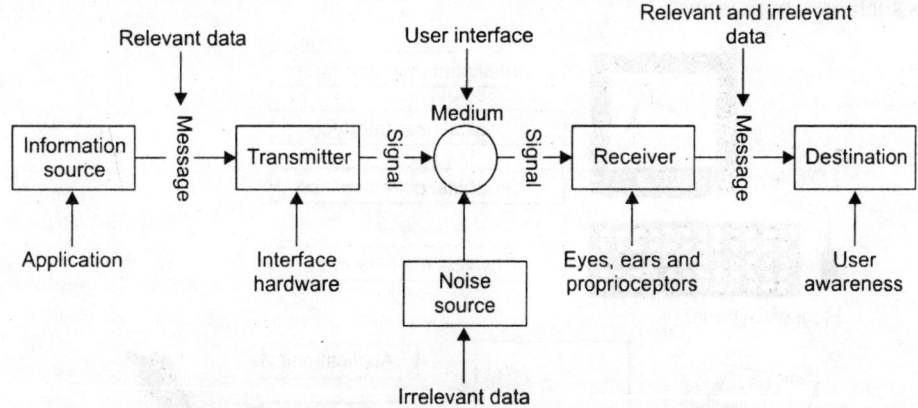

Fig. 13.4. The user interface and information theory.

One purpose of the user interface is to simplify and focus the user's attention—superfluous data detracts from this purpose. The receiver in the Information Theory model is the user's perceptual apparatus, including eyes for visual content, ears for audio content and proprioceptors for tactile or haptic content. Finally, the message, now containing relevant and irrelevant data, reaches the ultimate destination—the user's awareness.

The user interface is the medium and therefore a major bandwidth-limiting element in the delivery of data from the application to the user; everything that affects the effectiveness of the user interface affects delivery of data. Regardless of the complexity and technical marvel of the underlying molecular biology database and any related visualisation tools, users see and interact with the user interface. This interaction with the user interface defines the utility of the 30 molecular models and other data displayed on the screen. Designing an interface to support bioinformatics or any niche area for that matter, involves more than simply deciding on the layout for buttons and check boxes on a display.

User Interface Components

Even the simplest user interface can be viewed as a complex, multi-tiered structure that supports a dialogue or a communications channel between the user and the computer and between the user and the concepts presented by the software executing on the computer. The user interface minimally consists of a physical interface between the user and the computer. The user interface may also include graphical, logical, emotional or intelligent interface components, as illustrated in Fig. 13.5.

This hierarchical model is especially relevant when discussing multimedia interfaces, which may incorporate graphics, video and tactile feedback. A user interface may support sound, but sound has limited applicability in making molecular biology data more understandable. The model reflects our heavy reliance on visual information for communications and most user interface work is graphical in nature. The hierarchical interface model also highlights the tactical aspects of human-computer interfaces, which may be critical in virtual reality presentation of data. Many concepts, such as energy wells, Van der Waals forces and structural stability can be perceived more naturally through haptic devices, negating the need for the user to interpret graphics and colours used to represent physical forces.

The low-level interface layer, the physical layer, is concerned with the physical input and more relevant as a component of visualisation, physical output. With virtual reality visualisation systems, this layer includes data gloves and other devices to manipulate synthetic 3D molecules or other objects. The physical layer also includes monitors of all types, haptic controls, speech synthesisers and complex mechanisms such as robotic arms.

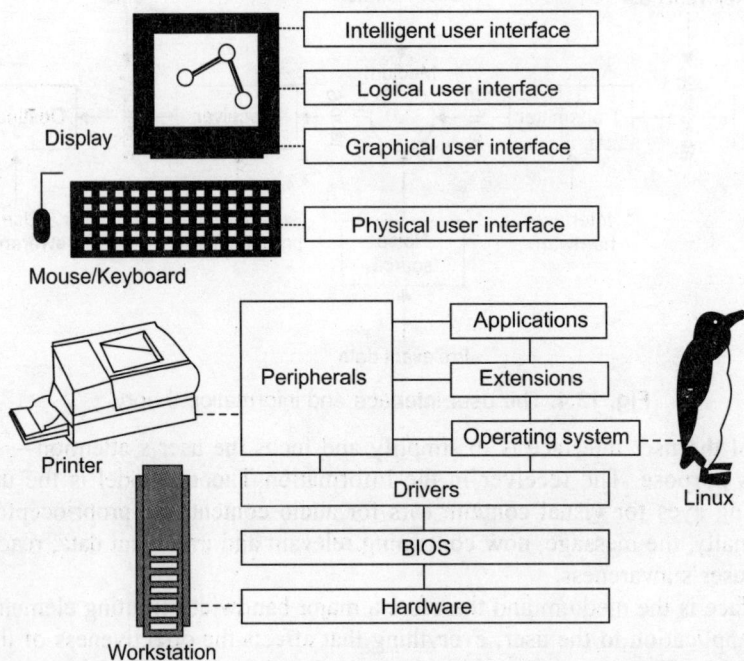

Fig. 13.5. User Interface Hierarchy. The typical user interface consists of four basic components: the physical, graphical, logical and intelligent interfaces. Higher-level components may be intentionally left out of the user interface in some systems.

A major component of the physical interface is the monitor. Traditional cathode ray tube (CRT) monitors and LCD panels limit the quality of graphics and text that can be displayed. Although LCD monitors are more space- and energy-efficient, higher-end CRT monitors are considered superior for extended use because of their higher maximum refresh rate and greater maximum resolution, brightness and contrast. LCD monitors are clearly superior as head-mounted displays because of their lighter weight and the safety afforded by their lower operating voltage. The most promising display technology for virtual reality applications in bioinformatics uses a low-powered laser to paint an image directly on the wearer's retina. The result is a virtual, wide-screen display in which protein molecules or other objects appear to float in space directly in front of the wearer.

One of the more intriguing physical interface components is the haptic controller, which is a specially constructed electromechanical mouse or joystick or other controller that provides the computer user with computer-mediated tactile sensations (Fig. 13.6). Haptic devices use electric motors to provide variable resistance to the movement of the controlling device, allowing users to experience the elasticity, the viscosity, the texture of surfaces and vibrations. In bioinformatics, the major use of haptics is in manipulating and testing protein binding sites in a virtual reality environment, with the amount of force provided by the interface used to provide an indication of the ease or difficulty in manipulating the quaternary structure of a protein introducing a molecule at a particular binding site.

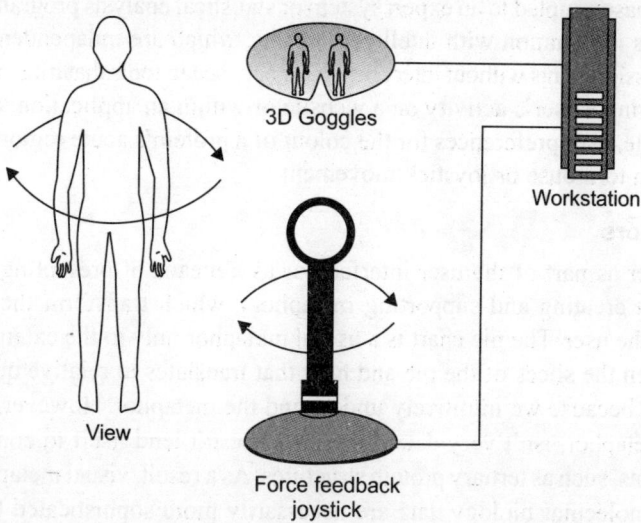

Fig. 13.6. Haptic joystick and part of a virtual reality workstation. Force feedback joysticks and 3D (stereo) goggles can be used to create virtual reality workstations in which proteins and other molecules exhibit attraction and repulsion as they are manipulated like physical objects.

Moving up the user interface hierarchy, the graphical user interface represents everything displayed on the computer display. Good graphical interface design is an art that's difficult to master. For example, even subtle differences in the relative size of objects displayed on the screen can profoundly affect how they are perceived. The graphical user interface typically makes use of mental models, which are the metaphors that give a graphical interface meaning. The desktop metaphor, with its desktop, trashcan, documents and file folders, exemplifies how a metaphor can be used to provide a large number of users who have diverse backgrounds with a conceptual model of how and where information in a computer operating system fits together. Graphical interface designers have to make assumptions about the previous experiences of the typical user for an interface to work. The level of graphic complexity most appropriate for a graphical interface balances the need to focus a user's attention on a 3D model or other data, with hardware limitations and the resources necessary to create a graphical interface.

The logical interface level is about rules, guidelines and standards of interface behaviour, such as how an interface should display the image of a molecule. A well-designed logical interface layer, like a properly executed graphical interface layer allows users to focus on the problem at hand, such as identifying the location of a specific gene on a physical map, rather than on the mechanics of operating the interface. Logical interface design relies heavily on the concept of information design, which deals with the organisation, presentation, clarity and complexity of information. Information design focuses on communications and on developing a framework for expressing information, not aesthetics. The primary metric for assessing the degree to which an interface supports a logical model is commonly referred to as cognitive ergonomics.

Intelligent interfaces rely on a variety of pattern-recognition techniques to adapt to the user's behaviour. Ideally, an intelligent interface learns user preferences by monitoring the user's responses to certain situations, tailoring the experience to the user's current interests and never demands that users explicitly state their preferences. The inner workings of an intelligent interface may be very complex and rely on an elaborate knowledge base coupled to an expert system or statistical analysis program. Intelligent interfaces share many properties in common with intelligent agents, which are independent programs capable of completing complex assignments without intervention, as opposed to tools that must be directly manipulated by a user. By monitoring a user's activity on a website or within an application, an intelligent interface may learn, for example, user preferences for the colour of a protein's acute region or the responsiveness of the protein rotation to mouse or joystick movement.

Alternative Metaphors

Visualisation, whether as part of the user interface or as a means of presenting structure or sequence data, is largely about creating and supporting metaphors, which transform the data into a form that means something to the user. The pie chart is a useful metaphor only to the extent that users understand the difference between the slices of the pie and how that translates to relative quantities. The pie chart works for most of us because we intuitively understand the metaphor. However, the pie chart, like the Windows desktop metaphor, isn't very data-dense and doesn't lend itself to communicating advanced biotechnology concepts, such as tertiary protein structures. As a result, visual metaphors for user interfaces intended to present molecular biology data are necessarily more sophisticated than ordinary business graphics, especially when the challenge is to present large volumes of complex data.

One of the challenges of creating a suitable metaphor for bioinformatics work is the variety of potential users of the applications and their level of expertise. For example, bioinformatics researchers, high-school and college students studying molecular biology, research fellows, clinicians and even the marketing departments of international pharmaceutical companies may use a given suite of applications. Devising a reasonable interface metaphor is therefore a compromise between information density, ease of use and power—the ability to quickly and easily manipulate data communicated through the interface.

Bioinformatics is pushing the metaphor component of visualisation technology to new levels. For example, even though the desktop, folder and trash can user interface—introduced by the Xerox Star, popularised by the Apple Lisa and Macintosh and fully exploited and commercialised by Microsoft— is the dominant metaphor on desktop computers, it fails to reflect the needs of bioinformatics. Many researchers in bioinformatics contend that a new user interface is in order, one not based on folders and trashcans, but on molecular biology metaphors such as the Central Dogma, where chromosomes and genes provide organisational hierarchies in which form and function are mapped.

Work on interface design in clinical medicine provides one model for how a niche-specific interface can become the *de facto* standard. In clinical medicine, the metaphor of a paper medical record is pervasive. Many clinicians interact with a patient's electronic medical record through the metaphor of a paper medical chart in which the data are arranged by the patient's chief complaint, medical history, review of systems, physical exam and laboratory results and never see or interact directly with the underlying operating system.

Whether a bioinformatics-centric user interface evolves out of academic or commercial molecular biology laboratories depends on the creativity and resources of those in the field.

Developing a completely new user interface from scratch is a formidable task. It's easier to extend current interfaces through commercial utilities or by writing browser extensions, than to specify a new interface. For example, eXtensible markup language (XML), virtual reality modelling language (VRML), PHP: hypertext processing (PHP) and similar high-level languages can be used to extend browser functionality to work with manipulating 3D images and to create a new interface metaphor. Another option is to select from commercial or shareware alternative front ends to desktop and web-based applications that use alternative metaphors. The Brain Technologies, illustrated in Fig. 13.7, is but one of many alternatives to the business-oriented desktop metaphor.

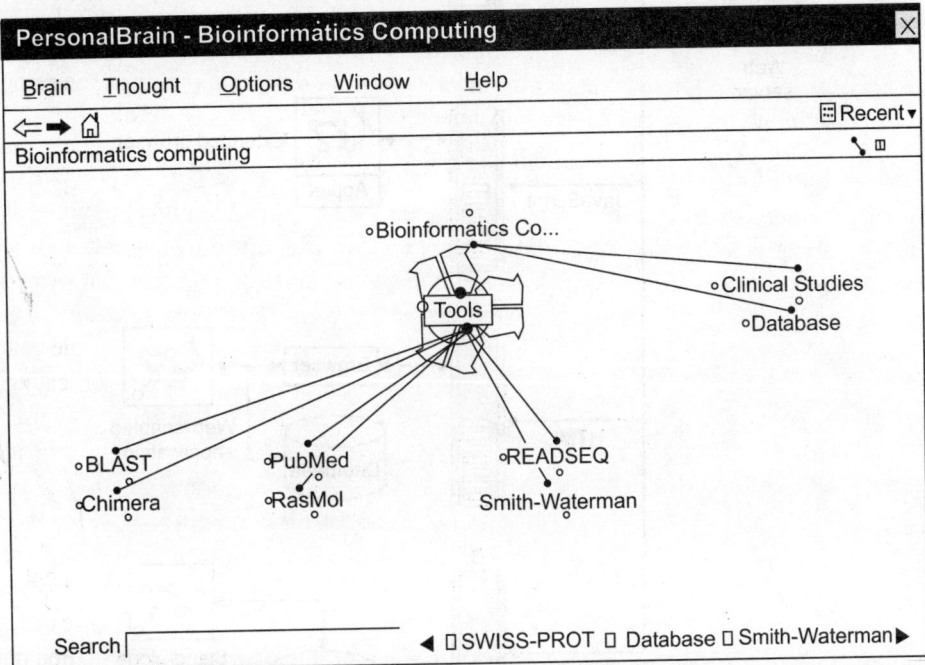

Fig. 13.7. Alternative user Interface. This example of an alternative desktop and web browser. The brain technologies corporation's personal brain, illustrates how an alternative metaphor can be used to provide access to computer and web-based bioinformatics applications and data.

It uses the metaphor of a nonhierarchical mesh of linked associations, in which concepts are related to each other through logical association. For example, a mesh of associations based on the Central Dogma can be established in which nucleotide sequences are associated with protein structures through an intermediary link that associates proteins with both 3D structures and with genes that code for the specific protein.

Often the task defines the most appropriate user interface. For example, if the data are from a DNA microarray device, then an interface that mirrors the array of florescent markers may be the most appropriate, especially if the user is the same person who works directly with the microarray equipment. However, if the user is removed from the device and works more closely with the binding sites, then an interface based on a metaphor of nucleotide sequences may be more effective in support of his work.

Display Architecture

The user interface is defined and limited by the overall system architecture, especially as it relates to how the data and interface are communicated to the workstation and its display. As illustrated in Fig. 13.8, system architectures range from standard Web-browser-based systems based on native web browsers to stand-alone systems that use the Internet only as an asynchronous data source.

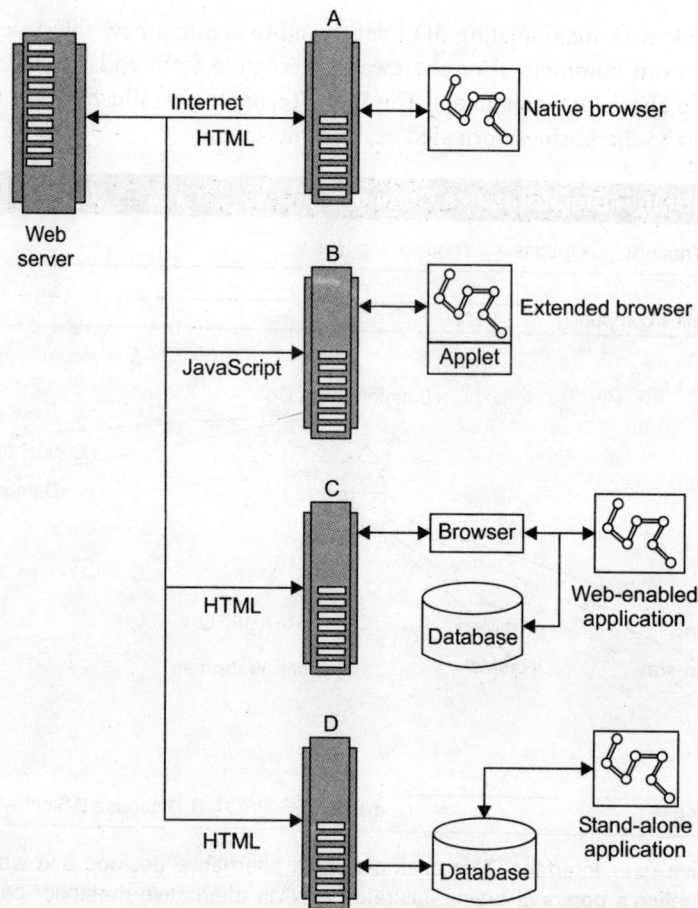

Fig. 13.8. Bioinformatics visualisation system architectures. (A) Native browser; (B) extended browser; (C) web-enabled application; (D) stand-alone-application.

In the native browser model (A), the user interface is defined by the application running on the server, within the constraints of the browser environment. The user interface to the application—a graphic sequence display, for example—can range from a simple, static line art display to an interactive, graphically rich environment with colour graphics and links to numerous web-based resources.

Furthermore, since the program actually executes on the server, the responsiveness of the application is a function of the server performance and the bandwidth of the communications link to the Internet.

In the model in which a Java applet is employed (B), the server sends Java script to the workstation browser environment, which interprets and executes the script locally. This approach, typified by the Chime plug-in, provides potentially greater interactivity and responsiveness because the code runs locally and can take advantage of local workstation's processing power. In addition, the bandwidth limitation of the Internet isn't normally an issue nor is the degree of interactivity possible because only data and Java strings are communicated from server to the workstation. The primary downside of this architecture is that the user must periodically download the latest version of the applet or plug-in.

In example (C), a web-enabled application interactivity makes use of data over the Internet, but the application runs locally and extends the browser environment. As exemplified by PyMol, high levels of user intractivity are possible with this approach and performance isn't affected by the potentially slow-speed Internet connection. The application can use any metaphor, input devices and user interfaces within the limits of the operating system, local hardware, programming language and the designer's skill and imagination. The other major approach to system architecture (D) is a stand-alone application, such as RasMol, that uses data from a local database. These data may be downloaded from local experiments or downloaded asynchronously from the public databases on the Internet.

Given this range of possible architectures, what remains to be defined are the implementation-specific capabilities that support visualisation of data, such as nucleotide sequence or protein structures and the format of the results of data analysis.

Due to the wide range of open-source tools available, the new tools underdevelopment and the additions being made to existing tools, selecting the best tool for a particular application generally begins with exploring the bioinformatics websites.

A summary of the characteristics of the four basic architectures is, provided in Table 13.3. Note that a native browser application, such as map viewer, generally has high marks for portability and ease of maintenance. Portability is not a concern because virtually every computer platform is compatible with netscape navigator and/or internet explorer. In addition, because the graphics-rendering program sits on the server, there is nothing to update on the workstation running map viewer—with the possible exception of the web browser if an application requires a later version than is installed on the workstation. The downside of this third-part maintenance of the application is that the user interface is limited to whatever the original designers defined; there isn't an easy way to alter how data are displayed in the map viewer program, for example. Similarly, the performance of map viewer is limited to that of the server, so there is little in the way that be done on the workstation to increase performance other than assuring a high-speed connection.

Table 13.3. Visualisation program architecture characteristics.

Architecture	Portability	Performance	User interface flexibility	Ease of maintenance
Native Browser	X			X
Extended Browser	X	X	X	
Web-enabled		X	X	
Stand-alone		X		

The extended browser model gets high marks for portability, performance and user interface flexibility and, compared to a native browser application, less than stellar marks for ease of, maintenance. Most, but not all, plug-ins are compatible with every platform that supports a web browser. Some plug-ins are optimised for netscape navigator and don't perform well or at all with Microsoft's internet explorer. The Chime plug-in, for example, requires a netscape browser. Moving from a native browser environment to a plug-in that executes on the local workstation means that local hardware can be used to improve program performance.

Most of this performance increase is due to support for high-performance OpenGL-compatible graphics cards. OpenGL is a cross-platform standard (Windows, MacOS 9 and X, Linux and UNIX) for 3D rendering and hardware acceleration. The underlying architecture of an OpenGL-compatible video card is usually some variation of that depicted in Fig. 13.9. An application communicates through the workstation bus to the controller hardware in the video card that drives a monitor.

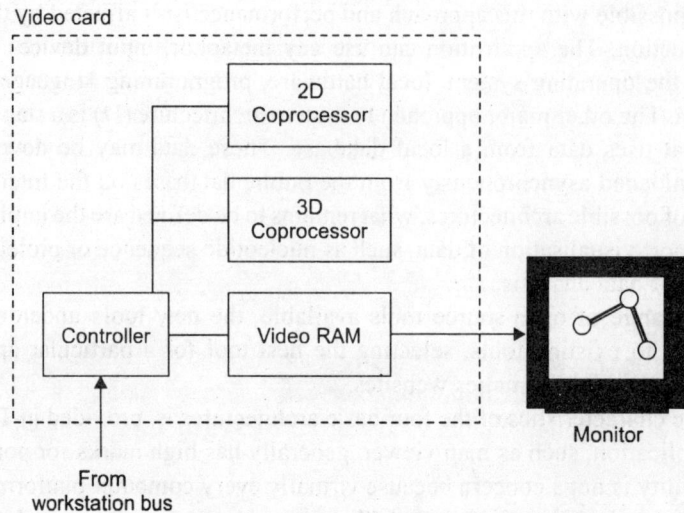

Fig. 13.9. Interface display architecture.

OpenGL-compatible video cards are designed to accelerate specific graphics procedures. These cards have their own high-performance microprocessor, high-speed video RAM and support programs stored in firmware that can be accessed through software drivers. Image data communicated to the video card from the workstation through the main bus are buffered and processed according to the type of content. Content such as windows, buttons and icons common to the Windows interface is sent to the 2D graphics coprocessor that contains instructions in firmware optimised for rendering these objects. These and other graphical interface elements are rendered to the Video RAM, which is configured as a frame buffer. In this way, the processor can be rendering the next frame or image while simultaneously driving the monitor with the current image, allowing a high-speed refresh rare that eliminates flicker.

In a similar way, 3D structures are rendered at high-speed by the dedicated 3D graphics coprocessor. The processor is optimised for making the many calculations required for rendering 3D images—including smoothing image edges, shading, applying texture maps to objects, providing perspective corrections and mapping polygons over wireframe skeletons—thereby freeing the computer's main CPU(s) to do other tasks. High-end, specialised workstations from Sun, Silicon Graphics, DEC and other manufacturers often use proprietary graphic support hardware that may not be OpenGL-compatible. Programs that work on these computers must use special video driver software in order to take full advantage of proprietary high-performance hardware.

Returning to the discussion of visualisation program architectures, both web-enabled and stand-alone applications receive high marks for performance, for the same reasons cited for extend browser applications. Web-enabled programs such as PyMol and stand-alone applications such as RasMol are designed to take advantage of local RAM and CPU power, as well as OpenGL-compatible video cards. Because updates to programs must be downloaded from the Web, maintenance is an issue and it's up to the user to maintain the latest version of the program and keep associated drivers up-to-date. Portability is also an issue for web-enabled and stand-alone programs because they have to be installed on every workstation that may be used for rendering. In addition, stand-alone applications tend to have a fixed user interface that can't be easily modified.

ANIMATION VERSUS SIMULATION

Visualisation tools can be grouped into three major categories: simulation, animation and static graphics. Simulation involves the dynamic, computationally intensive interaction of the user with a program that reevaluates the underlying data and renders the results. Animation, in contrast, involves the display of pre-computed data that can be accessed and analysed as needed to illustrate certain findings or relationships. The data in the PDB, for example, serves as the data for a rendering program such as Swiss-PDBViewer that can be used to create animations of rendered molecules from various perspectives. Rotating a protein structure, doesn't result in a change in the underlying data. Static graphics, like animations, use fixed data. As in animations, viewing an image from different perspectives doesn't modify the underlying data.

Some of the rendering packages provide limited simulation capabilities. For example, SWISS-PDBViewer allows the user to create point mutations along a molecule and then visualise the results. This is a limited form of simulation, in that a more powerful system can compute the 3D interaction of multiple proteins as well as alter underlying sequences.

GENERAL-PURPOSE TECHNOLOGIES

The bioinformatics research community is characterised by cooperation in the sharing of data and in application development. Thanks to the efforts of thousands of researchers in laboratories around the world, there are libraries of bioinformatics-specific applications that are freely shared among members of the community. Many of these applications deal with visualisation, given the overwhelming need to have an intuitive means of manipulating the vast amounts of molecular biology data being generated daily worldwide. Many general-purpose data-analysis programs provide reasonable visualisation capabilities that can be used in bioinformatics work. The challenge is identifying a proprietary or open-source software package that either accepts standard bioinformatics data formats or that uses a utility to convert bioinformatics data into a format suitable for the package.

When it comes to hardware, few laboratories can afford high-end, dedicated visualisation workstations from Silicon graphics and other manufacturers, much less develop custom hardware to supplement their visualisation needs. The problem with high-end commercial visualisation hardware—from 3D or stereo goggles, data gloves, 3D displays and haptic devices—is a lack of standards. A visualisation system designed around a particular model of stereo goggles likely won't work with other hardware because the proprietary software drivers may require a specific operating system and the display drivers may be incompatible with displays from other manufactures. As a result, sharing research findings with others is more difficult. The more standard the general-purpose hardware and software used to support visualisation in a laboratory, the more easily the system can be shared with others. In addition, using a general-purpose tool shifts the maintenance and standards challenge to the hardware vendors, allowing R&D teams to focus on their own work.

ON THE HORIZON

Virtual reality—the use of computers to immerse the user in a multimedia environment that's rich enough in synthetic cues to make the simulated environment seem real—has great potential in bioinformatics R&D. In the general marketplace, the commercial uses of virtual reality technology include virtual prototyping, museum displays, design evaluation, architecture trade show displays, engineering, aerospace simulation, collaborative engineering, game development and education. Most of these applications of the technology translate directly to bioinformatics applications. For example, the virtual prototyping of the functionality of running shoes or tractors isn't conceptually different from prototyping drugs and their effects on different human protein binding sites. Just as many of the traditional museums have been placed online to allow access to those who don't have museums in their communities, so virtual tours of protein molecules allow researchers and students access to data in a form that they couldn't otherwise access.

Design evaluation, which involves illustrating how a device or apparatus will look, can also be applied to protein structures. Virtual reality visualisation methods can illustrate, for example, the different shapes that a protein molecule might assume with changes in local pH or temperature. Similarly, just as virtual architecture applications allow potential clients to experience the finished product before it's built, a virtual reality model of a protein structure allows researchers to work with 3D images of molecules before they're actually synthesised. The advantage of this approach is that it allows potential problems to be identified before resources are invested in developing the molecule.

To date, the greatest commercial use of virtual reality in molecular biology is in the form of booth attractions at trade shows. The pharmaceutical industry spends several hundred-million dollars annually on the marketing of drugs at major medical conferences and virtual reality and other forms of visualisation technology are commonly used to attract future prescribers to their booths and to quickly communicate the mechanism of action and relative efficacy of their drugs.

Similarly, in the aerospace industry, the practical application of virtual reality includes everything from turbine design to flight simulation training for pilots and support personnel. Much of this is in the form of collaborative engineering, where engineers share models and interact online. Collaborative engineering has been used for years in the automotive and aerospace industries to design subsystems and test their functionality before actually creating them. The result is that ineffective designs are disposed of before they make it to the prototyping stage, saving the companies time and money.

Closely related to virtual reality entertainment systems in which combatants donning virtual reality helmets immerse themselves in battle situations is the use of virtual reality in education. Several medical boards have invested heavily in virtual patient encounter systems in which physicians interact with animated, talking 3D patient simulations. These virtual reality systems allow medical students, residents and physicians to develop their clinical pattern-recognition skills before interacting with patients suffering from the conditions being studied.

These and other applications of virtual reality have obvious application in molecular biology and bioinformatics research. For example, in the area of education, there is a significant gulf in what traditionally educated health care professionals and researchers understand about the bioinformatics arena. Similarly, virtual reality technologies can be used to enable students, researchers and professionals in other fields to understand and help address the challenges in bioinformatics.

To sum up visualisation is one of the most active areas of R&D in bioinformatics. One reason that visualisation technology is so advanced today is the huge investment over the past several decades in the area by the military establishment. Consider that the development of the first bitmapped screens were supported by the military because the screens could track the trajectory of missiles more precisely than a simple grid of 'Xs' on a character-oriented screen. Another reason for the rapid advances in the field is the parallel work in visualisation being conducted in fields as diverse as the military, medicine and weather forecasting. For example, based on the interfaces developed for use in clinical medicine, such as fMRI, the next generation of user interfaces used in bioinformatics will likely inherit some of this higher-level biological focus.

Bioinformatics visualisation requirements, especially those related to 3D rendering of protein structures and modelling protein-protein interactions in real time, will certainly drive development in high-end computing, including supercomputer and grid computing. The challenge for the bioinformatics community is to devise visualisation techniques and related technologies that are easily shared, capable of being supported in the long-term and ones that provide developers of next-generation hardware and software with a viable target to support.

Bioinformatics visualisation programs, espescially those related to 3D rendering of protein structures, modelling protein-protein interactions in cell functional networks drive the elegance in advanced computing, including advance matrix and grid computing. This challenge for the bioinformatics domain is to develop visualisation to high quality and standard of molecules that are easily shared, capable of being saved on multiprocessing machines. The emergence of next generation hardware and software with every effort is right to support.

Chapter 14

Sequence Alignment and Analysis

INTRODUCTION

Given the nucleotide or amino acid sequence of a biological molecule, what do we know about that molecule? We can find biologically relevant information in sequences by searching for particular patterns that may reflect some function of the molecule. These can be catalogued motifs and domains, secondary structure predictions, physical attributes such as hydrophobicity or even the content of DNA itself as in some of the gene-finding techniques.

What about comparisons with other sequences? Can we learn about one molecule by comparing it to another? Yes, naturally we can; inference through similarity is fundamental to all the biological sciences. We can learn a tremendous amount by comparing our sequence against others.

The comparative method is a cornerstone of the biological sciences. Multiple sequence alignment is the comparative method on a molecular scale and is a vital prerequisite to some of the most powerful biocomputing techniques available. Many methods are available for aligning more than two sequences. Understanding the algorithms and the program parametres of each is the only way to rationally know what is appropriate. Several methods are even available on the Internet over www servers. Knowing and staying well within the limitations of this route will avert much frustration. However, realising these limitations and being able to do something about them are very different things.

The power and sensitivity of sequence based computational methods dramatically increases with the addition of more data. More data yields stronger analyses if carefully carried out! Otherwise, it can confound the issue. The patterns of conservation become clearer by comparing the conserved portions of sequences among a larger and larger dataset. As in pairwise comparisons and database searching, those areas most resistant to change are functionally the most important to the molecule. The basic assumption is that those portions of sequence of crucial functional value are most constrained against evolutionary change. They will not tolerate many mutations. Not that mutations do not occur in these portions, just that most mutations in the region are lethal and thus not observed. Other areas of sequence are able to drift more readily being less subject to evolutionary pressure. Therefore, sequences become a mosaic of quickly and slowly changing regions over evolutionary time. We can use those constrained portions as anchors to create a sequence alignment allowing comparison. It is easy to see that two sequences are aligned when they have identical symbols at identical positions, but what happens when symbols are not identical or the sequences are not the same length? How can we know that the most similar portions of the sequences are aligned, when is an alignment optimal and does optimal mean biologically correct? Part of the solution is the dynamic programming algorithm.

Although it is not possible to completely predict the function or shape (structure) of a protein from its sequence *de novo*, some useful inferences about structure and function can be drawn, especially by comparing the sequence of a protein of unknown structure and function to sequences of proteins with known structure and function. Second, if the goal of structure/function prediction is to be reached in the future, it will be because of partial analyses done in the present. Third, by comparing the sequence of equivalent proteins from different species of animals (such equivalent proteins are called 'homologs'), one can draw inferences about the evolution of these species from their common ancestors.

One of the most useful things people do with sequences is to compare them to other sequences. However, such comparisons are not as easy to make as one might first think. One factor that complicates analysis is that the sequences biologists need to compare are usually not identical, but only similar. In addition to having a small number of substitutions (e.g. a Guanine for an Adenine at one position in a DNA sequence) there will be insertions and deletions in one sequence relative to the other. Also, depending on what you are comparing and what you want to learn from the comparison, how you do the comparison will be different. For these reasons, there have been many different kinds of programs written to compare sequences.

PRINCIPLE OF MULTIPLE SEQUENCE ALIGNMENT

Once a sequence search is completed, the question arises whether the found similarities do share similarity amongst each other. This can be achieved either automatic or manual fashion by using programs which will align the sequences of interest.

If you painted a map from the result of your sequence search as described earlier, it might be obvious that sequences do usually share similarity only in parts. This will leave the ends or over hang parts of two sequences badly aligned due to low similarity, therefore before alignments are attempted, it is a good practice to create sequence fragments of approximately the same length which will allow programs to operate more easily. If sequences are not specifically tailored for multiple sequence alignment programs, they might fail to report alignments unreliably.

Finding the Best

The approach used for automatic sequence alignment can be described as 'clustering', of the most similar sequences. In a first step, the program will need to find the sequence pairs which shares the most obvious similarity. To achieve this, each sequence is compared to each, which results in $(n \times n)/2$ comparison if we have n sequences to compare. As in rigorous sequences searching, a comparison is made using sequence comparison tables to compute the best possible alignment and score this appropriately. Note that the score will be not as desired if the sequences have not been tailored as mentioned above.

Grouping

Once the comparison for each possible sequence pair has been completed, the best candidates serve as nuclei and additional sequences are aligned to the already existing alignment. This will work well with similar proteins but too many gaps, in particular on DNA level, will most probably not yield the desired result. The largest errors will occur if regions with low similarity are used as 'closest' set, as this will cause trouble for additional sequences to be matched.

If problems are encountered because similarity cannot be determined well enough automatically, either manual alignment is required or the selection of sequences must be improved by tailoring or omission of very remotely related fragments.

Result Evaluation

The result of a multiple sequence alignment will be a block of sequences, which are nicely painted on top of each other. Programs exist which will plot the degree of similarity along the sequence coordinate. Other programs allow to print or paint the output nicely. The GCG programs also produce a figure which schematically displays the level of similarity as a dendrogram.

Limitation

Multiple sequence alignment is not the tool for you if you are working on fragment assembly or shortgun sequencing. In order to align multiple sequences reliably, the similarity amongst the members of the alignment should be extensive along the entire length rather than only overlapping fragments.

MULTIPLE SEQUENCE DYNAMIC PROGRAMMING

As seen in pairwise dynamic programming, a brute force approach, looking at every possible position by sliding one sequence along every other sequence, is just not practical for alignment. Even without considering the introduction of gaps, the computation required to compare all possible alignments between just two sequences requires time proportional to the product of the lengths of the two sequences. Therefore, if the two sequences are approximately the same length (N), this is a N^2 problem. To include gaps, the calculation would be repeated $2N$ times to examine the possibility of gaps at each position within the sequences. This is now a $N4^N$ problem! Dynamic programming reduces the problem to N^2.

How do you work with more than just two sequences at a time? You could painstakingly manually align all your sequences using some type of editor and many people do that, but an automated solution is desirable, at least as a starting point to manual alignment. However, solving the dynamic programming algorithm for more than just two sequences rapidly becomes intractable. Dynamic programming's complexity and hence its computational requirements, increases exponentially with the number of sequences in the dataset being compared [complexity = (sequence length)$^{\text{number of sequences}}$]. Mathematically this is an N-dimensional matrix, quite complex indeed. As we have seen, pairwise dynamic programming solves a two-dimensional matrix and the complexity of the solution is equal to the length of the longest sequence squared. A three-member standard dynamic programming sequence comparison would be a matrix with three axes, the length of the longest sequence cubed and so forth. You can at least draw a three-dimensional matrix, but more than that becomes difficult, if not impossible, to even visualise. It quickly boggles the mind.

Several different heuristics have been employed over the years to simplify the complexity of the problem. One program, MSA, attempts to globally solve the N-dimensional matrix equation using a bounding box trick. However, the algorithm's complexity precludes its use in most situations, except with very small datasets. One way to globally solve the algorithm and yet reduce its complexity is to restrict the search space to only the most conserved local portions of all the sequences involved. This approach is used by the program PIMA. MSA and PIMA are both available through the Internet.

How the Algorithm Works

The most common implementations of automated multiple alignment modify dynamic programming by establishing a pairwise order in which to build the alignment. This modification is known as pairwise progressive dynamic programming. Originally attributed to Feng and Doolittle, this variation of the dynamic programming algorithm generates a global alignment, but restricts its search space at any one time to a local neighbourhood of the full length of only two sequences. Consider a group of sequences. First, all pairs are compared to each other, using normal dynamic programming. This establishes an order for the set, most to least similar. Similarly, subgroups are clustered together. Then, take the top two most similar sequences and align them using normal dynamic programming. Now create a consensus of the two and align that consensus to the third sequence using standard dynamic programming. Now create a consensus of the first three sequences and align that to the forth most similar. This process continues until it has worked its way through all sequences and/or sets of clusters. The pairwise, progressive solution is implemented in several programs including Des Higgins' and Julie Thompson's Clustal.

As seen with pairwise alignments and sequence database similarity searching, all of this is much easier with protein sequences vs nucleotide sequences. Twenty symbols are easier to align then only four; the signal-to-noise ratio is far better. Furthermore, the concept of similarity applies to amino acids but generally not to nucleotides. If at all possible, multiple sequence alignment should always be carried out at the protein level. Therefore, translate nucleotide sequences to their protein counterparts if you are aligning coding sequences before performing multiple sequence alignment. The process is much more difficult if you are forced to align nucleotides because the region does not code for a protein. Automated methods may be able to provide a starting point, but there is no guarantee that the alignment will be biologically correct. The resulting alignment will probably require extensive editing, if it works at all. Success will largely depend on the similarity of the nucleotide dataset.

One liability of the global progressive pairwise methods is they are entirely dependent on the order in which the sequences are aligned. Fortunately, ordering them from most similar to least similar usually makes biological sense and works very well. However, the techniques are very sensitive to the substitution matrix and specified gap penalties.

Programs that allow fine-tuning areas of an alignment by realignment with different scoring matrices and/or gap penalties can be extremely helpful. However, any automated multiple sequence alignment program should be thought of as only a tool to offer a starting alignment that can be improved upon, not the end-all-to-meet all solution, guaranteed to provide the one-true answer.

Reliability

To help assure the reliability of the sequence alignment, always use comparative approaches. A multiple sequence alignment is a hypothesis of evolutionary history. To insure that you have prepared a reasonable alignment, be sure it makes sense. Think about it, a sequence alignment is a statement of positional homology. It establishes the explicit homologous correspondence of each individual sequence position, each column in the alignment. Therefore, devote considerable time and energy toward developing the most satisfying multiple sequence alignment possible. Editing alignments is encouraged. Specialised sequence editing software helps achieve this, but any editor will do as long as the sequences are properly formatted. After some automated solution has offered its best guess, go into the alignment and use your own brain to improve it. Use all available information and understanding to insure that all columns are homologous. Look for conserved functional sites to help guide your judgement. Assure that known enzymatic, regulatory and structural elements all align. The results of subsequent analyses are absolutely dependent on the alignment.

Researchers have successfully used the conservation of covarying sites in ribosomal and other structural RNA alignments to assist refinement. That is, as one base in a stem-structure changes the corresponding

Watson-Crick paired base will change in a corresponding manner. The ribosomal database project at the centre for microbial ecology at Michigan State University has used this process extensively to help guide the construction of their rRNA alignments and structures (Website: http://rdp.cme.msu.edu/html/index.html).

Be sure an alignment makes biological sense. Beware of comparing apples and oranges. If creating alignments for phylogenetic inference, either make paralogous comparisons (i.e. evolution via gene duplication) to ascertain gene phylogenies within one organism or orthologous (within one ancestral loci) comparisons to ascertain gene phylogenies between organisms, which should imply organismal phylogenies. Try not to mix them up without complete data representation. A substantial amount of confusion can arise, especially if you do not have all the data and/or if the nomenclature is contradictory; extremely misleading interpretations can result. Be wary of trying to align genomic sequences with cDNA when working with DNA, the introns will cause all sorts of headaches. Similarly, do not align mature and precursor proteins from the same organism and loci. It does not make evolutionary sense, as one has not evolved from the other, rather one is the other. These are an easy mistakes to make, try your best to avoid them. Some general guidelines to remember include the following:

1. If the homology of a region is in doubt, then throw it out (or mask it).
2. Avoid the most diverged parts of molecules, they are the greatest source of systematic error.
3. Do not include sequences that are more diverged than necessary for the analysis at hand.

Practical consideration: remember the old adage; 'garbage in—garbage out'!

Applicability

The question arises, what are the uses of multiple sequence alignments? They are:

1. Very useful in the development of PCR primers and hybridisation probes.
2. Great for producing annotated, publication quality, graphics and illustrations.
3. Invaluable in structure/function studies through homology inference.
4. Essential for building 'Profiles' for remote homology similarity searching.
5. Required for molecular evolutionary phylogenetic inference programs such as those from phylogenetic analysis using parsimony (and other methods) (PAUP) and PHYLogeny inference package (PHYLIP).

The results from a multiple sequence alignment are useful for probe and primer design. They allow you to visualise the most conserved regions of an alignment. This technique is invaluable for designing phylogenetic specific probes as it clearly localises areas of high conservation and high variability in an alignment. Depending on the dataset that you analyse, any level of phylogenetic specificity can be achieved. Areas of high variability in the dataset can be used to differentiate between universal and specific probe sequences. After localising these general target areas, you can then use any of a number of primer discovery programs to find the best primers within those regions and to test those potential probes for common PCR conditions and problems.

Graphics prepared from multiple sequence alignments can dramatically illustrate functional and structural conservation. These can take many forms of all or portions of an alignment, shaded or coloured boxes or letters for each residue, cartoon representations of features, running line graphs of overall similarity, overlays of attributes, various consensus representations. All can be printed with high-resolution equipment, in colour or gray tones. These can make a big difference in a poster or manuscript presentation.

Conserved regions of an alignment are functionally important. In addition to the conservation of primary sequence and function, structure is also conserved in these crucial regions. In fact, recognisable structural conservation between true homologs extends way beyond statistically significant sequence similarity. An often-cited example is in the serine protease superfamily. *S. griseus* protease A demonstrates remarkably little similarity when compared to the rest of the superfamily (Expectation-values E $\geq 10^{1.8}$ in a typical search) yet its three-dimensional structure clearly shows its allegiance to the serine proteases. These principles are the premise of homology modelling and it works remarkably well.

As originally described by Michael Gribskov, profiles are a position specific weight matrix description of an alignment or a portion of an alignment. Gap insertion is penalised more heavily in conserved areas than in variable regions and the more highly conserved a residue is, the more important it becomes. Later refinements have added more statistical rigour. Generally, a profile is created from an alignment of related sequences and then used to search databases for remote sequence similarities. Profile searching is tremendously powerful and can provide the most sensitive, albeit extremely computationally intensive, database similarity searches possible.

We can use multiple sequence alignments to infer phylogeny. Based on the assertion of homologous positions in an alignment, several algorithms can estimate the most reasonable evolutionary tree for that alignment. Always remember that regardless of the algorithm used, parsimony, any distance method, or even maximum likelihood, all molecular sequence phylogenetic inference programs make the absolute validity of your input alignment their first and most critical assumption.

The most important factor to infer reliable phylogenies is the accuracy of the multiple sequence alignment. The interpretation of your results is utterly dependent on the quality of your input. In fact, many experts advice against using any parts of the sequence data that are at all questionable. Only analyse those portions that assuredly align.

As a general rule, if any portions of the alignment are in doubt, throw them out. This usually means trimming down or masking the alignment's terminal ends and may require internal trimming or masking as well. Biocomputing is always a delicate balance—signal against noise—and sometimes it can be quite the balancing act.

GLOBAL ALIGNMENTS

The Needleman and Wunsch algorithm for finding the best global alignment of two sequences can readily be extended to multiple sequences. The problem is that the time the computer needs for such a job is roughly proportional to the product of the sequence lengths. So, if aligning two sequences of 300 positions takes 1 second, aligning 3 sequences takes 300 seconds and aligning 10 sequences would take 300^8 seconds, which is longer than the lifetime of the universe!

Since searching for a best global alignment using a rigorous algorithm is not realistic for more than three sequences, a number of strategies have been developed to carry out a multiple global alignment in a reasonable amount of time with a reasonable chance of finding the best alignment. The GCG program pileup first aligns all possible pairs of sequences according to Needleman and Wunsch [for *n* sequences, this makes $n \times (n-1)/2$ alignments]. Then it uses the pairwise similarity scores to construct a tree using the UPGMA method. Finally, this tree serves as a guide for a progressive multiple alignments starting from the tips. Once two sequences have been aligned, their relative alignment is no longer changed. Clusters of previously aligned sequences are treated as a linearly weighted profile when they are subsequently aligned with another sequence or another cluster.

LOCAL ALIGNMENTS

There are cases where sequences share a similar region but are otherwise completely different. Take, for example, the amino acids in the active site of an enzyme or transcription factor binding sites in a DNA sequence. To handle these cases local multiple alignment algorithms have been developed. Usually they only look for ungapped alignments thereby avoiding the problem of choosing the optimal gap penalty. Two such programs have been developed at the NCBI:

MACAW by Schuler, Altschul and Lipman first tries to find high scoring segment pairs (HSPs) for each possible pair of sequences using the BLAST algorithm (with the sensitivity set high). It then assembles overlapping HSPs into blocks. An interesting feature of MACAW is that it does not try to align all sequences, but can pick out only those that share similar regions. There are versions of MACAW for the PC under Windows and for the Mac.

The MACAW distribution also contains Gibbs and a pattern searcher.

The Gibbs sampler algorithm involves iteratively making a profile with stretches of n-bases or amino acids, selected from the sequences and then searches this profile against one of the sequences. The result of the search is used to weight the selection of the stretches at the next run. A drawback is that the user must choose the width n and the number of elements in each sequence and thus must have a certain idea of the outcome or run the program several times. An interesting feature is that the Gibbs sampler algorithm avoids the choice of an externally added scoring scheme since it derives the highest scoring profile, in a self-consistent manner, from the data. Gibbs is available for UNIX.

WHAT IS A MULTIPLE ALIGNMENT?

The purpose of multiple sequence alignment is to bring the large number of similar features into register in the same column of the alignment optimally.

If the sequences in the MSA (Multiple sequence alignment) align well, they are likely to be derived from a common ancestor sequence presence of several similar domain in several sequences suggests a biochemical function, this may become the basis of further experimental investigation.

Based on similarities obtained by MSA. Similar proteins have been organised into databases of protein families—multiple sequence alignment of a set of sequences can provide information as to the most alike regions in the set. In proteins such regions may represent conserved functional or structural domains. A good alignment is that which includes a series of columns where majority of sequences have same amino acid or an amino acid that is a conservative substitution for that amino acid. In the same column very few examples of other substitutions or gaps may be present. These columns should be present throughput the alignment, often clustered into domains. In case of Nuclei acids, multiple sequence alignment can reveal structural and functional relationships. In case when promoter regions of a set of similar sequences aligned well, they may represent consensus binding sites for regulatory proteins.

Classes of Multiple Sequence Alignment

Global alignment

Global sequence alignment is the entire length sequence alignment. It is an extension of dynamic programming global alignment algorithm.

Sequence block

Sequence block is a common pattern of alignment in a group of sequence where matches, mismatches but no gaps are included. Sequence block can be found by pattern matching/pattern finding algorithms.

Profile

A profile is a type of scoring matrix which is produced from an alignment of common patterns in protein sequences that includes matches, mismatches, insertions and deletions.

Scoring Multiple Sequence Alignments

SP Model for Scoring MSA:

SP stands for sum of pairs.

MSA-Multiple Sequence Alignment.

With SP model we can score the MSA by adding all the possible combination of pairs scores of amino acids in a column of a MSA. This model assumes that any sequence could be ancestor of the other sequence. When the number of mismatched residues pairs increases, scores in the MSA column decreases rapidly. This decrease should be greater for a large number of sequences say more than five sequences with all R or with one or two S substitutions, because there will be more R–R matched pairs relative to mismatched R–S pairs. However, the opposite is true with the SP method of scoring. We can understand it more clearly from the below mentioned illustrations in Fig. 14.1.

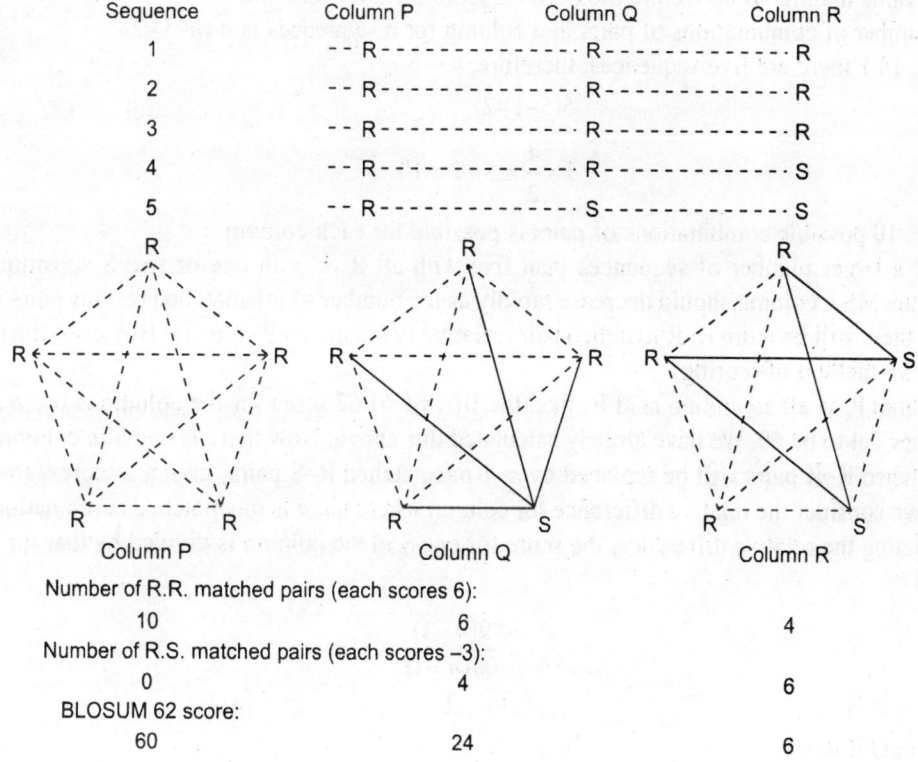

Fig. 14.1. The SP model for scoring a MSA.

SP method is an optimisation method where maximisation of number of matched pairs score is performed by minimising the cost or number of mismatched pairs in all columns in the MSA.

Figure 14.1 there are three columns of a five sequence MSA. In column P all residues, i.e. R are matched, in column Q four R are matched and one S is mismatched, whereas in column R three R are matched and two S mismatched. With SP method cumulative scores for columns of a MSA can be calculated. SP method can be illustrated by means of graph with five sequences as vertices and representing the ten possible sequence pairwise sequence comparisons as shown Fig. 14.1. Solid lines represents a matched pair and dotted liner a mismatched pairs.

BLOSUM 62 scores are calculated as shown in last row.

$\longrightarrow$ Solution for calculating Blosum 62 scores.

1. For column P.

The number of R–R matched pairs for column P is 10. For each match pair the score is 6.

The number 6 is by our convention we can put any score the first column P has no R–S matched pair therefore score is zero. Therefore, the effective score of the column is $10 \times 6 = 60$ (Blosum score 62). Similarly the blossum score for column Q is calculated as below:

The number of matched pairs of R–R in column Q is 6 each pair has score 6, i.e. $6 \times 6 = 36$

However, the number of R–S matched pairs in same column is 4 each with a score of –3, i.e.

$$4 \times -3 = -12.$$

The effective score or the Blosum 62 score for the same column is $36 - 12 = 24$.

In the same manner as above the blossum 62 score for the R column is 6.

The number of combinations of pairs in a column for n sequences is $n(n-1)/2$.

In Fig. 14.1 there are five sequences, therefore, $n = 5$.

$$5(5-1)/2$$

$$5 \times \frac{4}{2} = 5 \times 2 = 10$$

Therefore, 10 possible combinations of pairs is possible for each column.

Note: For a larger number of sequences than five with all R or with one or two S substitutions, the scores in the MSA column should decrease rapidly as the number of mismatched residue pairs increases (Because there will be more R–R matched pairs relative to mismatch R–S pairs. However, the reverse is true with SP method of scoring).

In column P, as all are amino acid R, then the BLOSUM 62 score for the column is $6 \times n(n-1)/2$.

It comes out to be 60. We have already calculated this above. Now there is one S in column Q. Then $(n-1)$ matched R–R pairs will be replaced by $n-1$ mismatched R–S pairs, giving a score $9(n-1)$ less.

Now we consider the relative difference for column where there is mismatched combinations of pair for calculating the relative difference, the score for one S in the column is divided by that for zero S in column, i.e.

$$\frac{9(n-1)}{\dfrac{6n(n-1)}{2}} = 3/n.$$

for column Q it is $3/n$.

where,

n = no. of sequences

For 3 sequences relative difference is 1 whereas for six sequences the relative difference is 2.

As more sequences are present in the column the relative difference increases, not in agreement with expectation. Hence, the SP method is not providing a reasonable result when this type of scoring matrix is used.

PAIRWISE SEQUENCE ALIGNMENT VERSUS MULTIPLE SEQUENCE ALIGNMENT

One of the important contributions of molecular biology to evolutionary analysis is the discovery that the DNA sequences of different organisms are often related. Similar genes are conserved across widely diverged species, often performing a similar or even identical function and at other times, mutating or rearranging to perform an altered function through the forces of natural selection. Thus, many genes are represented in highly conserved forms in organisms.

Through simultaneous alignment of the sequences of these genes sequence patterns that have been subject to alteration may be analysed. Because the potential for learning about the structure and function of molecules by multiple sequence alignment (MSA) is so great, computational methods have received a great deal of attention. In MSA sequences are aligned optimally by bringing the greatest number similar characters into register in the same column of the alignment of more than two sequences that includes matches, mismatches and gaps and that takes into account the degree of variation in all of the sequences at the same time poses a very difficult challenge. The dynamics programming algorithm used for optimal sequence alignment of pairs of sequences can be extended to three sequences, but for more than three sequences, only small number of relatively short sequences may be characterised. Thus approximate methods are used, including:

Progressive global alignment of the sequences starting with an alignment of the most alike sequences and then building an alignment by adding more sequences.

Iterative methods that make an initial alignment of group of sequences and then revise the alignment to achieve a more reasonable result.

Alignment based on locally conserved patterns found in the same order in the sequences. Use of statistical methods and probabilistic models of the sequences.

Just now we discussed about statistical method. A second computational challenge is identifying a reasonable method of obtaining a cumulative score for the substitution in the column of a MSA. Finally, the placement and scoring of gaps in the various sequences of an MSA presents an additional challenge.

The MSA of a set of sequences may also be viewed as an evolutionary history of the sequences. If these sequences in the MSA align very well, they are likely to be recently derived from a common ancestor sequence.

Conversely a group of poorly aligned sequences share a more common complex and distant evolutionary relationship. The task of aligning a set of sequences, some more closely and other less closely related is identical to that of discovering the evolutionary relationship among the sequences.

As with aligning a pair of sequence the difficulty in aligning a group of sequences varies considerably with sequence similarity. On the one hand, if the amount of sequence variation is minimal, it is quite straightforward to align the sequences, even without the assistance of a computer program. On the other hand, if the amount of sequence variation is great, it may be difficult to find an optimal alignment of the sequences because so many combinations of substitutions, insertions and deletions, each predicting a different alignment, are possible.

The availability of a subset of the many MSA programs are shown below:
CLUSTALW or CLUSTALX; MSA; PRALINE; DIALIGN; MULTALIN PRRP; SAGA; HMMER; MACAW; SAM;
Websites: clustal W   www.ebi.ac.vk/clustalw or clustalx
              clustal X   available at Ebi or Expary websites

When dealing with a sequence of unknown function the presence of similar domains in several similar sequences implies a similar biochemical function or structural fold that may become the bias of further experimental investigation. A group of similar sequences may define a protein family that may share a common biochemical function or evolutionary origin. Similar proteins have been organised into databases of proteins families, which will be discussed later.

One application MSA is in genome sequencing projects. Instead of cloning and arranging a very large number of fragments of a large DNA molecule and then moving along the molecule and sequencing the fragments in order, random fragments of the large molecules are sequenced and those that overlap are found by the MSA program. This approach enables automated assembly of large sequences. Bacterial genome has been quite readily sequenced by this method.

Just as the alignment of a pair of nucleic acid or protein sequences can reveal whether or not there is an evolutionary relationship between the sequences, so can the alignment of three or more sequences reveal relationship among multiple sequences. MSA of a set of sequences can provide information as to the most alike regions in the set.

In proteins, such regions may represent conserved functional or structural domains. If the structure of one or more members of the alignment is known it may be possible to predict which amino acids occupy the same spatial relationship in other proteins in the alignment. In nucleic acids, such alignments also reveal structural and functional relationships. For example, aligned promoters or set of similarity-regulated genes may reveal consensus-binding sites for regulatory proteins.

Another use of consensus information retrieved from a MSA is for the prediction of specific probes for other members of the same group or family of similar sequences in the same or other organisms. There are both computer and molecular biology applications. Once a consensus pattern has been found database-searching programs may be used to find other sequences with a similar pattern. In the laboratory a reasonable consensus of such patterns may be used to define polymerase chain reaction (PCR) primers for amplification of related sequences.

Once MSA has been found, the number or types of changes in the aligned sequence residues may be used for a phylogenetic analysis. The alignment provides a prediction as to which sequence character corresponds. Each column in the alignment predicts the mutations that occurred at one site during evolution of the sequence family.

The close relationship between MSA and evolutionary tree construction shown is a short section of one MSA of four protein sequences including conserved and substituted positions, an insertion (of K) and a deletion of L below MSA shown as hypothetical evolutionary tree that could have generated these sequence changes.

Each outer branch in the tree represents one of the sequences. The outer branches are also referred to as leaves. The deepest, oldest branch is that of the sequence D, followed by A, then by B and C. The optimal alignment of several sequences can thereby be thought of as minimising the number of mutational steps in an evolutionary tree for which the sequences are the outer branches or leaves. The mathematical solution to this problem was first outlined by Sankoff.

Fast MSA programs that are tree based have since been developed. However, such an approach depends on knowing the evolutionary tree to perform an alignment. Often this is not the case. Usually, pairwise alignments are generated first and then used to predict the tree. In this example, the alignment could be explained by several different trees including the one shown in Fig. 14.2.

Within the column are original characters that are present early, as well as other derived characters that appeared later in evolutionary time. In some cases the position is so important for function that mutational changes are not observed. In other cases the position is less important and substitutions are observed.

Deletions and insertions may also be present in some regions of the alignment. Thus, starting with the alignment one can hope to dissect the order of appearance of the sequences during evolution.

Seq A	N	•	F	L	S
Seq B	N	•	F	•	S
Seq C	N	K	Y	L	S
Seq D	N	•	Y	L	S

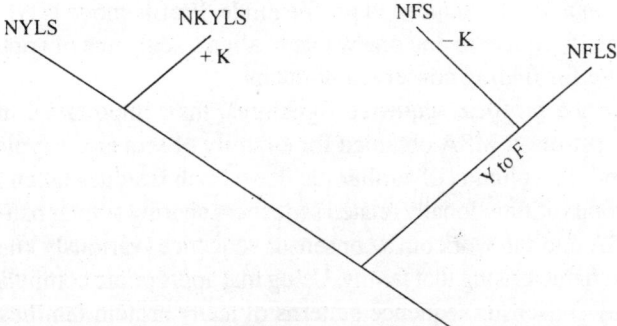

Fig. 14.2. Tree diagram.

PHYLOGENETIC TREES

Ideally a researcher would like to have a black box in which to throw sequences and get out a fully annotated phylogenetic tree. This is, however, not possible for two reasons. First, an algorithm that considers all possible multiple sequence alignments and then, for each alignment, all possible phylogenetic trees and picks out the best one, would take too much time. That is why most phylogenetic programs work on previously aligned sequences. Second, the result is always strongly influenced by the criteria that are used to define the best tree. Phylogenetic analysis will be the subject of a separate chapter. However, a few remarks seem appropriate here. There are three main kinds of tree building methods: Distance matrix, maximum likelihood and parsimony.

Distance matrix methods first estimate the pairwise distances between the sequences (which means that the information in the alignment of two sequences is reduced to one number) while the other methods construct many trees from all the information in the multiple alignments and decide which is best.

The simplest distance based method is UPGMA (unweighted pair-group method using arithmetic averages) which involves iteratively taking together the two sequences that have the shortest distance from each other, placing them at the end of branches on a node of the tree and replacing their distances from the other sequences by an average value.

The guide tree used by pileup and CLUSTAL should never be used to infer phylogeny. It has been derived from the distances between pairwise aligned sequences and these distances are not necessarily the same as the distances between sequence pairs taken from the multiple sequence alignment.

TOOLS USED SUCH AS CLUSTAL X

CLUSTAL X provides graphical interface to the program CLUSTAL X. Clustal was developed by Higgins and Sharp in 1988 and much improved versions were developed later. CLUSTAL W is the more recent version of CLUSTAL with W standing for weighing to represent the ability of the program to provide weights to the sequence and program parametres.

CLUSTAL performs a global-multiple sequence alignment by a stepwise process. In step I it performs pairwise alignments of all the sequences provided by the user. In step II the scores obtained for the pairwise alignment are used to produce a phylogenetic tree and in step III the phylogenetic tree is used as a guide to align sequences sequentially thus the most closely related sequences are aligned first, and then additional sequences are added one by one to a profile of an existing MSA. The scoring of gaps is done in a manner different from that followed for a pairwise alignment. CLUSTAL W calculates gaps in a novel way. The graphical version of CLUSTALX provides a versatile environment for doing MSA of sequences. Alignments can also be produced in profile mode. Profile mode is typically used when MSA is already known for a set of sequences and one wants to align a sequence of another MSA to that MSA. This is very useful feature for finding conserved domains.

Family specific sequence profiles, sequence signatures, their importance in sequence alignments and homology searches, psi-blast; MSA obtained for a family of sequences typically contains columns of conserved residues and the columns of similar residues. Such residues taken together may specify a pattern or signature or groups of functionally related sequences sharing similar patterns. From the columns of the residues in the MSA one can work out a consensus sequence (variously known as a pattern, motif, signature or finger print) characterising that family. Using that appropriate computational tools, PROSITE is a database where many consensus sequence patterns of many protein families have been deposited.

MULTIPLE SEQUENCE ALIGNMENTS USING CLUSTAL X (PRACTICAL)

Clustal X can be obtained from the following website:

www.ebi.ac.uk/clustal X

Clustal X is a graphical version of the clustal program that not only aligns sequences but also draws pretty pictures of the alignments.

1. Convert your sequences, which are probably in Fasta format, into 'PIR' format, which is only slightly different. If Fasta format is:
2. >SequenceName1
3. GSAVVALTNDRDTSYFGEIGIGTPPQKFTV
4. IFDTGSSVLWVPSSKCINSKACRAHSMYES
5. >SequenceName2
6. GNTTSSVILTNYMDTQYYGEIGIGTPPQTF
7. KVVFDTGSSNVWVPSSKCSRLYTACVYHKL

...Then PIR format is...

>SequenceName1 /
GSAVVALTNDRDTSYFGEIGIGTPPQKFTV
IFDTGSSVLWVPSSKCINSKACRAHSMYES
*

>SequenceName2
GNTTSSVILTNYMDTQYYGEIGIGTPPQTF
KVVFDTGSSNVWVPSSKCSRLYTACVYHKL
*

8. To keep Clustal happy, make sure the first word of the header line is unique for each sequence. If
9. >1hrn A
10. GSAVVALTNDRDTSYFGEIGIGTPPQKFTV

11. IFDTGSSVLWVPSSKCINSKACRAHSMYES
    *
12. >1hrn B
13. GNTTSSVILTNYMDTQYYGEIGIGTPPQTF
14. KVVFDTGSSNVWVPSSKCSRLYTACVYHKL
    *

... Change to...
    >1hrnA
    GSAVVALTNDRDTSYFGEIGIGTPPQKFTV
    IFDTGSSVLWVPSSKCINSKACRAHSMYES
    *

    >1hrnB
    GNTTSSVILTNYMDTQYYGEIGIGTPPQTF
    KVVFDTGSSNVWVPSSKCSRLYTACVYHKL
    *

... else clustal will think there are two sequences for 1hrn.

15. Load your sequences into ClustalX by typing:
    /usr/local/apps/clustalx/clustalx my_alignment.pir &
16. Align the sequences by clicking the 'Alignment' menu and selecting 'do complete alignment'.
17. Save the alignment in PIR format by selecting 'file'/'save sequences as' and checking the appropriate format on the dialog box.
18. Save a picture of the alignment by choosing 'file'/'write alignment as postscript' and checking the options in the 'write postscript' dialog box. Dismiss any printing-related error or warning messages (these are unimportant) then close the dialog box once clustalX has saved the .ps file. Postscript (abbrev. 'ps') is a printer language and postscript files can be viewed or printed under unix. View the postscript file by typing:
    gs my_alignment_pic.ps &
    Ask a demonstrator to print this picture out in colour.
19. Multiple sequence alignments can indicate which positions or regions are important for the structure and/or function of a protein, and which regions may vary with little consequence.
    Look at your alignment. Are there any positions that are completely conserved? Are there any positions that show only conservative substitutions, i.e. like substituting for like? Are there any regions of one sequence unmatched by the other sequences? If the proteins in your alignment have identical functions, what does this suggest about the relative importance of these unmatched regions? Which regions of sequence might correspond to loops in the structure?
20. When all the sequences in an alignment are highly similar it can be difficult to distinguish important from unimportant positions; the sequences may be so closely related that less important regions have not had time to diverge and so appear conserved.
    Look at the BLAST outputs for the sequences in your alignment. How similar are your sequences to each other? If you have time, add some of the lower scoring BLAST hits to your alignment, i.e. sequences in the 30–40 per cent identity range (no lower, else they may not be genuine relatives). Make another alignment with this larger set. How does this alignment differ from your original?
    Note: Blast can be found at www.ncbi.n/m.nih.gov/blast.

USE OF SEQUENCE PATTERNS

It is often observed that a new protein is too distantly related to any protein of known structure to detect its resemblance by overall sequence alignment. But it can be identified by the occurrence in its sequence of a particular motif. These motifs arise because of particular requirement on the structure of specific regions of a protein, which may be important for example for the binding properties or for their enzymatic activity. These requirements impose very tight constraints on the evolution of those limited in size but important portion of a protein sequence. The use of protein sequence patterns (or motifs) to determine the function of proteins is becoming very rapidly one of the essential tools of sequence analysis.

As it is clear now from the above discussion that MSA of proteins can be used to develop sequence pattern. The first and the most important criterion is that a good signature pattern must be as short as possible, should detect all or most of the sequences it is designed to describe and should not give too many false positive results. In other words it must exhibit both high sensitivity and high specificity. Therefore, while deriving a motif particular attention is paid to the residues and regions thought or proved to be important to the biological function of the group of Proteins. These biologically significant regions or residues are generally:

Enzyme catalytic sites; prosthetic group attachment sites (heme, pyridoxal phosphate, biotin, etc.).

Amino acids involved in binding a metal ion.

Cysteine involved in disulphide bonds.

Regions involved in binding a molecule (ADP/ATP, GDP/GTP, CALCIUM, DNA).

Or another protein.

For example from the following MSA one can derive a sequence pattern a [R, T or D]-[D, A or Q]-[F, E or A]-A-T-H-[D or E]. Please note the shorter motif, viz. the conserved A-T-H could have been sufficient. However, in order to increase the specificity the sequence pattern in the flanking regions have also been taken.

ALRDFATHDDF

SMTAEATHDSI

ECDQAATHEAS

There are a number of protein families as well as functional or structural domains that cannot be detected using patterns due to their extreme sequence divergence. But by using family specific sequence profiles it is possible to detect such proteins or domains.

A profile (also called, as weight matrix) is a table of position specific amino acid weights and gap costs. These numbers (also referred to as scores) are used to calculate a similarity score for any alignment between a profile and a sequence or parts of a sequence and a profile. An alignment with a similarity score higher than or equal to a given cut off value constitutes a motif occurrence. As with patterns, there may be several matches to a profile in one sequence, but multiple occurrences in the same sequences must be disjoint (nonoverlapping) according to a specific definition included in the profile.

Profile can be constructed by a large variety of different techniques. The classical method developed by Gribskov and coworkers requires a multiple sequence alignment as input and uses a symbol comparison table to convert residue frequency distribution into weights.

Unlike patterns, profiles are usually not confined to small regions with high sequence similarity. Rather they attempted to characterise a protein family or domain over its entire length. This can lead to specific problems not arising with PROSITE patterns. With a profile covering conserved as well as diverged sequence regions, there is a chance to obtain a significant similarity score even with a partially incorrect alignment. This possibility is taken into account by our quality evaluation procedures. In order to be acceptable, a profile must not only assign high similarity scores to true motif occurrences and low scores to false matches. In addition it should correctly align those residues having analogues functions or structural properties according to experimental data.

Profiles are supposed to be more sensitive and more robust than patterns because they provide discriminatory weights not only for the residues already found at a given position of a motif but also for those not yet found. The weights for those not yet found are extrapolated from the observed amino acid compositions using empiric knowledge about amino acid substitutability.

PSI-BLAST

As mentioned earlier it is quite advantageous to use a sequence profile that represents a sequence pattern in a protein family instead of a single query sequence to search a database. The search of database thereby will be expanded to identify additional related sequences that might otherwise be missed. A new version of blast called Position specific iterated blast has been designed to build profiles iteratively and then to do blast search. As name itself indicate the methods of Psi-Blast involves a series of repeated steps or iterations. First a database search of protein sequence database is performed using query sequence. Second the results of the search are checked to include only the convincing hits in other words only the high scoring sequence matches. These sequences are aligned and a weigh matrix is produced from the alignment. The database is again searched with this scoring matrix. Again the hits are aligned and the weight matrix is updated. This type of database search and updating of weight matrix are repeatedly carried out until no new hits are found (converged).

PSI-BLAST is highly sensitive as well as specific due to the use of family specific profile which gets updated iteratively and that is used as the scoring matrix for next database search. An analysis on the performance of PSI-BLAST has demonstrated that BLAST can detect weak similarities that exist between distant homologs.

PSI-BLAST can be accessed from the following website:

www.ncbi.nlm.nih.gov/BLAST.

STRUCTURE-BASED SEQUENCE ALIGNMENT—COMPARER

So far we discussed about alignment of sequences using some scoring matrices. It is also possible to align sequences of proteins based on their structures. Such alignments are called as structure-based sequence alignments. In fact structure-based sequence alignments more accurately represents the similarities between the Proteins than the alignments purely based on sequence scoring matrices. The basic underlying fact is that even the proteins, which have diverged very much with respect to their amino acid sequences, still retain their overall 3D structure. The fact has led to the development of many computational algorithms.

The basic prerequisite to carry out structure-based alignments is that the 3D structures of the proteins in the form of brookhaven protein data bank (PDB) files are known. A PDB file contains Cartesian coordinates of all the amino acids residue of a protein. Using the atomic coordinate the protein 3D structures are superimposed on to each other. After the best superposition the residues that are within a distance usually 3 Angstroms are listed. Such residues are called as topologically equivalent residues. The topologically equivalent residues have similar structural environment. From topologically equivalent residues an unequivocal sequence alignment is worked out.

COMPARER is a computational tool developed by Sali and Bundall to carry out structural-based sequence alignments of Proteins. The underlying idea in this method is that the protein is not only viewed as a string of amino acids which makes its primary structure but also additionally as string of structural features such as secondary structures, the degree of residue solvent accessibilities and hydrogen bonds. All these structural features along with the residues are used and an alignment is produced using dynamic programming algorithms.

Other Approaches Include

1. The very popular CLUSTAL program differs only from pileup in that it performs the initial pairwise alignments using the fast algorithm of Wilbur and Lipman.
   CABIOS 8:189. You can obtain versions of CLUSTAL for UNIX.

2. Starting with a search for words of n bases or amino acids that are common between the sequences. An example is Martin Vingron's program MALI.
   CABIOS 5:115. MALI is not distributed freely but may be obtained from its author Martin Vingron (vingron@embl-heidelberg.de).

3. PIMA uses pattern matching, rather than profile matching, while making the progressive alignment. PNAS 87:118.
   PIMA can be obtained for UNIX.

4. Building a phylogenetic tree, using a more elaborate algorithm, as the sequences are progressively aligned. An example is Jotun Hein's program Tree Align.
   Meth.Enzymol. 18:626.
   TreeAlign can be obtained for UNIX from the same address as given for clustalw.

5. Making the best multiple alignments in a limited area of alignment space. This can only realistically be performed with eight to ten sequences.

BLAST 3

It is also worth mentioning the program blast 3. This searches a protein against a protein databank using the BLAST algorithm (with the sensitivity set high) and then makes threefold alignments between the query sequence and each possible pair of databank sequences that have been found. Only the statistically significant threefold alignments which are made from three nonsignificant pairwise alignments are retained. Blast 3 is useful in finding proteins that share a region of only weak similarity. Occasionally it can show that a query sequence makes the bridge between two databank sequences whose relationship had not yet been suspected. It is possible to access a BLAST (including blast 3) server at the NCBI, either through WWW or with a specific blast Internet client that you can install on your computer.

Note: www.ncbi.nlm.nih.gov/BLAST.

MULTIPLE SEQUENCE ALIGNMENTS AND PATTERNS

Multiple sequence alignment is the process of aligning several related sequences, showing the conserved and unconserved residues across all of the sequences simultaneously. These conserved/unconserved residues form a pattern that can often be used to retrieve sequences that are distantly related to the original group of sequences. These distant relatives are extremely helpful in understanding the role that the groups of sequences play in the process of life.

GLOBAL MULTIPLE SEQUENCE ALIGNMENTS

Global multiple sequence alignments are sequence alignments that require the participation of all sequence residues. A multiple sequence alignment shows the residue juxtaposition across the entire set of sequences; thus showing the conserved and unconserved residues across all of the sequences simultaneously.

DYNAMIC PROGRAMMING APPROACH

In order to understand the multiple sequence alignment algorithms, we first, need to review aligning two sequences using the dynamic programming approach. In a straightforward implementation, this problem would require memory proportional to the lengths of the sequences. Thus, if sequence A had length L and sequence B had length M this problem could be solved using $N \times M$ cells of memory. For example if sequence A was 8 residues long and sequence B were 5 residues long, 40 memory cells would be needed (Fig. 14.3).

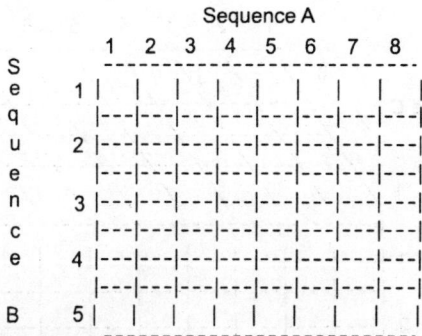

Fig. 14.3. Dynamic programming approach.

If we were to align 3 residue third sequence, sequence C, with the original two sequences we would need $8 \times 5 \times 3 = 120$ memory cells: shown in Fig. 14.4.

This approach is not practical for more than three average sized protein sequences. Let's look at the memory required to align average sized (300 residue) protein sequences:

Sequences	Cells	Memory (4 bytes/cells)
2	$300^2 = 90000$	351Kb
3	$300^3 = 27000000$	105Mb
4	$300^4 = 8.1 \times 10^9$	31640Mb

PROGRESSIVE PAIRWISE APPROACH

The progressive pairwise approach relies on exhaustive pairwise alignments between all of the sequences to produce a measure of sequence relatedness. From this measure, an algorithm (UPGMA in Pileup, Neighbour Joining in Clustalw) is used to develop a joining order. This joining order corresponds to a tree that is used to produce the multiple sequence alignment. It should be noted that this tree is not an evolutionary tree—do not make the mistake of using it as one. The tree is shown in Fig. 14.5.

After the joining order has been determined, sequences close to each other are aligned first. In the example above, SEQ#01 and SEQ#04 are the first two sequences to be aligned. The third sequence, SEQ#05, is then aligned with the two previously aligned sequences, SEQ#01 and SEQ#04. SEQ#02 is then aligned, followed by SEQ#03.

While this approach produces adequate results for many sets of sequences, the alignment produced by the procedure will vary depending on the joining order.

Thus, joining the sequences in this order:

[[[[SEQ#03 + SEQ#02] + SEQ#05] + SEQ#04] + SEQ#0l]

may not produce the same alignment as joining the sequences in the original order:

[[[[SEQ#0l + SEQ#04] + SEQ#05] + SEQ#02] + SEQ#03]

The advantages to this approach are that it requires only modest computer resources and that it is capable of aligning hundreds of sequences.

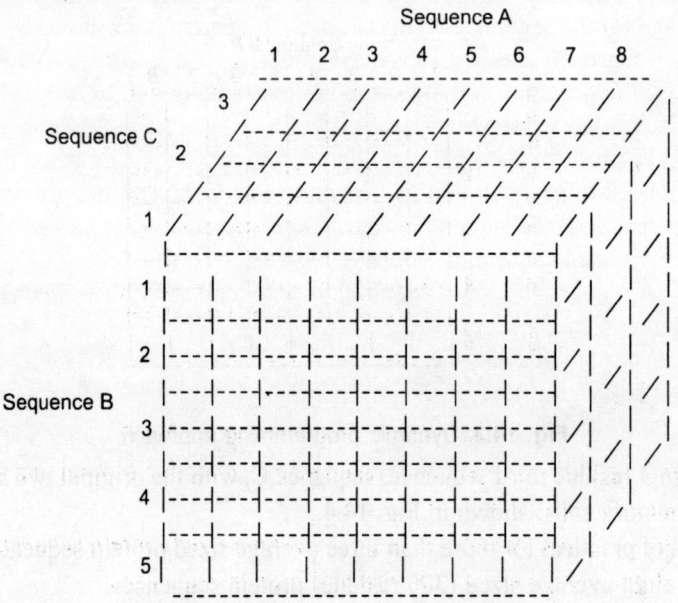

Fig. 14.4. Memory cells representation.

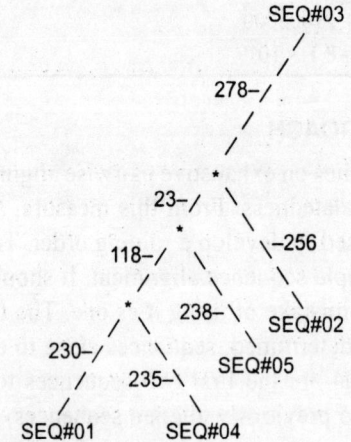

Fig. 14.5. Tree of multiple sequence alignment (progressive pairwise approach).

MODIFIED DYNAMIC PROGRAMMING APPROACH

If we had a good global alignment between two related sequences, the memory cells that contain this alignment would be near the centre diagonal of the two dimensional grid. Likewise if we had a good global alignment between three related sequences we would expect its alignment path to make use of the memory cells near the centre of the cube. The MSA program uses a clever approach to restrict the amount of memory by computing bounds that approximate the centre of a multi-dimensional hypercube. The first bound is produced by computing pairwise alignments between the set of sequences. Weights are usually applied to this value to produce the lower bound used by the program. Next a heuristic alignment is produced for the sequences. This heuristic alignment is produced by a procedure similar to progressive pairwise approach outlined above. Weights are usually applied to this value to produce the upper bound used by the program. A delta value is then computed to be the difference between these two values. The epsilon values shown by the program is the computed delta value broke down per pairwise alignment. To produce good optimal alignments, epsilon and delta are the two most important parametres that you need to pay attention to. The delta and epsilon values are preliminary measures of the divergence between the set of sequences. Thus, closely related sequences will have low epsilons and deltas while distantly related sequences will have high epsilons and deltas.

Even though MSA reduces the space required to produce a multiple alignment dramatically, it still uses much more memory than the progressive pairwise technique. Generally speaking, MSA will produce better alignments than most multiple sequence alignment programs such as clustal or pileup. The drawback with using MSA is that it requires an enormous amount of both computer time and memory to align more than a few distantly related sequences. However, we have been able to use MSA to optimally align 20 Phospholipase A2 sequences (approximately 130 residues), 14 Cytochrome C sequences (approximately 110 residues), 6 aspartal proteases (approximately 350 residues) and 8 lipid binding proteins (approximately 480 residues) on our computers. All of these problems approached the limits of the problems that can be solved optimally by the MSA program. The size of the problems solved by MSA are directly related to the sequence lengths, the number of sequences and the amount of sequence diversity.

An example for best results running the program, first produce only a heuristic alignment with your set of sequences. Examine the alignment and the epsilons. If you are only using a few short sequences and the computed epsilons are relatively low (epsilons < 50) then the sequences are closely related. Continue on to produce an optimal alignment. If you are using a more complicated set of sequences, a ramping strategy is suggested. First, align three of your sequences optimally, then four, then five..., etc. until you exceed 32 Mb of memory. Then double, triple or quadruple the memory requirements and add one last sequence. You may or may not be able to get this last sequence to align. If you are dealing with long sequences, you may want to divide your sequences into two or three sub regions and align the sub regions separately. The Table 14.1 illustrates using this strategy.

Table 14.1. Strategy for using this modified programming approach.

#	Sequences	Elapsed	CPU time	Memory
1	humcetp	na	na	na
2	hupltp	00:00:00	00:00:00	608056
3	rrrya3	00:00:24	00:00:24	632863
4	bovbpi	00:01:53	00:01:53	20432143
5	ratlbp	00:20:52	00:20:51	75296490
6	rry2g5	16:48:04	16:04:10	10129449583

PATTERNS

Patterns Derived from Aligned Families

Early patterns were first reported as consensus sequences. These patterns were essentially composite sequences consisting of the most common residue occurring at a position in an alignment. Today, these patterns are of little use unless if the sequences are highly conserved. A later approach stored the pattern as a regular expression. A regular expression is much more flexible than a consensus sequence because more than one residue can be stored at each position. There are many patterns that can be described as regular expressions. Many of these excellent patterns can be found in the PROSITE dictionary of sites and patterns. The GCG program motifs make use of this data. The findpatterns program can be used to search a database for an ambiguous pattern. A more recent approach is to use a weight matrix to represent the pattern. This approach is much more sensitive to patterns that are not strongly conserved. The profile analysis method can be used to create a weight matrix patterns from a sequence alignment. These patterns, (called profiles) can then be used to search the sequence databases for additional sequences that contain the pattern. The profilemake program can be used to create a profile, with the profile search or PROFILE-SS programs can be used to scan a database for a profile. The profilescan program can be used to see if a sequence contains a pattern placed in the profile library.

Patterns Derived from Unaligned Sequences

Deriving patterns from unaligned sequences is a new area of research. One successful method uses an information content measure to discover patterns. This approach is incorporated into the MEME program. MEME essentially finds a position-dependent letter frequency matrix that is similar to a gapless profile. This gapless profile can then be used to search a database for copies of the profile. An experimental approach being used today is that of a hidden markov model. At the current time software using this technique is still very experimental. We anticipate that in a few years this approach may become useful technique.

OPTIMAL AND SUB-OPTIMAL ALIGNMENTS

We discussed about optimal alignment between two sequences and how to achieve it using dynamic programming method. In several instances especially when the two sequences are highly diverged, there can be alternative alignments with nearly same probability or more generally the same score as the optimal alignment. Such alternative alignments that are worthy of examination are known as sub-optimal alignments.

There are two classes of sub-optimal alignments. One class where the scores are closer to that of optimal alignment but differ in a few positions from the optimum alignment. The second class is of sub-optimal alignments.

Chapter 15

Data Mining

INTRODUCTION

Getting at the hard-won sequence and structure data in molecular biology databases and the functional data in the online biomedical literature is complicated by the size and complexity of the databases. Often, it's assumed—sometimes incorrectly—that certain data are contained in a database. However, exhaustively searching for the raw data and performing the transformation and manipulations on the data through manual operations is often impractical. Similarly, in cases where it isn't certain what relationships can be garnered from searching through a database, the odds of finding every biologically relevant relationship through manually authored query statements are low. When it's known in general what resides in a database and there is a need to extract it, the challenge is more of a translation problem. Conversely, when, very little is known about what resides in the database, the work is primarily data discovery. In either case, the time and computational resources required to locate and manipulate the data are limiting factors.

Camouflaged by the size and complexity of a database, the millions of data points from genomic or proteomic studies are of little value. Only when these data are categorised according to a meaningful theme are they useful in furthering our understanding of sequence, structure or function. Regardless of whether this categorisation is at the base pair, chromosome or gene level, an organising theme is critical because it simplifies and reduces the complexity of what could otherwise be a flood of incomprehensible data. For example, the individual databases managed by the NCBI represent generally recognisable organisational themes that facilitate use of their contents. At a higher level, our understanding of health and disease is facilitated by the organisation of clinical research data by organ system, pathogen, genetic aberration or site of trauma.

Ideally, the creator and the users of the database share an understanding of the underlying organisational theme. These themes, and the tools used to support them, determine how easily databases created for one purpose can be used for other purposes. For example, in a relational database of gene sequences, the data may be arranged tables and the user may need to construct structured query language (SQL) statements to search for and retrieve data. However, if inherited diseases organise the relational database, it may not readily support an efficient search by protein sequence.

The challenge for researchers looking in the exponentially increasing quantities of microbiology data for assumed and unknown relationships can be formidable, even if the number of data elements and dimensionality are relatively small. For example, a relational database with a few hundred records (rows) and a small number of fields per record (low dimensionality) can probably be searched manually for new interrelationships in the data. However, the task may involve creating relatively complicated, computationally intensive joins in order to create views that support a given hypothesis of how data are related. In addition, even within a relatively small database, it may be practically impossible to specify a relationship query exactly. At issue is how best to support the formulation of a hypothesis-based query. In addition, even if the technology is available that allows a researcher to specify any hypothetical query, the potential for discovering new relationships in data is a function of the insights and biases imposed by the researcher. While these limitations may be problematic in relatively small databases, they may be intolerable in databases with billions of interrelated data elements. To avoid the computational constraints imposed by these large molecular biology databases, researchers frequently turn to biological heuristics to avoid exhaustive searches or processes with a low likelihood of success. For example, in hunting for new genes, a good place to start, from a statistical perspective, is near sequences that tend to be found between introns and exons. However, even with heuristics, user-directed discovery is inherently limited by the time required to manually search for new data.

An alternative to manual searching—and one that has had considerable success in the travel, banking and telecommunications industries—is to use computer-mediated data mining, the process of automatically extracting meaningful patterns from usually very large quantities of seemingly unrelated data. Unlike human-directed exploration of databases, data mining can initiate queries that aren't limited to the user's fluency in authoring effective database queries. This isn't to say that data mining reduces the need for the researcher to establish a strategy or to evaluate the results of a data-mining session. When used in conjunction with the appropriate visualisation tools, data mining allows the researcher to use her highly advanced pattern-recognition skills and knowledge of molecular biology to determine which results warrant further study. For example, mining the millions of data points from a series of microarray experiments might reveal several clusters of data, as visualised in a 3D cluster display. The researcher could then select data belonging to one or more of the clusters and use a variety of tools to determine the parametres that distinguish it from the other data.

Given the ever-increasing store of sequence and protein data from several worldwide genome projects, data mining the sequences has become a major research focus in bioinformatics. This is in part because molecular biologists can now conduct basic bioinformatics research from their desktop workstation, without the overhead of establishing a wet lab. The aim of this chapter is to explore data-mining techniques as an automated means of reducing the complexity of data in large bioinformatics databases and of discovering meaningful, useful patterns and relationships in data. The 'methods' section explores data mining from the perspective of the process of knowledge discovery. 'Technology overview' reviews the underlying computer infrastructure and algorithms that make data mining a practical endeavour. 'Infrastructure' reviews the hardware and software requirements of an efficient data-mining operation. 'Pattern recognition and discovery' explores the basic pattern recognition process and how it can be extended to pattern discovery.

The 'machine learning' section reviews the numerous technologies that can be applied to support data mining, from neural networks to hidden markov models. 'Text mining' focuses on the importance of mining the biomedical literature for data on functions to complement the sequence and structure data mined from nucleotide and protein databases. The 'tools' section introduces some of the practical general-purpose and bioinformatics-specific tools available for data mining. The 'On the horizon' section looks at the leading-edge data-mining technologies, especially real-time transaction monitoring that promises to decrease the infrastructure requirements. The 'Endnote' section explores the long-term role of machine learning versus human-directed data-mining efforts.

METHODS

Data mining isn't an endpoint, but is one stage in an overall knowledge-discovery process. It is an iterative process in which preceding processes are modified to support new hypotheses suggested by the data.

As illustrated in Fig. 15.1, given a data warehouse or separate databases, the knowledge-discovery process involves:

1. Selection and sampling of the appropriate data, from the database(s).
2. Preprocessing and cleaning of the data to remove redundancies, errors and conflicts.
3. Transforming and reducing data to a format more suitable for the data mining.
4. Data mining.
5. Evaluation of the mined data.
6. Visualisation of the evaluation results.
7. Designing new data queries to test new hypotheses and returning to step 1.

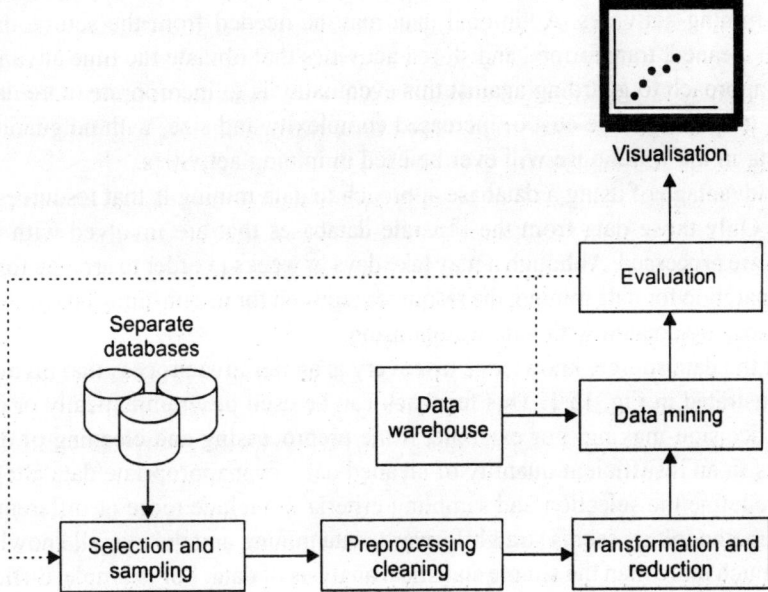

Fig. 15.1. Data mining. Data mining operations are shown here in the context of a larger knowledge-discovery process.

The relative timing of sequences in the knowledge-discovery process depends on whether the source of data is a data warehouse or one or more separate databases. A data warehouse is a central database in which data have been combined from a variety of noncompatible sources, such as sequencing machines, clinical systems, textual bibliographic databases or national genomic databases. In the process of combining data from disparate sources, the data are selected, cleaned, and transformed to support user-driven analytical and data-driven mining tools.

Whereas a data warehouse is a ready store of data to be mined at any time, using separate databases requires much more work on an as-needed basis. The processing up to the point of data mining may take hours or weeks, depending on the complexity and size of the databases involved in the process.

The advantage of using a data warehouse approach to data mining is time-savings. Assuming that everything needed for data mining is available in the data warehouse, a typical mining operation may be able to be completed in a matter of hours, depending on the processing power available, the size of the data warehouse, and the complexity of the mining operation.

However, this ability to begin mining operations at any time comes at a cost. A data warehouse that is capable of efficiently supporting data mining is significantly larger and the associated data processing takes much longer than in a simple database, one designed to provide a central, unified data repository that can be accessed through a single user interface. The reason for the increased data warehouse size and increase in complexity of associated processing is the increasingly fine-grained data required for data-mining support, as well as the need to incorporate contextual or metadata to support the data-mining process. For example, data mining requires a controlled vocabulary, usually implemented as part of a data dictionary, so that a single word can be used to express a given concept. Similarly, the extra attention to cleaning the data and other processing is necessary to maximise the odds that the conclusions based on data mining are valid.

What's more, there is no guarantee that the data in the data warehouse will be sufficient to support the desired data-mining activities. Additional data may be needed from the source databases, which then must also be cleaned, transformed and stored activities that obviate the time advantage of the data warehouse. One approach to guarding against this eventuality is to incorporate more data into the data warehouse when it is built, at the cost of increased complexity and size, with no guarantee that any of the additional data in the warehouse will ever be used in mining activities.

The primary advantage of using a database approach to data mining is that resources are used on an as-needed basis. Only those data from the separate databases that are involved with a specific data-mining operation are processed. Although it may take days or weeks in order to arrange for the appropriate processing in preparation for data mining, the resources required for just-in-time data mining are generally much less than those associated with data warehousing.

Regardless of the data source, knowledge discovery is an iterative process that involves feedback at each stage, as illustrated in Fig. 15.1. This feedback can be used programmatically or can serve as the basis for human decision-making. For example, if the preprocessing and cleaning of data from a data warehouse results in an insufficient quantity of cleaned data, or inappropriate data altogether, then the researcher may redefine the selection and sampling criteria to include more or different data.

Although the methodology seems straightforward, data mining and the overall knowledge-discovery process involve much more than the simple statistical analysis of data. For example, difficult-to-describe metrics, such as novelty, interestingness and understandability, are often used to define data-mining parametres for data discovery. Similarly, each phase of the knowledge-discovery process has associated challenges, as outlined here.

Selection and Sampling

Because of practical computational limitations and a prior knowledge, data mining isn't simply about searching for every possible relationship in a database. In a large database or data warehouse, there may be hundreds or thousands of valueless relationships. For example, a researcher interested in the relationship of SNPs with clinical findings can reasonably ignore the zip code of the tissue donors or the dates that the tissue samples were obtained. There are exceptions, of course, such as if there is a concentration of a specific ethnicity in a geographical area defined by a zip code.

Because there may be millions of records involved and thousands of variables, initial data mining is typically restricted to computationally tenable samples of the holding in an entire data warehouse. The evaluation of the relationships that are revealed in these samples can be used to determine which relationships in the data should be mined further using the complete data warehouse. With large, complex databases, even with sampling, the computational resource requirements associated with nondirected data mining may be excessive. In this situation, researchers generally rely on their knowledge of biology to identify potentially valuable relationships and they limit sampling based on these heuristics.

Preprocessing and Cleaning

The bulk of work associated with knowledge discovery is preparing the data for the actual analysis associated with data mining. The major preparatory activities, listed in Table 15.1, are normally performed to some extent in the creation of a data warehouse. However, data mining may be performed on one or more independent databases or the data in the warehouse may not have been cleaned initially, at least to the degree necessary for optimum data-mining results. In either case, these activities need to be performed as part of the preprocessing and cleaning phase of the overall knowledge-discovery process.

Table 15.1. Data mining preparatory activities.

Data characterisation
Consistency analysis
Domain analysis
Data enrichment
Frequency and distribution analysis
Normalisation
Missing value analysis

Data characterisation involves creating a high-level description of the nature and the content of the data to be mined. This stage in the knowledge-discovery process is primarily for the programmers and other staff involved in a data-mining project. It provides a form of documentation that can be referred to by those who may not be familiar with the underlying biology represented by the data.

Consistency analysis is the process of determining the variability in the data, independent of the domain. Consistency analysis is primarily a statistical assessment of data, based solely on data values. Outliers and values determined to be significantly different from other data may be automatically excluded from the knowledge-discovery process, based on predefined statistical constraints. For example, data associated with a given parametre that is more than three standard deviations from the mean might be excluded from the mining operation.

Domain analysis involves validating the data values in the larger context of the biology. That is, domain analysis goes beyond simply verifying that a data value is a text string or an integer or that it's statistically consistent with other data on the same parametre, to ensure that it makes sense in the context of the biology. For example, values for physiological parametres can be validated to the extent that they are within physiologically possible ranges consistent with life. A blood pH of 13, a body temperature of 45°C, a protein with molecular weight of 20 milligrams and a patient age of 120 would be flagged as invalid values that should be excluded from the knowledge-discovery process. Domain analysis requires that someone familiar with the biology create the heuristics that can be applied to the data.

Data enrichment involves drawing from multiple data sources to minimise the limitations of a single data source. For example, two databases on inherited diseases might each be sparsely populated in terms of proteins that are associated with particular diseases. This deficit could be addressed by incorporating data from both databases, assuming only a moderate degree of overlap in the content of the two databases. Data enrichment may be tied to consistency analysis, so that outliers that would skew knowledge-discovery results aren't included in the final analysis.

Frequency and distribution analysis places weights on values as a function of their frequency of occurrence. The effect is to maximise the contribution of common findings while minimising the effect of rare occurrences on the conclusions made from the data-mining output. For example, a clinical database of genetic diseases might contain 500 entries for one disease and only 1 entry for another, based on the number of patients with each disease who were admitted to a given hospital or clinic. Ignoring the relative frequency of each disease in the database could lead a researcher to conclude that the odds of patients expressing either disease is the same.

The normalisation process involves transforming data values from one representation to another, using a predefined range of final values. For example, qualitative values, such as 'high' and 'low' and qualitative values from multiple sources regarding a particular parametre might be normalised to a numerical score from 1 to 10.

The major issues in normalisation are range, granularity, accuracy, precision, scale and units. Range is the difference between the highest and lowest values that are represented, whereas granularity is a static property of the scale. For example, length might be measured with a granularity of either nanometres or millimetres. Accuracy is a measure of how close measurements come to actual values, and precision is a measure of the repeatability of the measurements.

The most common scales used in the normalisation process are listed in Table 15.2. Absolute scales are based on quantities, such as the number of amino acids in a protein. Nominal scales are based on unique identifiers, such as names and descriptions. Categorical scales assign data to numerical or textual categories. Ordinal scales put things in order, according to some organisational theme. For example, proteins can be ordered according to molecular weight. Rank scales are like ordinal scales with the addition of a natural ranking, such as 'more stable' and 'less stable' protein configurations. Interval scales have a natural ordering, such as time. Ratio scales are expressed as a multiple or a fraction of a unit or interval, such as micrometres and milligrams.

Table 15.2. Scales used in normalisation.

Scale	Example
Absolute	Count (3 amino acids)
Nominal	List of protein names (lysine, arginine, tyrosine)
Ordinal	Process phase (first, second, third)
Categorical	Types of amino acids (essential, nonessential)
Rank	Protein folding (primary, secondary, tertiary)
Interval	Time (seconds)
Ratio	Weight (micrograms)

With the exception of absolute scales, these scales can be converted to another scale if they are the same type and measure the same attribute. When data are defined with the same scale, the normalisation process depends on the type of data. For example, nominal scales are converted to other nominal scales by a mapping function. However, mapping can introduce errors when there is a one-to-many mapping or many-to-one mapping between the two nominal scales. For example, the name of an amino acid can be mapped to a triplet of base pairs, but if there are multiple possible base pairs that code for a given amino acid, then the alternative base pair sequences are lost in the translation.

Both ordinal and rank order scales are translated by a function that maintains their relative order. As in the mapping of nominal scales, errors of omission are introduced by the conversion process when there isn't a one-to-one mapping between the two scales. Interval scales are converted to other interval scales through linear functions that preserve the ordering but shift the relative values, as in the conversion of degrees Fahrenheit to degrees Celsius. Ratio scales are converted to another ratio scale by a constant multiplier. For example, a ratio scale of 0 to 2 metres could be multiplied by a factor of 100 to provide a scale of 0 to 200 centimetres. The units used in the process of normalisation may be primary, such as seconds of time or micrograms of mass, or derived, such as density (grams per cubic centimetre) or volume (cubic millimetres). The standard systeme international (SI) measurement units for primary units include metre for length, kilogram for mass, second for time, ampere for electrical current, degree Kelvin for temperature and the mole for molecules.

The final preprocessing and cleaning activity, missing-value analysis, involves detecting, characterising and dealing with missing data values. One way of dealing with missing data values is to substitute the mean, mode or median value of the relevant data that are available.

Transformation and Reduction

In the transformation and reduction phase of the knowledge-discovery process, data sets are reduced to the minimum size passible through sampling or summary statistics. For example, tables of data may be replaced by descriptive statistics, such as mean and standard deviation. Transformation involves translating one type of data to another through mathematical or mapping operations that, for example, map numerical data onto textual data (or *vice versa*). Transformation differs from the normalisation process in the preprocess and cleaning phase of knowledge discovery in that the purpose of the transformation isn't to allow the combination of data from multiple sources, but rather to directly support the data-mining and knowledge-discovery process. For example, normalised data may be transformed from floating-paint to integer data to increase computer processor performance.

Data-Mining Methods

The process of data mining is concerned with extracting patterns from the data, typically using classification, regression, link analysis, segmentation or deviation detection (Fig. 15.2). Classification involves mapping data into one of several predefined or newly discovered classes. In the former case, a set of predefined examples is used to develop a model that can be used to classify data culled from the data warehouse or database. In the latter case, the system develops its own models that it uses to classify data according to analysis of the data. In the illustration, there are three groups or classes of data, (A), (B) and (C). The classification rule may specify minimum proximity to the centre of a particular group, as defined by numerical range or statistical spread, for example.

Data mining based on regression methods involves assigning data a continuous numerical variable based on statistical methods. One goal in using regression methods is to extrapolate trends from a few samples of the data. In the example in Fig. 15.2, the extrapolation formula is a simple linear function of the farm:

$$y = mx + b$$

where, x and y are coordinates on the plot, m is the slope of the line and b is a constant. In practice, more complex extrapolation formulas are used to describe data trends.

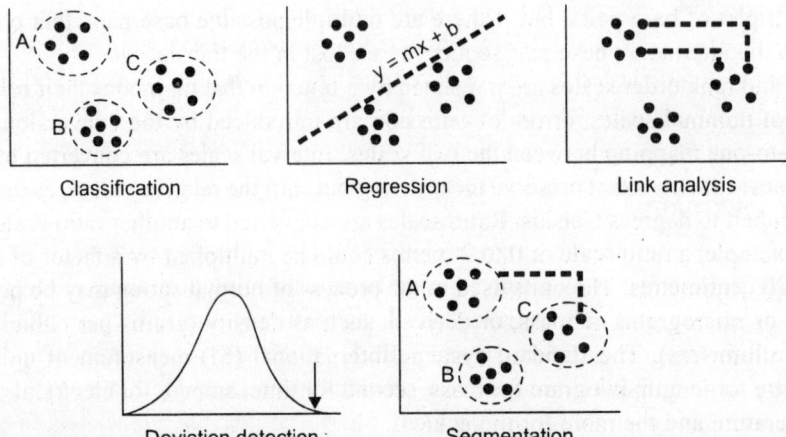

Fig. 15.2. Data mining methods. Classification—mapping to a class or group. Regression—statistical analysis. Link analysis—correlation of data. Deviation detection—difference from the norm. Segmentation—similarity function.

Link analysis evaluates apparent connections or links between data in the database or data warehouse. Link analysis highlights correlations in data that can suggest linkage, but not causality. In the illustration, the two pairs of data paints are apparently linked, in that the value of one data element in the pair can be predicted by the value of the other data paint in the pair.

Deviation detection identifies data values that are outside of the norm, as defined by existing models or by evaluating the ordering of observations. The outlier in the illustration is an example of a data value outside of the expected spread of data in a sample. The data may represent a particular sequence of amino acids or the molecular weight of a protein or a vital sign, for example.

Segmentation-based data mining identifies classes or groups of data that behave similarly, according to some metric. Segmentation is akin to link analysis applied to groups of data instead of individual data points. In the figure, groups (A) and (C) behave similarly.

These methods of data mining are typically used in combination with each other, either in parallel or as part of a sequential operation. For example, segmentation requires classes to be defined through a classification process. Similarly, link analysis assumes that statistical analysis, including correlation coefficients, are available. Likewise, deviation detection assumes that the data have been properly classified and evaluated statistically to define the 'normal' model. As described later in this chapter, there are a variety of technologies available to support these methods.

Evaluation

In the evaluation phase of knowledge discovery, the patterns identified by the data-mining analysis are interpreted. Typical evaluation ranges from simple statistical analysis and complex numerical analysis of sequences and structures to determining the clinical relevance of the findings.

Visualisation

Visualisation of evaluation results is an optional stage in the knowledge-discovery process, but one that typically adds considerable value to the overall system. Visualisation can range from converting tabular listings of data summaries to pie charts and similar business graphics, to using real-time data to create 3D virtual reality displays that can be manipulated by haptic controllers.

Designing New Queries

Data mining is an iterative continual activity, in that there are always new hypotheses to test. Sometimes the new hypotheses are suggested by the data returned by the mining process, and other times the hypotheses originate from other research. In either case, testing the new hypotheses requires formulating new queries and revisiting the selection and sampling stage of the data-mining process.

TECHNOLOGY OVERVIEW

The remainder of this chapter provides an overview of the key technologies that can be applied to data mining, especially those capable of supporting the basic data-mining methods outlined earlier. As a prelude to this discussion, it's important to note that an efficient and effective data-mining system requires, above all, an experimental design that reflects the biology of the data being mined. In this regard, technology is an empowering agent that provides leverage to facilitate a well-designed data-mining initiative-technology isn't a solution in itself. Simply connecting a black box to a database with hopes of it turning up fruitful information on previously hidden relationships in the data is unlikely at best.

Given this caveat, data mining requires a hardware and software infrastructure capable of supporting high-throughput data processing and a network capable of supporting data communications from the database to the visualisation workstation. With a robust hardware and software infrastructure in place, processes such as machine learning can be used to automatically manage and refine the knowledge-discovery and data-mining processes. This work can be performed with minimal user interaction once a knowledgeable researcher has established the basic design of the system.

The core technologies that actually perform the work of data mining, whether under computer control or directed by users, provide a means of simplifying the complexity and reducing the effective size of the databases. This focus isn't limited to genome sequences and protein structures, but extends to the wealth of data hidden in the online literature. Advanced text-mining methods are used to identify textual data and place them in the proper context.

Finally, as discussed later in this chapter, although data mining was once relegated to internal research groups, the technology is readily available today through a variety of commercial and academic shareware tools. These tools range from shrink-wrapped, general-purpose software tools to bioinformatics-specific commercial and academic systems designed for highly specific data-mining applications.

INFRASTRUCTURE

At first glance, data mining can be performed with little more than a laptop and a connection to the internet. Although it's possible to work with such a system, serious data-mining work typically requires much more in terms of infrastructure. As illustrated in Fig. 15.3, a typical laboratory data-mining infrastructure includes high-speed internet and intranet connectivity, a data warehouse with a data dictionary that defines a standard vocabulary and data format, several databases and high-performance computer hardware. Not shown are the software tools, including the database management system (DBMS) software that supports queries and searching and ensures data integrity and the data mining software.

In the example in Fig. 15.3, the data-mining operations take place on a workstation with a high-speed connection to the data warehouse. However, this centralised data-mining infrastructure is only one of several configurations possible.

For example, a competing infrastructure involves distributing the data-mining operation to process-specific workstations, as illustrated in Fig. 15.4. In this configuration, a server doles out data in a format appropriate to the process performed by a particular workstation. In this way, greater overall throughput can be achieved, using inexpensive desktop hardware that is configured with the appropriate hardware and software tools to support a specific process. A distributed architecture also supports parallel processing, so that intermediate results from one workstation can be fed to another workstation. For example, link analysis performed on one workstation can be fed the regression analysis results from another workstation.

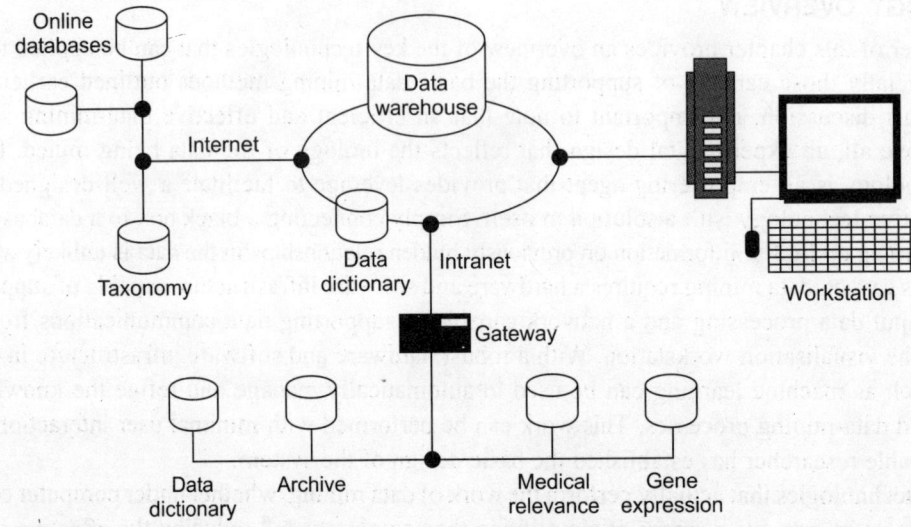

Fig. 15.3. Centralised data-mining infrastructure. In this example, a data warehouse, data dictionary, high-bandwidth access to data on the internet and a high-performance workstation form the basis for an effective data-mining operation.

The trend of distributed data mining using relatively inexpensive desktop hardware is largely a reflection of the economics of modern computing. Not only is the price-performance ratio of desktop hardware superior to that of mainframe computers, but the cost of desktop software licenses is typically several orders of magnitude less than that for mainframe computer systems. Of course, if time is the primary issue, then a mainframe computer optimised for data mining can provide superior performance compared to small networks of desktop computers.

PATTERN RECOGNITION AND DISCOVERY

Data mining is the process of identifying patterns and relationships in data that often are not obvious in large, complex data sets. As such, data mining involves pattern recognition and by extension, pattern discovery. In bioinformatics, pattern recognition is most often concerned with the automatic classification of character sequences representative of the nucleotide bases or molecular structures and of 3D protein structures.

As illustrated in Fig. 15.5, the pattern-recognition process starts with an unknown pattern, such as a potential protein structure, and ends with a label for the pattern. From an information-processing perspective, pattern recognition can be viewed as a data simplification process that filters extraneous data from consideration and labels the remaining data according to a classification scheme.

The major steps in the pattern recognition and discovery process are:

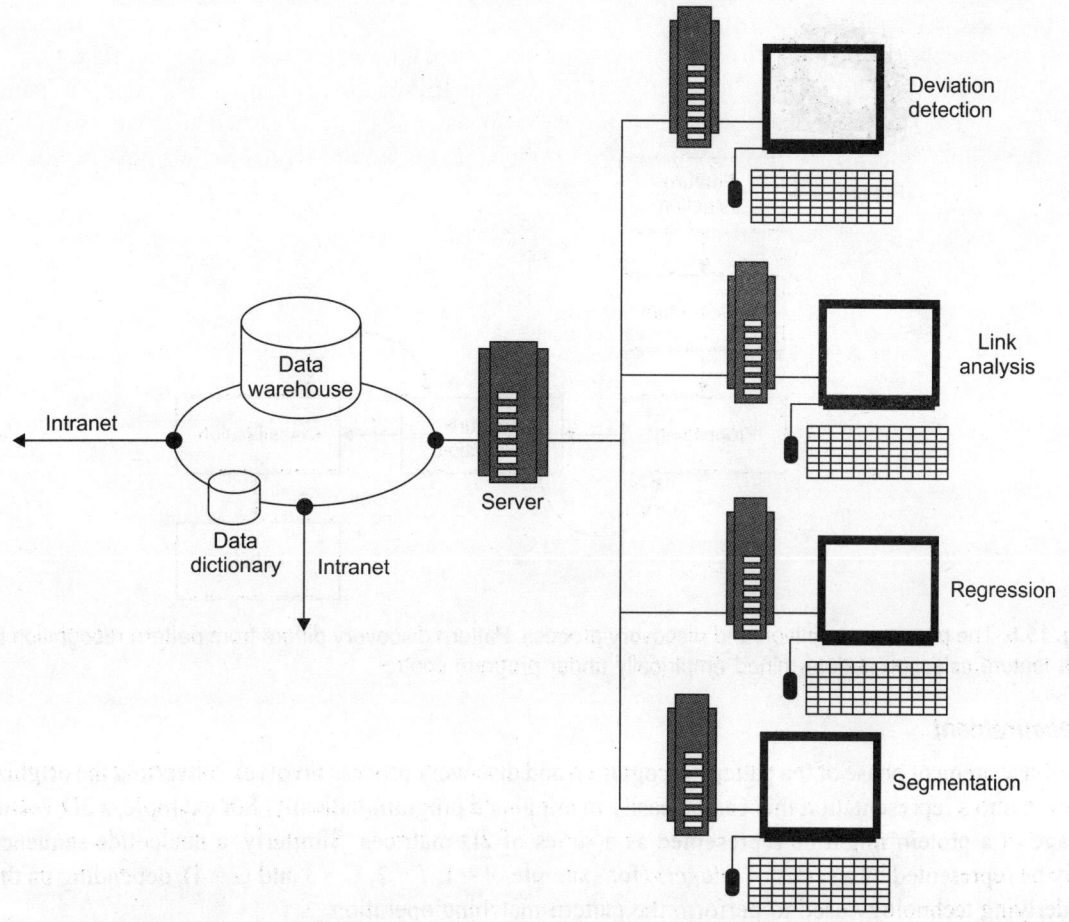

Fig. 15.4. Distributed data-mining infrastructure. A server to specialised workstations distributes data from a central data warehouse or single database. The distribution refers to the processing, not the data source.

Feature selection

Given a pattern, the first step in pattern recognition is to select a set of features or attributes from the universe of available features that will be used to classify the pattern. When pattern recognition is directed at known patterns, the researcher defines *a priori* the features that will be used to distinguish the pattern from other data. Feature selection often takes the form of exemplars or representative examples of the features that will be measured, such as the tertiary geometry of a protein. In pattern discovery, which is more complex than simple pattern recognition, feature selection is under program control. Instead of an *a priori* definition of pattern attributes defining a class or group of data that are similar or equivalent in some way, samples are classified programmatically into empirically established groups, based on groups or clusters in the unlabelled collection of samples. That is, simple pattern recognition is assumption-driven, in that a hypothesis is developed and tested against the data. In pattern discovery, the extracted data serve as the seed of a new hypothesis. Clustering techniques are used to group samples that are more similar to each other than to other groups and that have a low internal cluster variability or scatter.

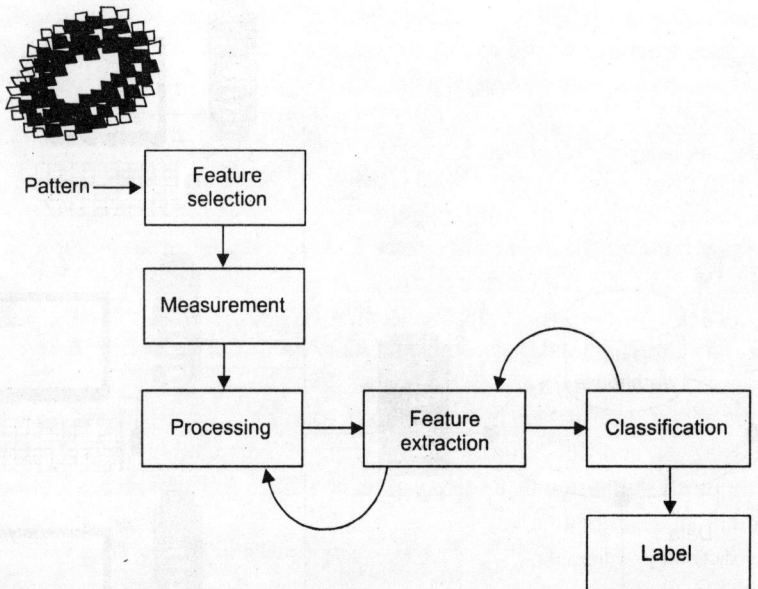

Fig. 15.5. The pattern-recognition and discovery process. Pattern discovery differs from pattern recognition in that feature selection is determined empirically under program control.

Measurement

The measurement phase of the pattern-recognition and discovery process involves converting the original pattern into a representation that can be easily manipulated programmatically. For example, a 3D vector image of a protein might be represented as a series of 2D matrices. Similarly, a nucleotide sequence may be represented by a series of integers (for example, $A = 1$, $T = 2$, $C = 3$ and $G = 4$), depending on the underlying technology used to perform the pattern-matching operation.

Processing

After the measurement process, the data are processed to remove noise and prepare for feature extraction. Processing typically involves executing a variety of error checking and correction routines, as well as specialised processes that depend on the nature of the data. For example, images may undergo edge enhancement and transformation to correct for size and orientation variations (normalisation) in order to facilitate feature extraction.

Feature extraction

Feature extraction involves searching for global and local features in the data that are defined as relevant to pattern matching during feature selection. Clustering techniques, in which similar data are grouped together, often form the basis of feature extraction.

Classification and discovery

In the classification phase of pattern recognition and discovery, data are classified based on measurements of similarity with other patterns. These measurements of similarity are commonly based on either a statistical or a structural approach. In the statistical approach, exemplar patterns are represented by points in a multidimensional space that is partitioned into regions associated with a classification. In the structural approach, the structures of the exemplar patterns are explicitly defined. In either case, the similarity of the data to be classified is compared with the exemplar data to assess closeness of association.

Labelling

The pattern-recognition process ends when a label is assigned to the data, based on its membership in a class. As illustrated in Fig. 15.5, the pattern-recognition process isn't unidirectional, but is iterative to the extent that failures at the classification and feature-extraction stages can be corrected by reevaluating the preceding phase. For example, if the feature-extraction phase fails to identify relevant data, then the processing of the original image may need to be modified by removing extraneous data from consideration and by taking other, more relevant data, into consideration.

Feature extraction and classification and discovery, which represent the core of the pattern-recognition and discovery process, are performed by using some combination of classification, regression, segmentation, link analysis and deviation detection methods, depending on the nature of the data. Similarly, these methods are supported by a variety of technologies and approaches, collectively referred to as machine learning, as described here.

MACHINE LEARNING

The pattern-matching and pattern discovery components of data mining are often performed by machine learning techniques. Machine learning isn't a single technology or approach, but encompasses a variety of methods that represent the convergence of several disciplines, including statistics, biological modelling, adaptive control theory, psychology and artificial intelligence (AI). Although many computer scientists consider the entire field of machine learning to be an outgrowth of traditional statistical methods, biological modelling is clearly a source of several machine learning approaches. These include genetic algorithms and neural networks. Similarly, adaptive control theory, in which system parametres change dynamically to meet the current conditions, and psychological theories, especially those regarding positive and negative reinforcement learning, heavily influence machine learning methods. AI techniques, such as pattern matching through inductive logic programming, are designed to derive general rules from specific examples. As illustrated in Table 15.3, the spectrum of machine learning technologies applicable to data mining includes inductive logic programming, genetic algorithms, neural networks, statistical methods, Bayesian methods, decision trees and hidden markov models.

Table 15.3. Machine learning technologies and their applicability to data-mining methods.

Machine learning technologies	Data mining methods				
	Classification	Regression	Segmentation	Link analysis	Deviation detection
Inductive logic programming	X	X			
Genetic algorithms	X	X	X		
Neural networks	X	X	X		
Statistical methods	X	X	X	X	X
Decision trees	X		X		
Hidden Markov models	X				

Regardless of the underlying technology, most machine learning follows the general process outlined in Fig. 15.6. Input data are fed to a comparison engine that compares the data with an underlying model. The results of the comparison engine then direct a software actor to initiate some type of change. This output, whether it takes the form of a change in data or a modification of the underlying model, is evaluated by an evaluation engine, which uses the underlying goals of the system as a point of reference. Feedback from the actor and the evaluation engine direct changes in the model. In this scenario, the goals can be standard patterns that are known to be associated with the input data. Alternatively, the goals can be stated, such as minimal change in output compared with the system's previous encounter with the same data.

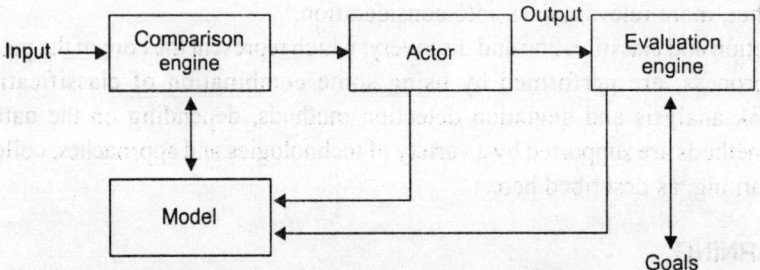

Fig. 15.6. The machine learning process.

The feedback loops and a mechanism capable of responding to feedback enable two types of machine learning: supervised and unsupervised. In supervised learning, the system is trained with a set of examples, called the training set. The goals are specific outputs that are associated with each input. For example, a specific amino acid sequence on the input can be associated with the name of a protein on the output. The performance of a supervised learning, system can be evaluated by presenting the system with a known testing set that is similar to the training set.

In unsupervised learning, there is no specific output associated with a given input, and the system must invent new categories and ways to classify the input data. In machine learning systems based on unsupervised learning, it isn't known *a priori* whether the input data contains a biologically significant pattern, where it is or even what it looks like.

One of the key issues in supervised learning is that the training set must be sufficiently large relative to the number of categories or different outputs provided by the machine learning system. When there are too many categories or recognised patterns that are consistent with the input data, the training data is said to be overfitted. That is, overfitting is the process of assigning undue importance to random variations in the data.

Whether supervised or unsupervised, the machine learning process requires bias. It isn't enough to simply open a database up to a machine learning algorithm and sit back while it automatically discovers all of the interrelationships in the data. Bias is created in a machine learning system by placing constraints on the data that can be examined, by using different underlying models and by altering the machine learning system goals. Bias can increase the efficiency of the machine language process and provide more meaningful results. For example, the process can probably ignore a correlation between the time of day a sample was evaluated and gene expression in a microarray. In practice, the bias can be a single heuristic, such as preferring the single, simplest rule that explains the data to a more complex solution.

This 'simplest solution' bias is often used with machine learning approaches to mining nucleotide sequence data.

Inductive Logic Programming

Inductive logic programming uses a set of rules or heuristics to categorise data. A common heuristic is to use change in entropy to iteratively choose an attribute of the data that will subset the data according to the attribute. That is, an entropy-based classification system based on an induction algorithm works by incrementally dividing the data into the largest possible spaces until all data has been assigned to a collection.

Consider the scenario depicted in Fig. 15.7, in which the data to be classified includes 20 circles and 10 squares, 16 of which are white and 14 of which are black. With two dimensions to compare—shape and colour—an entropy-based inductive classifier bifurcates the space first according to colour because it provides the maximum change in entropy, resulting in one group of 14 black circles and squares and one group of 16 white circles and squares. After dividing the space by colour, it's further subdivided by shape, as shown in the figure.

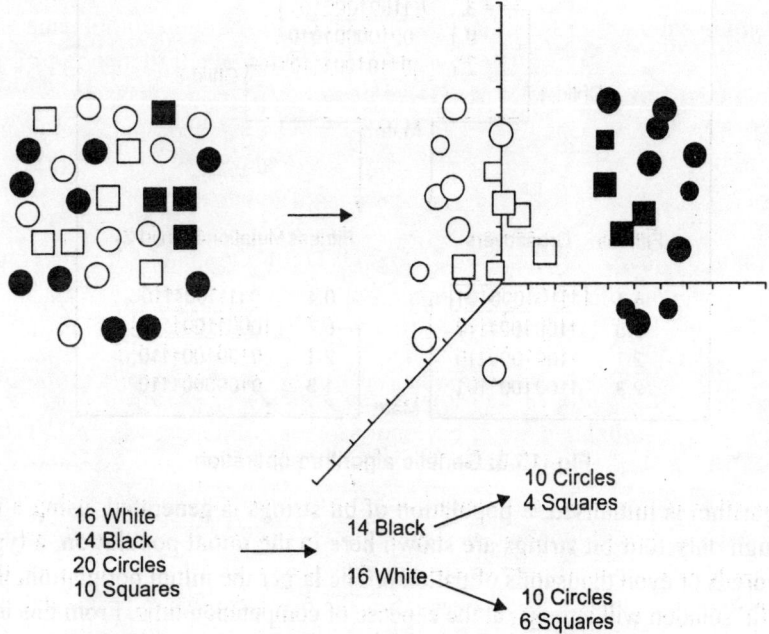

Fig. 15.7. Induction-based classification. Using changes in entropy (a measure of disorder) as an organisational heuristic, the induction algorithm divides the unorganised data (top left) first by colour and then by shape.

The alternative, bifurcating the circles and squares initially by shape would have resulted in a split of 10 to 20, which is less than the spread (increase in entropy) associated with a 14-to-16 split. In a typical bioinformatics data-mining problem, there may be 10 or more attributes to consider, according to entropy change or some other driving heuristic.

Genetic Algorithms

Genetic algorithms are based on evolutionary principles wherein a particular function or definition that best fits the constraints of an environment survives to the next generation and the other functions are eliminated. This iterative process continues indefinitely, allowing the algorithm to adapt dynamically to the environment as needed. Genetic algorithms evaluate a large number of solutions to a problem that are generated at random. The members of the solution population with the highest fitness scores are allowed to 'mate' with crossovers and mutations, creating the next generation.

Figure 15.8 illustrates the typical operation of a genetic operation. In this example, the possible solutions to a problem defined by the fitness function are represented by bit strings. Each bit represents the presence or absence of some quality that is mapped to the real-world solution. If there is a need to represent gradations of quantities, then integers or floating-point variables could be used instead of bit strings. However, in this example, 12 bits are used to represent the problem matrix.

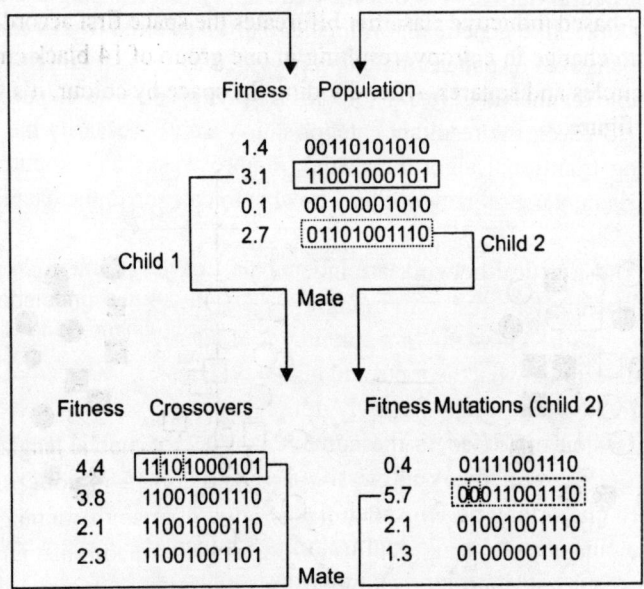

Fig. 15.8. Genetic algorithm operation.

When the algorithm is initialised, a population of bit strings is generated, using a random number generator. Although only four bit strings are shown here in the initial population, a typical population may include hundreds or even thousands of patterns. The larger the initial population, the more likely a high-scoring or 'fit' solution will emerge, at the expense of computation time. From this initial population, two children are selected, based on the two highest-scoring patterns. All other bit strings are discarded. These children are then allowed to 'mate' with crossovers (bottom, left) and point mutations (bottom, right).

As in the initial population, there are hundreds or even thousands of crossovers and mutations created, and each resulting bit string is ranked by the fitness function to identify two new children. There are various combinations of crossover and mutations possible. For example, the fittest two children from the crossover population can each be subject to point mutations at each position in their strings, and the fittest children with mutations can be mated with the highest-ranking crossover children or with the parents. In this way, the string with the highest score from the fitness function is iteratively generated. The process can continue indefinitely or as is normally done, terminated after a set number of generations.

Both the encoding of bit strings and the fitness function are domain-specific. For example, the first position in the bit string might represent the presence of a particular amino acid in a protein, the presence of a start codon in a nucleotide sequence or the presence of a hydrogen bond at a position on an alpha helix. Similarly, the fitness function can be as simple as positive and negative weightings for each of the

12 bits (for example, 1s at odd positions are weighted with −1 and 1s at even positions are weighted with +1) for a sequence analysis problem or as a complex trigonometric function for a structure prediction problem.

Neural Networks

Neural networks are simulations loosely patterned after biological neurons. They are said to learn or be trainable. In molecular biology, they learn to associate input patterns with output patterns in a way that allows them to categorise new patterns and to extrapolate trends from data. In operation, a neural network is presented with a pattern on its input nodes and the network produces an output pattern, based on this learning. The power of neural networks is that they can apply this learning to new input patterns. For this reason, neural networks, like genetic algorithms, are often referred to as a form of 'soft' or 'fuzzy' computing because the answers or pattern matching provided by these methods represent best guesses, based on the data available for analysis. Neural networks always produce an output pattern when presented with an input pattern. However, the resultant categorisation isn't necessarily the best answer. The best answer, computed using traditional algorithms, may require weeks of computing time on a desktop workstation. In comparison, a neural network may be able to categorise the data in a few seconds using the same hardware.

The inner workings of a neural network are independent of the problem domain, in that the same neural network configuration (with different training) can be used to recognise a nucleotide triplet or a critical pattern on a patient's EKG tracing or a potential mid-air collision when used with radar data. It's up to the researcher to determine what the input and output patterns represent: That said, neural networks, like other fuzzy systems, work best in a narrowly defined domain in which input patterns are likely to follow the same progression or logic. As the number and complexity of the possible input patterns increases, the ability of a neural network to classify input patterns deteriorates. For example, a neural network that works well classifying proteins within a given protein family will likely fail to classify the universe of known proteins, despite additional training. An increase in the number and complexity of input patterns typically requires reconfiguring or rewriting a neural network with more layers and different interconnections. For example, the simple three-layer neural network shown in Fig. 15.9 may have to be replaced by a four-layer neural network with double the number of interconnections.

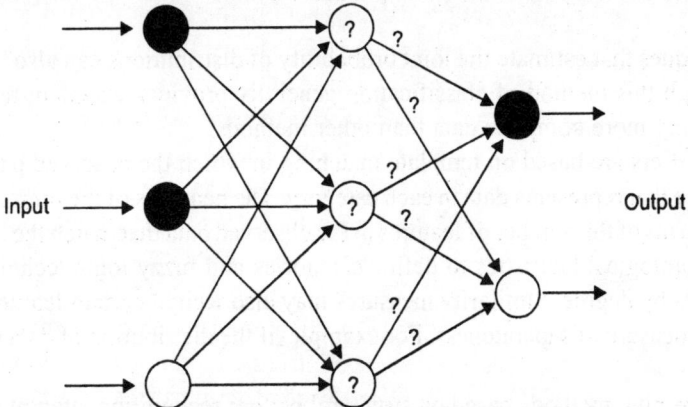

Fig. 15.9. Neural network. One of the limitations of a neural network is that the significance of the strength of the internal interconnections is unknown. As a result, as a pattern recogniser or categoriser, the neural network can be treated as a black box.

As a result, training time the time required for a neural network to consistently associate an input pattern with an output pattern correctly may be extended from a few minutes to several hours, even on high-performance hardware. Recognition time should be relatively unaffected.

The challenge of using a neural network to recognise and categorise data, especially novel data that haven't been presented to the system before, is that of validating the results and of communicating the rationale behind the results to the user. The greatest drawback of neural networks is that it's practically impossible to assess the significance of what's happening inside of a complex network. Even though the 'wiring' of the nodes may be known, the relevance of changes in the strength of the connections is difficult to assess, even when the strengths are known. As a result, the inner workings of a neural network are difficult to validate.

Because a pure neural network presents such a formidable validation challenge, many neural network data-mining systems are used in conjunction with rule-based expert systems that contain human-readable rules in the form:

IF condition THEN outcome.

These hybrid systems can categorise novel patterns and provide researchers with insight into the operation of the biological system. The challenge in creating hybrid classification systems is integrating the neural networks and rule-based expert systems in a way that doesn't compromise classification performance while providing enough information on internal operation to allow the user to assess the validity of the classification results. One approach to maximising performance is to develop a neural network and then use a tool that converts the network into a rule base that can be compiled in C++ or Assembly language.

Statistical Methods

The statistical methods used to support data mining are generally some form of feature extraction, classification or clustering. Statistical feature extraction is concerned with recovering the defining data attributes that may be obscured by imperfect measurement, improper data processing, or noise in the data.

A variety of statistical pattern-classification methods may be applied to data mining. For example, probabilistic classifiers are based on the principle that a pattern should be assigned to the class that is most probable.

Bayesian techniques that estimate the joint probability of distributions can also be used to assess this probability. Although this method of classification generally provides excellent results, it has a major drawback of requiring more complete data than other methods.

Geometric classifiers are based on template matching in which the observed pattern is compared to a geometric template that represents data in each category. The nearness of the mined data to the template can be assessed in terms of the number of features in the observed data that match the template. Conceptual classifiers rely on biological heuristics to define categories and fuzzy logic techniques can be used to assign data to a class by degree. Similarity measures may also weight certain features more than others, according to some measure of separateness. For example, if the distribution of data is spherical, the data mean may be used.

Statistical data-mining methods based on structural pattern recognition attempt to describe complex patterns in terms of simpler patterns. They extract features from the data and represent the structural features as vectors that are used with statistically determined discriminant functions. They use a rule base to define structural features in a given class or transform the data into a descriptive language based on pattern primitives. The descriptions are then analysed syntactically to provide the classification.

Predictive modelling, which uses data within a database to predict other missing data, can be based on continuous numerical variables (regression) or more frequently, on categorical data (classification). The major challenge in predictive modelling is to select the input criteria that are most influential in defining missing data and in identifying the most appropriate transformation. With continuous numerical variables, nonlinear transformations on the input data are often used. With categorical data, feature extraction serves the same purpose.

Cluster analysis, also known as data segmentation, groups data into subsets that are similar to each other. Cluster analysis is a technique that can take a large amount of data about a number of objects and construct a simple, unique tree diagram that expresses those objects' similarities and differences. Cluster analysis involves sorting data so that members of the same cluster are most alike and members of different clusters are least alike. In this way, each cluster describes the class to which its members belong.

The results of cluster analysis are commonly reported in human-readable form as a dendogram, illustrated in Fig. 15.10.

In this dendogram, groups (D) and (E) are the most alike, as indicated by the shortest bracket. The next level of similarity is between (F) and the (D)-(E) complex. In addition, Groups (A) and (B) are similar. Group (G) shares the least similarity with the other groups.

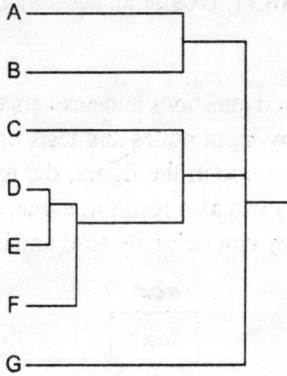

Fig. 15.10. Dendogram showing the results of a cluster analysis. Groups (D) and (E) show the greatest similarity, whereas Group (G) shows the greatest differences between groups, based on cluster analysis criteria.

Cluster analysis may reveal associations and structure in data that, though not previously evident, are sensible and useful once found. The results of cluster analysis may contribute to the definition of a formal classification scheme, such as a taxonomy for related bacteria. It may suggest statistical models with which to describe population or indicate rules for assigning new cases to classes for identification and diagnostic purposes.

Cluster analysis includes metric, model and partition-based methods (Fig. 15.11). In metric-based clustering, the data are partitioned so that they are closer to the centroid or centre of mass than they are to other data in the cluster. In model-based clustering, a hypothetical model for each cluster is defined and the data that best fit the model are considered part of that cluster.

A problem with model-based approaches is overfitting-by chance, a model may fit data that is irrelevant to it. Partition-based methods, which are general cases of metric and model-based methods, use an ad hoc method of dividing the data space.

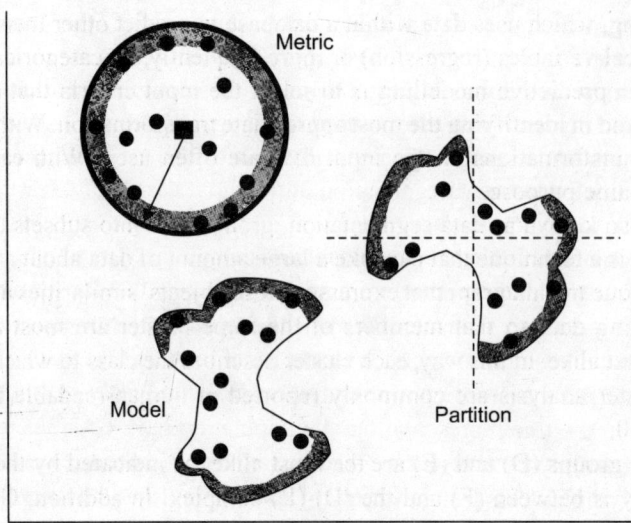

Fig. 15.11. Cluster analysis methods.

Decision Trees

Decision trees are hierarchically arranged questions and answers that lead to classification. As shown in Fig. 15.12, decision trees are formed by input nodes and tests on input data and whose leaf nodes are categories of those data. In the decision tree in the figure, the tests (Test 1 to Test 8) result in textual categories [categories (A)-(H)] but they can also result in numerical categories. An advantage of using decision trees in data mining is that they can be easily read and modified by humans.

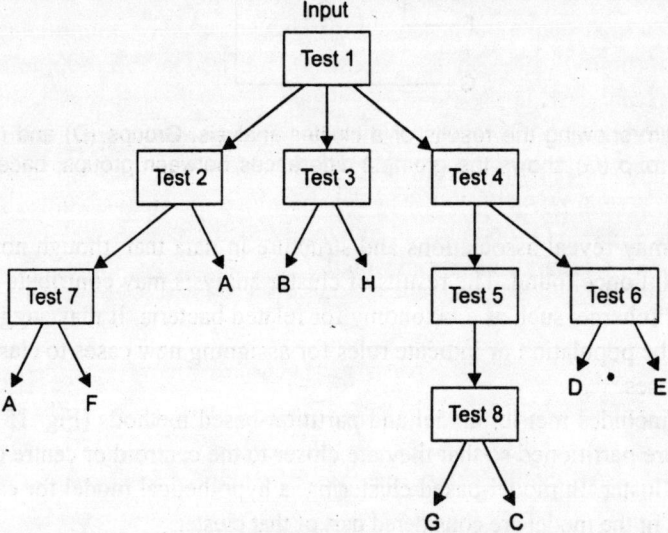

Fig. 15.12. Decision trees. A decision tree categorises a pattern by filtering it down through the tests in a tree.

For example, the results of Test 1 may lead to Test 2, 3 or 4. Once Test 2 is selected, the only options are to characterise the input as belonging to category (A), or to select Test 7. Category (A) can represent a particular family of proteins, for example. The only options from Test 7 are to place the data into category (A) or category (F).

The tests can be binary (yes/no) as in Test 2 or multi-variant (high, medium, low) as in Test 1. For example, in operation, a decision tree can be used to categorise a protein based on a combination of molecular weight, length and configuration. As illustrated in the figure, the terminal or leaf nodes needn't result in mutually exclusive categorisation of the input data. Both Test 2 and Test 7 classify the input into category (A), for example.

A potential limitation of using decision trees is related to their inability to represent relative occurrence frequencies. For example, with a very small training set, it's likely that the terminal leaves of a complex tree are defined by chance alone. Consider the typical evolutionary tree that represents the speciation over the past several hundred-million years. A single fossil may be responsible for a bifurcation in the tree, even though the fossil may represent a relatively small, insignificant mutation in a much larger population. However, in the tree representation, the population have equal weights.

In some cases, this inability to represent the relative frequency of occurrence can be used to advantage. For example, in classifying globins from a variety of species, multiple samples from the same or closely related species may skew the relative abundance of some properties over others. However, if these properties are represented as a decision tree, then the skew due to sample anomalies can be avoided.

Hidden Markov Models

A powerful statistical approach to constructing classifiers that deserves a separate discussion is the use of hidden markov modelling (HMM). A hidden markov model is a statistical model for an ordered sequence of symbols, acting as a stochastic state machine that generates a symbol each time a transition is made from one state to the next. Transitions between states are specified by transition probabilities. A Markov process is a process that moves from state to state depending on the previous 'n' states. The process is called an order 'n' model where 'n' is the number of states affecting the choice of the next state. The Markov process considered here is a first order, in that the probability of a state is dependent only on the directly preceding state.

In order to understand HMMs, consider the concept of a Markov Chain, which is a process that can be in one of a number of states at any given time (Fig. 15.13). Each state generates an observation, from which the state sequence can be inferred. A Markov Chain is defined by the probabilities for each transition in state occurring, given the current state. That is, a markov chain is a nondeterministic system in which it is assumed that the probability of moving from one state to another doesn't vary with time. A HMM is a variation of a markov chain in which the states in the chain are hidden.

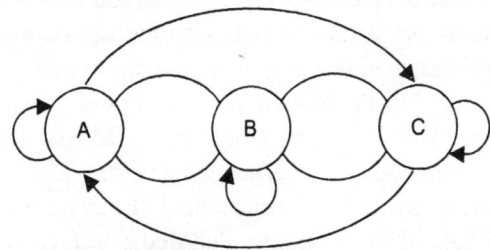

Fig. 15.13. Markov Chain. (A), (B) and (C) represent states, and the arrows connecting the states represent transitions.

Like a neural network classifier, a HMM must be trained before it can be used. Training establishes the transition probabilities for each state in the markov chain. When presented with data in the database, the HMM provides a measure of how close the data patterns—sequence data, for example—resemble the data used to train the model. HMM-based classifiers are considered approximations because of the often unrealistic assumptions that a state is dependent only on predecessors and that this dependence is time-independent.

TEXT MINING

For mankind to benefit from bioinformatics research, the sequence and structure of proteins and other molecules must be linked to functional genomics and proteomics. The primary store of functional data that links clinical medicine, pharmacology, sequence data, and structure data is in the form of biomedicine documents in online bibliographic databases such as PubMed. Mining these databases is expected to reveal the relationships between structure and function at the molecular level and their relationship to pharmacology and clinical medicine.

Text mining—automatically extracting this data from documents, which is published in the form of unstructured free text, often in several languages—is a nontrivial task. Although computer languages such as LISt processing (LISP) have been developed expressly for handling free text, working with free text remains one of the most challenging areas of computer science. This is primarily because, unlike the analysis of the sequence of amino acids in a protein, natural language is ambiguous and often references data not contained in the document under study. For example, a research article on the expression of a particular gene in PubMed may contain numerous synonyms, acronyms and abbreviations. Furthermore, despite editing to constrain the sentences to proper English (or other language), the syntax— the ordering of words and their relationships to other elements in phrases and sentences—is typically author-specific. The article may also reference an experimental method that isn't defined because it's assumed as common knowledge in the intended readership. In addition, text mining is complicated because of the variability of how data are represented in a typical text document. Data on a particular topic may appear in the main body of text, in a footnote, in a table or embedded in a graphic illustration.

Natural Language Processing

The most promising approaches to text mining online documents rely on natural language processing (NLP), a technology that encompasses a variety of computational methods ranging from simple keyword extraction to semantic analysis (Fig. 15.14). The simplest NLP systems work by parsing documents and identifying the documents with recognised keywords such as 'protein' or 'amino acid'. The contents of the tagged documents can then be copied to a local database and later reviewed.

More elaborate NLP systems use statistical methods to recognise not only relevant keywords, but their distribution within a document. In this way, it's possible to infer context. For example, an NLP system can identify documents with the keywords 'amino acid', 'neurofibromatosis' and 'clinical outcome' in the same paragraph. The result of this more advanced analysis is document clusters, each of which represents data on a specific topic in a particular context.

This capability of identifying documents or document clusters is used by the typical Web search engines, such as Google or Yahoo! or the native PubMed interface. This approach is also used in commercial bibliographic database systems, such as EndNote, ProCite and Reference manager, which create a local subset of PubMed data by capturing the native field definitions, such as author name, publication title and MESH keywords. However, these products don't support the automatic integration of structure and sequence data with functional data. Their support for text mining of the data within a document is limited to simple user-directed keyword search.

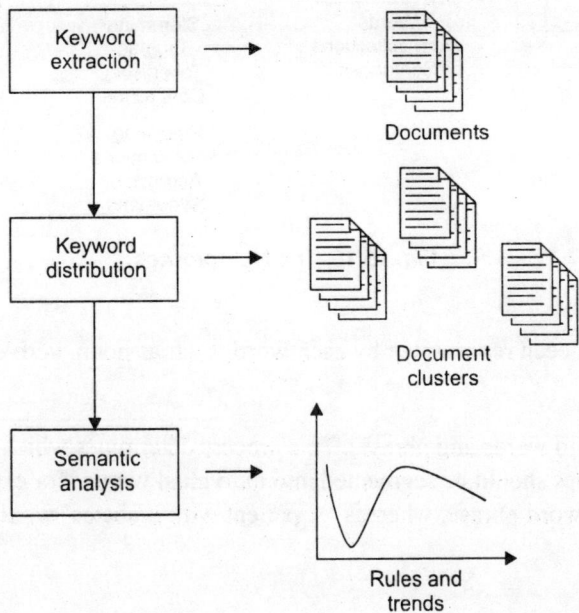

Fig. 15.14: Text mining with NLP. Simple keyword extraction is useful in identifying documents, analysis of keyword distribution identifies document clusters and semantic analysis can reveal rules and trends.

The most advanced NLP systems work at the semantic level—the analysis of how meaning is created by the use and interrelationships of words, phrases and sentences in a sentence. Unlike a typical search engine, these advanced systems attempt to automatically populate a database with, for example, functional genomic and proteomic data relevant to a specific gene, protein or disease, including rules and trends not explicitly stated or defined in the documents.

These systems, which represent the leading edge of NLP R&D, are less reliable than systems based on keyword extraction and distribution techniques in that they sometimes formulate incorrect rules and trends, resulting in erroneous search results.

Regardless of the level of NLP, most systems follow the basic process outlined in Fig. 15.15. Online documents are first parsed into words, word collections, or sentences, depending on the NLP method used. The simplest systems simply look at individual words, whereas systems that support mining of document clusters focus on word collections to establish context.

The most advanced NLP systems, which attempt to extract meaning from words and word order, parse the documents at the sentence level.

The processing phase of NLP involves one or more of a variety of the following techniques:

Stemming

Identifying the stem of each word. For example, 'hybridised', 'hybridising' and 'hybridisation' would be stemmed to 'hybrid'. As a result, the analysis phase of the NLP process has to deal with only the stem of each word and not every possible permutation.

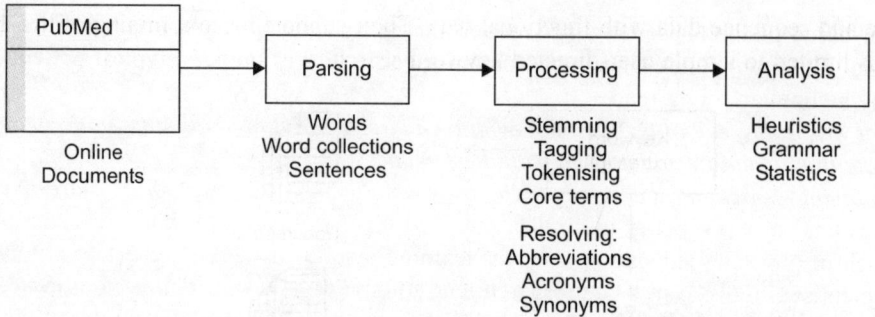

Fig. 15.15. The NLP process.

Tagging

Identifying the part of speech represented by each word, such as noun, verb or adjective.

Tokenising

Segmenting sentences into words and phrases. This process determines which words should be retained as phrases, and which ones should be segmented into individual words. For example, 'Type II Diabetes' should be retained as a word phrase, whereas 'A patient with diabetes' would be segmented into four separate words.

Core terms

Significant terms, such as protein names and experimental method names, are identified, based on a dictionary of core terms. A related process is ignoring insignificant words, such as 'the', 'and' and 'a'.

Resolving abbreviations, acronyms and synonyms

Replacing abbreviations with the words they represent and resolving acronyms and synonyms to a controlled vocabulary. For example, 'DM' and 'Diabetes Mellitus' could be resolved to 'Type II Diabetes', depending on the controlled vocabulary.

The analysis phase of NLP typically involves the use of heuristics, grammar or statistical methods. Heuristic approaches rely on a knowledge base of rules that are applied to the processed text. Grammar-based methods use language models to extract information from the processed text. Statistical methods use mathematical models to derive context and meaning from words. Often these methods are combined in the same system. For example, grammar-based methods and statistical methods are frequently used in NLP systems to improve the performance of what could be accomplished by using either approach alone.

Heuristic or rule-based analysis uses IF-THEN rules on the processed words and sentences to infer association or meaning. Consider the following rule:

> IF <protein name>
>   AND <experimental method name> are in the same sentence
>   THEN the <experimental method name> refers to the <protein name>

This rule states that if a protein name, such as 'haemoglobin', is in the same sentences as an experimental method, such as 'microarray spotting', then microarray spotting refers to haemoglobin. One obvious problem with heuristic methods is that there are exceptions to most rules. For example, using the preceding rule on a sentence starting with 'Microarray spotting was not used on the haemoglobin molecule because...' would improperly evaluate the sentence.

Grammar-based methods use language models that serve as templates for the sentence and phrase-level analysis. These templates tend to be domain-specific. For example, a typical patient case report submitted by a clinician might read:

'The patient was a 45-year-old white male with a chief complaint of abdominal pain for three days'.

A template that would be compatible with the sentence is:

<patient> <patient age> <race> <sex> <chief complaint> <complaint duration>

Templates tend to work better in clinical publications than they do in basic research publications because much of physician education involves learning a strict method of reporting clinical findings. However, scientists involved in basic research tend to have less indoctrination in a particular way of revealing their findings and so the statement of findings doesn't follow a syntactic formula.

Most statistical approaches to the analysis phase of NLP include an assessment word frequency at the sentence, paragraph and document level. Word frequency is relevant because words with the lowest frequency of occurrence tend to have the greatest meaning and significance in a document. Conversely, words with the highest frequency of occurrence, such as 'and', 'the' and 'a', have relatively little meaning.

In one statistical approach based on word frequency, a document is represented as a vector of word frequency, with the individual words or phrases forming the axes of the multi-dimensional space. This vector can be compared to a library of standard vectors, each of which represents a particular concept. Because the closeness of the two vectors represents similarity in concepts or at least content, this method can be used to automatically classify the contents of the document under analysis. For example, in Fig. 15.16, a document represented by a vector is compared with a vector that represents the use of microarray spotting of the haemoglobin extracted from patients with sickle-cell anemia. Similarly, documents dealing with other proteins and experimental processes can be identified by comparing their vectors with a library of vectors representing other concepts.

Text Summarisation

In addition to NLP, text mining is facilitated by text summarisation, a process that takes a page or more of text as its input and generates a summary paragraph as the output. Because each summary paragraph represents a sample of the source document, analysis of the summaries can be used as an initial screen for data on a particular topic described in documents or document clusters. In effect, text summarisation utilities, such as the 'AutoSummarise' feature within Microsoft Word, are useful in creating a rough abstract of a document when none has been provided by the author. Like semantic-level NLP, text summarisation is an imperfect, evolving technology that works well in niche areas, but not universally.

TOOLS

For most applications, data mining needn't involve writing neural networks or genetic algorithms in a traditional programming language. Instead, it can make use of a variety of general purpose and bioinformatics-specific tools, as well as several high-level languages (Table 15.4).

The most common languages used to perform data mining in bioinformatics are Perl, Python and SQL. Perl and Python are scripting languages that are useful for implementing custom character and string-based data mining for textual and sequence data. As true programming languages, they are flexible and powerful. The greatest limitation of Perl and Python is that they are interpreted scripting languages. That is, unlike C++ or other high-performance languages, the scripts are not compiled, but instead execute at runtime in an interpreter. As a result, data mining with Python or Perl is slower than using a well-written program using the same algorithms in C++. The time penalty associated with Python is considerably less than that associated with Perl, however, because it is based primarily on modules written in C++. Using either Perl or Python, a script defining a data-mining routine can be modified and executed within a few seconds without taking the time to compile source code. This advantage often outweighs the runtime speed penalty of using an interpreted language. In addition, Python and Perl are open-source, free programs.

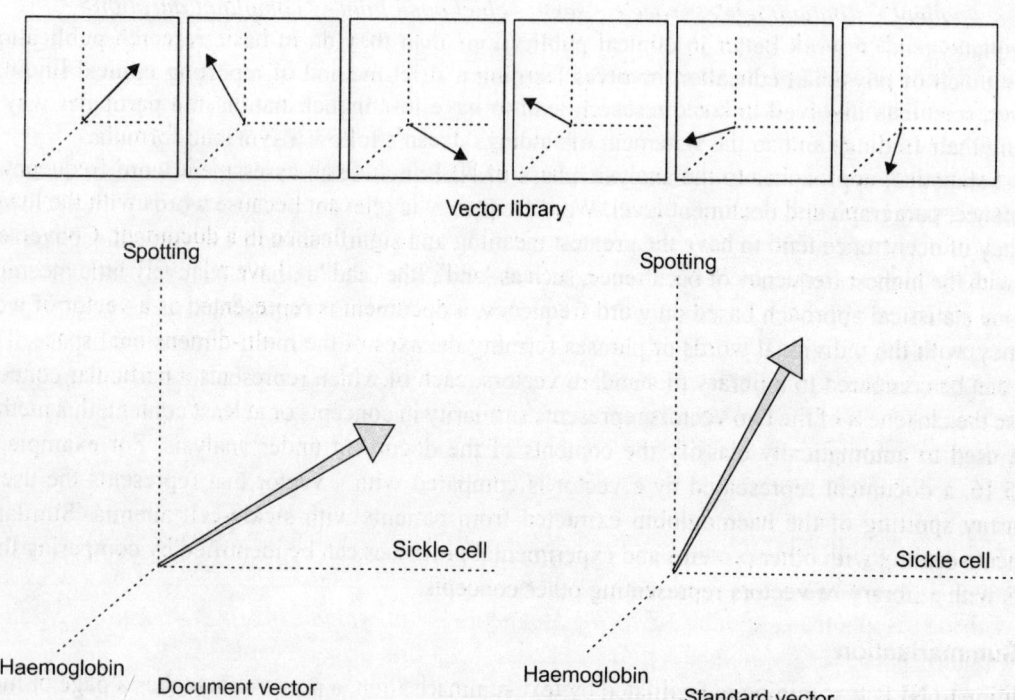

Fig. 15.16. Documents represented as word frequency vectors. The vector of a document under analysis (left) is compared to the standard vector (right) that represents spotting of haemoglobin from patients suffering from sickle-cell anemia. A vector library (top) contains vectors representing a variety of concepts relevant to the researcher.

Table 15.4. Examples of data mining tools.

Tool	Examples
Languages	Perl, Python, SQL, XML
General-purpose	Angoss, Clustran, Cross-graph, Cross-z, Daisy, Data distilleries, Database marksman, DataMind, GVA, IBM intelligent, Miner, Insightful miner, Integral solutions, KXEN, Magnify, MatLab, NeoVista solutions, Oracle Darwin, Quadstone, SAS, Spotfire, SPSS Clementine, StatPac, Syllogic, Think Analytics, Thinking Machines, Weka
Bioinformatics-specific	MEME, PIMA, Pratt, PrattWWW, SPEXS

SQL is also an interpreted language. However, SQL lacks the flexibility of Perl or Python, in that it's useful only for querying a relational database. This specificity results in high performance, even as an interpreted language. In addition, SQL isn't a stand-alone application, but is normally part of a vendor-specific DBMS. The advantage of using SQL is that the language is portable from one relational database system to the next, independent of the vendor, allowing a researcher to query different database systems without having to learn a new query language. The SQL commands are identical, regardless of whether the database is manufactured by Oracle, Microsoft, or IBM. Although SQL statements can be manually submitted in real-time, they are frequently embedded in another language, such as Perl, so that the other language can perform operations on the returned data, such as writing the data to a new database, plotting the data, or translating it to a new format.

XML is a data format that's the current darling of online database development because of its extensibility and use of tags that can provide contextual clues helpful in data mining. A database or data warehouse built around XML can more readily support data mining than one that only supports standard relational tables and SQL database queries. A major disadvantage of XML is the lack of constraints on how it can be extended. Unless external standards are used, databases written by different programmers using XML may bear little resemblance to each other.

In addition to programming languages, there are hundreds of general-purpose stand-alone and Web-based data-mining applications. Of the commercial data-mining applications, many of the more popular offerings are listed in Table 15.4. Some of these applications, such as Oracle Darwin, are tied to specific database products, whereas others, such as SAS, can be used with any major database system. Similarly, some of these applications, such as MatLab, support a wide variety of data-mining capabilities. MatLab is an example of a commercial application that can be extended through a variety of commercial and public-domain add-ons. If performance isn't a primary concern, then a researcher with knowledge of Perl or Python, SQL and MatLab can probably handle any data-mining challenge.

A sampling of the many academic bioinformatics-specific data-mining tools available include MEME, Pratt, PIMA and SPEXS. Multiple em for motif elicitation (MEME) is a motif discovery tool. Pratt, a stand-alone pattern discovery tool, is designed to uncover patterns conserved in sets of unaligned protein sequences. The user can specify what kind of patterns should be searched for, and how many sequences should match a pattern to be reported. The web-based version of Pratt, PrattWWW, includes a visualisation tool written as a Java applet to display patterns discovered in different sequences. Pattern-induced multi-sequence alignment program (PIMA) can be used to perform a multi-sequence alignment of a set of sequences. All pairwise comparisons between sequences in the set are performed and the resulting scores clustered into one or more families. Sequence pattern eXhaustive search (SPEXS) is a sequence pattern discovery tool. Because most of the other bioinformatics-specific data-mining tools tend to be optimised for a specific data-mining application, they tend to be very efficient. The downside of using these specific tools is the need to learn several different packages if data mining extends from nucleotide sequences to protein structures.

ON THE HORIZON

Real-time data mining, sometimes referred to as transaction monitoring, is rapidly gaining in popularity because of its increased value over the traditional mining of a data warehouse or database. In many industries, just-in-time analysis of data is much more valuable than analysis of data dredged up from the past—even if the past is only an hour or two removed from the present. For example, transaction monitoring is used by the credit card industry to detect fraud. As soon as a questionable transaction—a major purchase from a vendor not frequented by the legitimate card holder, for example—is detected, the system flags the point-of-sale system and the retailer has to call the credit card company for authorisation. Mining the data even 30 seconds after the transaction is complete is of relatively little value, especially if the thief disposes of the card after the purchase.

In clinical medicine, real-time data mining is being used to detect potential drug-drug interactions, allergic reactions and other side effects at the time a prescription is ordered. In some instances, a drug already in the body can potentiate another drug, causing the patient to overdose on the second drug, even though the dosage would be therapeutic without the other drug in the body. An overdose may result, for example, because both drugs are eliminated by the same pathway in the liver, and one drug completely saturates the metabolic pathway for drug elimination. Obviously, data on possible interactions is pertinent only before a patient is accidentally given the wrong drug or wrong dose of the appropriate drug.

The same technology can be extended to provide real-time analysis of drugs against a patient's genome, enabling the just-in-time delivery of custom drugs or as a means of detecting likely side effects of standard drugs on a given patient. In the bioinformatics laboratory, real-time data mining of results as they are generated by a sequencing machine or microarray reader can provide researchers with indicators as to the value of the data, error rate and relatedness of the data to previous studies.

Three technologies that support real-time data mining are real-time capture, message-oriented middle-ware and rule-based systems. Real-time data capture intercepts data from the source, before it is written to the database or data warehouse. This allows comparison of data to be made without a time-consuming data extraction process. Similarly, message-oriented middle-ware captures transactions, takes them off-line in batches, and stores the data in high-speed RAM (Fig. 15.17). While in RAM, the data are mined using a high-performance database manager with powerful RAM-based data handling features. The third technology, rule-based systems, can be used to create filters that intercept only those real-time transactions fitting a profile defined in easily edited rules. The data selected by the filter can then be rapidly mined using conventional processors or RAM-based technologies, as dictated by the performance limitations of the system.

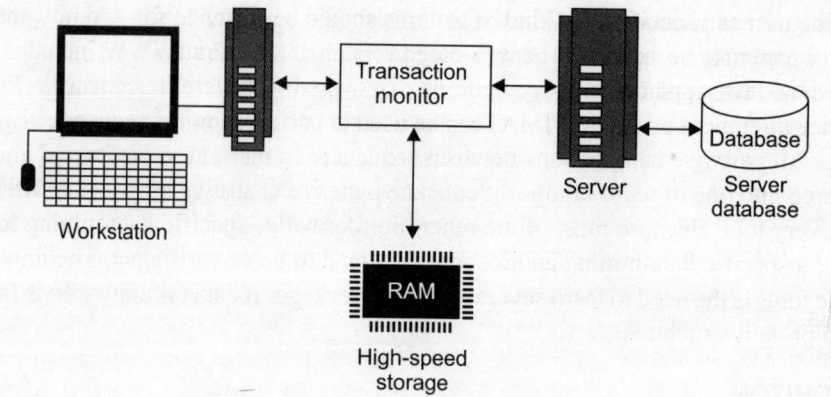

Fig. 15.17. Real-time data mining.

Each of these technologies supports different levels of data mining and has unique architectural limitations, such as the maximum number of transactions that can be monitored per minute. Overcoming these limitations at a reasonable cost is the focus of many computer scientists and corporations involved in data mining R&D.

ENDNOTE

The technologies and methodologies associated with data mining and knowledge discovery, while mature in areas such as fraud detection in credit card use, are not yet fully developed for bioinformatics applications. One issue is that, while fraud can be defined on an intuitive basis—sudden expenditure for luxury goods, transactions through vendors not frequented in the past, out-of-state transactions and the like—much of the nature of genetic material under scrutiny is unknown.

Because researchers provide the final filtering in the knowledge-discovery process, it's likely that unfamiliar concepts—truly new discoveries—will more likely be attributed to chance clustering than to some underlying process.

What's more, labels such as 'junk DNA', for example, influences the amount of time and energy that a researcher will invest in applying data-mining tools to the noncoding regions of a genome, in favour of areas more likely to provide meaningful results. Similarly, for years scientists took for granted that there were only 20 genetically coded amino acids. When additional amino acids were discovered, they were first verified by arduous wet-lab work that required several years of work. For example, it took scientists over two years to crystallise and determine the structure of pyrrolysine, the 22nd amino acid. Given the existence of an additional amino acid, however, searching through a database for occurrences ignored in the past is comparatively trivial.

Despite the effects of bias, humans are an indispensable part of the data-mining process. One reason for their continued inclusion in what would otherwise be an automated process is that current technologies assume uniform and relatively simple data structures. Very large, complex databases, replete with multiple potential relationships present scalability issues that may require significant computational time on powerful computer systems. In addition, many of the traditional data-mining methods were developed for homogenous numerical data. However, bioinformatics databases increasingly hold text sequences protein structure and other data sets that are anything but homogeneous.

The technical challenges associated with data mining are compounded by the lack of statistical methods that can adequately assess the significance of figures calculated from very large database sets. Similarly, because few bioinformatics databases are static, but are growing exponentially with time, the statistical concept of a fixed population from which samples are drawn is violated. As a result, a statistical analysis of a particular relationship at one point in time may provide a different result a month or two later. These and similar challenges remain for those in the bioinformatics arena to solve.

## Chapter 16

Pattern Matching

INTRODUCTION

Automated pattern matching—the ability of a program to compare novel and known patterns and determine the degree of similarity—forms the basis for automated sequence analysis, modelling of protein structures, locating homologous genes, data mining, internet search engines and dozens of other activities in bioinformatics. Some of the key bioinformatics applications of pattern recognition and matching—often referred to as simply pattern matching—are listed in Table 16.1. For example, as already discussed in 'data mining', data mining relies on heuristic and algorithmic pattern matching to locate patterns in online and local databases, using a variety of technologies, from simple keyword matching to rule-based expert systems and artificial neural networks.

Table 16.1. Pattern-matching applications in bioinformatics.

Constructing controlled vocabularies

Data mining

Functional genomics

Functional proteomics

Genome sequencing

Homologous gene identification

Homologous protein identification

Natural language processing

Neural network-based structure classifiers

Nucleotide sequence alignment

Protein sequence alignment

Protein structure prediction

Rule-based structure classifiers

One of the major challenges associated with using pattern matching in bioinformatics is that, in most cases, the task isn't simply one of finding a match for a given pattern, but finding one or more matches quickly from large databases using affordable and readily available hardware. In addition, the task is often complicated by the need to identify patterns that are 'similar' to a target pattern, but the concept of similarity isn't well-defined from a programmatic and biological sense. Not only is the degree of similarity defined in part by the technology underlying a particular software tool, but the relationship of a technology based on mathematical principles to the biological reality is often unclear. This ambiguity is common in the bioinformatics literature in the confusion of homology with similarity, for example.

This challenge of relating computational methods in pattern matching to our knowledge of the real world isn't limited to bioinformatics. For example, it's been a major focus of artificial intelligence (AI) research for several decades. Consider the illusion in Fig. 16.1. We can quickly decide that this picture could not denote a real object because of our knowledge of what constitutes the fundamental physical properties of objects. Even so, it has taken decades to formulate this knowledge into algorithms that confer the same capabilities on computer-based pattern-matching devices. Now, consider the challenges of extending this example to a complex protein-protein interaction, in which physical principles that act at an atomic level must be considered in systems designed to automatically classify proteins and other complex molecular structures. Despite these and other hurdles, pattern matching has been applied with varying degrees of success in areas as diverse as voice, image and optical character recognition, as well as the monumental task of sequencing the human genome.

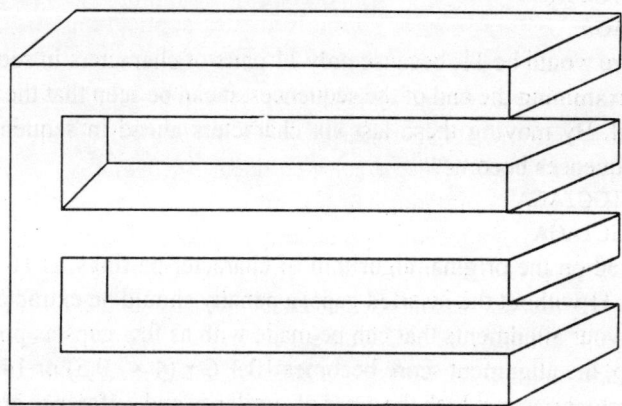

Fig. 16.1. Three or Four-prong illusion. Endowing computational pattern-recognition systems with knowledge of physical reality remains a challenge in AI and in other fields that rely on pattern-recognition methods.

This chapter explores the application and methodology behind pattern matching, with a focus on nucleotide and protein sequence alignment. The fundamentals section explores the challenges of sequence alignment and the following five sections, from 'dot matrix analysis' to 'Bayesian methods' review the key pairwise sequence alignment approaches. 'Multiple sequence alignment' extends the discussion to more challenging multiple sequence alignment tasks. The 'tools' section examines the more popular of the web-based tools available for sequence alignment. 'On the horizon' explores the future of pattern matching, given the surge in proteomic research and 'endnote' considers the ultimate fate of user-directed pattern recognition, given the move to intelligent agents and other technologies.

FUNDAMENTALS

Sequence alignment is fundamental to inferring homology (common ancestry) and function. For example, it's generally accepted that if two sequences are in alignment—part or all of the pattern of nucleotides or polypeptides match—then they are similar and may be homologous. Another heuristic is that if the sequence of a protein or other molecule significantly matches the sequence of a protein with a known structure and function, then the molecules may share structure and function. The issues related to single pairwise sequence alignment, global versus local alignment and multiple sequence alignment are introduced here.

Pairwise Sequence Alignment

Pairwise sequence alignment involves the matching of two sequences, one pair of elements at a time. The challenge in pairwise sequence alignment is to find the optimum alignment of two sequences with some degree of similarity. This optimum condition is typically based on a score that reflects the number of paired characters in the two sequences and the number and length of gaps required to adjust the sequences so that the maximum number of characters are in alignment. For example, consider the ideal case of two identical nucleotide sequences, (A) and (B):

(A) ATTCGGCATTCAGTGCTAGA

(B) ATTCGGCATTCAGTGCTAGA

Assuming that the alignment scoring algorithm counts one point per pair of aligned characters, then the score is one point for each of the 20 pairs or 20 points. Now, consider the case when several of the character pairs aren't aligned:

(C) ATTCGGCATTCAGTGCTAGA

(D) ATTCGGCATTGCTAGA

In this case, the score would be 11, because only 11 pairs of characters in sequences (C) and (D) are aligned. However, by examining the end of the sequences, it can be seen that the sequence of the last six characters are identical. By moving these last six characters ahead in sequence (D) by adding four spacers or gaps, the sequences become:

(E) ATTCGGCATTCAGTGCTAGA

(F) ATTCGGCATT- - - -GCTAGA

Now the score, based on the original algorithm of character pairings, is 16. However, because the score would have been 11 without the inserted gaps, a penalty should be extracted for each gap inserted into the sequence to favour alignments that can be made with as few gaps as possible. Assuming a gap penalty of –0.5 per gap, the alignment score becomes $10 + 6 + (4 \times -0.5)$ or 14.

A more likely scenario is one in which the areas of similarity and difference are not obvious. Consider the sequences (G) and (H):

(G) ATTCGGCATTCAGAGCGAGA

(H) ATTCGACATTGCTAGTGGTA

Unlike the previous cases, there are no relatively long runs of character pairings, and the matching pairs are separated by unaligned characters. The alignment score is 1 point per aligned pair or 13. One attempt at visual alignment by adding four gaps into sequence (H) results in:

(G) ATTCGGCATTCAGAGCTAGA

(I) ATTCGACATT----GCTAGTGGTA

This alignment results in a score of 12 or 14 alignments minus 2 points for the 4 gaps introduced into sequence (H), transforming it to sequence (I). In addition, a penalty of –0.5 per character pair is scored for an inexact match. In the case of sequences (G) and (I), there are 6 inexact matches, for a penalty of $(6 \times -0.5 = -3)$. Using this new alignment-scoring algorithm and ignoring the length difference between the two sequences, the alignment score for the (G)–(I) alignment becomes:

$$\text{Alignment Score} = 14 \text{ alignments} + 4 \text{ gaps} + 6 \text{ inexact matches}$$
$$= 14 + (4 \times -0.5) + (6 \times -0.5)$$
$$= 14 - 2 - 3$$
$$= 9$$

In this example, adding gaps results in a lower alignment score, illustrating how the relative worth of exact matches, inexact matches and gaps determines the eventual alignment of two sequences. For example, if gaps are penalised heavily and inexact matches are minimally counted, then sequences will have few gaps. Although a simple gap penalty of −0.5 point per gap has been used to illustrate the role of alignment scores on sequence alignment, gap penalty is typically calculated as:

$$Penalty_{gap} = Cost_{opening} + Cost_{extension} \times Length_{gap}$$

In this formula, $Penalty_{gap}$ is the total gap penalty, $Cost_{opening}$ is the cost of opening a gap in a sequence, $Cost_{extension}$ is the cost of extending an existing gap by one character, and $Length_{gap}$ is the length of the gap in characters. The minimum value of $Length_{gap}$ is one. Returning to the sequence pair (E)–(F), assuming that $Cost_{opening}$ is (−0.5) and $Cost_{extension}$ is (−0.5), the gap penalty becomes:

$$Penalty_{gap} = Cost_{opening} + Cost_{extension} \times Length_{gap}$$
$$= -0.5 + (-0.5 \times 4)$$
$$= -2.5$$

With the expanded method of computing gap penalty, the score becomes $10 + 6 - 2.5 = 13.5$ points. The gap penalty formula can be extended to include a penalty for alignments for the gaps at the end of a sequence to make the sequences of equal length. However, if the sequences are of very different lengths, then it probably doesn't make sense to penalise for these end gaps. It's important to realise that picking arbitrary gap opening and extension costs typically has no real relationship to the underlying biology of the protein or DNA involved. One solution is to use gap penalty values that relate to biologically relevant data, as described in the 'Substitution Matrices' section later in this chapter.

Local Versus Global Alignment

Sequence pair (E)–(F) is an example of a global alignment—that is, an attempt to line up the two sequences matching as many characters as possible, for the entire length of each segment. Global alignment considers all characters in a sequence, and bases alignment on the total score, even at the expense of stretches in the sequence that share obvious similarity (Fig. 16.2). Global alignment is used to help determine whether two protein sequences are in the same family, for example.

There are several methods of performing local sequence alignment, each of which has particular uses, advantages and computational overhead. For example, the Smith-Waterman dynamic programming method, which uses a scoring system that penalises the total score for a mismatch, is a computationally intensive sequence alignment method that favours local over global alignment.

Multiple Sequence Alignment

Multiple sequence alignment, in which three or more sequences must be aligned, is useful in finding conserved regulatory patterns in nucleotide sequences and for identifying structural and functional domains in protein families. Unfortunately, multiple sequence alignment is much more challenging than single pairwise alignment. For nucleotide sequences, the problem appears as:

(J) TCAGAGCGAGA
(K) ATCCGGCCCGGCAGCGAGA
(L) CAAAATTCAGAGCGAGA
(M) ATCCGCAGAGCCCGGGGAGA
(N) CCCGGCAGCGAGA
(O) ATCCGTTTTTTTTTTGAGA

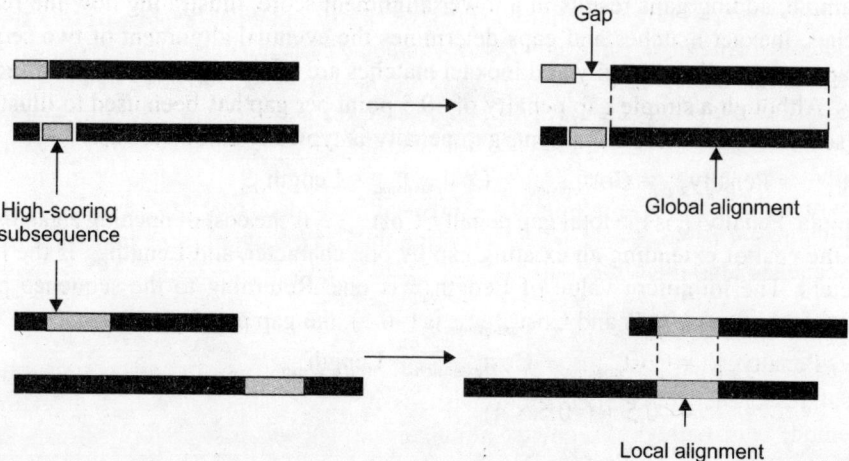

Fig. 16.2. Local (top) versus global (bottom) alignment. In local alignment, the alignment of local, high-scoring sequences takes precedence over the overall alignment. In global alignment, the best overall alignment is sought, regardless of whether local, high-scoring subsequences are in alignment or not.

Instead of simply considering gaps, inexact matches and global-versus-local alignment for a pair of sequences, multiple sequences must be considered—in this example, six sequences. Of course, in an actual multiple sequence alignment, each sequence may consist of several hundred characters, making manual gap insertions and other noncomputational methods infeasible. Although most of the following discussion deals with single pairwise alignment, multiple alignment is an area of active research in bioinformatics because of the computational challenges involved.

Computational Methods

Fortunately, a variety of computational methods is available for sequence alignment, whether single, multiple, global or local. A sampling of major computational approaches to pattern matching and sequence alignment is listed in Table 16.2.

Table 16.2. Computational methods of sequence alignment.

Bayesian methods
Dot matrix
Dynamic programming
Genetic algorithms
Hidden Markov models
Neural networks
Scoring matrices
Word-based techniques

Of the methods listed in Table 16.2, word-based techniques, followed by dynamic programming methods, are used most often. The popularity of word-based techniques is in part because of the ready availability of Web-based tools that use these methods, such as fast alignment (FASTA) and basic local alignment and search tool (BLAST). Similarly, dynamic programming techniques, such as the Smith-

Waterman algorithm, while computationally expensive, are also popular because of free access to Web-based tools. Dot matrix methods, once a mainstay of manual and computer-enabled sequence alignment, have become less popular since the advent of BLAST and its derivatives. However, dot matrix methods are still studied because of the insight they provide into other techniques, including dynamic programming.

Many of the other approaches to sequence alignment, such as the use of artificial neural networks, genetic algorithms, Bayesian approaches and hidden markov models (HMMs), are either experimental or combined with dynamic programming or word-based methods to provide users with practical tools. Similarly, many adjunct technologies, such as scoring matrices, have become integral to the operation of the major sequence alignment methods.

DOT MATRIX ANALYSIS

Because alignment by visual inspection of linear sequences hundreds of characters or more in length was impractical, researchers developed a more visually intuitive method of pattern detection called the dot matrix method. This method of sequence alignment, which was first performed manually and then computerised, makes the similarities in patterns more obvious to visual inspection. Using this method, one sequence appears along the top and one along the side of the matrix, and a dot is placed at the intersection of matching character pairs. Contiguous diagonal rows of dots indicate sequences of matching pairs, as in the dot matrix plot of sequences (G) and (H) in Fig. 16.3.

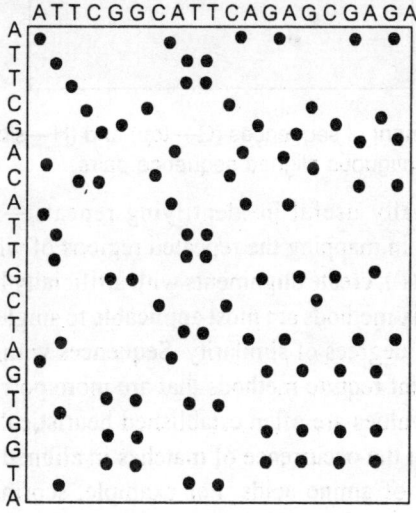

Fig. 16.3. Dot matrix pairwise alignment of nucleotide sequences (G—top) and (H—side). Diagonal sequences of dots indicate areas of contiguous sequences of aligned pairs. In a typical plot, there may be hundreds of characters in each sequence.

The dot matrix pattern for a pair of perfectly matching sequences would include a contiguous sequence of dots running down the centre diagonal of the matrix. However, this pattern is rarely seen in practice. Most often, the diagonal patterns are difficult to discern without additional processing. In addition to the use of colour and other methods of highlighting matching sequences, a variety of filters are often applied to the data. For example, a common filter is a combination of window and stringency. The window refers to the number of data points examined at a time, while the stringency is the minimum number of matches required within each window.

With a filter in which the window size is set to 2 and the stringency to 1, a dot is printed at a matrix position only if 1 out of the next 2 positions is identified, as in Fig. 16.4. Similarly, with a window size of 6 and a stringency of 3, a dot would be printed at a matrix position only if 3 of the next 6 positions in the sequences are identified. A typical window-stringency combination is $^{15}\!/_{10}$ for nucleotide sequences and much narrower combinations for polypeptide sequences, such as $^1\!/_1$ or $^3\!/_2$.

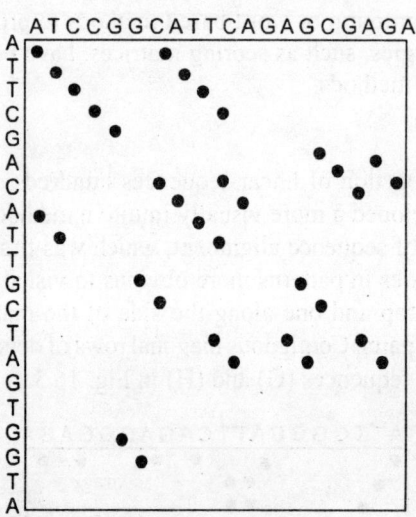

Fig. 16.4. Dot Matrix Pairwise Alignment of sequences (G—top) and (H—side). The filter, with a window of 2 and stringency of 1, emphasises contiguous aligned sequence pairs.

Dot matrix analysis is especially useful in identifying repeats—repeating characters or short sequences—within a sequence, as in mapping the repeated regions of whole chromosomes. Repeats of the same character, as in sequence (P), create alignments with artificially high scores and make sequence alignment more difficult. Dot matrix methods are most applicable to single pairwise alignment problems, especially those with relative high degrees of similarity. Sequences with lower degrees of similarity as well as multiple sequence alignment require methods that are more powerful.

Although window-stringency values are often established heuristically, they may also be based on dynamic averages, scores based on the occurrence of matches in aligned protein families or on various methods of scoring the similarity of amino acids. For example, scoring matrices provide scores for alignment based on their statistical occurrence in aligned protein families. Using these matrices, described in the following section, a sliding window feature can be implemented, in which only dots above a certain average score can appear in the matrix.

SUBSTITUTION MATRICES

Protein structure and function are surprisingly resistant to polypeptide substitution, to the degree that the substitutions don't alter the chemistry of the protein. Substitutions are common over large expanses of time and from one species to the next. In many cases, the substitution of polypeptides through evolution can be predicted. In this way, a matrix of likely polypeptide substitutions can be constructed. As in a dot matrix analysis, the amino acids are listed across the top and side of a matrix, typically using the amino acid code letters listed in Table 16.3. At each intersection, the matrix is filled with a score that reflects how often one polypeptide would have been paired with the other in an alignment of related protein sequences. An underlying assumption is that this association is symmetrical, in that either polypeptide can be substituted for the other.

Table 16.3. Amino acid code letters.

Code	Meaning
A	Alanine
B	Aspartate or Asparagine
C	Cysteine
D	Aspartate
E	Glutamic Acid
F	Phenylalanine
G	Glycine
H	Histidine
I	Isoleucine
K	Lysine
L	Leucine
M	Methionine
N	Asparagine
P	Proline
Q	Glutamine
R	Arginine
S	Serine
T	Threonine
V	Valine
W	Tryptophan
X	Unknown
Y	Tyrosine
Z	Glutamate or Glutamine

Two popular substitution matrices are percent accepted mutation (PAM) and blocks amino acid substitution matrix (blosum), examples of which are shown in Figs. 16.5 and 16.6, respectively. Unlike dot matrix analysis, these matrices are static. Furthermore, these matrices aren't mere mathematical constructs designed simply to facilitate computational sequence alignment, but they reflect the biology of the molecules represented by the sequences. For example, matrix in the series is named after the level of change assumed by the matrix. For example, the commonly used PAM-250, shown in Fig. 16.5, assumes a 250 per cent change in the probability matrix. A matrix value of '0' signifies that a substitution typically occurs at a random base rate, whereas a negative matrix value infers that the substitution is less likely than by chance alone. A positive matrix value means that the substitution occurs more often than suggested by chance. For example, in the PAM-250 matrix, A and N (Alanine and Asparagine) substitute for each other at a rate (0) that is expected by chance alone. Conversely, A and W (alanine and tryptophan) substitute for each other at a rate (–6) much lower than expected for a random substitution.

PAM-250 SUBSTITUTION MATRIX																						
	A	R	N	D	C	Q	E	G	H	I	L	K	M	F	P	S	T	W	Y	V	B	Z	X
A	2																						
R	-2	6																					
N	0	0	2																				
D	0	-1	2	4																			
C	-2	-4	-4	-5	12																		
Q	0	1	1	2	-5	4																	
E	0	-1	1	3	-5	2	4																
G	1	-3	0	1	-3	-1	0	5															
H	-1	2	2	1	-3	3	1	-2	6														
I	-1	-2	-2	-2	-2	-2	-2	-3	-2	5													
L	-2	-3	-3	-4	-6	-2	-3	-4	-2	2	6												
K	-1	3	1	0	-5	1	0	-2	0	-2	-3	5											
M	-1	0	-2	-3	-5	-1	-2	-3	-2	2	4	0	6										
F	-4	-4	-4	-6	-4	-5	-5	-5	-2	1	2	-5	0	9									
P	1	0	-1	-1	-3	0	-1	-1	0	-2	-3	-1	-2	-5	6								
S	1	0	1	0	0	-1	0	1	-1	-1	-3	0	-2	-3	1	2							
T	1	-1	0	0	-2	-1	0	0	-1	0	-2	0	-1	-3	0	1	3						
W	-6	2	-4	-7	-8	-5	-7	-7	-3	-5	-2	-3	-4	0	-6	-2	-5	17					
Y	-3	-4	-2	-4	0	-4	-4	-5	0	-1	-1	-4	-2	7	-5	-3	-3	0	10				
V	0	-2	-2	-2	-2	-2	-2	-1	-2	4	2	-2	2	-1	-1	-1	0	-6	-2	4			
B	0	-1	2	3	-4	1	2	0	1	-2	-3	1	-2	-5	-1	0	0	-5	-3	-2	2		
Z	0	0	1	3	-5	3	3	-1	2	-2	-3	0	-2	-5	0	0	-1	-6	-4	-2	2	3	
X	0	0	0	0	0	0	0	0	0	0	0	0	0	0	0	0	0	0	0	0	0	0	0

Fig. 16.5. The per cent accepted mutation substitution matrix 250 (PAM-250).

BLOSUM62 SUBSTITUTION MATRIX																						
	A	R	N	D	C	Q	E	G	H	I	L	K	M	F	P	S	T	W	Y	V	B	Z	X
A	4																						
R	-1	5																					
N	-2	0	6																				
D	-2	-2	1	6																			
C	0	-3	-3	-3	9																		
Q	-1	1	0	0	-3	5																	
E	-1	0	0	2	-4	2	5																
G	0	-2	0	-1	-3	-2	-2	6															
H	-2	0	1	-1	-3	0	0	-2	8														
I	-1	-3	-3	-3	-1	-3	-3	-4	-3	4													
L	-1	-2	-3	-4	-1	-2	-3	-4	-3	2	4												
K	-1	2	0	-1	-3	1	1	-2	-1	-3	-2	5											
M	-1	-1	-2	-3	-1	0	-2	-3	-2	1	2	-1	5										
F	-2	-3	-3	-3	-2	-3	-3	-3	-1	0	0	-3	0	6									
P	-1	-2	-2	-1	-3	-1	-1	-2	-2	-3	-3	-1	-2	-4	7								
S	1	-1	1	0	-1	0	0	0	-1	-2	-2	0	-1	-2	-1	4							
T	0	-1	0	-1	-1	-1	-1	-2	-2	-1	-1	-1	-1	-2	-1	1	5						
W	-3	-3	-4	-4	-2	-2	-3	-2	-2	-3	-2	-3	-1	1	-4	-3	-2	11					
Y	-2	-2	-2	-3	-2	-1	-2	-3	2	-1	-1	-2	-1	3	-3	-2	-2	2	7				
V	0	-3	-3	-3	-1	-2	-2	-3	-3	3	1	-2	1	-1	-2	-2	0	-3	-1	4			
B	-2	-1	3	4	-3	0	1	-1	0	-3	-4	0	-3	-3	-2	0	-1	-4	-3	-3	4		
Z	-1	0	0	1	-3	3	4	-2	0	-3	-3	1	-1	-3	-1	0	-1	-3	-2	-2	1	4	
X	0	-1	-1	-1	-2	-1	-1	-1	-1	-1	-1	-1	-1	-1	-2	0	0	-2	-1	-1	-1	-1	-1

Fig. 16.6. The blocks amino acid substitution matrix 62 (Blosum62).

The figures used to populate the matrices are based on the formula:

$$\text{Matrix value} = \log\left[\frac{\text{frequency}_\text{Observed}}{\text{frequency}_\text{Expected}}\right]$$

From the perspective of supporting sequence alignment, the main diagonal reveals the relative value of maintaining matches in the pairwise sequence alignment process. For example, in the PAM-250 substitution matrix, given a choice of shifting a sequence by adding gaps or other means that affect either an A-A (Alanine-Alanine) alignment or a C-C (Cysteine-Cysteine) alignment, the C-C alignment should not be disturbed. This is because the C-C alignment is rated at 12, compared to only 2 for the A-A alignment.

Although the values in the Blosum matrix mean the same as in a PAM matrix, the Blosum, matrices incorporate substitution scores that encompass a range of evolutionary periods and in some cases provide greater sensitivity over PAM matrices. Blosum takes its name from the blocks—areas of conserved amino acids—used to define substitution patterns. Unlike PAM, which is based on a relatively small set of closely related proteins, Blosum is based on a large-scale analysis of over 500 families of related proteins. Similarly, Blosum doesn't explicitly consider evolutionary factors.

Matrices aren't necessarily symmetric or based on the same alphabet. For example, it's possible to relate polypeptides to experimental or environmental conditions. Furthermore, although this discussion of matrices has centred on polypeptides, they can also be designed for use with nucleic acids. The matrix values of these matrices are necessarily different from those used with polypeptides.

As noted in the earlier discussion of gap penalties, arbitrarily selecting opening and extension costs so that the output 'looks nice' from a mathematical perspective likely has no relevance to the actual biology of the protein under study. It's commonly assumed that a better approach is to assign gap extension and opening costs relative to the substitution matrix used for a given protein. If the gap penalty figures are too high relative to the matrix scores, the gap penalty figures will override the matrix scores, and gaps will never appear in the sequence alignment.

Conversely, if gap penalty figures are too low relative to the matrix scores, gaps will be used wherever possible in order to align the sequences. That is, simply because a substitution matrix is used doesn't guarantee biologically relevant results. The matrices and related calculations must be used appropriately and in consideration of the underlying biology.

DYNAMIC PROGRAMMING

One way to be certain that the solution to a sequence alignment is the best alignment possible is to try every possible alignment, introducing one or more gaps at every position and computing an alignment score based on aligned character pairs and inexact matches. However, the computational overhead of evaluating all possible alignments of one sequence against another grows exponentially with the length of the two sequences. For reasonable length sequences of several hundred characters each, an exhaustive evaluation of potential alignments could take days of computer time without using specific algorithms developed for sequence alignment, such as dynamic programming.

Dynamic programming is a form of recursion in which intermediate results are saved in a matrix where they can be referred to later by the program. The comparison can be likened to solving a series of complex mathematical equations, with the results of one equation feeding the input of another, with and without the benefit of pen and paper or other temporary storage and retrieval mechanism. With pen and paper (as with dynamic programming), the intermediate results can be recorded and the next equation can be solved without regard to the previous or following equation. Without the pen and paper, it may be impossible for some people to solve the series of equations. Dynamic programming is processor and RAM-intensive, but the technique of storing intermediate values in a matrix can transform an otherwise intractable problem requiring immense computational capabilities into one that is computationally feasible.

To illustrate the value of dynamic programming in sequence alignment, consider the function:

$$MaxValue = f(A_i, B_j)$$

In this equation, MaxValue is some function of variables A_i and B_j, where i and j are indices to the variables defined in the tree structure illustrated in Fig. 16.7. That is, the possible values of A_i are represented by A_1 through A_5 and the possible values of B are represented by B_1 through B_{11}. The best solution to MaxValue depends on the equation that defines MaxValue. For example, consider the following possible definition of MaxValue:

$$MaxValue = (A_i \times B_j)$$

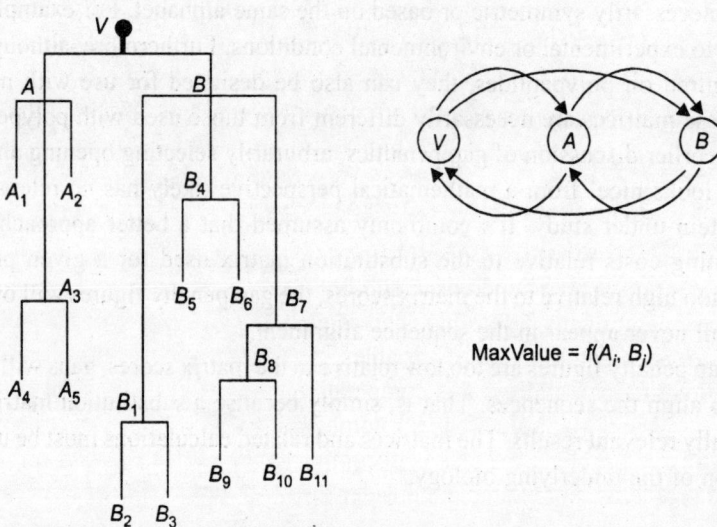

Fig. 16.7. Dynamic programming problem. Values for A and B are defined in the tree structure. Maximising maxvalue requires evaluating the equation for every combination of i and j.

In this example, the solution is simply the largest value of A and the largest value of B. However, consider the following definition of MaxValue:

$$MaxValue = \sqrt[3]{\frac{14 \times A^2}{\log(A^2 + B^2)}}$$

In this example, the solution to MaxValue is less obvious and much more computationally intensive.

The brute-force method of solving for MaxValue is to recursively walk down each of the trees and try the various combinations of A and B in the MaxValue equation. However, as illustrated in the upper-right of Fig. 16.7, evaluating every value of B in the MaxValue equation entails evaluating every value of A.

For example, assume that the values for A_i and B_j are defined as:

$$A = \begin{bmatrix} 2 \\ 3 \\ 8 \\ 4 \\ 1 \end{bmatrix} \qquad B = \begin{bmatrix} 9 \\ 11 \\ 1 \\ 0 \\ 3 \\ 8 \\ 1 \\ 7 \\ 5 \\ 3 \\ 2 \end{bmatrix}$$

Solving for the first value of A_i ($A_1 = 2$) and ignoring the specific equation for MaxValue for clarity:

$\text{MaxValue}_{1,1} = f(A_1, B_1) = f(2, 9) = 5$

$\text{MaxValue}_{1,2} = f(A_1, B_2) = f(2, 11) = 3$

$\text{MaxValue}_{1,3} = f(A_1, B_3) = f(2, 1) = 0$

$\text{MaxValue}_{1,4} = f(A_1, B_4) = f(2, 0) = 2$

$\text{MaxValue}_{1,5} = f(A_1, B_5) = f(2, 3) = 8$

$\text{MaxValue}_{1,6} = f(A_1, B_6) = f(2, 8) = 0$

$\text{MaxValue}_{1,7} = f(A_1, B_7) = f(2, 1) = -2$

$\text{MaxValue}_{1,8} = f(A_1, B_8) = f(2, 7) = 1$

$\text{MaxValue}_{1,9} = f(A_1, B_9) = f(2, 5) = 2$

$\text{MaxValue}_{1,10} = f(A_1, B_{10}) = f(2, 3) = 8$

$\text{MaxValue}_{1,11} = f(A_1, B_{11}) = f(2, 2) = 4$

If the branches of A and B have hundreds of sub-branches, representing hundreds of values, then the problem is likely computationally infeasible. This is especially true if the MaxValue function, which must be evaluated for each combination of variables, is also computationally intensive.

Dynamic programming can address this computational and time dilemma by creating a matrix to store the values for A_i, B_j and MaxValue for each combination of i and j. Instead of solving one complex CPU and RAM-intensive problem, the task is decomposed into hundreds or even thousands of easily and quickly solved problems. For example, consider the solution matrix for MaxValue in Fig. 16.8.

A_i \ B_j	1	2	3	4	5	6	7	8	9	10	11
1	5	3	0	2	8	0	-2	1	2	8	4
2	0	3	0	6	11	0	-6	5	7	4	0
3	9	0	(12)	2	0	0	0	5	0	0	0
4	1	7	5	5	11	0	-1	1	7	5	4
5	9	0	0	2	5	0	-2	5	1	4	1

Fig. 16.8. Solution matrix for maxvalue for A_i and B_j. The solution to maxvalue is A_3 and B_3 with MaxValue = 12.

The solution set to MaxValue computed earlier for A_1 appears in the first row of the matrix. Examining only this first row, it can be seen that there are two solutions to MaxValue, B_5 and B_{10}, each of which results in a value of 8.

With the completed solution matrix available for examination, it's a trivial matter to locate the best values for i and j, second-best and so on. The same approach can be extended to any number of dimensions. For example, consider adding a third variable, as in Fig. 16.9. The equation for MaxValue now takes the form:

$$\text{MaxValue} = f(A_i, B_j, C_k)$$

In this new equation, MaxValue is some function of variables A_i, B_j and C_k, where i, j and k are indices to the variables defined in the tree structure illustrated in Fig. 16.9. The best solution to MaxValue is in the form $[i = 3, j = 3, k = 2]$, for example. As in the simpler 2D problem, a matrix of solutions can be constructed. However, the matrix of solutions is now much larger and is better represented as a 3D structure, as in Fig. 16.10.

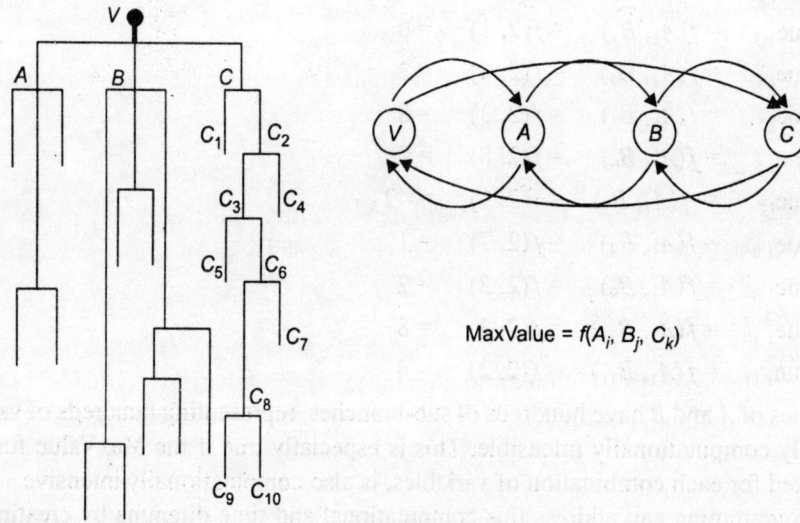

Fig. 16.9. Dynamic programming problem with added dimensionality. Values for A_i, B_j and C_k are contained in the tree structure (left). The exhaustive solution to maxvalue involves evaluating every combination of i, j, and k.

$$\text{MaxValue} = f(A_i, B_j, C_k)$$

		1	2	3	4	5	6	7	8	9	10	11
	1	5	3	0	2	8	0	–2	1	2	8	4
	2	0	3	0	6	11	0	–6	5	7	4	0.
	3	9	0	12	2	0	0	0	5	0	0	0
	4	1	7	5	5	11	0	–1	1	7	5	4
	5	9	0	0	2	5	0	–2	5	1	4	1

Fig. 16.10. Solution matrix for maxvalue = $f(A_i, B_j, C_k)$. Only one value for k ($k = 0$) is shown here for clarity.

Even though there are now many more solutions to consider, the process of evaluating MaxValue for three variables and saving intermediary results in the 3D matrix is the same as in the previous 2D example. Adding additional dimensions, although computationally intensive, makes it possible to evaluate all possible ways of aligning the three sequences against each other in a reasonable time, even though the number of such possible alignments grows exponentially with the length of the two sequences. Similarly, just as adding a dimension to the problem doesn't fundamentally change the evaluation process, the alignment of multiple strings can be evaluated using this process as well.

To bring the power of dynamic programming into the realm of pairwise sequence alignment, consider MaxValue to be the alignment score for pairwise alignment of two sequences. MaxValue takes into account gap penalties, correct alignments, and imperfect alignments. After the matrix is filled in using the alignment score to determine MaxValue, the highest scoring path is followed back to the beginning of the alignment to define the best alignment of elements in the sequence, including gaps.

Graphically, this approach to the local alignment of two sequences is illustrated in Fig. 16.11. The starting point is the best score in the matrix, the C-C alignment with a value of 11. Working backwards to the row and column to the upper left, step (1), the best score is for the G-G alignment, with a score of 10. Because the value is on the diagonal immediately adjacent to the value for the C-C alignment, there is no gap penalty. Now, moving to step (2), the highest score, 8, is also immediately adjacent and therefore free of a gap penalty. In step (3), there are three high scores, each of which has a gap penalty. The minimum gap penalty is associated with the closest alignment with a score of 5, the A-A alignment. Continuing to step (4), there are two competing high scores. Because there is no penalty for the C-C alignment that is diagonally adjacent to the A-A alignment, with a value of 6, the process continues to the G-G bond with a value of 8, to completing the local alignment. That is, the local alignment appears as:

(Q) ATCGAGCA–GCATG...

(R) ------ --GCATGCT...

In this example, sequence (Q) appears across the top and sequence (R) is listed across the side of Fig. 16.11. The characters involved in the local alignment appear in bold.

Mathematically, the algorithm for this form of local alignment, known as the Smith-Waterman algorithm, is defined as:

$$H_{ij} = \max \begin{cases} H_{i-1,j-1} + s(A_i B_j) \\ \max(H_{i-x,j} - w_x, \\ x \geq 1 \\ \max(H_{i,j-y} - w_y, \\ y \geq 1 \\ 0 \end{cases}$$

where, A_i and B_j are the two sequences to be aligned; H_{ij} is the score at position A_i, B_j; $s(A_i B_j)$ is the score for aligning the characters at positions i and j; w_x is the penalty of a gap of length x in sequence A and w_y is the penalty for a gap of length of y in sequence B.

The three special provisions of this algorithm that favours local alignments are:

1. Negative numbers are not allowed in the scoring matrix.
2. Inexact matches are penalised.
3. The best score is sought any where in the matrix, and not simply in the last column or row.

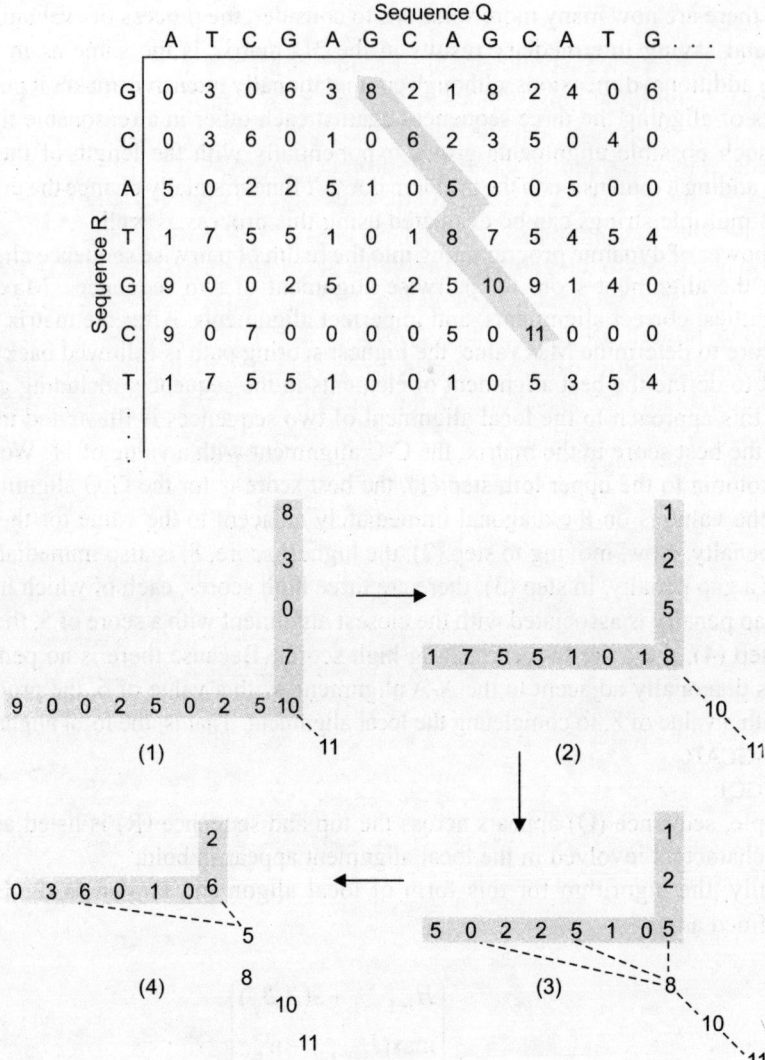

Fig. 16.11. Matrix scores and optimum local alignment for two sequences.

Even though dynamic programming guarantees to find the best local or global alignment because the technique considers all possible alignments, the technique is computationally intensive. Short pairwise comparisons using the Smith-Waterman algorithm can require several hours of workstation processing. High-end parallel processing hardware, such as the UCSC Kestrel server, which provides the equivalent of 40 times the processing power of a desktop workstation, requires several minutes for pairwise alignment using the Smith-Waterman algorithm.

Given the computational overhead of dynamic programming, a variety of first-pass, heuristic-based methods have been developed to support alignment on the desktop workstation. These techniques, often referred to as word methods, include the ubiquitous FASTA and BLAST algorithms, as described in the next section.

WORD METHODS

BLAST and FASTA are called word methods of sequence alignment because these algorithms work at the level of words—multiple polypeptides or nucleic acids—instead of with individual polypeptides or nucleic acids. Both methods of sequence alignment are fast enough to support searching for alignments of query sequences against entire nucleotide or protein databases.

The high-level flow of the FASTA algorithm, which predates BLAST, is shown in Fig. 16.12. The first step in the FASTA algorithm is to create a hash table of words from the query sequence. Hashing is a function that maps words to integers to get a smaller set of values so that the search space is minimised, for example. A hash table, such as the one in Fig. 16.13, maps words to array positions, based on the hash function. For proteins, word length is typically one or two amino acids long. For nucleic acid sequences, the word length is usually from four to six characters. In either case, the longer the word length, the more rapid and the less thorough the search.

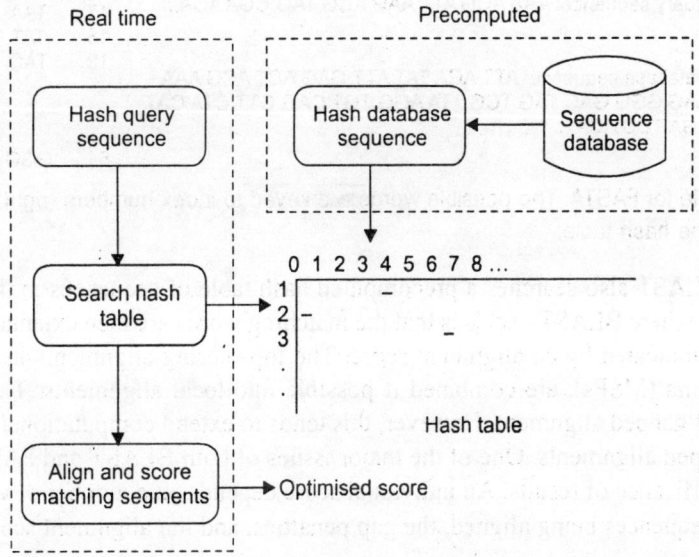

Fig. 16.12. FASTA algorithm flowchart.

Next, the characters are compared to those in the database, which has previously been processed into words of the same length. FASTA uses the Blosum50 substitution matrix to score the top-10 alignments (without gaps) that contain the most similar words. These words are then merged into a gapped alignment, which is scored, producing an 'optimised score'. FASTA produces an expectation score, E, which represents the expected number of random alignments with z-scores greater than or equal to the value observed, thereby providing an estimate of the statistical significance of the results.

Although FASTA was the first widely used program for sequence alignment against genome-length sequences and is still actively supported in both Web and workstation versions, BLAST is by far the more popular of the word-based algorithms for sequence alignment. Like FASTA, BLAST is a heuristic approach to sequence alignment that provides speed through a hashing technique. BLAST also differs from FASTA in that words are typically 3 characters long for proteins and 11 characters in length for nucleotide sequences.

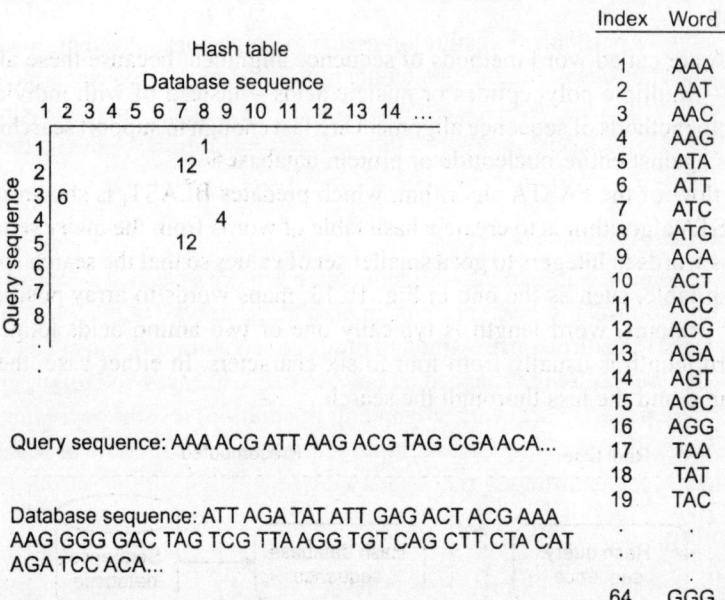

Query sequence: AAA ACG ATT AAG ACG TAG CGA ACA...

Database sequence: ATT AGA TAT ATT GAG ACT ACG AAA
AAG GGG GAC TAG TCG TTA AGG TGT CAG CTT CTA CAT
AGA TCC ACA...

Fig. 16.13. Hash table for FASTA. The possible words are keyed to index numbers (right), which are used to represent words in the hash table.

Like FASTA, BLAST also searches a precomputed hash table of sequences in the protein or DNA database. However, where BLAST excels is that the matching words are then extended to the maximum length possible, as indicated by an alignment score. The top-scoring alignments in a sequence, called maximal-scoring pairs (MSPs), are combined if possible into local alignments. The latest version of BLAST can attempt gapped alignment. However, this tends to extend computational time significantly, compared to ungapped alignments. One of the major issues of both BLAST and FASTA results is how to interpret the significance of results. An individual score depends on a number of variables, including the lengths of the sequences being aligned, the gap penalties, and the alignment scoring system used.

BAYESIAN METHODS

Although not considered mainstream by many researchers in the bioinformatics field, Bayesian statistical methods can be used to determine pairwise sequence alignment and to estimate the evolutionary distance between DNA sequences. Bayesian methods involve examining the probabilities of all possible alignments, gap scores and substitution matrix values (the prior probabilities) to assess the probability of an alignment (the posterior probability). Proponents of the Bayesian approach to sequence alignment cite as advantages over the limitations of dynamic program the method's ability to fully and exactly describe uncertainty, derive exact significance measures and eliminate the need to specify all parametres.

In practice, Bayesian-based tools, such as the Bayes Block Aligner, a workstation-based tool available from the Centre for Bioinformatics at Rensselaer and Wadsworth Centre of the New York Department of Health, performs better than dynamic programming in some cases and not as well in others. The block aligner manipulates two sequences to find the highest-scoring contiguous regions (blocks), which are then joined in various combinations to form alignments. Unlike a dynamic programming or word-based approach, the Bayes block aligner, which works with both DNA and protein sequences, doesn't require the user to specify a particular substitution matrix or gap scoring system. Instead, it bases the posterior probability distributions of alignments on the number of blocks expected in an alignment and a range of substitution matrices. A Web-based Bayesian analysis tool, the Bayesian algorithm for local sequence alignment (BALSA) is also available from the centre. BALSA is described in the 'tools' section later in this chapter.

MULTIPLE SEQUENCE ALIGNMENT

Applications of multiple sequence alignment—aligning three or more sequences—range from suggesting homologous relationships between several proteins to predicting probes for other members of the same family of similar sequences in a proteome. Although multiple sequence alignment can be performed on nucleotide sequences, it's more often performed on polypeptide sequences and draws upon many of the techniques used for single pairwise sequence alignment. In addition, several novel methods have been devised to deal with the challenge of aligning multiple sequences. An overview of several key multiple sequence alignment technologies follows.

Dynamic Programming

Dynamic programming methods used for pairwise sequence alignment are easily extended to encompass multiple sequences, at least in theory. Algorithmically, there is little difference between a two or three dimensional alignment problem, as discussed earlier. However, the computational requirements for 10 or more relatively short polypeptide sequences are beyond the reach of most research laboratories. Three or four-sequence alignment is the limit for workstation-class hardware. As a result, for desktop work in multiple sequence alignment, several heuristic methods have been developed that provide results in reasonable time, even though it's usually impossible to prove that the results achieved through these methods are the best attainable.

Progressive Strategies

Progressive strategies take the salami-slice approach to multiple sequence alignment. Instead of addressing the multidimensional problem head-on, progressive strategies break the multiple sequence alignment challenge into a series of pairwise alignment problems. The first pair of sequences is aligned and then that result is aligned with the third sequence and so on, aligning each subsequent search with the previous alignment. Alternatively, the first pair of sequences can serve as the basis for aligning all subsequent sequences, which are then combined at the end of the process. Other alignment schemes are possible as well.

For example, the approach used by the PILEUP program is to start with pairwise alignments that score the similarity between every possible pair of sequences. These similarity scores are used to define the order of alignment. That is, PILEUP first aligns the two most-related sequences to each other in order to produce the first alignment. It then aligns the next most-related sequence to this alignment or the next two most-related sequences to each other in order to produce another alignment. A series of such pairwise alignments that includes increasingly dissimilar sequences and alignments of sequences at each iteration eventually creates the final alignment.

The problem with progressive methods is that the validity of the result varies greatly as a function of the order in which pairs of sequences are aligned. Errors in the earlier alignments are propagated to the later alignments. In addition, progressive strategies are a heuristic approach in that they don't necessarily return best possible alignment. In addition to PILEUP, programs that use a progressive strategy are CLUSTALW, CLUSTALX, MSA and PRALINE.

Iterative Strategies

Because of the limitation of progressive strategies due to sensitivity to errors introduced by early alignments, iterative methods have been developed that correct for the problem by repeatedly realigning subgroups of sequences. Iterative methods include the use of genetic algorithms and HMMs.

Approaches based on genetic algorithms generally start with a random definition of gap insertions and deletions and use the alignment score as the fitness function. The pattern that defines the gaps and the relative position of each sequence is allowed to mutate and mate with other patterns. Offspring of these original patterns that maximise the alignment score are in turn allowed to mate and mutate, creating other patterns. In this way, an optimal—but not the optimal—multiple alignment solution is obtained.

Multiple alignment methods based on HMMs have been incorporated into a variety of tools. As introduced in Chapter 15 on, 'Data Mining', a HMM is a statistical model for an ordered sequence of symbols, acting as a stochastic state machine that generates a symbol each time a transition is made from one state to the next. A limitation of a HMM approach is that the model must be trained before it can be used. As such, HMMs tend to be problem-specific, albeit powerful.

Other Strategies

There are dozens of approaches to multiple sequence alignment, some relegated to specific laboratories, and others vying for use as a standard in the bioinformatics arena. Many of these methods are highly specialised at solving specific types of multiple sequence alignment problems. For example, the eMOTIF Method is optimised for identifying motifs in protein sequences. Profile analysis is used for localised alignments in multiple sequence analysis. BLOCK analysis is used for working with conserved regions (blocks) in a multiple sequence alignment. Expectation maximisation (EM) is used to perform local multiple sequence alignment (as in Multiple EM for Motif Elicitation or MEME). These and other approaches are constantly evolving, thanks to feedback and support from the worldwide bioinformatics user community.

TOOLS

Although general-purpose pattern-matching tools can be used in search engines and data-mining applications, nucleotide and polypeptide sequence alignment applications generally dictate the use of bioinformatics-specific tools. As illustrated in Table 16.4, in addition to the sequence alignment tools designed for nucleotide and polypeptide pattern alignment, there are support utilities for format conversion, sequence editors and protein and nucleotide databases.

Table 16.4. Sequence alignment tools. These examples typify the dozens of pattern-matching tools available to the bioinformatics community.

Tool	Examples
Nucleotide pattern alignment	BLASTN, BLASTX, TBLASTX, DotLet, BALSA
Polypeptide pattern alignment	BLASTP, PHI-BLAST, PSI-BLAST, Smith-Waterman, ScanPROSITE, ExPASy, DotLet, BALSA
Utilities	READSEQ, Text Editors
Protein sequence databases	SWISS-PROT, TrEMBL, PROSITE, BLOCKS
Nucleotide sequence databases	GenBank, Entrez Nucleotide Database
Sequence editor	CINEMA, GeneDoc, MACAW

Nucleotide Pattern Matching

BLAST

The best known and most used nucleotide pattern-matching programs are the original Nucleotide-Nucleotide BLAST—sometimes referred to as BLASTN—and its derivatives. In addition to the most recent version of BLAST, two popular derivatives are BLASTX (Nucleotide Query BLAST) and TBLASTX (Nucleotide Query-Translated Database).

The search string representing the nucleotide sequence to be searched for is entered, in FASTA format, in the 'Search' field. The entire string can be used in the search or only a subset of the string. To use a subset, the researcher enters the subset sequence locations in the 'From' and 'To' fields of the 'Set subsequence' area. For example, to limit matches to the region in the search string from nucleotide 10 to nucleotide 20, the researcher would enter 'From' = 10 and 'To' = 20. The default search includes the entire search string.

The only other parametre that must be defined for a basic BLAST search is the database to use for the search. Database options available through a pull-down menu include, among others, 'nr' (all GenBank, EMBL, DDBJ and PDB sequences), 'est' (GenBank, EMBL and DDBJ sequences from EST Divisions), 'pat' (nucleotides from the Patent division of GenBank), 'pdb' (sequences derived from the 3D structures in the Protein Data Bank) and 'month' (all new or revised GenBank, EMBL, DDBJ and PDB sequences released in the last 30 days).

The 'limit by entrez query' option allows BLAST searches to be limited to the results of an entrez query against the selected database. Because entrez supports a powerful query engine, 'the search can be significantly narrowed through an entrez query'. Alternatively, the search can be limited to one of several dozen organisms from a pull-down menu.

The 'choose filter' option enables masks for low compositional complexity, human repeats, lookup table and lowercase characters in the search sequence; all or none of these options can be selected. The low complexity filter masks off the regions of the query sequence (the sequence entered in the 'Search' field) that have low compositional complexity. Areas of low complexity, such as those composed of only a few characters repeated, are not likely to be biologically interesting. The 'Human repeats' option masks repeating sequences, speeding the search, especially against databases containing sequences with large numbers of repeats. The 'mask for lookup table only' option is an experimental mask that eliminates hits based on low-complexity sequences. The 'mask lower case' option causes only the uppercase sequences in the 'search' field to be executed.

The 'expect' field represents the statistical significance threshold for reporting matches against database sequences. The lower the threshold, the more stringent the alignment criteria, resulting in fewer chance matches being reported. The default value is '10'; meaning that of the reported match values, 10 will occur by chance alone. In comparison, a search with an 'expect' value of '1' would likely return only 1 result by chance alone. Too small a value in the 'expect' field will result in too few search results. 'Word size' can be set to 7, 11 or 15 nucleotides through a pull-down menu.

In addition to the pull-down menu and checkbox options, the 'other advanced' field accepts command-line entry of advanced options, including the cost to open and extend gaps, the specification of penalties for nucleotide mismatch, the reward for a match and the ability to adjust output formatting. The 'other advanced' field can also be used to override many of the program default settings. For example, the command '-W12' sets the word size to 12, an option not available through the pull-down menus.

The other major options of BLAST deal with formatting the output. Formatting options range from colour graphics in which the colours represent alignment scores to page formatting. Perhaps the most useful output utility is a Database Linkout feature, which provides reference links from the BLAST Results to various NCBI databases and other resources.

BALSA

The BALSA tool, from the Centre for Bioinformatics at Rensselaer and Wadsworth Centre of the New York Department of Health, provides web based access to Bayesian-based sequence alignment. A virtually identical tool, BALSA database query, is available for database queries using either the PDB or the structural classification of proteins (SCOP) databases.

BALSA determines the probability that a given pair of sequences should be aligned by sampling alignments in proportion to their joint posterior probability. Probabilities are based on alignments produced by specific combinations of substitution matrix, gap penalty and gap extension. In operation, the two sequences to be aligned are entered in FASTA format. BALSA supports copy-paste as well as local file retrieval to populate the query and comparison sequences.

Up to four sets of scoring matrix, gap penalty and gap extension penalty combinations can be specified. The PAM-250 as well as Blosum30 to Blosum80 scoring matrices are available. Output, which consists of the posterior probability for each scoring matrix/gap penalty/gap extension combination, is sent to the E-mail address entered on the form. A separate output is provided for each matrix-gap entry specified.

Polypeptide Pattern Matching
BLASTP

Protein-protein BLAST (BLASTP) shares many of the features and options of BLASTN, with a focus on polypeptide sequences instead of nucleotide sequences. The BLASTP interface is similar to the interface used with BLASTN. The major differences are in the databases available and in the advanced options available in BLASTP. For example, the peptide parallels to the nucleotide sequence databases are available to BLASTP, including 'nr' (nonredundant GenBank CDS translations, PDB, SWISS-PROT, PIR and PRF), 'swissprot' (SWISS-PROT protein sequence database), and 'month' (the GenBank CDS translation, PDB, SWISS-PROT, PLR and PRF data released in the last 30 days).

A feature in the basic BLASTP search is the 'Do CD-Search' option, which is checked to compare protein sequences to the conserved domain (CD) database maintained by NCBI. The 'Do CD-Search' option may be used to identify the conserved domains (modules with distinct evolutionary origin and function) present in a protein sequence.

Advanced options include the ability to specify a substitution matrix and gap costs. The substitution matrix is used to assign a score for aligning residue pairs, and should reflect the types of sequences being searched. The default matrix is BLOSUM62, which assigns a probability score for each position in an alignment that is based on the frequency with which that substitution is known to occur among related proteins. The 'Gap Costs' field allows the penalties to be specified for opening and extending a gap. Increasing the gap costs results in alignments with fewer gaps.

The PSSM field holds the matrix automatically computed by PSI-BLAST (position-specific iterative BLAST). A position-specific scoring matrix (PSSM) is a matrix of scores representing a locally conserved-region of a sequence of motif. A PSSM is used in the scoring of multiple alignments with sequences. A PSSM plots the probability score for the occurrence of each amino acid along the length of a motif.

PSI-BLAST, which is based on the BLAST, algorithm, is enhanced to be more sensitive than BLASTP. This sensitivity comes from the use of a profile of the position-specific scores for every position in the alignment that is constructed from a multiple alignment of the highest-scoring hits in the initial BLAST search. The profile or matrix created by PSI-BLAST can be formatted, saved and then pasted into the PSSM field of BLASTP.

A-feature recently added to BLASTP is the ability to specify a PHI pattern, which is used by PHI-BLAST (Pattern Hit Initiated BLAST) to search for similarities that are presumably also homologs. PHI-BLAST, which expects as input a protein query sequence and a pattern contained in that sequence, searches the current database for other protein sequences that also contain the input pattern and have significant similarity to the query sequence in the vicinity of the pattern occurrences. PHI-BLAST filters out cases where the pattern occurrence is probably random and not indicative of homology.

Smith-Waterman

The Smith-Waterman dynamic programming algorithm is available on the UCSC Kestrel Server, which is an experimental, high-performance, 512-processor system. As compared to the BLASTP interface with its array of options, the interface presented by the Kestrel Server appears somewhat limited. The parametres are simply costs to open and extend gaps, the substitution matrix, the database to search and the number of alignments to report.

The Kestrel implementation of Smith-Waterman supports the use of PAM-10 through PAM-500 and BLOSUM30 through BLOSUM100 substitution matrices against the SWISS-PROT or NR protein databases or a nucleotide search against the dbEST part 1 database. A maximum of 40 alignments can be E-mailed to the address specified in the query form.

DotLet

The DotLet dot matrix analysis program, available on the expert protein analysis system (ExPASy) server, is one of the most popular of the web-based dot matrix analysis programs. The program—a Java applet—supports the pairwise analysis of nucleotide or polypeptide sequences that are pasted into the pop-up input fields accessed by the 'input' button. DotLet also supports a variety of matrices (Blosum30 to Blosum100 and PAM-30 to PAM-250), sliding window size (1 to 15) and zoom (1:1 to 1:8) through pull-down menus along the top of the screen.

Each pixel in the main display (centre, left) corresponds to a residue in the horizontal and vertical sequences, with the darker pixels representing higher scores. The histogram window to the right of the main display window supports the interactive adjustment of the display. The height of the histogram peak indicates the quality of data, in that the higher the peak, the greater the signal-to-noise ratio. The alignment panel along the bottom of the figure shows the actual sequence alignment and supports interactive manipulation of the sequence positions.

Utilities

Most pattern-matching programs accept data in the FASTA format. Format conversion can be performed manually with a text editor or a sequence editing utility such as READSEQ. A web-based version of READSEQ is available through the bioinformatics and molecular analysis section (BIMAS) of the National Institutes of Health.

READSEQ accepts and automatically recognises 16 different input formats, including IG/Stanford, GenBank/GB, NBRF, EMBL, Plain/Raw, Fitch and Pearson/FASTA. Output formats include support for the major formats, including ASN.1, EMBL, PAUP/NEXUS, DNAStrider, GenBank/GB, Phylip and IG/Stanford. READSEQ, like most file translation utilities, doesn't handle every format conversion. This is in part due to the hundreds of application-specific file formats used in bioinformatics work.

Sequence Databases

The key protein sequence databases used for sequence alignment are SWISS-PROT, TrEMBL and PROSITE. These and other databases and tools are available through the ExPASy server of the Swiss Institute of Bioinformatics. SWISS-PROT is a highly annotated protein sequence database that is highly integrated with other databases in the ExPASy system. The TrEMBL database is a supplement of SWISS-PROT that also contains translations of the EMBL nucleotide database that have not yet been integrated into the latest official release of SW1SS-PROT. PROSITE is a database of protein families and domains that contains high-level profiles such as categories of toxins, inhibitors, chaperone proteins and hormones. The major source of nucleotide sequence data for alignment research is NCBI's integrated entrez system, which contains data from GenBank, RefSeq and PDB. BLOCKS is a database of ungapped multiple protein sequence alignments. Finally, SCOP, which incorporates all PDB entries, is a structural classification database expressly designed for the investigation of protein sequences and structures.

ON THE HORIZON

The latest version of BLAST available from the NCBI illustrates movement toward integration of methodologies within the same toolset. As in other areas of computing, the hundreds of bioinformatics methods and tools have grown out of niche areas to address specific needs of investigators. However, as the field of bioinformatics matures and methodologies are extended out from their original niche areas, researchers are clustering around standards and a small subset of the many tools that have been developed, and rely less and less on translation utilities such as READSEQ. Similarly, whether traditional methods, such as dot matrix analysis and still-experimental methods, such as genetic algorithms, survive into the next generation of tools depends on how these techniques can be adapted to support current challenges in a computationally robust and user friendly manner.

Web portals, such as Entrez and, to a lesser extent, ExPASy, represent the first level of integration of bioinformatics data, methodologies and tools. They also illustrate the central role that funding from the government and academic institutions plays in the continued development and maintenance of tools to support the bioinformatics community.

Thus, the pattern-matching approaches using scores for gaps and inexact matching or black-box neural network technology discussed here are statistically valid for assessing the degree of string similarity. However, in selecting gaps and other methods to make the matches 'look good', it's important to remember that these techniques don't necessarily relate to the biology of the nucleotide or polypeptide chains represented by the symbols manipulated by BLAST or other algorithms. It's easy to rationalise the need for gaps because of the computational infeasibility of solving long string comparisons without the provision for gaps. However, even a short gap in a polypeptide sequence can disrupt the secondary and tertiary structures of a protein and probably alter its function as well.

Heuristic approaches, such as match matrices, attempt to add some sense of biological relevance to the mathematical equations that define the relative similarity of nucleotide and polypeptide sequences. It's up to individual researchers to consider the biological implications of the techniques and assumptions they make in simply filling out a form on a Web page during the course of their daily work.

## Chapter 17

Information Retrieval from Biological Databases

INTRODUCTION

As already discussed, GenBank was created in response to the explosion in sequence information resulting from a panoply of scientific efforts, such as the Human Genome Project. To review, GenBank is an annotated collection of all publicly available DNA and protein sequences. GenBank contains 2 million sequence (year 2004) records covering over 1.4 billion nucleotide bases. Sequences find their way into GenBank in one of two ways: by direct submission through tools such as Sequin and BankIt or through a data-sharing agreement conducted between GenBank, EMBL and DDBJ as part of the international nucleotide sequence database collaboration.

GenBank or any other biological database for that matter, serves little purpose unless the database can be easily searched and entries retrieved in a usable, meaningful format. Otherwise, sequencing efforts serve no useful end, since the biological community as a whole cannot make use of the information hidden within these millions of bases and amino acids. Much effort has gone into making such data accessible to the average user and the programs and interfaces resulting from these efforts are the focus of this chapter. The discussion centres on querying the NCBI databases, since these more 'general' repositories are far and away the ones most often accessed by biologists, but attention also is given to a number of smaller, specialised databases that provide information not necessarily found in GenBank.

RETRIEVING DATABASE ENTRIES: THE RETRIEVE SERVER

Perhaps the easiest way to retrieve entries from an NCBI database is by using an e-mail server called retrieve. The Retrieve server retrieves records through a simple keyword search. Available databases can be searched one at a time and searches may be simple (consisting of a single keyword) or complex (with multiple keywords strung together by Boolean operators). The address for the server is simply retrieve@ncbi.nlm.nih.gov. As with most e-mail servers, sending a mail message to the server with just the word help in the body of the message will return a detailed explanation of how to use the Retrieve service. Whenever an e-mail server is used, the message sent to the server needs to be precisely formatted so that the server can understand the instructions being conveyed by the user.

Consider the following example:

    To: retrieve@ncbi.nlm.nih.gov
    Subject: Complex query
    DATALIB swiss-prot
    BEGIN
    'histone H1' AND (Saccharomyces OR Schizosaccharomyces)

Here, the subject of the message is irrelevant to the server. However, since the subject is echoed back by the server when it returns the results, providing a descriptive subject allows the user to keep track of results when multiple messages are sent to retrieve. The body of the message begins with a DATALIB search parametre, indicating which of the available databases should be searched (here, SWISS-PROT). The BEGIN flag indicates that there are no more search parametres, and the words that follow are all search terms. The Boolean operators AND, OR and NOT can be used to join terms together; parentheses can be used to separate the terms into subsets; and quotation marks can be used to indicate a phrase that must be kept together. In the example, the server will return all entries containing the phrase 'histone H1' and either the word Saccharomyces or Schizosaccharomyces. If no Boolean operators or delimiters were indicated (i.e. if the search terms read histone H1 Saccharomyces Schizosaccharomyces), a default OR would have been placed between terms, which is most likely not what the user intended the server to do. The results from this complex query are shown in Fig. 17.1.

Often, when searches are submitted, the search is too general, returning many more entries than can be of use to the requester. For example, the foregoing search would have failed if the species names had been left out, because the phrase 'histone H1' appears in many entries. Moreover, the phrase may appear in the entry even though it is not the actual subject of the entry: for example, although the phrase was part of the title of the paper, the sequence might be of something else. When an unmanageable number of entries is found, an error is generated to that effect. Limits are placed on the numbers of printed lines and entries that can be retrieved, primarily because many e-mail systems cannot handle inordinately large e-mail messages and too many unfocused queries simply slow down the system. To help refine searches, users can specify additional search parametres, which can be used to change the number of lines or entries or to return only the titles of the entries rather than the complete listings. Users can also restrict the fields that are actually searched. Returning to the example, if the search terms instead began as 'histone H1' [DEF], only the definition line of entries would be searched for the presence of the phrase. The complete list of search parametres and field restrictions, as well as a list of searchable databases, can be found in the Retrieve Help document.

INTEGRATED INFORMATION RETRIEVAL: THE ENTREZ SYSTEM

While the retrieve server allows targeted retrieval of records, its main drawback is that records may be retrieved from only one database at a time; a user who wishes to poll a number of databases must send a separate request to the Retrieve server for each target database. It should be immediately apparent, though, that there are preexisting logical relationships between the individual entries in these numerous public databases. For example, a paper in MEDLINE may describe the sequencing of a gene whose sequence appears in GenBank. The nucleotide sequence, in turn, codes for a protein product whose sequence is stored in the protein databases. The three-dimensional structure of that protein may be known, and the coordinates for that structure may appear in the structural database. Finally, the gene may have been mapped to a specific region of a given chromosome, with that information being stored in a mapping database.

The existence of such natural connections, mostly biological in nature, argued for the development of a method through which all the information about a particular biological entity could be found without having to sequentially visit and query disparate databases. The answer to this need lies in a molecular retrieval system known as entrez.

Database: Swiss-Prot Updates (33.0+, 4/19/96)
Query: 'histone h1' AND (saccharomyces OR schizosaccharomyces)
Parse status: Ok: 0 documents retrieved.

Database: Swiss-Prot (34.0, 10/96)
Query: 'histone h1' AND (saccharomyces OR schizosaccharomyces)
Parse status: OK: 1 document retrieved.
Documents selected: 1–1 (up to 1000 lines)

>> Document 1 <<
[HIL_YEAST] HISTONE H1–LIKE PROTEIN.

ID [LOC]
     H1L_YEAST STANDARD; PRT; 258 AA.

ACCESSION [ACC]
     P53551;

DATES [DAT]
     01–OCT–1996 (REL. 34 CREATED)
     01–OCT–1996 (REL. 34 LAST SEQUENCE UPDATE)
     01–OCT–1996 (REL. 34 LAST ANNOTATION UPDATE)

KEYWORDS [KEY]
     CHROMOSOMAL PROTEIN; NUCLEAR PROTEIN; DNA-BINDING.

GENE NAME [GEN]
     YPL127C OR LPI17C.

SOURCE [SRC]
     SACCHAROMYCES CEREVISIAE (BAKER'S YEAST).

ORGANISM CLASSIFICATION [CLS]
     EUKARYOTA; FUNGI; ASCOMYCOTINA; HEMIASCOMYCETES.

CROSS REFERENCE [DCR]
     EMBL; U43730; G1244786;

REFERENCE [REF]
     [1]
     SEQUENCE FROM N.A.
     HALL J., DEPAULO T., AHMED A., BUSSEY H., FORTIN N., FRIESEN J.D.,
     STORMS R.K., VO D.H., WANG Y., WINNETT E.;
     SUBMITTED (DEC–1995) TO EMBL/GENBANK/DDBJ DATA BANKS.
     [2]
     POSSIBLE FUNCTION.
     MEDLINE; 96368276.
     LANDSMAN D.;
     TRENDS BIOCHEM. SCI. 21:287–288 (1996).

COMMENT [COM]
     –1– FUNCTION: COULD ACT AS AN H1-TYPE LINKER HISTONE. HAS BEEN SHOWN
          TO BIND DNA.
     –1– SUBCELLULAR LOCATION; NUCLEAR (POTENTIAL).
     –1– SIMILARITY: TO HISTONE H1.

FEATURES [FEA]
     DOMAIN   38   130   H1–LIKE, GLOBULAR.
     DOMAIN   148   258   H1–LIKE, GLOBULAR.

SEQUENCE DATA [BAS]
     SEQUENCE   258 AA;   27803 MW;   CE87A12B CRC32;

SEQUENCE
     MAPKKSTTKT TSKGKKPATS KGKEKSTSKA AIKKTTAKKE   EASSKSYREL IIEGLTALKE
     RKGSSRPALK KFIKENYPIV GSASNFDLYF NNAIKKGVEA   GDFEQPKGPA GAVKLAKKKS
     PEVKKEKEVS PKPKQAATSV SATASKAKAA STKLAPKKVV   KKKSPTVTAK KASSPSSLTY
     KEMILKSMPQ LNDGKGSSRI VLKKYVKDTF SSKLKTSSNF   DYLFNSAIKK CVENGELVQP
     KGPSGIIKLN KKKVKLST

Fig. 17.1. Results of a complex query submitted to the retrieve server. Note that the search was done against both SWISS-PROT and SWISS-PROT Updates (the latter contains new entries since the last major release of the database). Here, the submitted search returned one and only one entry.

Developed at and maintained by NCBI, entrez software is freely available for all the major computer platforms and allows for integrated access to PubMed (MEDLINE) records, nucleotide and protein sequence data, three-dimensional structure information and mapping information—all by issuing a single query. Entrez is able to offer integrated information retrieval through the use of two types of connection between database entries: neighbouring and hard links.

Neighbouring

Neighbouring connects entries within a given database. A user who is looking at a MEDLINE entry can ask entrez to 'find all papers that are like this one'. Similarly, a user who is looking at a sequence entry can ask entrez to 'find all sequences that are similar to this one'. The establishment of neighbouring relationships within a database is based on statistical measures of similarity.

BLAST

Sequence data are compared to one another using the basic local alignment search tool (BLAST). This algorithm attempts to find 'high-scoring segment pairs' (HSPs), which are pairs of sequences that can be aligned without gaps and meet certain scoring and statistical criteria. Chapter 15 on 'Data mining' discusses at length the family of BLAST algorithms and their application.

VAST

Sets of coordinate data are compared using a vector-based method known as VAST, for Vector Alignment Search Tool. There are three major steps in a VAST comparison:

1. First, based on the coordinate data, all of the α helices and β sheets that comprise the core of the protein are identified. Straight-line vectors are then calculated based on the position of these secondary structure elements and subsequent steps use these vectors rather than the entire coordinate set for comparison.

2. Next, the algorithm attempts to optimally align these vectors, looking for pairs of structural elements that are of the same type and relative orientation and have the same connectivity between elements. The object is to identify highly similar 'core substructures', pairs that represent a statistically significant match above that which would be obtained by comparing randomly chosen proteins to one another.

3. Finally, a refinement is done using Monte Carlo methods at each residue position in an attempt to optimise the structural alignment.

Through this method, it is possible to find structural (and presumably, functional) relationships between proteins in cases that may lack overt sequence similarity. The resultant alignment need not be global; matches may be between individual domains of different proteins.

It is important to note here that VAST is not the best method for determining structural similarities. More robust methods, such as homology model building, provide much greater resolving power in determining such relationships, since the raw information within the three-dimensional coordinate file is used to perform more advanced calculations regarding the positions of side chains and the thermodynamic nature of the interactions between side chains. Reducing a structure to a series of vectors necessarily results in a loss of information. However, considering the magnitude of the problem here— that is, the number of pairwise comparisons to be made—and both the computing power and time needed to employ any of the more advanced methods, VAST provides a simple and fast first answer to the question of structural similarity.

Weighted key terms

The problem of comparing sequence-data-somewhat pales next to that of comparing MEDLINE entries, free text whose rules of syntax are not necessarily fixed. Entrez employs a method known as the relevance pairs model of retrieval to make such comparisons, relying on what are known as weighted key terms. This concept is best described by example. Consider two manuscripts with the following titles:

BRCA1 as a Genetic Marker for Breast Cancer

Genetic Factors in the Familial Transmission of the Breast Cancer BRCA1 Gene

Both these titles contain the terms BRCA1, Breast and Cancer and the presence of these common terms may indicate that the manuscripts are similar in their subject matter. The proximity between the words is also taken into account, so that words common to two records that are closer together are scored higher than common words that are further apart. In the current example, the terms Breast and Cancer would score higher based on proximity than either of those words would against BRCA1, since the words are next to each other.

Common words found in a title are scored higher than those found in an abstract, since title words are presumed to be 'more important' than those found in the body of an abstract. Overall weighting depends on the frequency of a given word among all the entries in MEDLINE, with words that occur infrequently in the database as a whole carrying a higher weight.

Regardless of the method by which the neighbouring relationships are established, the ability to actually code and maintain these relationships are based in the format underlying all of the constituent databases. This format, called abstract syntax notation (ASN.1), provides a format in which all similar fields (e.g. those for a bibliographic citation) are all structured identically regardless of whether the entry is in a protein database, nucleotide database and so forth.

Hard Links

The hard link concept is much easier conceptually than neighbouring. Hard links are applied between entries in different databases and exist everywhere there is a logical connection between entries. For instance, if a MEDLINE entry talks about the sequencing of a cosmid, a hard link is established between the MEDLINE entry and the corresponding nucleotide entry. If an open reading frame in that cosmid codes for a known protein, a hard link is established between the nucleotide entry and the protein entry. If, by sheer luck, the protein entry has an experimentally deduced structure, a hard link would be placed between the protein entry and the structural entry.

The relationship between neighbours and hard links is best illustrated by Fig. 17.2. Each of the constituent databases or divisions (MEDLINE, protein, nucleotide, structure and genomes) is represented by a pentagon. The curved lines leading out of and back into any given pentagon represent the neighbouring relationships, which allow related entries within the same database to be found. The straight-line connections at the centre of the figure, going from pentagon to pentagon, represent the hard link relationships, which allow related entries between databases to be found. Wise use of both these types of relationship allow the user to amass an incredibly large amount of information based on just a single query, in much less time than queries of the individual databases would take.

Search Entry Points

As indicated by Fig. 17.2, searches can, in essence, begin anywhere within entrez—the user has no constraints with respect to where the foray into this information space must begin. However, depending on which database is used as the jumping-off point, different fields are available for searching.

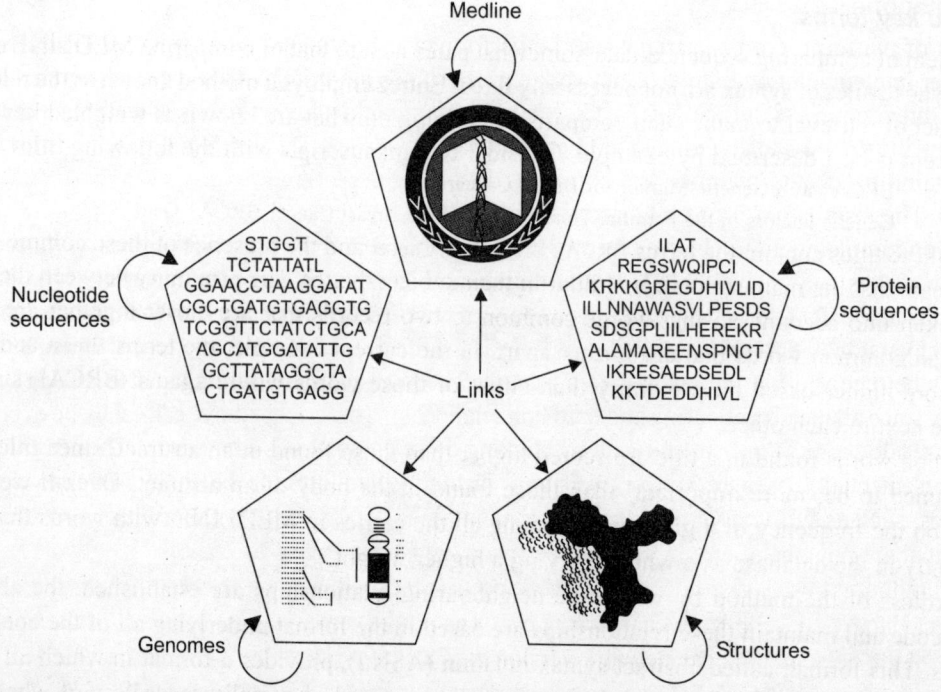

Fig. 17.2. Overview of the relationships in the Entrez integrated information retrieval system. Each pentagon represents one of the component databases; the curved lines pointing back toward each pentagon represent neighbouring relationships and the straight-lines in the centre of the figure represent hard links.

This stands to reason, in as much as the entries in databases of different types are necessarily organised differently, reflecting the biological nature of the entity they are trying to catalogue. A list of searchable fields for each of the Entrez divisions is given in Table 17.1.

Table 17.1. Searchable fields for the five Entrez divisions.

Category	MEDLINE	Nucleotide	Protein	Structure	Genome
Plain text	•	•	•	•	•
Author name	•	•	•	•	•
Journal title	•	•	•	•	•
Accession number		•	•	•	•
Date of publication	•	•	•	•	•
Medical subject heading (MeSH)	•				
Organism name		•	•	•	•
Gene symbol or gene name		•	•		•
Protein name		•	•		•
EC number		•	•		•
Chemical substance name	•	•	•	•	
Sequence database keywords		•	•		•
Feature key (e.g. CDS)		•			•
Properties (e.g. partial)		•			•

Implementations

Regardless of platform, entrez searches can be performed using one of two interfaces. The first is a client-server implementation known as network entrez. This is the fastest of the entrez programs in that it makes a direct connection to an NCBI 'dispatcher'. The graphical user interface features a series of windows, as illustrated shortly. Since the client software resides on the user's machine, it is up to the user to obtain, install and maintain the software, downloading periodic updates as new features are introduced. The installation process is fairly trivial.

The second implementation is over the world wide web and is known as www entrez or web entrez. This option makes use of available web browsers, such as internet explorer or netscape, to deliver search results to the desktop. The use of a web browser relieves the user of having to make sure that the most current version of entrez is installed—as long as the browser is of relatively recent vintage, results will always be received via the latest entrez release. The Web naturally lends itself to an application such as this, since all the neighbouring and hard link relationships described above can easily be expressed as hypertext, allowing the user to navigate by clicking on selected words in an entry. The advantage of the Web implementation over the network version is that the Web allows for the ability to link to external data sources, such as full-text versions of papers maintained by a given journal or press or specialised databases that are not part of entrez proper. The speed advantage that is gained by the network version causes its limitation in this respect; the direct connection to the NCBI dispatcher means that the user, once connected to NCBI, cannot travel anywhere else. The other main difference between the two methods lies simply in the presentation: the network version uses a series of windows, while the web version is formatted as sequential pages, following the standard web paradigm. The final decision is one of personal preference, for both methods will produce the same results within the entrez search space.

Entrez Discovery Pathway: Examples

The best way to illustrate the integrated nature of the entrez system and to drive home the power of neighbouring is by considering a biological example, using the web version of entrez as the interface. Starting at the entrez home page on the NCBI Web site, the user can select one of the five component entrez databases as the initial point of entry for a query. In this case, the search will be performed against MEDLINE. First, the user must select a Search field, which allows searches to be restricted to a particular field within a database entry (e.g. biological species or subject heading). Second, the user must select a search mode, which refers to the method of interaction between the user and the server. In automatic mode, the server will look at the term that has been entered in the query box and look for the closest match that exists in the database. In list terms mode, which provides finer control over the final search results, the user is returned a list of terms that most closely match the one the user requested. While automatic and list terms modes frequently return the same results, use of list terms is highly recommended, since terms may be indexed in anyone of a number of ways that may not be apparent to the user at the start of a search.

Suppose one wishes to retrieve abstracts on human immunodeficiency virus 1. Using the entrez query window, one could enter hiv 1 in the query box, text word as the field (so that the titles and abstracts are searched for the occurrence of HIV 1) and list terms as the mode (Of course, organism could have been used as the field; a good exercise would be to perform the search both ways to see how the output would differ). Hitting the search key then generates a new web page. This page contains a term selection window that allows the user to browse the closest matches to the original query (HIV 1). Notice that the Select window shows a number of entries following HIV 1 that are catalogued slightly differently. If the user had chosen automatic as the search mode, these extra entries would have been missed, and possibly important information as well. With list terms, however, the user is guaranteed to see all variations of the original search term.

To this point, no entries have actually been retrieved. To retrieve the entries, the user must highlight the desired term from the Term selection box (here, hiv 1) and then click the select button.

The individual entries in this window each have several elements: a checkbox, the name of the first author with the year of publication and the title and citation information. Focusing on the Jacobo-Molina 1998 entry at the bottom of the window and clicking on the author's name brings up yet another window, this one containing the citation information, the name of the paper, a list of all the authors, their affiliation and the abstract (Fig. 17.3) in standard citation format. A number of alternate formats are available and can be selected using the pulldown menu next to the display button. Switching to abstract format would produce a very similar-looking entry, the difference being that cataloguing information such as MeSH terms and indexed substances relating to the entry are shown after the abstract. MEDLINE format produces the MEDLINE/MEDLARS layout, with two-letter codes corresponding to the contents of each field going down the left-hand side of the entry (e.g. the author field is denoted by the code AU). Entries in this format can be saved and easily imported into third-party bibliography management programs, such as EndNote and Reference manager.

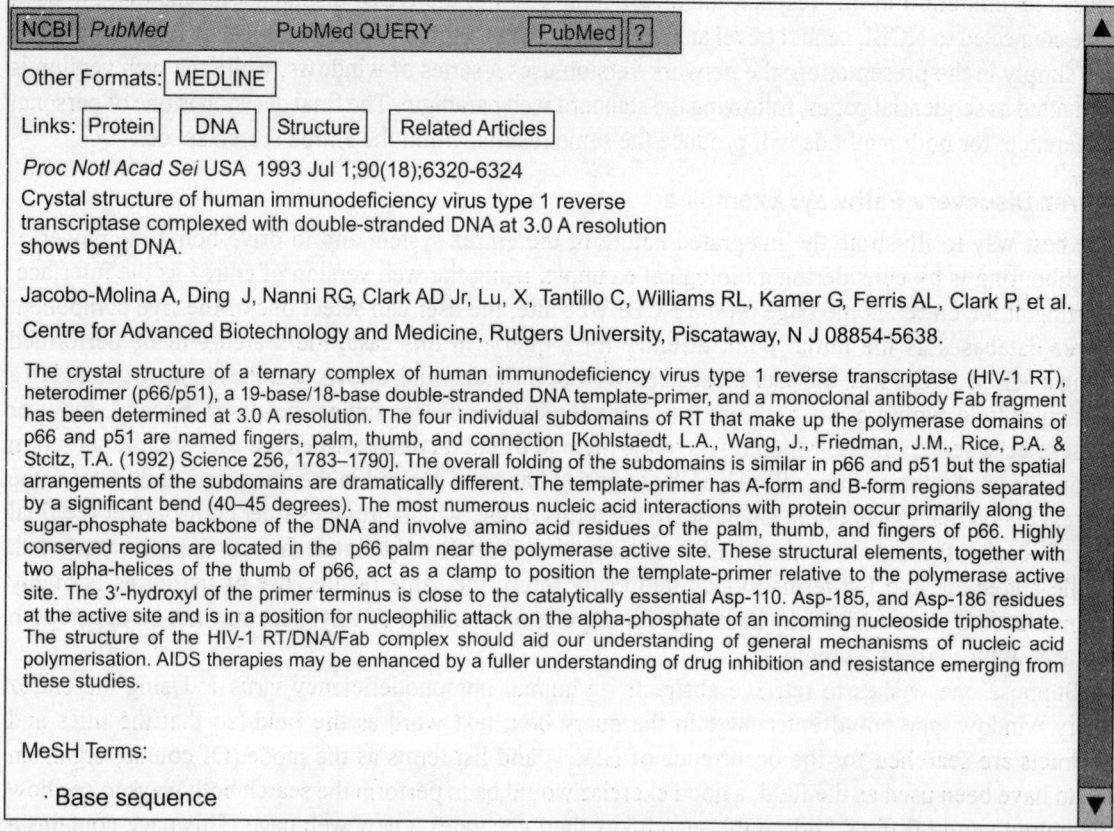

Fig. 17.3. Example of a MEDLINE record in citation format as returned using Entrez. Links to neighboured and hard-linked entries, as well as other format options, are available through buttons at the top of the window.

At the top of Fig. 17.3 is a series of buttons labelled links. This is one of the entry points from which the user can take advantage of the neighbouring and hard link relationships described earlier. If the user clicks on related articles, entrez will indicate that there are 133 neighbours associated with the Jacobo-Molina reference—that is, 133 references of similar subject matter.

Thus from above, one can summon up hard-linked entries using the checkboxes next to each entry in the list. Continuing with the example, changing the pulldown menu next to the display button to protein links and then clicking the display button, will produce a list of 19 entries from the protein databases associated with the MEDLINE entries on that page; six of these are shown in Fig. 17.4. This page generally has the same format as those already seen for MEDLINE, except that a number of hyperlinks follow each entry, corresponding either to different available formats or providing paths to neighbours and hard-linked entries. One of the more useful formats is FASTA, which provides the format needed for import into most other sequence analysis programs. The output that would be produced by clicking on any of the protein neighbours hyperlinks would represent, in essence, the results of precomputed BLAST searches of that individual protein sequence. At this point, one could follow similar steps to get to the nucleotide databases.

▦ 1HNV-A
   Chain A, Hiv-1 Reverse Transcriptase (Hiv-1 Rt) (E.C.27.7.49) Mut ant With Cys 280 Replaced By Ser (C280s), Hiv-1 (Bh10 Isolate) Expressed In (Escherichia Coli)
   gi½1065293½pdb½1HNV ½A (1065293)
   (View GenP ept Report, FASTA report, ASN.1 report, Graphical view, 7 MEDLINE links, 1700 protein neighbours, or 1 structure link)

▦ 1HNI-B
   Chain B, Human Immunodeficiency Virus Type 1 Reverse Transcript ase (Hiv-1rt) (E.C.2.7.7.49) Mut ant With Cys 280 Replaced By Ser (C280s), Hiv-1 (Bh10 Isolate) Expressed In (Escherichia Coli)
   gi½1065288½pdb½1HNI ½B (1065288)
   (View GenP ept Report, FASTA report, ASN.1 report, Graphical view, 9 MEDLINE links, 1683 protein neighbours, or 1 structure link)

▦ 1HNI-A
   Chain A, Human Immunodeficiency Virus Type 1 Reverse Transcriptase (Hiv-1rt) (E.C.2.7.7.49) Mut ant with Cys 280 Replaced By Ser (C280s), Hiv-1 (Bh10 Isolate) Expressed IN (Escherichia Coli)
   gi½1065287½pdb½1HNI ½A (1065287)
   (View GenP ept Report, FASTA report, ASN.1 report, Graphical view, 9 MEDLINE links, 1700 protein neighbours, or 1 structure link)

▦ 3HVT-B
   Chain B, Reverse Transcriptase (E.C.2.7.7.49), Hiv-1 (Bh10 Isolate)
   gi½640349½pdb½3HVT ½B (640349)
   (View GenP ept Report, FASTA report, ASN.1 report, Graphical view, 4 MEDLINE links, 1678 protein neighbours, or 1 structure link)

▦ 3HVT-A
   Chain A, Reverse Transcriptase (E.C.2.7.7.49), Hiv-1 (Bh10 Isolate)
   gi½640348½pdb½3HVT ½A (640348)
   (View GenP ept Report, FASTA report, ASN.1 report, Graphical view, 4 MEDLINE links, 1700 protein neighbours, or 1 structure link)

▦ 1RDH-B
   Chain B, Hiv-1 Reverse Transcriptase (Ribonuclease H Domain) (E.C.2.7.7.49), Human Immunodeficiency Virus Type 1 Recombinant Form Expressed In (Escherichia Coli)
   gi½576256½pdb½1RDH ½B (576256)
   (View GenP ept Report, FASTA report, ASN.1 report, Graphical view, 2 MEDLINE links, 287 protein neighbours, or 1 structure link)

Fig. 17.4. Partial Entrez output produced by requesting protein neighbours from the previous screen. See text for details.

In the list of protein entries obtained for this query were entries for 1HNV-A and 1HNV-B, an HIV-1 reverse transcriptase mutant with a point mutation (Cys 280 → Ser). Clicking on the Graphical View link produces a graphical view of all the information in that entry's Feature table (Fig. 17.5). In this case, the protein has a large number of secondary structure elements and this type of view makes it much easier to sort out exactly where those elements fall along the length of the protein. If the hyperlink labelled 1 structure link is clicked instead, a Structure summary page will be produced.

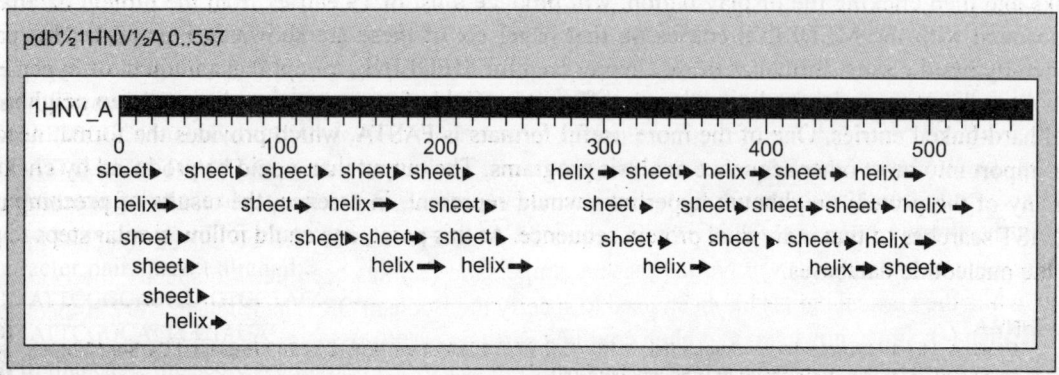

Fig. 17.5. Graphical view of a protein entry, showing all the information available in that entry's feature table. Any details known about this protein that can be attributed to particular locations along the primary sequence are shown in this view.

INTEGRATED INFORMATION ACCESS: THE QUERY SERVER

When an entrez platform is not available, as sometimes happens, a user will be restricted to performing searches via e-mail. Or, a user who can access entrez from the lab through a Tl connection may not have a fast enough internet connection at home to make using the world wide web practical. Query, the e-mail alternative to entrez, fills the gap. The idea behind query is very similar to that of retrieve, but instead of querying just one database at a time, query can search a given database domain (protein, nucleotide, structure or MEDLINE) and is capable of returning both neighbours and hard-linked entries.

As with retrieve, query users must follow a defined format when sending a search request to the server. The simplest type of search is done by search term. To perform such a search, the user merely specifies the target database and one or more search terms. As with retrieve and Entrez, term-based searches can be restricted to particular fields in a database entry, which should yield more refined results. To show the differences between query and retrieve, we will begin with the example considered in Fig. 17.6, formulated for the query server.

```
To:          query@ncbi.nlm.nih.gov
Subject:     Simple query
DB p
TERM histone H1 [PROT]
        & (Saccharomyces [ORGN] | Schizosaccharomyces [ORGN])
```

The query begins with the line DB p, which signifies that the protein databases are to be searched. Recall that Retrieve allowed users to search only one database at a time; query allows searching of all like databases at once [here, the protein databases making up the nonredundant (*nr*) *set*]. Databases are specified by a single-letter code: p for protein, n for nucleotide, m for MEDLINE, t for structure and s to search both protein and nucleotide databases at once.

Database	DB [m½p½n½t½s]
Search type–	UID [MUID½gi½acc½FASTA–spec]
use one of:	or
	TERM term field_spec

Options–	DOPT display_option
use any or all:	HTML
	DISPMAX n
	PATH address

Fig. 17.6. Generalised format for requests sent to the *Query* server. For bracketed items, users must select one of the variables in the brackets to execute the search. More detailed information on structuring query searches can be found in the text and on the *Query* documentation web page at NCBI.

The search space, then, is the same as that used during an entrez search. Unlike the original retrieve search, discrete fields have been specified to restrict the search: the histone H1 term will be looked for only in the Protein name field ([PROT]), whereas the organism names will be looked for only in the Organism name field ([ORGN]). Notice that the ampersand (&) has been used to specify the Boolean AND, while the vertical bar (|) has been used to specify the Boolean OR. The Boolean NOT is specified by a hyphen (-); since, however, a hyphen could be part of a search term as well, a hyphen representing a Boolean operator must have at least one space on either side of it, to separate it from the actual search terms.

Up to this point, query does not seem to differ much from retrieve. In fact, the foregoing search will produce the same results as retrieve. However, use of the DOPT (display options) flag can drastically change the nature of the returned results, to the user's advantage. Continuing with the example, perhaps the user wants to have the results returned in FASTA format rather than the standard entrez document summary format. Additionally, rather than seeing the protein entries themselves, the user wants the nucleotide links to those entries. To produce that result, the preceding search would be refined as follows:

DB P
TERM histone H1 [PROT]
    & (Saccharomyces [ORGN] | Schizosaccharomyces [ORGN])
DOPT fn

The fn in the DOPT statement signifies that nucleotide records (n) linked to the protein records specified by the TERM command be displayed in FASTA format (f). The results of this particular search are shown in Fig. 17.7.

Requested WWW query:

http: //www.ncbi.nlm.nih.gov/htbin-post/Entrez/query?db=p&form=4&term=
histone+H1+[PROT] ++AND++(Saccharomyces+[ORGN] ++OR++schizosaccharomyces
+ [ORGN]) &dopt=fn&dispmax=200&html=no

Content–type: text/html

Entrez reports

>gi½2131283½pir½|½S69056 histone H1 – yeast (saccharomyces cerevisiae)

MAPKKSTTKTTSKGKKPATSKGKEKSTSKAAIKKTTAKKEEASSKSYRELIIEGLTALKERKGSSRPALK
KFIKENYPIVGSASNFDLYFNNAIKKGVEAGDFEQPKGPAGAVKLAKKKSPEVKKEKEVSPKPKQAATSV
SATASKAKAASTKLAPKKVVKKKSPTVTAKKASSPSSLTYKEMILKSMPQLNDGKGSSRIVLKKYVKDTF
SSKLKTSSNFDYLFNSAIKKCVENGELVQPKGPSGIIKLNKKKVKLST

Fig. 17.7. Results of a complex query submitted to the query server. Notice that the original request sent to the server has been reformatted as a URL that can be directly opened using a web browser.

The versatility of the DOPT statement make query very useful in amassing information that is to be handled off to other programs, such as sequence alignment editors or predictive tools, particularly when the results are obtained in FASTA format.

Finally, three additional flags are available to query users. HTML will return the results in HTML format, so that the results can be viewed using any web browser. DISPMAX controls the number of entries returned; if DISPMAX is not invoked, the default is 200, but with an overriding e-mail line limit of 1,00,000. Finally, PATH can be used to return the results to an e-mail address different from the one that sent the request.

SEQUENCE DATABASES BEYOND NCBI

While it may appear from this discussion that NCBI is the centre of the sequence universe, many specialised sequence databases throughout the world serve specific groups in the scientific community. Often, these databases provide additional information such as phenotypes, experimental conditions, strain crosses, and map features. The data is of great importance to these subsets of the scientific community, in as much as they can influence rational experimental design, but such types of data do not fit neatly within the confines of the NCBI data model. Development of specialised databases necessarily ensued, but they are intended to be used as an adjunct to GenBank, not in place of it.

Two such specialised databases are the *Saccharomyces* genome database (SGD) and the *Arabidopsis thaliana* database (AtDB), both housed at the Stanford human genome centre. Focusing on SGD because the entire *Saccharomyces* genome has been sequenced, the database provides a very simple search interface that allows text-based searches by gene name, gene information, clone, protein information, sequence name, author name or full text. For example, using Gene name as the search topic and hho1 as the name of the gene to be searched for produces a SacchDB information window showing all known information on locus HHO1. The Locus window provides jumping-off points to other databases, such as MEDLINE and the yeast protein database (YPD). Following the link to Sacch3D for this entry provides information on structural homologs of the HHO1 protein product found in PDB, links to secondary and tertiary structure prediction sites and precomputed BLAST reports against a number of query databases.

Returning to the Locus window and clicking on the Seq & Display link, the user finds a graphical view of the area surrounding the locus in question. Available views include physical maps, genetic maps and chromosomal features maps, among others. The physical map view for HHO1 is shown in Fig. 17.8. Note the thick yellow bar at the top of the figure, which gives the position of the current view with respect to the centromere. Clicking on the yellow bar allows the user to move along the chromosome and clicking on individual gene, clone or sequence names gives more detailed information about that particular region.

Another example of an organism-specific database is FlyBase, whose goal is to maintain comprehensive information on the genetics and molecular biology of *Drosophila*. Access to FlyBase is available through the world wide web, gopher and FTP and by e-mail. The information found in FlyBase includes an extensive drosophila bibliography, addresses of researchers involved in drosophila projects, a compilation of information on over 38000 aileles of over 11000 genes, descriptions of over 13000 chromosomal aberrations, mapping information, functional information on gene products, lists of stock centres and genomic clones, and information from allied databases. Searches on any of these 'fields' can be done through a simple search mechanism.

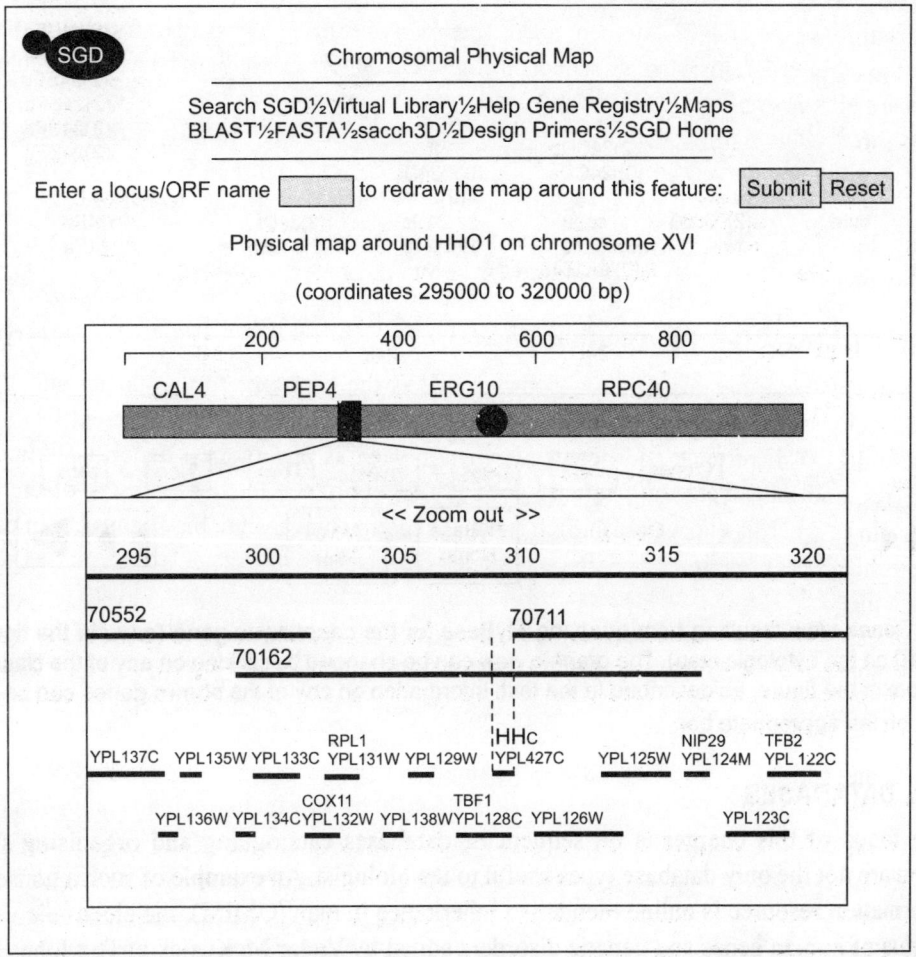

Fig. 17.8. Physical map resulting from the query generates the Locus view. Chromosome XVI is shown at the top of the Figure, with the exploded region. If an ORF has been defined, the gene name is shown in maroon, above the corresponding ORF name. Most items are clickable, returning detailed information about that particular entity.

For example, searching by gene symbol using capu as the search term brings up a record for a gene named *cappuccino*, which is required for the proper polarity of the developing drosophila oocyte. Calling up the graphical view generates a map showing the gene and cytologic location of cappuccino and other genes in that immediate area, and users can click on any of the gene bars to bring up detailed information on that particular gene (Fig. 17.9).

Information on overlaps become obvious in this view; here, cappuccino is seen to overlap with *slp1* and *slp2*, which code for transcription factors.

The view can be changed by selecting one of the class buttons at the bottom of the window, so that a graphical view of clones, deficiencies, duplications, inversions, transpositions, translocations or other aberrations can be examined instead.

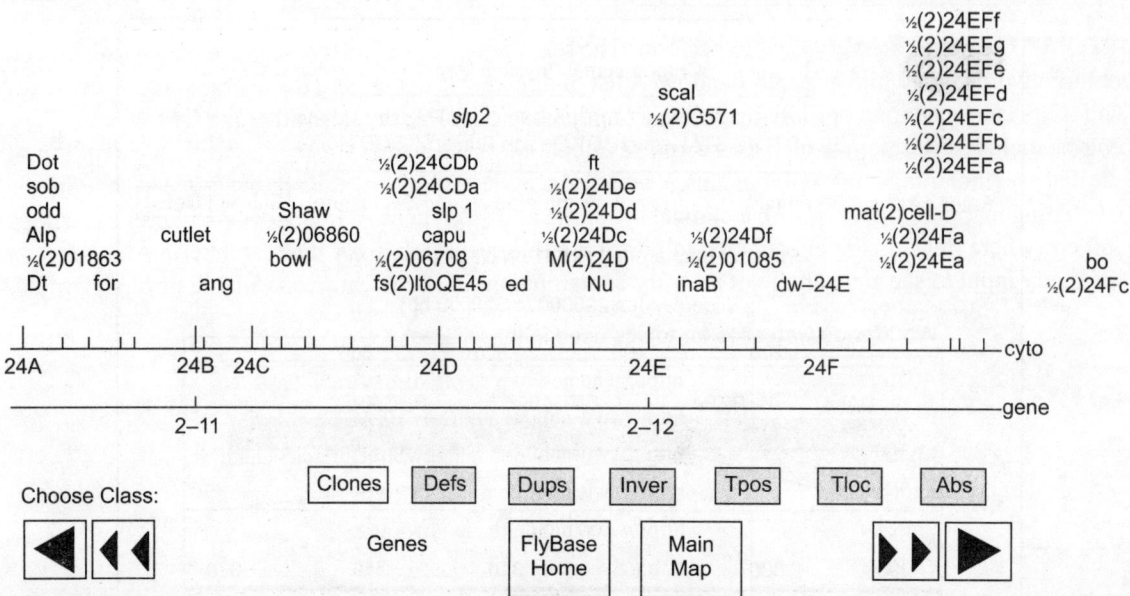

Fig. 17.9. Genes view resulting from querying FlyBase for the *cappuccino* gene (*capu* in the figure, near position 24D on the cytologic map). The graphic view can be changed by clicking on any of the class buttons at the bottom of the figure, as described in the text. Information on any of the shown genes can be obtained by clicking on the appropriate bar.

MEDICAL DATABASES

While the focus of this chapter is on sequences, databases cataloguing and organising sequence information are not the only database types useful to the biologist. An example of such a nonsequence-based information resource is online mendelian inheritance in man (OMIM), the electronic version of the catalogue of human genes and genetic disorders edited by Victor McKusick at The Johns Hopkins University. OMIM provides concise textual information from the literature published on most human conditions having a genetic basis, as well as pictures illustrating the condition or disorder where appropriate and full citation information. Since the online version of OMIM is housed at NCBI, links to entrez are provided from all references cited within each OMIM entry.

OMIM has a defined numbering system in which each entry is assigned a unique number, similar to an accession number, but certain positions within that number indicate information about the genetic disorder itself. For example, the first digit represents the mode of inheritance of the disorder: 1 stands for autosomal dominant, 2 for autosomal recessive, 3 for X-linked locus or phenotype, 4 for Y-linked locus or phenotype, 5 for mitochondrial and 6 for autosomal locus or phenotype (The distinction between 1 or 2 and 6 is that entries catalogued before May 1994 were assigned either a 1 or 2, whereas entries after that date were assigned a 6 regardless of whether the mode of inheritance was dominant or recessive). An asterisk preceding a number indicates that the phenotype caused by the gene at this locus is not influenced by genes at other loci; however, the disorder itself may be caused by mutations at multiple loci. Disorders for which no mode of inheritance has been determined do not carry asterisks. Finally, a pound sign (#) indicates that the phenotype is caused by two or more genetic mutations.

OMIM searches are very easy to perform. The search engine performs a simple query based on one or more words typed into a search window. A list of documents containing the query words is returned, and users can select one or more disorders from this list to look at the full text of the OMIM entry. The entries include information such as the gene symbol, alternate, names for the disease, a description of the disease (including clinical, biochemical and cytogenetic features), details on the mode of inheritance (including mapping information), a clinical synopsis, and references. While space precludes showing a full entry here, readers are encouraged to perform a sample search using the search term Alzheimer as the query input to see an example of an entry containing most of the features available through OMIM.

World wide web sites for topics used in this chapter.

AtDB	http://genome-www.stanford.edu/Arabidopsis/
BLAST	http://www.ncbi.nlm.nih.gov/BLAST/
Cn3D	http://www.ncbi.nlm.nih.gov/Structure/cn3d.html
EndNote	http://www.niles.com/
Entrez	http://www.ncbi.nlm.nih.gov/Entrez/
FlyBase	http://flybase.bio.indiana.edu
Kinemage	http://www.umass.edu/microbio/rasmol/mage.htm
MIPS	http://speedy.mips.biochem.mpg.de/mips/yeast/
OMIM	http://www.ncbi.nlm.nih.gov/Omim
Query	http://www.ncbi.nlm.nih.gov/Web/Search/query.txt
PDB	http://www.pdb.bnl.org
RasMol	http://www.umass.edu/microbio/rasmol/
Reference manager	http://www.risinc.com/
Retrieve	http://www.ncbi.nlm.nih.gov/Web/Search/retrieve.txt
Sacch3D	http://www-genome.stanford.edu/Sacch3D/
SGD	http://genome-www.stanford.edu/Saccharomyces/
VAST	http://www.ncbi.nlm.nih.gov/Structure/vast.html
YPD	http://quest7.protease.com/YPDhome.html

SECTION V

APPLICATIONS OF BIOINFORMATICS IN INDUSTRY AND RESEARCH

## Chapter 18

Innovations of Bioinformatics

INTRODUCTION

Bioinformatics technology uses computational tools provided by the information technology revolution, such as statistical software, graphics simulation and database management, to organise and analyse information about biological systems, which, for biotechnology, is information about cells and biological molecules.

Using another product of the information revolution, the Internet, scientists broadcast this information around the world.

Bioinformatics technology provides us with tools and methods for consistently organising, accessing, processing and integrating data from different sources.

This uniformity, in conjunction with the universal language of life at the molecular level, enables international collaboration among scientists studying any plant, animal or microbe. Bioinformatics technology helps in following ways:

1. Map genomes and identify genes.
2. Determine protein structure and simulate protein interactions.
3. Discover new therapeutic targets and design medicines aimed at the targets.
4. Assess the effects of virtual mutations on gene function.
5. Study of phylogenetics.
6. Issues and initiatives:
   (a) Prescription coverage and reimbursement.
   (b) Food and agriculture.
   (c) Industrial and environmental.
7. Bioethics and biomedical research:
   (a) Intellectual property.
   (b) Tax and fiscal policies.
   (c) Regulatory policies.
8. Media centre:
   (a) Press releases.
   (b) Industry statistics.
   (c) Bio speeches.
   (d) Site guide.

APPLICATIONS OF BIOINFORMATICS

Use in Nucleic Acid Sequence Databases

Of special importance to the progress of biological research and biotechnology are the nucleic acid and protein sequence databases. These databases have proved to be a valuable resource for the planning and evaluation of the results of sequencing experiments. They have also provided the basis for statistical analysis and the comparison of large numbers of sequences.

The availability of sequence databases has helped further biological knowledge in a number of areas. In oncogene research, for example, the complete sequences with similar ones of genes present in certain RNA tumour viruses that are implicated in case of cancer in mice and chickens. In 1985 it was discovered that one of these oncogenes, v-sis, found in a simian sarcoma virus, is very similar to a human gene gives rise to the growth factor PDGR, of platelet-derived growth factor. In the body, PDGR stimulates epithelial cells to grow, thereby playing an important role in wound heating. PDGR also plays a role in the proliferation of cells that clog blood vessels, creating the conditions that may lead to a heart attack. The computerised comparison established a surprising link between heart disease and cancer. This demonstrates that information of the function in a database.

The availability of sequence data has also furthered out understanding of evolutionary relationships among many forms of life. Using the aligned RNA or certain enzymes, biologists have been able to infer the phulogenetic relatedness of different organisms. These approaches are helping to develop more stable systems of classification, particularly with regard to prokaryotic organisms.

There are other areas of biotechnology and the life sciences that are growing as sequence information are accumulated. One area involves protein structure determinations. The elucidation of the structure and/or function of a protein often begin with the direct determination of its amino acid sequence or buy inferring the sequence from the corresponding nucleated sequence (cDNA) of the gene that encodes the protein. This capability has assisted the growth of the kind of protein engineering where the structure of proteins is determined through X-ray crystallographic studies. These studies generated and require large quantities of data-amino acid sequence, crystallisation conditions and coordinates of the 3-D representation of the protein, among them—that are analysed by elaborate computer programs. Much of this data is being stored in large databases such as the protein identification resource or the protein Data Bank of the Brookhaven National Laboratory which includes the result of structural studies of proteins, tRNAs, polynucleotides and polysaccharides. Atomic coordinates and structure factor-phase data are collected, stored and distributed.

The growth in sequence data has arisen as a result of technological breakthroughs occurring in the 1970s. Advances in sequencing made it clear that sequencing had become an important tool of the life sciences. After these developments came a rapid increase in the number of sequences. Nucleic acid sequences are now being reported for a range of known functions such as protein coding, RNA-coding, regulatory region of both DNA and mRNA and also for structural region of RNA. Rapid growth in the volume of data has led to numerous problems that demand the scientific community attention. For example, there are long lags in the submission and entry of data; there are problems ensuring sufficient review and quality control and whole more documentation on data is often needed.

GenBank

It provides a computer database of all published (and increasingly, unpublished) DNA and RNA sequences and related bibliographic and biological information. The project is funded through an NIGMS contract with Intelli Genetics, Inc. (IG) which, in turn contracts with the DOC acting on behalf of Los Alms National Laboratory (LANL). The project is funded with cosponsorship from other institutes of the National Institutes of Health, National Library of Medicine (NLM), DRR, USAA, NSF, DOE and dod. Data collection and distribution are carried out in collaboration with the EMBL data library and the DNA data bank of Japan (DDBJ).

The database provides the bibliographic context of the sequence. This is most often represented by a specific journal citation, although GenBank accepts and cites submissions of original data published in books, thesis and other sources. Increasingly, unpublished nucleated sequences are appearing in the database, although most often indirectly tied to a publication that describes the sequence without presenting it explicitly. Unpublished submissions are cited as such.

The physical context of a sequence, that is the organism, chromosome, map position, etc. describes their origin. Official nomenclature lists and map assignments are beginning to be made available to us in a form that allows GenBank to dramatically maintain proper, uniform values for these data items. The functional context of a sequence (or parts of a sequence) is also annotated in the database. A good example is protein-coding regions, which are annotated to support automatic extrication of the coding regions from the sequences in which they are embedded (GenBank uses such a tool for checking the intergrity of coding regions in the database).

EMBL Data Library

The EMBL data library was established in 1980 to collect, organise and distribute a database of nucleotide sequences and related descriptive information extracted from publication in scientific journals. Since 1982 this work has been done in collaboration with GenBank and recently the DNA Data Bank of Japan joined the colouration. Each of the three groups collects a portion of the total reported sequence data and exchanges it with the others on a regular bases. Since 1987, the Data library has begun to provide additional data sets useful to molecular biologists, including the Eukaryotic Promoter Database and the Restriction enzyme database.

Data Nucleotide Sequence

Presently distributed as flat text files where each entry comprises a single contiguous sequence and accompanying descriptive information (annotation). Different line types, each with their own two-letter code are used to make up an entry.

Although the EMBL and GenBank databases regularly exchange data, the problem has existed that the content of the two databases does not completely overlap. Unfortunately for the user, this has meant that a complete collection of nucleated sequences was obtainable only using both the EMBL and GenBank databases.

Protein Sequence Database

The Protein Sequence Database has been maintained by researchers at the national biomedical research foundation (NBRF) since the early 1960s. The database was originally completed by the late Margaret O. Dayhoff as a collection of sequences for the study of evolutionary relationship between operations and it continues to be maintained by a scientific staff as research database. The database has become truly international with the recent establishment of-PIR-International, an association of protein sequence data collection centres including NBRF (Martinsried Institute for protein sequences MIPS) and the International Protein Information Database, Japan (JIPID). All three centres are working cooperatively to produce a single protein sequence database.

Currently the NBRF effort is supported as part of the protein identification resource (PIR) project founded by the NIH division of research resources, the national library of medicine and the national institute for general medical sciences. The main purpose of this resource is to aid the research community in the identification and interpretation of protein graded computer system composed of a number of protein and nucleic acid sequence databases and software designed for the identification and analysis of protein sequences.

Currently the NBRF effort is supported as part of the protein identification resource (PIR) project founded by the NIH division of research resources, the national library of medicine and the national institute for general medical sciences. The main purpose of this resource is to aid the research community in the identification and interpretation of protein sequence information. The PIR consists of an integrated computer system composed of a number of protein and nucleic acid sequence databases and software designed for the identification and analysis of protein sequences.

A sequence entry consists of an entry identification code, an entry title containing the name of the protein its biological source, a block of text consisting of citations of summarising the experimental details of the sequence determinations, a block of descriptive information concerning the properties of the molecule and the protein sequence. The amino acid composition and molecular weight are calculated from the sequence.

SWISS-PROT Protein Sequence Database

The SWISS-PORT database, maintained collaboratively by the EMBL data library and Amos Bairoch (University of Geneva), is a collection of amino acid sequences from the protein identification resource collection along with translations of coding sequence in the EMBL nucleated sequence database. The releases are coordinated with those of the nucleated Sequence Database such that they include translation of the newest data. SWISS-PORT is essentially identical in format to the nucleated sequence database and therefore the two collections can easily be used together.

Protein Engineering Technology

Protein engineering technology will often be used in conjunction with genetic modification to improve existing proteins, usually enzymes and to create proteins not found in nature. These new and improved proteins will encourage the development of ecologically sustainable industrial processes because they are renewable, biodegradable resources.

Unlike other catalysts used in industrial manufacturing processes, enzymes, as biocatalysts, dissolve in water and work best at neutral pH and comparatively low temperatures. Because biocatalysts are more specific than chemical catalysts, they also produce fewer unwanted by-products.

The chemical, textile, pharmaceutical, pulp and paper, food and feed and energy industries are all benefiting from cleaner, more energy-efficient production made possible by incorporating biocatalysts into their production processes. The traits that make biocatalysts environmentally advantageous may, however, become detrimental in certain industrial processes. Most enzymes fall apart at temperatures above 100°F. Scientists are circumventing these limitations by using protein engineering to increase enzyme stability under harsh manufacturing conditions.

Hybrid Technologies

The biotechnologies described above, which rely almost exclusively on knowledge of cells and biological molecules, have provided us with an extraordinary array of new options. We are also combining our understanding of biological processes with scientific advances and technological innovations in other disciplines, which gives birth to a synergistic set of new technologies.

Biosensor Technology

Biosensor technology couples our knowledge of biology with advances in microelectronics. A biosensor is composed of a biological component, such as a cell or antibody, linked to a tiny transducer. Biosensors are detecting devices that rely on the specificity of cells and molecules to identify and measure substances at extremely low concentrations. When the substance of interest collides with the biological component, the transducer produces a digital electronic signal proportional to the concentration of the substance. Biosensors can measure the nutritional value, freshness and safety of food provide emergency room physicians with bedside measures of vital blood components locate and measure environmental pollutants, etc.

Animal Tissue Engineering Technology

Tissue engineering technology combines advances in cell biology and materials science, allowing us to create semi-synthetic tissues and organs in the laboratory. These tissues consist of biodegradable scaffolding material plus living cells produced through cell culture.

The most basic forms of tissue engineering use natural biological materials, such as collagen, for scaffolding. For example, two-layer skin is made by infiltrating a collagen gel with connective tissue cells, then creating the outer skin with a layer of tougher protective cells. In other methods, the scaffolding, made of a synthetic polymer, is shaped and then placed in the body where new tissue is needed. Adjacent cells invade the scaffolding, which eventually degrades and is absorbed. At other times, the biodegradable implant is spiked with cells grown in the laboratory.

Simple tissues, such as skin and cartilage, were the first to be engineered successfully. Ultimately the goal is to create complex organs, consisting of a number of tissue types that can replace diseased or injured organs.

DNA Chip Technology

DNA chip technology, a marriage of the semiconductor manufacturing industry and molecular genetics, will transform genetic analysis because it allows us to analyse tens of thousands of genes simultaneously on a single chip. The manufacturing process of microchips and DNA chips is similar, in principle; but instead of shining light through a series of masks to etch circuits into silicon, automated DNA chipmakers use a series of masks to lay down an array of DNA fragments on a glass slide.

DNA chip technology is being used to detect mutations in disease-causing genes, monitor gene activity, diagnose infectious diseases and identify the best antibiotic treatment, identify genes important to crop productivity and improve screening for microbes used in bioremediation.

DNA chips will be essential for converting the raw genetic data provided by the Human Genome Project into useful products. Sequencing the human genome, while a remarkable achievement, provides only the first milestone in the upcoming medical revolution. The gene sequence and mapping data mean little until we determine what those genes do? This field of study, known as functional genomics, helps us translate gene identification and DNA sequence data into biological functions.

Any study of gene function is, at its core, a study of proteins. Each cell produces thousands of proteins, each with a specific function. This collection of proteins in a cell is known as the proteome and unlike the genome, which is constant irrespective of cell type, the proteome varies from one cell type to the next. The science of proteomics attempts to identify the protein profile of each cell type, assess protein differences between healthy and diseased cells and uncover not only a protein's specific function but also how it interacts with other proteins.

Neither functional genomics nor proteomics is an end in itself. Their medical value will be in identifying specific therapeutic targets and helping us understand the complex biochemistry of disease processes. For more information on the exciting advances spawned by genomics and proteomics.

The technologies described above (from monoclonal antibody technology to DNA chips) have provided us with massive amounts of information, in addition to useful products. Without methods for organising and analysing the raw data, however, we will not be able to turn it into knowledge, understanding and ultimately, products. Bioinformatics technology provides us with tools and methods for consistently organising, accessing, processing and integrating data from different sources. This uniformity, in conjunction with the universal language of life at the molecular level, enables international collaboration among scientists studying any plant, animal or microbe.

Study of Phylogenetics

Similarities and differences can be observed among species because, if two species are very similar, they are likely to have shared a recent common ancestor. Phylogenetic analysis of various kinds of character can be used for such studies e.g. nucleic acid and protein sequences. These biomolecules are the most common to all life forms and allow both closely and distantly related taxa under study and they can be compared objectively. However, caution must be exercised when inferring phylogenies from sequences because the rate of mutation may not be constant and sequences may be subject to differential selection. Evolutionary relationships is generally represented by a special type of graph called a tree. It has n nodes and $n-1$ links. A phylogenetic tree is a simple way to show evolutionary relationships, with species represented by nodes and lines of descent represented by links. Such tree may be unrooted or rooted (the position of the last common ancestor of each tree member). A phylogenetic tree that shows the evolution of species as a series of bifunctions is a cladogram (binary tree). The links in a cladogram may vary in length and convey a sense of evolutionary period. Classification systems of biological organisms are arbitrary in nature because there is no standard measure of difference that can define a species, genus, family or order.

Bioinformatics helps in building phylogenetic trees

Percentage of matches (similarity table) or percentage of differences (distance table) are being prepared which are used for construction of a phylogenetic tree. Distance tables are used for the analysis of macromolecular sequence data.

Methods used for construction of phylogenetic trees

Several methods are being used for construction of a phylogenetic tree; these are as follows:

Distance matrix methods

These methods work by selecting the two most closely related taxa in a distance matrix and clustering them. The operation is then repeated until there is only one cluster left.

Maximum parsimony methods

In these methods, sequences are compared and clustered on the basis of the minimum number of mutations required to convert one sequence into another at any given position. The final phylogenetic tree is based on the overall number of changes required throughout the whole sequence.

Maximum likelihood methods

These are similar to maximum parsimony methods but include a user-defined model that allows the probability of a given substitution occurring at any given position in the sequence to be built into the algorithm. The likelihood of a given sequence change is calculated for each position in the sequence and the most reliable tree is that with the maximum overall likelihood.

Phylogenetic software available for phylogenetic analysis like PAUP and PHYLIP. These are suitable for distance matrix, maximum parsimony and maximum likelihood analysis.

Bioinformatics and molecular phylogeny

DNA accumulates mutations over evolutionary time, leading to divergence in DNA, RNA and protein sequences in different lines of descent. This principle can be used to construct phylogenetic trees. Due to differences in intrinsic mutation rate and selective constraints, different macromolecular sequences evolve at different rates, allowing the phylogenetic analysis of both closely related and distantly related organisms.

Choice of macromolecular sequences for a particular evolutionary study

The macromolecular sequence chosen for this purpose reflects the biological diversity exists in nature. Mitochondrial DNA is a rapidly evolving molecule used for such studies. For those organisms who have more diverse phylogenies, molecule of ribosomal RNA is used. Care should be taken while interpreting apparent phylogenies from poorly selected macromolecules. A few RNA viruses have rapidly evolving sequences whose repication enzymes are error-prone. Human immunodeficiency virus is an example, where up to 30 genotypes can evolve during a single infection. Rooted tree is shown in Fig. 18.1.

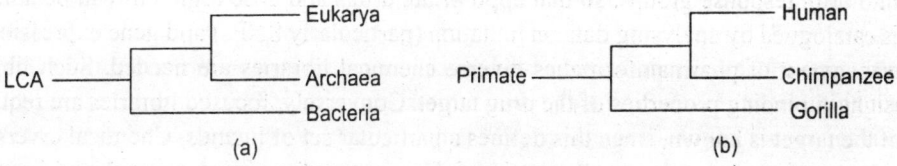

Fig. 18.1. Presentation of rooted tree. (a) Tree of major forms on this planet. (b) Three great apes with an unspecified primate ancestor.

Bioinformatics in Discovery of Drugs

Any substance, which enters human body and can change either the function or structure of the human organism is a drug. It interacts with targets, usually proteins, in the body and through such interactions cause physiological responses. The pharmaceutical industry aims to discover drugs with specific beneficial effects to treat human diseases. At first stage, for development of a new drug the basic requirement is the identification of a suitable target, which must contribute significantly to a human disease. Ideally, altering the activity of this target should have a beneficial effect thus showing its potential for therapeutic intervention. At second stage the process is lead discovery. The compounds show some of the desired activity of an ideal drug. Optimisation of lead compounds results in drug candidates that may be registered and submitted for clinical trials, which establish their safety and metabolic behaviour in human subjects.

Bioinformatics plays important role in drug development. Pharmaceutical industry have developed massive amount of data using various techniques of genomics, proteomics, combinatorial chemistry and HTS. The role of bioinformatics is to store, track and provide tools for the analysis of these data. The large-scale functional annotation of genes is known as functional genomics and incorporates areas such as homology searching, structural analysis, expression analysis, large-scale mutagenesis and the analysis of protein interactions. All of these areas are important in drug development. Genome-scale mutagenesis is a rich source of animal disease models for target identification and validation, and large mutant collections in simple organisms can be used for the rapid high-throughout screening of potential lead compounds.

Specific applications are modelling of protein interactions with small molecules allowing rational drug design, the association of genotype and drug response patterns (pharmacogenomics), the design and assessment of chemical diversity in combinatorial libraries and the processing and storage of data from high-throughout screens of lead compounds.

Computational screening

Software applications such as DOCK and Autodock match potential ligands to binding sites by calculating steric constraints and bond energies. These help in searching chemical databases of potential drugs. Some applications consider the ligand and binding site as inflexible structures, rather like pieces of a jigsaw, while others can incorporate flexibility into the molecules by calculating allowable and compatible bond torsions.

Pharmainformatics

Pharmacogenomics is the study of how variation in the human population correlates with drug response patterns. It is the study of combination of biology, chemistry, mathematics and information technology that is essential for efficient data management, processing and analysis in the pharmaceutical industry.

The analysis of genomic data and its comparison with drug response data allows patients to be clustered into drug response groups, so that appropriate drugs and dose regimens can be administered. Variation is catalogued by analysing data on mutation (particularly SNPs) and gene expression profiles.

For advancement of pharmainformatics diverse chemical libraries are needed. Such libraries will provide insight in binding properties of the drug target. Conversely, focused libraries are required if the structure of the target is known, since this defines a particular set of ligands. Chemical diversity can be defined by comparing molecules on the basis of descriptors (functional groups) and how these fill chemical space. A number of software tools are available for the design and assessment of diverse of focused chemical libraries and virtual screening against drug targets.

Cheminformatics

The study of cheminformatics is a combination of chemistry and information technology, is required for the processing and analysis of chemical data. Cheminformatics is relevant to biologists because chemistry data are important in many areas of molecular biology, for example in the study of protein interactions and metabolism.

Molecular formulae

Molecules can be represented in the form of simple formulae. They represent the number and type of atoms. However, this does not show how they are connected. Structural formulae provide some information about the arrangement of atoms in a molecule and thus allow isomers to be distinguished. Molecules are represented by using simple graphs. They show atoms as nodes and bonds as links. For organic molecules, further simplification is achieved by assuming that carbon atoms make up the molecular backbone and that the valency of four is satisfied by hydrogen atoms unless otherwise shown.

Such diagrams present all molecules as planar shapes and do not indicate the spatial distribution of atoms in three dimensions.

If four different groups are coordinated around a central carbon atom, the molecule is described as chiral and the concept is known as chirality.

Chiral molecules

Chiral molecules exist in two conformations:

1. Enantiomers (mirror-images of each other). Although enantiomers have the same chemical properties, many enzymes and other proteins show chiral selectivity, which is important in drug development and related fields.
2. Diastereoisomers (molecules may contain any number of chiral centres and a series of forms).

These may have different chemical properties because of the way different groups interact within the molecule. The absolute configuration of groups around a chiral carbon atom is described by using a number of conventions.

In the DL system, molecules are named D or L according to whether the coordinated groups are arranged in a similar fashion to those in D-glyceraldehyde or L-alanine. In the RS system, molecules are named R (*rectus*) or S (*sinister*) according to the size of the chemical groups surrounding the carbon atom.

Resources of chemoinformatics

SMILES

This system represents chemical formulae as strings, based on a valence model in which all valencies are considered to be satisfied by hydrogen atoms unless otherwise shown. The system has conventions for representing different bond types, cyclic molecules, branches, *cis/trans* isomers and chirality.

RasMol and chime

There are several specialised data formats for chemical structures based on the principle of a molecular formula and associated table of connections. Viewing utilities such as RasMol and Chime can interpret these file formats and display interactive molecular structures in a variety of user-defined schemes and colours.

Chemical structure databases

A number of comprehensive WWW resources, including chemical abstracts on-line, chemfinder and MedChem are available. Each resource provides a chemical database that can be searched using a variety of query formats, for example systematic name, nonsystematic name, formula, molecular weight or CAS registry number. Search results provide physical, chemical and biomedical information with links to other databases and resources. MedChem also provides the SMILES string.

QSAR

It is a statistical method used to determine how the structural features of a molecule are related to biological activity. The QSAR approach is particularly useful for categorising the activities of related molecules with multiple functional groups. Each molecule is broken down into a series of descriptors (molecule properties) and the QSAR determines which descriptors are most likely to promote biological activity. This gives rise to a set of rules that can be used to evaluate the potential activity of new molecules.

Protein Interaction Informatics

Proteins that physically interact with each other may be involved in the same molecular pathway or network or may form part of a multisubunit complex. Using this principle, pathways can be reconstructed based on evidence of protein interactions. However, information from other sources—for example gene expression patterns and mutant phenotypes may also be useful.

Handling Y2H data

Yeast two-hybrid (Y2H) screens produce large amounts of protein interaction data, but there is a relatively high level of spurious results (false positives and false negatives). This problem can be addressed by scoring interactions for reliability, based either on the repeatability of interactions over multiple experiments or by the number of times a given bait will trap independent clones representing the same prey. Even so, similar large-scale screen tend to identify different (although overlapping) sets of interactions.

Protein interaction databases

Several databases have been set up to store the interaction data arising from large-scale Y2H screens. However, much more information on protein interactions is available in the scientific literature and a current challenge in bioinformatics is the assimilation of these interaction data from diverse sources.

Interactome

The interactome is the sum of all protein interactions in the cell. The simplest way to represent protein interactions is a graph with proteins as nodes and interactions as links. However, when large numbers of proteins are considered, the graphs become too complex. They can be simplified by clustering functionally similar proteins, resulting in a functional interaction map that links fundamental cellular processes.

SECTION VI

PREDICTIVE METHODS AND ANALYSIS

## Chapter 19

Predictive Methods Using Nucleotide Sequences

INTRODUCTION

This chapter discusses DNA sequence interpretation methods that rely primarily on detection of functional patterns rather than on comparison with other individual sequences. For the most part, such methods are intended to first find/mask repeats and other low-complexity sequences, and then find the genes and their associated regulatory regions. These methods play a major role both in intensive investigation of individual sequences and in rapid scanning, for the preliminary inventorying of possible genes, of whole genomes or of large regions thereof. As a result of rapid progress in algorithm development, there is no single tool that can perform all the relevant sequence analysis. Thus, to make use of the best computational techniques, it is necessary to submit one's sequence to the analysis of several different software packages. To make the process as efficient as possible, this chapter provides a concise guide to current tools.

The chapter first, a description of a conceptual framework, to help put the different tools in context; next, a review of the main types of computer tool and for each, a discussion of the underlying logic and use of example programs. Current tools are useful, but by no means infallible. One limitation of current development, for example, is that many descriptions of prototype functional domains are derived, by software developers, from the domains annotated in the DDBJ/EMBL/GenBank international sequence database. However the annotation in that database can itself be derived in part from sequence analysis, leading to circularity. The strengths and limitations of individual analysis methods receive special attention in what follows. Some of the most commonly used, network-available tools are listed in this chapter.

FRAMEWORK

Whether an overall gene-finding protocol is carried out by one integrated program or by a person using several specialised programs, the basic information flow is the same. First, evidence is gathered from several sources:

1. A map of repeat locations shows where regulatory and protein-coding regions are unlikely to occur.
2. Sequence similarity to other genes or gene products provides strong positive evidence for exons.
3. Statistical regularity evincing apparent 'codon bias' over a region is one of the clearest indicators of protein-coding regions.
4. Matches to template patterns may indicate the locations of functional sites on the DNA. Such analysis can be based on very simple patterns (e.g. the well-known consensus sequences for the

TATA box and splice junctions) or on much more complex reasoning (e.g. in promoter-finding algorithms described below).

Next, all the information so gathered is integrated to make as coherent a picture as possible of the overall situation. The rules applied at the integration stage are basically common sense: for example, an exon boundary found by a codon bias analysis may be adjusted slightly to take advantage of a better splice site; and codon bias is to be taken more seriously if there is also similarity to a known protein sequence.

For any particular inquiry, only a few of the many programs for gene identification are relevant. In setting up a protocol, certain main points need to be considered: (i) for eukaryotic sequences, screening for repeats should precede all other analysis, (ii) most programs are organism specific, (iii) many programs are specific for either genomic or cDNA data, and (iv) the length of the sequence is a major factor. For example, single reads from shotgun sequencing seldom can be analysed by the more sophisticated programs designed to find whole genes in the sequence.

MASKING REPETITIVE DNA

It is best to locate and remove interspersed and simple repeats from eukaryotic sequences as the first step in any gene identification analysis. Although such repeats may well overlap regions transcribed by RNA polymerase II, they rarely overlap promoters or the coding portions of exons. Thus their locations can provide important negative information on the location of gene features. Also, repeats can often confuse other analysis, especially database searches.

For occasional analyses of single sequences, an e-mail or web-based server is adequate. CENSOR and RepeatMasker are such servers, which provide annotation and masking of both interspersed and simple repeats, through either an E-mail or a World Wide Web interface (see end-of-chapter list). Figure 19.1 shows an example of repeat analysis and masking by CENSOR.

For high-volume analysis, installation of software locally may be necessary for efficiency. Of course privacy is also enhanced by carrying out the analysis locally. The source code for XBLAST (not to be confused with BLASTX) is available on the internet. Several collections of repeats are provided by J. Jurka in the Repbase collection. J.-M. Claverie also provides a curated Alu collection in association with the XBLAST software. For local installation it may also be useful to add cloning vector sequences to these sequence collections, to allow vectors to be masked out in the same step with repeat masking.

DATABASE SEARCHES

Searching for a known homolog is perhaps the oldest and most widely understood means of identifying new protein-coding genes, as well as snRNA and rRNA genes. Such searches depend only on evolutionary relatedness, and so are widely applicable. This section comments only on 'database searching techniques' and their specific application to finding genes.

Integrated gene-finding services are beginning to include database searches as part of the analysis. However, in some cases, the database search step still needs to be done separately by the user. For protein-coding genes, translating the sequence in all six possible reading frames and using the result as a query against databases of amino acid sequences and functional motifs is usually the best first step for finding important matches. Once a homolog has been found, procrustes may be used to make an optimal alignment between the known gene product and the new gene.

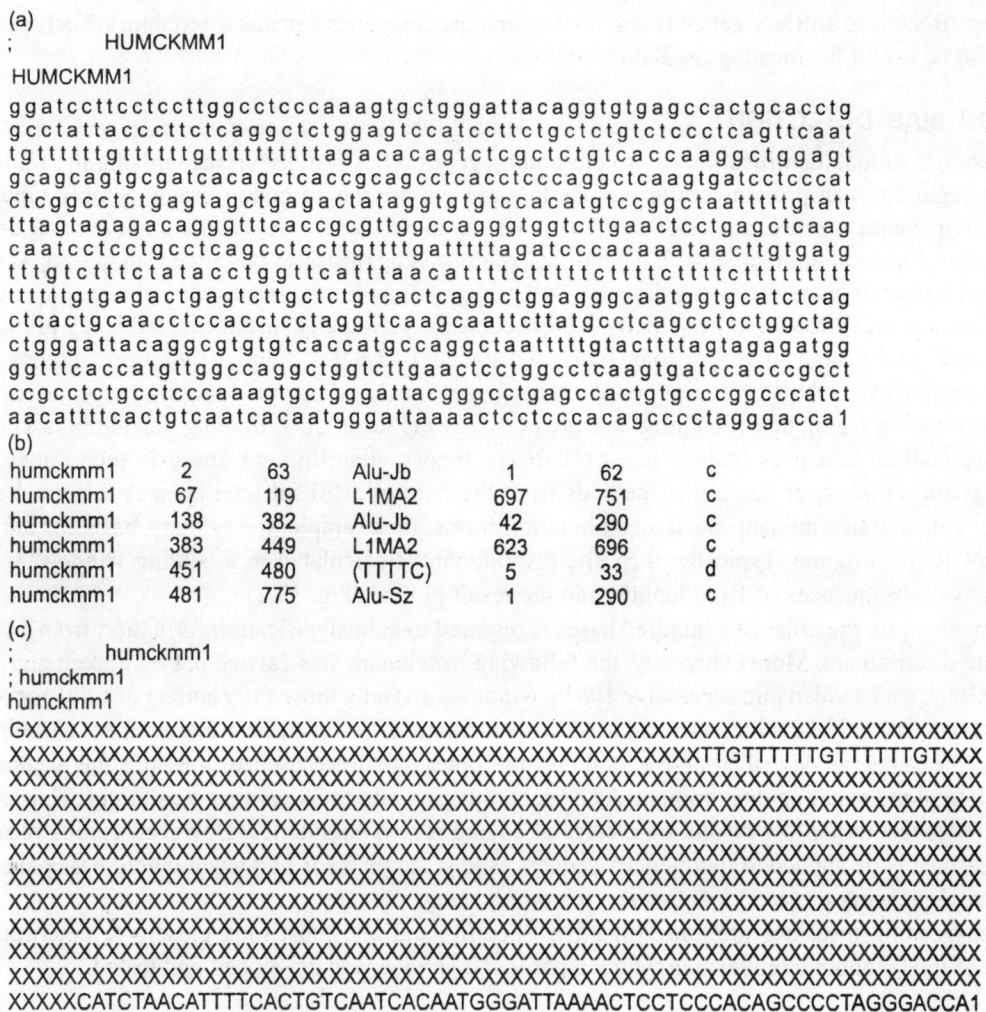

Fig. 19.1. Repeat analysis by CENSOR: (a) the input sequence; (b) the Feature table produced by CENSOR; and (c) the output sequence, with the repeats masked.

A major advantage of finding a homologous product is of course that some of the biology of the gene may be already elucidated. But there are two caveats. First, annotation by similarity may merely propagate errors. Second, only about half the new proteins being discovered have a homolog already in the databases, and this fraction seems to be increasing rather slowly. Green found that: (i) most ancient conserved regions (or ACRs, roughly defined as regions of protein sequences showing highly significant homologies across phyla) of the protein universe are already known and may be found in current databases; (ii) roughly 20–50 per cent of newly found genes contain an ACR that is represented in the databases; and (iii) rarely expressed genes are less likely to contain an ACR than moderately or highly expressed ones.

A direct search of nucleotide sequence databases will also be valuable. The EST (partial cDNA sequence) databases probably contain fragments of a majority of all genes. Thus they are an important resource for locating some part of most genes. However, it is not yet clear to what extent they are useful for delimiting gene structure. It is well known that nucleotide database searches are a valuable means of locating rRNA and snRNA genes (though of course pseudogenes remain a problem). Such searches may also be useful for locating regulatory regions.

CODON BIAS DETECTION

Most computational identification of protein-coding genes relies heavily on recognising the somewhat diffuse regularities in protein-coding regions that are due to bias in codon usage. Simply tabulating codon frequencies is one example of a coding measure, that is, a rule for calculating a number or table of numbers, meant to summarise such regularities. Many coding measures have been suggested; probably the most informative are dicodon counts (i.e. frequency counts for the occurrence of successive codon pairs), some direct measure of periodicity (in this context, 'periodicity' means the tendency of multiple occurrences of the same nucleotide to be found at distances of 3,6,9, . . . , bp), a measure of homogeneity versus complexity (such as counting long homopolymer runs) and open reading frame occurrence.

Many coding region detection programs are primarily the result of combining the numbers from one or more coding measures (using, e.g. probability theory, discriminant analysis techniques from multivariate statistics, or neural net methods from the field of artificial intelligence) to form a single number called a discriminant. Such a combination forms, for example, the primary basis for the well-known GRAIL program. Typically, then, the discriminant is calculated in a 'sliding window' (i.e. for successive subsequences of fixed length) and the result plotted (Fig. 19.2).

Something on the order of a hundred bases is required to gain significant information from a coding measure discriminant. More concretely, the following benchmark was carried out by Fickett and Tung: (i) GenBank was divided into successive 108 bp windows, (ii) only those fully coding or fully noncoding were saved, (iii) half the windows were used to set the parametres in a linear discriminant combination of four measures, as described above, and (iv) the other half were used to measure the accuracy of prediction of the resulting discriminant. A correct prediction rate of 88 per cent was found. Thus coding measures give a rather low-resolution picture of coding region boundaries. However, coding measures may reasonably be applied to fragmentary sequences (e.g. single reads of a few hundred base pairs from shotgun sequencing projects) and this is a major advantage.

Many coding measures are quite organism specific, and one must look closely to determine the subset of the taxonomic universe in which a particular service was developed and tested.

DETECTING FUNCTIONAL SITES IN THE DNA

Coding measures probably have little in common with the way a cell recognises and expresses genes. It will be more enlightening (and accuracy probably will improve) when we are able to recognise those locations, such as transcription factor binding sites and exon/intron junctions, where the gene expression machinery interacts with the nucleic acid.

One way to summarise the essential information content of these locations (typically called 'signals' by those who develop gene identification algorithms) is to give the consensus sequence, consisting of the most common base at each position of an alignment of specific binding sites. Consensus sequences are very useful as mnemonic devices but are typically not very reliable for discriminating true sites from pseudosites, in part because they contain no information on how often the other three bases can occur at each position. Many algorithms using more sophisticated techniques can give better discrimination. One technique with a basis in physical chemistry is that of the position weight matrix (PWM). A score is assigned to each possible nucleotide at each possible position of the signal. For any particular sequence, considered as a possible occurrence of the signal, the appropriate scores are summed to give a score to a potential site. Under some circumstances this score may be approximately proportional to the energy of binding for a control (ribonucleo) protein.

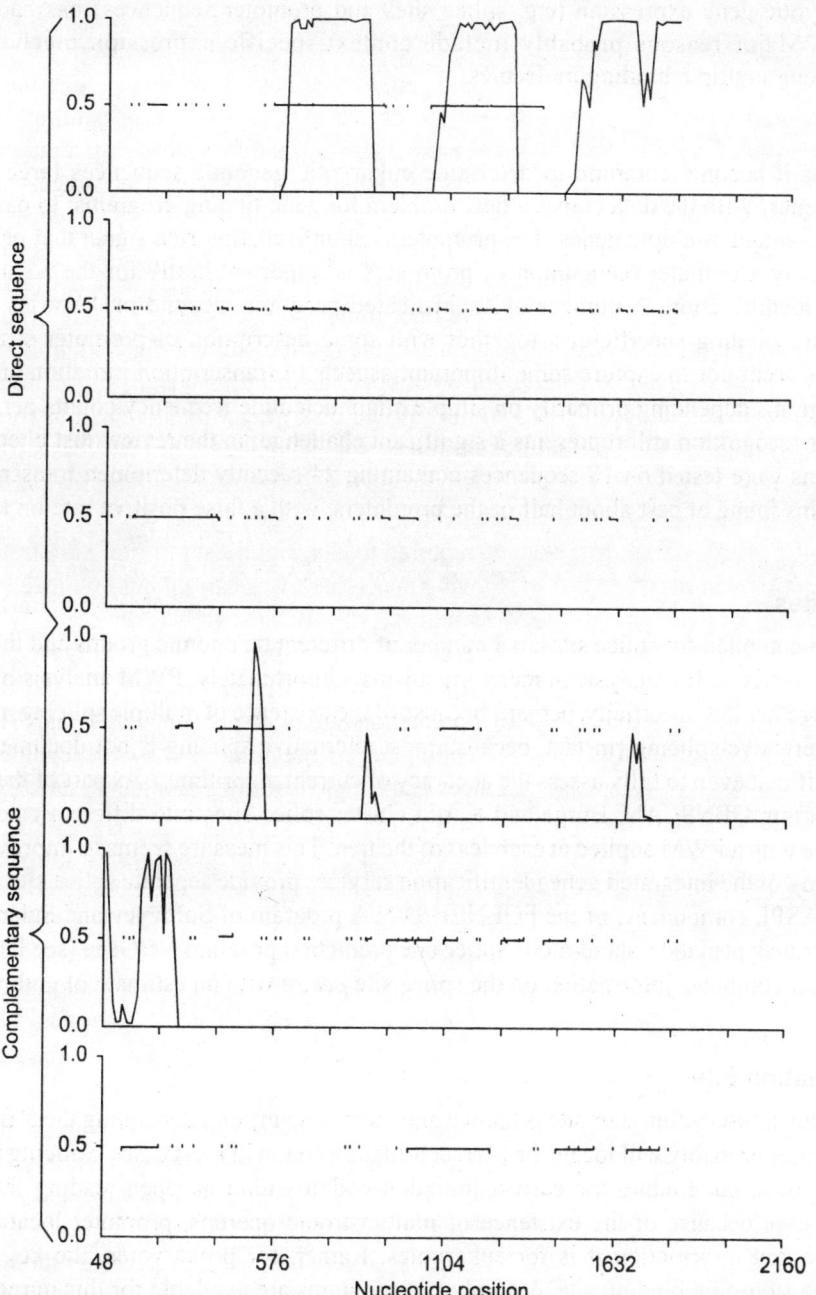

Fig. 19.2. Partial sample output from GenMark, an e-mail service for coding region identification. GenMark has seven probabilistic models of DNA, based on counts of hexamers in noncoding regions and in each of the six possible reading frames of coding regions. The program calculates the probability that windows of DNA are noncoding or should be read in one of the six reading frames.

There have been a few studies showing that a PWM works well to evaluate individual binding sites of a particular kind. Unfortunately, however, using PWMs in isolation for recognising complex elements of general eukaryotic gene expression (e.g. splice sites and promoter sequences) has had relatively limited success. Major reasons probably include context-specific expression mechanisms and cooperativity among multiple binding molecules.

Promoters

Only recently has it become common to determine eukaryotic genomic sequences large enough to contain several genes. With the data comes a new problem for gene finding programs: to partition a set of exons correctly among multiple genes. The promoter is an information-rich signal that performs this function biologically. Computer recognition of promoters is important partly for the advance it may provide in gene identification. A number of sophisticated programs depend on libraries describing transcription factor binding specificities, together with some description of promoter structure. But these descriptions seem not to capture some important aspects of transcription initiation and, perhaps surprisingly, programs depending primarily on simple oligonucleotide frequency counts perform about as well. Promoter recognition still represents a significant challenge: in the review just cited, currently available programs were tested on 18 sequences containing 24 recently determined transcription start sites. The programs found at best about half of the promoters, with a false positive rate on the order of one per kilobase.

Intron Splice Sites

PWMs have been compiled for splice sites in a number of different taxonomic groups and these may be the best resource available for analysis in many organisms. Unfortunately, PWM analysis of the splice junction provides rather low specificity, perhaps because of the existence of multiple splicing mechanisms and regulated alternative splicing (in fact, because most alternative splicing is not documented in the databases, it is difficult even to fully assess the accuracy of current algorithms). As part of the integrated gene-finding program GENSCAN, Burge and Karlin cluster splice sites into different categories and use a decision tree with a PWM applied at each leaf of the tree. This measure seems to improve accuracy significantly. Many of the integrated gene identification services provide separate splice site predictions (e.g. the H/D/N/ASPL components of the FGENEH/D/N/A program of Solovyev and Salamov).

In addition, Brunak provide a stand-alone splice site prediction program NetGene (see list at the end of the chapter) that combines information on the splice site *per se* with an estimate of coding potential on either side.

Translation Initiation Site

In eukaryotes, if the transcription start site is known and there is no intron interrupting the 5' untranslated region, Kozak's rules probably will locate the correct initiation codon in most cases. Splicing is normally absent in prokaryotes, but finding the correct initiation codon within an open reading frame is still difficult. In this case because of the existence of multicistronic operons, promoter location, though useful, is not the key information it is for eukaryotes. Rather, for prokaryotes, the key is reliable localisation of the ribosome binding site. A number of programs are available for this purpose.

Termination Signals

The polyadenylation and translation termination signals seem to be much less informative than the signals at the beginnings of genes, but these can nevertheless also help to demarcate the extent of a gene.

INTEGRATED GENE PARSING

The first generation of computational aids for gene identification treated mainly the recognition of isolated aspects of genes—for example, splice sites alone, or the regularities of coding regions without reference to signals.

But if, for example, a splice site interrupts a coding region, it will help in detection to look for coding region on one side and noncoding on the other. It has been shown that taking into account the overall consistency of putative features significantly increases prediction accuracy. For example, 60 per cent of exons under 50 bp missed by the original GRAIL E-mail program may be detected when a simple logical analysis of splicing and frame is added.

Integrated gene-finding programs begin by searching for signals and performing a coding region analysis (and sometimes doing homology searches as well). Then, by optimising some scoring function, they attempt to define exons and to give one or more tentative gene structures that seem most consistent with all the data at hand. Increased accuracy and user convenience are the primary forces behind the development of these programs.

Several such integrated algorithms are now available (Table 19.1) and at least in some circumstances can give a good idea of gene structure. The results of analysing the human enolase gene sequence (HSEN03; accession X56832) with GENSCAN (after masking repeats) are shown in Fig. 19.3.

Table 19.1. Internet tools for identification of protein-coding genes.

Service	Organism(s)	E-mail address and/or web site
EcoParse	*Escherichia coli*	e-mail: ecoparse@cse.ucsc.edu
FGENEH/D/N/Y/A	Mammalian, *Drosophila*	e-mail: analysis@theory.bchs.uh.edu
CDSB	nematode, yeast, plant and bacteria	http://defrag.bcm.tmc.edu:9503/ltp.html
GeneID	Vertebrate	e-mail: geneid@darwin.bu.edu
GeneMark	Many individual species	e-mail: genemark@ford.gatech.edu
		http://intron.biology.gatech.edu/~genmark
GeneParser	Human	http://beagle.colorado.edu/~eesnyder/GeneParser.html
Genie	Human	http://www-hgc.lbl.gov/inf/genie.html
GenLang	Dicotyledons, *Drosophila*, vertebrates	e-mail: genlang@cbil.humgen.upenn.edu
		http://cbil.humgen.upenn.edu/~sdong/genlang_home.html
GENSCAN	Vertebrate, *Caenorhabditis*, maize, *Arabidopsis*	e-mail:genscan@gnomic.stanford.edu
		http://genomic.stanford.edu/~chris/GENSCANW.html
Gen View	Human, mouse, Diptera	http://www.itba.mi.cnr.it/webgene
GRAIL/GAP/	Human	e-mail: grail@ornl.gov
XGRAIL		http://avalon.epm.ornl.gov/gallery.html
MZEF	Human, mouse, *Arahidopsis*, fission yeast	http://www.cshl.org/genefinder
Procrustes	Any	http://www-hto.usc.edu/software/procrustes

For comparison, the GenBank annotation reads:

CDS join (1579. .1663, 2540. .2635, 2796. .2854, 3016. .3085, 3455. .3588, 4820. .5042, 5153. .5350, 5688. .5889, 6318. .6426, 6576. .6634, 6723. .6792)

Predicted genes/exons:

Gn. Ex	Type S	.Begin	...End	.Len	Fr	Ph	I/Ac	Do/T	CodRg	P....	Tscr..
1.01	Init +	1579	1663	85	0	1	114	54	131	0.741	13.24
1.02	Intr +	2540	2635	96	0	0	1	100	134	0.698	6.38
1.03	Intr +	3455	3588	134	0	2	101	81	136	0.999	15.07
1.04	Intr +	4820	5042	223	1	1	85	56	432	0.998	37.93
1.05	Intr +	5153	5350	198	0	0	73	81	371	0.999	34.74
1.06	Intr +	5688	5889	202	1	1	53	69	378	0.979	31.27
1.07	Intr +	6318	6426	109	0	1	62	80	20	0.843	−0.61
1.08	Intr +	6576	6634	59	2	2	105	77	51	0.888	3.87
1.09	Term +	6723	6792	70	0	1	63	54	98	0.785	1.61
1.10	PlyA +	6853	6858	6							1.05

Predicted peptide sequence(s):

>gi ½ GENSCAN_predicted_peptide_1 ½ 391_aa

```
MAMQKIFAREILDSRGNPTVEVDLHTAKGRFRAAVPSGASTGIYEALELRDGDKGRYLGK
AKFGANAILGVSLAVCKAGAAEKGVPLYRHIADLAGNPDLILPVPAFNVINGGSHAGNKL
AMQEFMILPVGASSFKEAMRIGAEVYHHLKGVIKAKYGKDATNVGDEGGFAPNILENNEA
LELLKTAIQAAGYPDKVVIGMDVAASEFYRNGKYDLDFKSPDDPARHITGEKLGELYKSF
IKNYPVVSIEDPFDQDDWATWTSFLSGVNIQIVGDDLTVTNPKRIAQAVEKKACNCLLLK
VNQIGSVTESIQACKLAQSNGWGVMVSHRSGETEDTFIADLVVGLCTGQIKTGAPCRSER
LAKYNQLMRIEEALGDKAIFAGRKFRNPKAK
```

Column	Description
Gn.Ex	gene number, exon number (for reference)
Type	Init = Initial exonIntr = Internal exon
	Term = Terminal exonSngl = Single-exon gene
	Prom = PromoterPlyA = poly-A signal
S	DNA strand (+ = input strand; − = opposite strand)
Begin	beginning of exon or signal (numbered on input strand)
End	end point of exon or signal (numbered on input strand)
Len	length of exon or signal (bp)
Fr	reading frame (a codon ending at x is in frame f = x modulo 3)
Ph	net phase of exon (exon length modulo 3)
I/Ac	initiation signal or acceptor splice site score (x 10)
Do/T	donor splice site or termination of signal score (x 10)
CodRg	coding region score (x 10)
P	probability of exon (sum over all parses containing exon)
Tscr	exon score (depends on length, B/Ac, Do/T and CodRg scores)

Fig. 19.3. Sample output from GENSCAN; see text for details.

Table 19.2 lists these results in more human-readable form.

The main limitations of the programs (in this first generation of a new technology) are these: (i) integrated algorithms are currently available for only a few organisms, (ii) for all but one (GENSCAN) of these programs, if the input includes multiple genes or partial genes, the predicted exons may still make sense, but predicted gene structures may not, (iii) for reasons that are not altogether clear, accuracy may be considerably lower than originally thought, particularly on genes recently discovered (when Burset and Guigó, benchmarked available programs on a few hundred simple cases, no program succeeded in correctly predicting more than about half the exons), (iv) most integrated algorithms are apparently quite sensitive to sequencing errors, and (v) such facets of gene syntax as alternative splicing, overlapping genes and promoter structure remain beyond the reach of current programs.

Since none of the integrated gene identification programs is perfect, all embody somewhat different algorithms and all are rapidly evolving, analysis of each sequence with, say, three or four programs and carefully comparing the results is very strongly suggested. If the tools are to be used often, it may be worthwhile to analyse a number of test sequences, where the answer is already known, to get a feeling for algorithm capabilities.

Table 19.2. Comparison of predicted and annotated gene.

Predicted exons	Annotated exons
1579–1663	1579–1663
2540–2635	2540–2635
	2796–2854
	3016–3085
3455–3588	3455–3588
4820–5042	4820–5042
5153–5350	5153–5350
5688–5889	5688–5889
6318–6426	6318–6426
6576–6634	6576–6634
6723–6792	6723–6792

FINDING tRNA GENES

Recognition of tRNA genes is easier than recognition of protein coding genes, in part because of the simpler structure of pol III promoters and the conserved secondary structure of tRNAs. The tRNA gene recognition problem has apparently been solved in tRNAscan-SE, which combines elements of several earlier programs. Lowe and Eddy found that over 99 per cent of true tRNA genes could be identified by taking the union of the predictions of tRNAscan, which relies on a secondary structure check and PWM detection of two conserved promoter elements, with those of the algorithm of Pavesi, which relies on an analysis of transcription control elements. This merged prediction list contains over 50 per cent false positives. A very selective algorithm, COVELS, was found to remove essentially all false positives from this list. The overall result is a method that reportedly identifies over 99 per cent of true tRNA genes with less than one false positive expected per genome. Both a server and the tRNAscan-SE software are available (see end-of-chapter list). Sample output is shown in Fig. 19.4.

Sequence name	tRNA #	tRNA begin	Bounds end	tRNA type	Anti codon	Intron begin	Bounds end	Cove score
Your-seq	1	2348	2420	Val	TAC	0	0	76.52
Your-seq	2	2440	2512	Thr	TGT	0	0	77.70
Your-seq	3	2522	2594	Lys	TTT	0	0	84.24
Your-seq	4	2627	2698	Gly	GCC	0	0	75.46
Your-seq	5	2709	2794	Leu	TAA	0	0	62.99
Your-seq	6	2803	2876	Arg	ACG	0	0	71.02
Your-seq	7	2900	2973	Pro	TGG	0	0	79.67
Your-seq	8	2997	3069	Ala	TGC	0	0	71.25
Your-seq	9	4841	4914	Ile	GAT	0	0	84.04

Fig. 19.4. Sample output from tRNAscan-SE. The sequence analysed was SA5SRR, accession L36472, from *Staphylococcus aureus*. The tRNA genes predicted coincide exactly with those annotated in DDBJ/EMBL/GenBank.

FUTURE PROSPECTS

In the recent past the best techniques often were not easily accessible to the average user. The situation is getting better, with a number of Internet services easily available and a WWW page that is continually providing more of these services through a single interface. Even so, a user wanting access to a suite of state-of-the-art algorithms still must be willing to submit the data to a number of programs and furthermore, to either send data over the Internet (a difficulty if privacy is essential) or hire a programmer to import and install various programs. In the case of large-scale sequencing, one must further devise a means to automatically submit the sequence to all the programs and distill all the results in a way that makes sense to the end user. A very valuable development would be a framework for tool integration allowing every member of the community to continue independent development and also allowing workers with relatively little training in programming to integrate any set of such programs into a protocol appropriate for a particular laboratory. Such a framework might be based on e-mail and the world wide web. A new and very exciting development is the attempt to capture current understanding of transcriptional regulatory mechanisms in software, so as to provide, by computational analysis, some idea of the context under which a gene is expressed. The specification of transcriptional context seems usually to depend on more complex patterns than the binding of a single factor. While practical tools do not yet exist for the prediction of gene expression patterns from DNA sequence, it is not unreasonable to hope that such tools will be available in next few years.

Internet resources for repeat analysis and other topics presented in chapter 19.

Service	Organism(s)	Address
Repeat analysis		
CENSOR: annotates repeats in sequence and masks them out	Human or rodent	e-mail: censor@sharon.lpi.org see also http://www.girinst.org
Repbase: repeat collections	Human and several other collections	ftp ncbi.nlm.nih.gov; repository/repbase/REF; also http://www.girinst.org
Repeat masker: annotates repeats in sequence and masks them out	Several subgroups of vertebrates	http://ftp.genome.washington.edu/index.html
XBLAST: tools to mask repeat occurrences	Any	ftp ncbi.nlm.nih.gov; pub/jmc
Other topics		
BCM search Launcher (interface to multiple analysis tools)	Any	http://gc.bcm.tmc.edu:8088/search-launcher/launcher.html
Bibliography for computational gene identification	All	http://linkage.rockefeller.edu/wli/gene/list.html
Netgene (splice site identification)	Human	e-mail: netgene@cbs.dtu.dk
Procrustes (gene delineation by alignment)	Any	http://www-hto.usc.edu/software/procrustes
tRNAscan-SE (tRNA gene identification)	Any	http://genome.wustl.edu/eddy/

## Chapter 20

Predictive Methods Using Protein Sequences

INTRODUCTION

The discussions of databases and information retrieval in earlier chapters of this book document the tremendous explosion in the amount of sequence information available in a variety of public databases. As we have already seen with nucleotide sequences, all protein sequences, whether determined directly or through the translation of an open reading frame in a nucleotide sequence, contain intrinsic information of value in determining their structure or function. Unfortunately, experiments aimed at extracting such information cannot keep pace with the rate at which raw sequence data is being produced. Techniques such as circular dichroism spectroscopy, optical rotatory dispersion. X-ray crystallography, and nuclear magnetic resonance are extremely powerful in determining structural features, but their execution requires many hours of highly skilled, technically demanding work. The gap in information becomes obvious in comparisons of the size of the protein sequence and structure databases; as on 2004 there were 428,814 entries in the nonredundant protein sequence database (nr), but only 5017 protein entries in PDB. Attempts to close the gap centre around predictive methods. These entries can provide insights as to the properties of a protein in the absence of biochemical data.

This chapter focuses on computational techniques that allow for biological discovery based on the protein sequence itself; most of these techniques do not rely on pairwise or multiple sequence alignments in the sense used in earlier chapters. Unlike nucleotide sequences, which are composed of four bases that are chemically rather similar (yet distinct), the alphabet of 20 amino acids found in proteins allows for much greater diversity of structure and function, primarily because the differences in the chemical makeup of these residues are more pronounced.

Each residue can influence the overall physical properties of the protein because these amino acids are basic or acidic, hydrophobic or hydrophilic, have straight chains, branched chains, or are aromatic. Thus each residue has certain propensities to form structures of different types in the context of a protein domain. These properties, of course, are the basis for one of the central tenets of biochemistry: that sequence specifies conformation.

The major precaution with respect to these or any other predictive techniques is that regardless of the method, the results are predictions. Different methods, using different algorithms, may or may not produce different results and it is important to understand how a particular predictive method works rather than just approaching the algorithm as a 'black box': one method may be appropriate in a particular case but totally inappropriate in another. Even so, the potential for a powerful synergy exists: proper use of these techniques along with primary biochemical data can provide valuable insights into protein structure and function.

PROTEIN IDENTITY BASED ON COMPOSITION

The physical and chemical properties of each of the 20 amino acids are fairly well understood and a number of useful computational tools have been developed for making predictions regarding the identification of unknown proteins based on these properties (and *vice versa*). Many of these tools are available through the ExPASy server at the Geneva University Hospital and the University of Geneva. The focus of the ExPASy tools is twofold: to assist in the analysis and identification of unknown proteins isolated through two-dimensional gel electrophoresis, as well as to predict basic physical properties of a known protein. These tools capitalise on the curated annotations in the SWISS-PROT database in making their predictions. While calculations such as these are useful in electrophoretic analysis, they can be very valuable in any number of experimental areas, particularly in chromatographic and sedimentation studies. In this and the following section, tools in the ExPASy suite are identified, but the ensuing discussion also includes a number of useful programs made available by other groups. Internet resources related to these and other tools discussed in this chapter are listed at the end of the chapter.

AACompIdent and AACompSim (ExPASy)

Rather than using an amino acid sequence to search SWISS-PROT, AACompIdent uses the amino acid composition of an unknown protein to identify known proteins of the same composition. As inputs, the program requires the desired amino acid composition, the pI and molecular weight of the protein (if known), the appropriate taxonomic class and any special keywords. In addition, the user must select from one of six amino acid 'constellations', which influence how the analysis is performed; for example, certain constellations may combine residues like Asp/Asn (D/N) and Gln/Glu (Q/E) into Asx (B) and Glx (Z) or certain residues may be eliminated from the analysis altogether.

For each sequence in the database, the algorithm computes a score based on the difference in compositions between the sequence and the query composition. The results, returned by E-mail, are organised as three ranked lists: first, a list based on all proteins from the specified taxonomic class without taking pI or molecular weight into account; second, a list based on all proteins regardless of taxonomic class without taking pI or molecular weight into account; and finally, a list, based on the specified taxonomic class, that does take pI and molecular weight into account. Since the computed scores are a difference measure, a score of zero implies that there is exact correspondence between the query composition and that sequence entry.

A variant of AACompIdent, AACompSim performs a similar type of analysis, but rather than using an experimentally derived amino acid composition as the basis for searches, the sequence of a Swiss-Prot protein is used instead. A theoretical pI and molecular weight are computed prior to computing the difference scores using Compute pI/MW. It has been documented that amino acid composition across species boundaries is well conserved and that by considering amino acid composition, investigators can detect weak similarities between proteins whose sequence identity falls below 25 per cent. Thus consideration of composition in addition to performing 'traditional' database searches may provide additional insight into the relationships between proteins.

Propsearch

Along the same lines as AACompSim, PROPSEARCH uses the amino acid composition of a protein to detect weak relationships between proteins, and the authors have demonstrated that this technique can be used to easily discern members of the same protein family. However, this technique is more robust than AACompSim in that 144 different physical properties are used in performing the analysis, among which are molecular weight, the content of bulky residues, average hydrophobicity and average charge.

This collection of physical properties is called the query vector and it is compared against the same type of vector precomputed for every sequence in the target databases (SWISS-PROT and PIR). Having this 'database of vectors' calculated in advance vastly improves processing time for a query.

The input to the PROPSEARCH Web server is just the query sequence and an example of the program output is shown in Fig. 20.1. Here, the sequence of human autoantigen NOR-90 was used as the input query. The results are ranked by a distance score, and this score represents the likelihood that the query sequence and new sequences found through PROPSEARCH belong to the same family, thereby implying common function in most cases. A distance score of 10 or below indicates that there is a better than 87 per cent chance that there is similarity between the two proteins. A score below 8.7 increases the reliability to 94 per cent and a score below 7.5 increases the reliability to 99.6 per cent. Examination of the results showed NOR-90 to be similar to a number of nucleolar transcription factors, protein kinases, a retinoblastoma-binding protein, the actin-binding protein radixin and RalBP1, a putative GTPase target. None of these hits would necessarily be expected, since the functions of these proteins are dissimilar; however, a good number of these are DNA-binding proteins, opening the possibility that a very similar domain is being used in alternative functional contexts. At the very least, a BLASTP search would be necessary to both verify the results and identify critical residues.

Mowse

The molecular weight search algorithm (MOWSE) capitalises on information obtained through mass spectrometric (MS) techniques. Using both the molecular weights of intact proteins and those resulting from digestion of the same proteins with specific proteases, an unknown protein can be unambiguously identified given the results of several experimental determinations. This approach substantially cuts down on experimental time, since the unknown protein does not have to be sequenced in whole or in part.

MOWSE input is a simple text file, containing a list of experimentally determined peptide masses in the range of 0.7 to 4.0 kDa. Calculations are based on information contained in the OWL nonredundant protein sequence database. Scoring is based on the how often a fragment molecular weight occurs in proteins within a given range of molecular weights and the output is returned as a ranked list of the top 30 scores, with the OWL entry name, matching peptide sequences and other statistical information. Simulation studies produced an accuracy rate of 99 per cent using five or fewer input peptide weights. Searches are performed by sending an e-mail message to mowse@daresbury.ac.uk. Detailed information on formatting a query can be obtained by sending a message to the same address, with the word help in the body of the message.

PHYSICAL PROPERTIES BASED ON SEQUENCE

Compute pI/MW (ExPASy)

Compute pI/MW is a tool that calculates the isoelectric point and molecular weight of an input sequence. Determination of pI is based on pK values found in an earlier study on protein migration in denaturing conditions at neutral to acidic pH. Because of this, author Bjellqvist's caution that pI values determined for basic proteins may not be accurate. Molecular weights are calculated by the addition of the average isotopic mass of each amino acid in the sequence plus that of one water molecule. The sequence can be furnished by the user in FASTA format or a Swiss-Prot identifier or accession number can be specified. If a sequence is furnished, the tool automatically computes the pI and molecular weight for the entire length of the sequence. If a Swiss-Prot identifier is given, the definition and organism lines of the entry are shown and the user may specify a range of amino acids so that the computation is done on a fragment rather than on the entire protein.

Fragment search: OFF (POS1 and POS2 are begin and end of sequence)

Rank	ID	DIST	LEN2	POS1	POS2	pI	DE
1	>p1; s18193	0.00	727	1	727	5.33	autoantigen NOR-90 - human
2	ubf1_human	1.36	764	1	764	5.62	NUCLEOLAR TRANSCRIPTION FACTOR 1 (UPSTREAM BINDING FACTOR 1) (UBF-1)
3	ubf1_mouse	1.40	765	1	765	5.55	NUCLEOLAR TRANSCRIPTION FACTOR 1 (UPSTREAM BINDING FACTOR 1) (UBF-1)
4	ubf1_rat	1.57	764	1	764	5.61	NUCLEOLAR TRANSCRIPTION FACTOR 1 (UPSTREAM BINDING FACTOR 1) (UBF-1)
5	ubf1_xenla	3.95	677	1	677	5.79	NUCLEOLAR TRANSCRIPTION FACTOR 1 (UPSTREAM BINDING FACTOR 1) (UBF-1)
6	ubf2_xenla	4.18	701	1	701	6.05	NUCLEOLAR TRANSCRIPTION FACTOR 2 (UPSTREAM BINDING FACTOR 2) (UBF-2)
7	>p1; s57552	7.72	606	1	606	6.63	hypothetical protein YPR018w - yeast (Saccharomyces cerevisiae)
8	>p1; i50463	8.49	772	1	772	5.71	protein kinase - chicken
9	>p1; h54024	8.83	768	1	768	5.27	protein kinase (EC 2.7.1.37) cdc2-related PITSLRE alpha 2-3 - human
10	>p1; b54024	8.87	777	1	777	5.27	protein kinase (EC 2.7.1.37) cdc2-related PITSLRE alpha 2-2 - human
11	>p1; g54024	8.90	766	1	766	5.21	protein kinase (EC 2.7.1.37) cdc2-related PITSLRE beta 2-2 - human
12	>p1; a55817	9.00	783	1	783	5.19	cyclin-dependent kinase p130-PITSLRE - mouse
13	>p1; f54024	9.11	777	1	777	5.30	protein kinase (EC 2.7.1.37) cdc2-related PITSLRE beta 2-1 - human
14	>p1; e54024	9.11	779	1	779	5.42	protein kinase (EC 2.7.1.37) cdc2-related PITSLRE alpha 2-1 - human
15	yaa5_schpo	9.45	598	1	598	4.78	HYPOTHETICAL 69.5 KD PROTEIN C22G7.05 IN CHROMOSOME I
16	>p1; s62449	9.45	598	1	598	4.78	hypothetical protein SPAC22G7.05 - fission yeast (Schizosaccharomyces pombe)
17	>f1; i58390	9.45	920	1	920	5.00	retinoblastoma binding protein 1 isoform I - human (fragment)
18	>p1; s63193	9.58	590	1	590	6.15	hypothetical protein YNL227c - yeast (Saccharomyces cerevisiae)
19	ynw7_yeast	9.58	590	1	590	6.15	HYPOTHETICAL 68.8 KD PROTEIN IN URE2-SSU72 INTERGENIC REGION
20	>p1; s49634	9.74	899	1	899	4.79	Hypothetical protein YML093w - yeast (Saccharomyces cerevisiae)
21	ymj3_yeast	9.74	899	1	899	4.79	HYPOTHETICAL 103.0 KD PROTEIN IN RAD10-PRS4 INTERGENIC REGION
22	radi_human	9.76	583	1	583	6.33	RADIXIN
23	radi_pig	9.81	583	1	583	6.21	RADIXIN (MOESIN B)
24	>f1; i78883	9.83	866	1	866	4.77	retinoblastoma binding protein 1 isoform II - human (fragment)
25	>p1; b42997	9.87	754	1	754	5.17	retinoblastoma-associated protein 2 - human
26	>p1; a57467	9.91	647	1	647	5.74	Ra1BP1 - raf

Fig. 20.1. Results of a PROPSEARCH database query based on amino acid composition. The input sequence used was that of the human autoantigen NOR 90. Explanatory material and a histogram of distance scores against the entire target database have been removed for brevity. The columns in the table give the rank of the hit based on the distance score, the SWISS-PROT or PIR identifier, the distance score, the length of the overlap between the query and subject, the positions of the overlap (from POS1 to POS2), the calculated pI and the definition line for the found sequence.

PeptideMass (ExPASy)

Designed for use in peptide mapping experiments, PeptideMass determines the cleavage products of a protein after exposure to a given protease or chemical reagent. The enzymes and reagents available for cleavage through PeptideMass are trypsin, chymotrypsin, Lys C, cyanogen bromide, Arg C, Asp N and Glu C (bicarbonate or phosphate). Cysteines and methionines can be modified prior to the calculation of the molecular weight of the resultant peptides. By furnishing a Swiss-Prot identifier rather than pasting in a raw sequence, PeptideMass is able to use information within the SWISS-PROT annotation to improve the calculations, such as by removing signal sequences or including known post-translational modifications prior to cleavage. The results are returned in tabular format, giving a theoretical pI and molecular weight for the starting protein, and then the mass, position, modified masses, information on variants from SWISS-PROT and the sequence of the peptide fragments.

Tgrease

TGREASE calculates the hydrophobicity of a protein along its length. Inherent in each of the 20 amino acids is its hydrophobicity: the relative propensity the acid to bury itself in the core of a protein and away from surrounding water molecules. This tendency, coupled with steric and other considerations, influence how a protein ultimately folds into its final three-dimensional conformation. As such, TGREASE finds application in the determination of putative transmembrane sequences as well as the prediction of buried regions of globular proteins. TGREASE is part of the FASTA suite of programs available from the University of Virginia and runs as a stand-alone application that can be downloaded and run on either Macintosh or DOS-based computers.

The method relies on a hydropathy scale, where each amino acid is assigned a score reflecting its relative hydrophobicity based on a number of physical characteristics (e.g. solubility, the free energy of transfer through a water-vapour phase transition). Amino acids with higher, positive scores are more hydrophobic; those with more negative scores are more hydrophilic. A moving average or hydropathic index, is then calculated across the protein. The window length is adjustable, with a span of 7 to 11 residues recommended to minimise noise and maximise information content. The results are then plotted as hydropathic index versus residue number.

The sequence for the human interleukin 8 receptor B was used to generate a TGREASE plot, as shown in Fig. 20.2. Correspondence between the peaks and the actual location of the transmembrane segments, while not exact, is fairly good; keep in mind that the method is predicting all hydrophobic regions, not just those located in transmembrane regions. The specific detection of transmembrane regions is discussed further below.

SAPS

The statistical analysis of protein sequences algorithm provides extensive statistical information for any given query sequence. When a protein sequence is submitted via the SAPS web interface, the server returns a large amount of physical and chemical information on the protein, based solely what can be inferred from its sequence. The output begins with a compositional analysis, with counts of amino acids by type. This is followed by a charge distribution analysis, including the locations of positively or negatively charged clusters, high-scoring charged and uncharged segments and charge runs and patterns. The final sections present information on high-scoring hydrophobic and transmembrane segments, repetitive structures and multiplets, as well as a periodicity analysis.

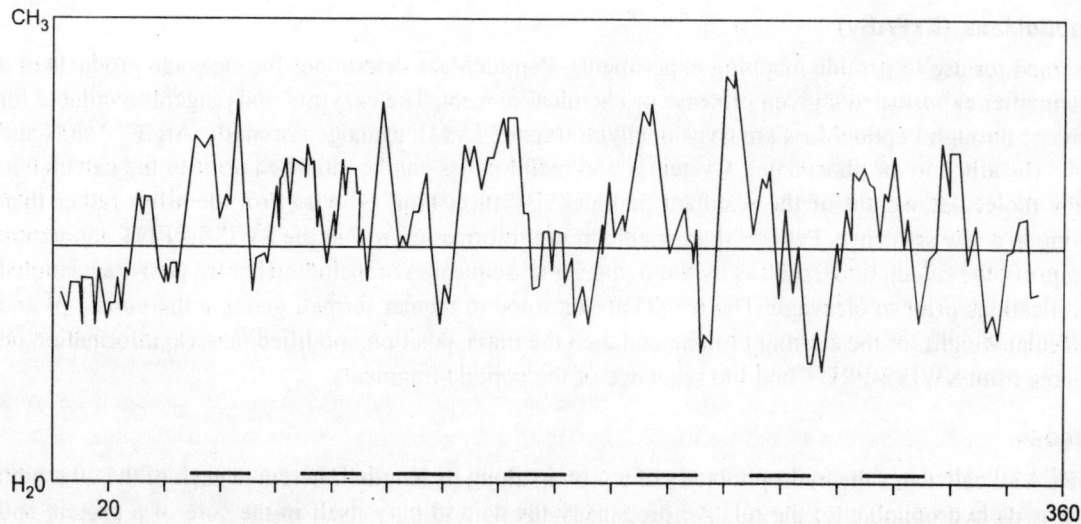

Fig. 20.2. Results of a Kyte-Doolittle hydropathy determination using TGREASE. The input sequence was of the high affinity interleukin 8 receptor B from human. Default window lengths were used. The thick, horizontal bars across the bottom of the figure were added manually and represent the positions of the seven transmembrane regions of IL-8R-B, as given in the SWISS-PROT entry for this protein (P25025).

SECONDARY STRUCTURE AND FOLDING CLASSES

The first step in the analysis of a newly discovered protein or gene product of unknown function is to perform a BLAST or other similar search against the public databases. However, such a search might not produce a match against a known protein; if there is a statistically significant hit, there may not be any information in the sequence record regarding the secondary structure of the protein, information that is very important in the rational design of biochemical experiments. In the absence of 'known' information, there are methods available for predicting the ability of a sequence to form α helices and β strands. These methods rely on observations made from groups of proteins whose three-dimensional structure has been experimentally determined.

A brief review of secondary structure and folding classes is warranted before the techniques themselves are discussed. As already alluded to, a significant number of amino acids have hydrophobic side chains, while the main chain or backbone, is hydrophilic. The required balance between these two seemingly opposing forces is accomplished through the formation of discrete secondary structural elements, first described by Linus Pauling and colleagues in 1951. An α helix is a corkscrew-type structure with the main chain forming the backbone and the side chains of the amino acids projecting outward from the helix. The backbone is stabilised by the formation of hydrogen bonds between the CO group of each amino acid and the NH group of the residue four positions C-terminal ($n + 4$), creating a tight, rodlike structure. Some residues form α helices better than others: alanine, glutamine leucine and methionine are commonly found in α helices, whereas proline, glycine, tyrosrine and serine usually are not. Proline is commonly thought of as a helix-breaker, since its bulky ring structure disrupts the formation of $n + 4$ hydrogen bonds.

In contrast, the β strand is a much more extended structure. Rather than having hydrogen bonds form within the secondary structural unit itself, stabilisation occurs through bonding with one or more adjacent β strands. The overall structure formed through the interaction of these individual β strands is known as a β-pleated sheet. These sheets can be parallel or antiparallel, depending on the orientation of the N- and C-terminal ends of each component β strand. A variant of the β sheet is the β turn, where the polypeptide chain makes a sharp, hairpin bend, producing an antiparallel β sheet in the process.

Levitt and Chothia proposed a classification system based on the order of secondary structural elements within a protein. Quite simply, an α structure is made up primarily from α helices and a β structure is made up of primarily β strands. Myoglobin is the classic example of a protein comprised entirely of α helices, falling into the α class of structures. Plastocyanin is a good example of the β class, where the hydrogen-bonding pattern between eight β strands form a compact, barrel-like structure. The combination class, α/β, is comprised primarily of β strands alternating with α helices. Flavodoxin is a good example of an α/β protein; its β strands form a central β sheet, which is surrounded by α helices.

An important term that appears repeatedly below is neural network. Basically, a neural network gives computational processes the ability to 'learn' in an attempt to approximate human learning, whereas most computer programs execute their instructions blindly in a sequential manner. The use of neural networks has found extensive application for problems that require analysis of patterns and trends, such as secondary structure prediction. Every neural network has an input layer and an output layer. In the case of secondary structure prediction, the input layer would be information from the sequence itself, and the output layer would be the probabilities of whether a particular residue could form a particular structure. Between the input and output layers would be one or more hidden layers in which the actual 'learning' takes place. This is accomplished by providing a training data set for the network. Here, an appropriate training set would be all sequences for which three-dimensional structures have been deduced. The network can process this information to look for what are possibly weak relationships between an amino acid sequence and the structures they can form in a particular context.

nnpredict

The nnpredict algorithm uses a two-layer, feed-forward neural network to assign the predicted type for each residue. In making the predictions, the server uses a FASTA format file with the sequence in either one-letter or three-letter code, as well as the folding class of the protein (α, β or α/β). Residues are classified as being within an α helix (H), a β strand (E) or neither (–). If no prediction can be made for a given residue, a question mark (?) is returned to indicate that an assignment cannot be made with confidence. If no information is available regarding the folding class, the prediction can be made without a folding class being specified; this is the default. For the best-case prediction, the accuracy rate of nnpredict is reported at over 65 per cent.

Sequences are submitted to nnpredict by sending an e-mail message to nnpredict @celeste.ucsf.edu. Using flavodoxin as an example, the format of the e-mail message would be as follows:

option: a/b
>flavodoxin–Anacystis nidulans

AKIGLFYGTQTGV'I'QTIAESIQQEFGGESIVDLNDIANADASDLNAYDYLIIGCPTWNVGELQSDWEGIY
DDLDSVNFQGKKVAYFGAGDQVGYSDNFQDAMGILEEKISSLGSQTVGYWPIEGYDFNESKAVRNNQFVG
LAIDEDNQPDLTKNRIKTWVSQLKSEFGL

The option line specifies the folding class of the protein: n uses no folding class for the prediction, a specifies α, b specifies β and a/b specifies α/β. Only one sequence may be submitted per e-mail message. The results returned by the server are shown in modified form in Fig. 20.3.

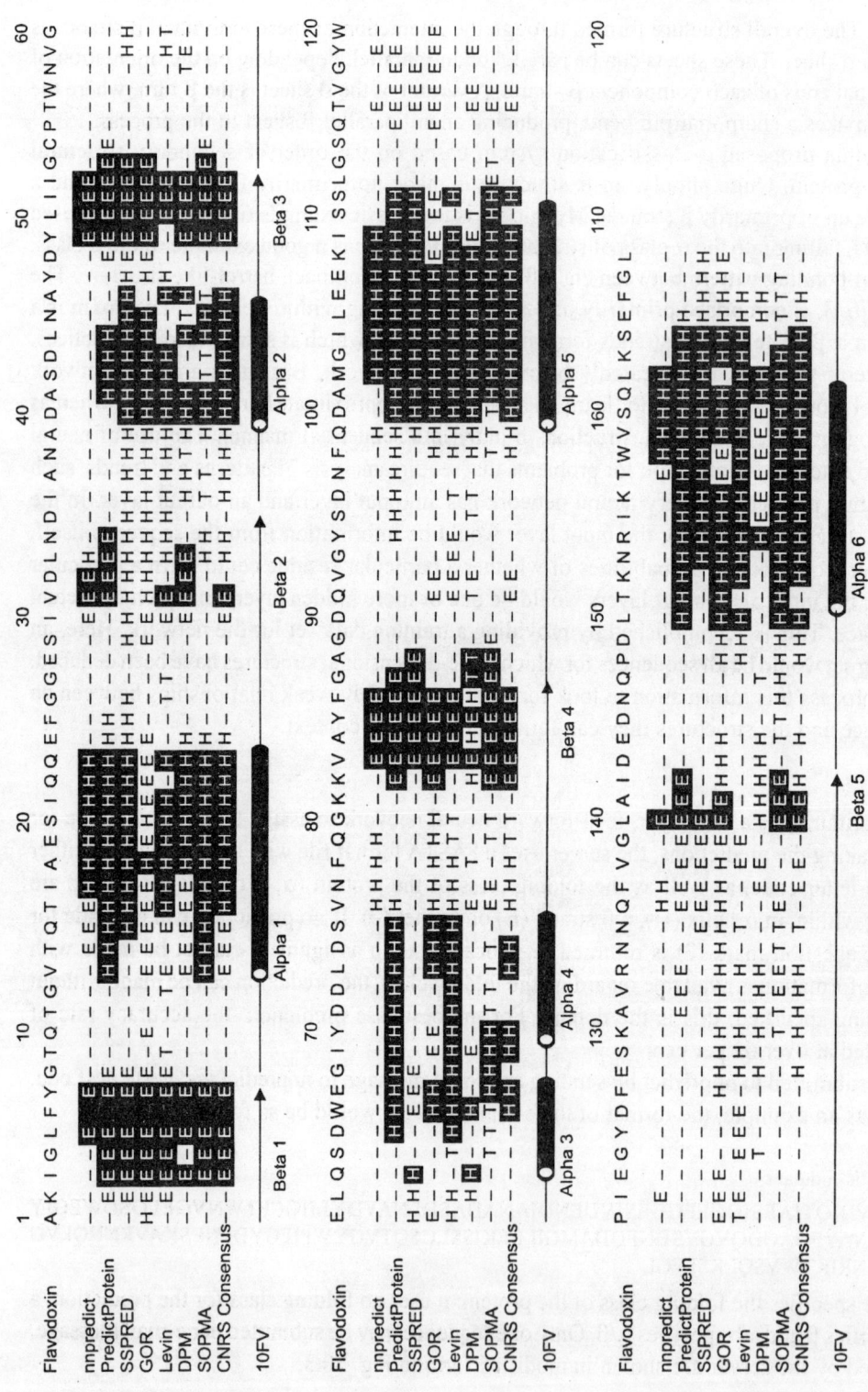

Fig. 20.3. Comparison of secondary structure predictions by various methods. The sequence of flavodoxin, an α/β protein, was used as the query and is shown on the first line of the alignment. For each prediction, H denotes an α helix, E a β strand, T a β turn; all other positions are assumed to be random coil. Correctly assigned residues are shown in inverse type. The methods used are listed along the left side of the alignment and are described in the text. At the bottom of the figure is the secondary structure assignment given in the PDB file for flavodoxin.

PredictProtein

PredictProtein uses a slightly different approach in making its predictions. First, the protein sequence is used as a query against Swiss-Prot to find similar sequences. When similar sequences are found, an algorithm called MaxHom is used to generate a profile-based multiple sequence alignment. MaxHom uses an iterative method to construct the alignment: After the first search of SWISS-PROT, all found sequences are aligned against the query sequence and a profile is calculated for the alignment. The profile is then used to search SWISS-PROT again to search for new, matching sequences. The multiple alignment generated by MaxHom is subsequently fed into a neural network for prediction by one of a suite of methods collectively known as PHD.

PHDsec, the method in this suite used for secondary structure prediction, not only assigns each residue to a secondary structure type, it provides statistics indicating the confidence of the prediction at each position in the sequence. The method produces an average accuracy of better than 72 per cent; the best-case residue predictions have an accuracy rate of over 90 per cent.

The input message, sent to predictprotein@embl-heidelberg.de, takes the following form:

Joe Buzzcut

National Human Genome Research Institute. NIH

buzzcut@baldguys. org

#flavodoxin – Anacystis nidulans

AKIGLFYGTQTGVTQTIAESIQQEFGGESIVDLNDIANADASDLNAYDYLIIGCPTWNVGELQSDWEGIY
DDLDSVNFQGKKVAYFGAGDQVGYSDNFQDAMGILEEKISSLGSQTVGYWPIEGYDFNESKAVRNNQFVG
LAIDEDNQPDLTKNRIKTWVSQLKSEFGL

After the Name, Affiliation and Address lines, the # signals to the server that a sequence in one-letter code follows. The sequence format is essentially FASTA, except that blanks are not allowed, and the standard > symbol is replaced by #. Nothing is allowed to follow the sequence.

The output from such a search is quite copious but contains a large amount of pertinent information. The results of the MaxHom search are returned, complete with a multiple alignment that may be of use in further study, such as profile searches or phylogenetic studies. If the submitted sequence has a known homolog in PDB, the PDB identifiers are furnished. Information follows on the method itself, finally followed by the actual prediction.

Unlike nnpredict, PredictProtein returns a 'reliability index of prediction' for each position ranging from 0 to 9, with 9 being the maximum confidence that a secondary structure assignment has been made correctly. The results returned by the server for this particular sequence, as compared to those obtained by other methods, are shown in modified form in Fig. 20.3.

Sspred

Like PredictProtein, the EMBL method for secondary structure prediction performs a search of the protein sequence databases for similar proteins, constructs a multiple sequence alignment and then performs the prediction. The method uses the alignment, paying particular attention to the nature of substitutions at nonconserved positions, to make an initial prediction. The initial prediction is then filtered to remove structural elements that are simply not plausible, either because of their length or because one structural type is interrupting a stretch of another (e.g. a prediction of HHHEHH would become HHHHHH). All α helices must be at least four residues long, while all β strands must be at least three residues long.

Again using flavodoxin as the example, the following is the format for an SSPRED search, submitted to sspred@embl-heidelberg.de:

SEQUENCE

TITLE flavodoxin – Anacystis nidulans

BLOSUM 62

ALIGN 50

INDEL 10

Z_SCORE 7. 0

SEQ

AKIGLFYGTQTGVTQTIAESIQQEFGGESIVDLNDIANADASDLNAYDYLIIGCPTWNVGELQSDWEGIY
DDLDSVNFQGKKVAYFGAGDQVGYSDNFQDAMGILEEKISSLGSQTVGYWPIEGYDFNESKAVRNNQFVG
LAIDEDNQPDLTKNRIKTWVSQLKSEFGL

END

The keyword SEQUENCE alerts the server that a single sequence is being submitted. The line TITLE allows a comment regarding the sequence to be entered and will appear in the results when returned. The command BLOSUM 62 instructs SSPRED to use that matrix when scoring alignments generated during the search. Both PAM and BLOSUM matrices are available, with the default being PAM 120. INDEL 10 is the value of the gap penalty. Users can leave this line out and allow SSPRED to predict a suitable default based on the scoring matrix used. Decreasing the value of INDEL makes the insertion of gaps more favourable. ALIGN 50 instructs the server to use the 50 best alignments in making the secondary structure predictions. The line Z_SCORE 7.0 allows users to increase or decrease the sensitivity of the BLITZ searches. Finally, the sequence is specified by a beginning keyword of SEQ and a termination keyword of END.

Upon completion of the analysis, a series of output files is returned to the user via e-mail. These include a message containing the multiple sequence alignment generated by BLITZ that was used in the prediction and a message containing the final results.

The e-mail message containing the prediction shows both the first prediction result and the final, filtered result. The final results of SSPRED on the query above are shown in relation to the outputs from the other algorithms in Fig. 20.3.

Sopma

The protein sequence analysis server at the centre national de la recherche scientifique (CNRS) in Lyons, France, takes a unique approach in making secondary structure predictions: rather than using a single method, it uses five, the predictions from which are subsequently used to come up with a 'consensus prediction'. The methods used are the Garnier-Gibrat-Robson (GOR) method, the Levin homolog method, the double-prediction method, the PHD method described above as part of PredictProtein and the method of CNRS itself, called SOPMA. Briefly, this self-optimised prediction method builds sub-databases of protein sequences with known secondary structures; each of the proteins in a sub-database is then subjected to secondary structure prediction based on sequence similarity. Then the information from the sub-databases is used to generate a prediction on the query sequence.

The method can be run by submitting just the sequence itself in single-letter format to deleage@ibcp.fr, using SOPMA as the subject of the mail message or by using the SOPMA web interface. The output from each of the component predictions, as well as the consensus, is shown in Fig. 20.3.

Comparison of Methods

Based on Fig. 20.3, it is immediately apparent that all the methods described above do a relatively good, but not perfect, job of predicting secondary structure. Flavodoxin was selected as the input query because it has a relatively intricate structure, falling into the α/β folding class with its six α helices and five β sheets. Some assignments were consistently made by all methods; for example, all the methods detected $\beta1$, $\beta3$, $\beta4$ and $\alpha5$ fairly well. However, some methods missed some elements altogether (e.g. nnpredict with $\alpha2$, $\alpha3$ and $\alpha4$) and some predictions made no biological sense (e.g. the double-prediction method and $\beta4$, where helices, sheets, and turns alternate, residue by residue). PredictProtein, which correctly found all the secondary structure elements and in several places, identified structures of the correct length, appears to have made the best overall prediction. This is not to say that the other methods are not useful or not as good; undoubtedly in some cases another method would have emerged as having made a better prediction. Where no other information is known, the best approach is to submit a query sequence to a number of these servers, compile the results, and then manually judge the validity of the predictions in comparison to one another (While the CNRS consensus sequence shown in Fig. 20.3 attempts to do this, the consensus in this case is not completely correct either). This approach does not provide a fail-safe method of prediction, but it does reinforce the level of confidence resulting from these predictions.

SPECIALISED STRUCTURES OR FEATURES

Just as the position of α helices and β sheets can be predicted with a relatively high degree of confidence, the presence of certain specialised structures or features, such as coiled coils and transmembrane regions, can be predicted. There are not as many methods for making such predictions as there are for secondary structure, primarily because the rules of folding that induce these structures are not completely understood. Despite this, when query sequences are searched against databases of known structure, the accuracy of prediction can be quite high.

Coiled Coils

The COILS algorithm runs a query sequence against a database of proteins known to have a coiled-coil structure. The program also compares query sequences to a PDB subset containing globular sequences, and based on the differences in scoring between the PDB subset and the coiled-coils database, determines the probability with which the input sequence can form a coiled-coil. COILS can be downloaded for use with VAX/VMS or may more easily be used through a simple web interface.

The program takes sequence data in GCG or FASTA format; one or more sequences can be submitted at once. In addition to the sequences, users may select one of two scoring matrices: MTK, based on the sequences of myosin, tropomyosin and keratin or MTIDK, based on myosin, tropomyosin, intermediate filaments types I–V, desmosomal proteins and kinesins. Smith cite a trade-off between the scoring matrices, with MTK being better for detecting two-stranded structures and MTIDK being better for all other cases. Users may invoke an option giving the same weight to the residues at the a and d positions of each coil (normally hydrophobic) as that given to the residues at the b, c, e, f and g positions (normally hydrophilic). If the results of running COILS both weighted and unweighted are substantially different, it is likely that a false positive has been found. Smith cautions that COILS is designed to detect solvent-exposed, left-handed coiled-coils and that buried or right-handed coiled-coils may not be detected. When a query is submitted to the web server, a prediction graph showing the propensity toward the formation of a coiled-coil along the length of the sequence is generated.

A slightly easier to interpret output comes from MacStripe, a Macintosh-based application that uses the Lupas COILS method to make its predictions. MacStripe takes an input file in FASTA, PIR and other common file formats and like COILS, produces a plot file containing a histogram of the probability of forming a coiled-coil, along with bars showing the continuity of the heptad repeat pattern. The following portion of the statistics file generated by MacStripe uses the complete sequence of GCN4 as an example.

```
89    89 L 5 a 0.760448 0.000047
90    90 D 5 b 0.760448 0.000047
91    91 D 5 c 0.760448 0.000047
92    92 A 5 d 0.760448 0.000047
93    93 V 5 e 0.760448 0.000047
94    94 V 5 f 0.760448 0.000047
95    95 E 5 g 0.760448 0.000047
96    96 S 5 a 0.760448 0.000047
97    97 F 5 b 0.760448 0.000047
98    98 F 5 c 0.774300 0.000058
99    99 S 5 d 0.812161 0.000101
100   100 S 5 e 0.812161 0.000101
101   101 S 5 f 0.812161 0.000101
102   102 T 5 g 0.812161 0.000101
```

The columns, from left to right, represent the residue number (shown twice), the amino acid, the heptad frame, the position of the residue within the heptad (a-b-c-d-e-f-g), the Lupas score and the Lupas probability. In this case, focusing on the fifth column, we can easily discern heptad repeat pattern. Examination of the results for the entire GCN4 sequence shows that the heptad pattern is fairly well maintained but falls apart in certain areas. While the statistics should not be ignored, the results are easier to interpret if the heptad pattern information is clearly presented. It is possible to get a similar type of output from COILS, but not through the COILS web server; instead, a C-based program must be installed on an appropriate Unix machine, a step that may be untenable for many users.

Transmembrane Regions

The Kyte-Doolittle TGREASE algorithm discussed above is very useful in detecting regions of high hydrophobicity, but as such it does not exclusively predict transmembrane regions, since buried domains in soluble, globular proteins can also be primarily hydrophobic. We consider first a predictive method specifically for the prediction of transmembrane regions. This method, TMpred, relies on a database of transmembrane proteins called TMbase. TMbase, which is derived from Swiss-Prot, contains additional information on each sequence regarding the number of transmembrane domains they possess, the location of these domains and the nature of the flanking sequences. TMpred uses this information in conjunction with several weight matrices in making its predictions.

The TMpred web interface is very simple. The sequence, in one-letter code, is pasted into the query sequence box and the user can specify the, minimum and maximum lengths of the hydrophobic part of the transmembrane helix to be used in the analysis. The output has four sections: a list of possible transmembrane helices, a table of correspondences, suggested models for transmembrane topology, and a graphic representation of the same results.

When the sequence of the G-protein-coupled receptor (P51684) served as the query, the following models were generated:

2 possible models considered, only significant TM-segments used

------> STRONGLY preferred model: N-terminus outside

7 strong transmembrane helices, total score: 14196

#	from	to length	score	orientation
1	55	74 (20)	2707	o-i
2	83	104 (22)	1914	i-o
3	120	141 (22)	1451	o-i
4	166	184 (19)	2155	i-o
5	212	235 (24)	2530	o-i
6	255	276 (22)	2140	i-o
7	299	319 (21)	1299	o-i

-----> alternative model

7 strong transmembrane helices, total score: 11974

#	from	to length	score	orientation
1	47	69 (23)	2494	i-o
2	84	104 (21)	1470	o-i
3	123	141 (19)	1352	i-o
4	166	185 (20)	1904	o-i
5	219	236 (18)	2453	i-o
6	252	274 (23)	1386	o-i
7	300	319 (20)	915	i-o

Each of the proposed models indicates the starting and ending position of each segment, along with the relative orientation (inside-to-outside or outside-to-inside) of each segment. The authors appropriately caution that the models are based on the assumption that all transmembrane regions were found in the course of the prediction. These models, then, should be considered in light of the raw data also generated by this method. The second predictive method, TMAP, takes an approach similar to that used by SSPRED in that it utilises a multiple sequence alignment to improve its accuracy of prediction. Considering again the G-protein-coupled receptor as the input sequence, a query would be formatted as follows and submitted to tmap@embl-heidelberg.de:

```
SEQUENCE
TITLE G protein-coupled receptor
BLOSUM 62
INDEL 10
ALIGN 50
Z_SCORE 4
SEQ
MSGESMNFSDVFDSSEDYFVSVNTSYYSVDSEMLLCSLQEVRQFSRLFVPIAYSLICVFGLLGNILVVIT
FAFYKKARSMTLVYLLNMAIADLLFVLTLPFWAVSHATGAWVFSNATCKLLKGIYAINFNCGMLLLTCIS
END
```

The line TITLE allows the sequence to be easily identified on output sent back to the user. The BLOSUM 62 command indicates the scoring matrix to be used in the performance of a BLITZ search against Swiss-Prot and any valid BLOSUM or PAM matrix may be specified here; INDEL, ALIGN and Z_SCORE all have the same meaning as with the SSPRED server described above.

The sequence is preceded by a beginning SEQ keyword, and the end of the query is signalled by the END keyword. Regardless of whether the e-mail server or Web interface is used, the results are returned by e-mail.

The messages returned include a multiple sequence alignment as generated by BLITZ for the query sequence, a prediction regarding the position of all the transmembrane regions and a PostScript file providing a graphical overview of the results. The prediction made on the G-coupled-protein receptor by TMAP is as follows:

PREDICTED TRANSMEMBRANE SEGMENTS FOR PROTEIN G protein-coupled receptor

TM	1:	46–74	(29)
TM	2:	82–108	(27)
TM	3:	117–145	(29)
TM	4:	159–187	(29)
TM	5:	212–24C	(29)
TM	6:	251–276	(26)

The output format is quite simple, giving the number of the transmembrane segment, the start and end points of each segment, and the length of the segment in parentheses. It is apparent that for the same protein, these two methods have produced significantly different results; TMpred predicts seven transmembrane regions and TMAP predicts six, with marginal overlap between the two sets. The Swiss-Prot entry for this sequence indicates seven transmembrane regions (43–69, 79–99, 115–136, 155–175, 206–233, 250–274 and 299–316) and the results from TMpred compare favourably to these positions: in most cases, TMpred predictions are either slightly longer than or slightly offset from the actual locations. The same is true for TMAP, except that TMAP failed to detect the final transmembrane region altogether. One can envision TMAP performing better than TMpred, however, again reinforcing the general strategy of using several algorithms to make predictions and then manually inspecting the results.

Signal Peptides

The Centre for Biological Sequence Analysis at the Technical University of Denmark has developed SignalP, a powerful tool for the detection of signal peptides and their cleavage sites. The algorithm is neural-network based, using separate sets of gram-negative prokaryotic. Gram-positive prokaryotic, and eukaryotic sequences with known signal sequences as the training sets. SignalP predicts secretory signal peptides and not those that are involved in intracellular signal transduction.

Using the Web interface, the sequence of the human insulin-like growth factor IB precursor (somatomedin C, P05019), whose cleavage site is known, was submitted to SignalP for analysis. The eukaryotic training set was used in the prediction, and the results of the analysis are as follows:

****************** SignalP predictions *********************

Using networks trained on euk data

>IGF–IB   length = 195

#	pos	aa	C	S	Y
	46	A	0.365	0.823	0.495
	47	T	0.450	0.654.	0.577
	48	A	0.176	0.564	0.369
	49	G	0.925	0.205	0.855
	50	P	0.185	0.163	0.376

< Is the sequence a signal peptide?

#	Measure	Position	Value	Cutoff	Conclusion
	max. C	49	0.925	0.37	YES
	max. Y	49	0.855	0.34	YES
	max. S	37	0.973	0.88	YES
	mean S	1–48	0.550	0.48	YES

Most likely cleavage site between pos. 48 and 49: ATA-GP

In the first part of the output, the column labelled C is a raw cleavage site score. The value of C is highest at the position C-terminal to the cleavage site. The column labelled S contains the signal peptide scores, which are high at all positions before the cleavage site and very low after the cleavage site. S is also low in the N-termini of nonsecretory proteins. Finally, the Y column gives the combined cleavage site score, a geometric average indicating when the C score is high and the point at which the S score shifts from high to low. The end of the output file asks the question, 'Is the sequence a signal peptide'? Based on the statistics, the most likely cleavage site is deduced. Based on the Swiss-Prot entry for this protein, the mature chain begins at position 49, the same position predicted to be the most likely cleavage site by SignalP.

Nonglobular Regions

In the use of the program SEG in the masking of low-complexity segments prior to database searches, the same algorithm can also be used to detect putative nonglobular regions of protein sequences by altering the trigger window length W, the trigger complexity K_1 and extension complexity K_2. Upon receiving the command seg sequence.txt 45 3.4 3.75, SEG will use a longer window length than the default of 12, thereby detecting long nonglobular domains. An example of using SEG to detect nonglobular regions is shown in Fig. 20.4.

TERTIARY STRUCTURE

By far the most complex and technically demanding predictive method based on protein sequence data has to do with structure prediction. The importance of being able to adequately and accurately predict structure based on sequence is rooted in the knowledge that while sequence may specify conformation, the same conformation may be specified by multiple sequences. The ideas that structure is conserved to a much greater extent than sequence and that there is a limited number of backbone motifs indicate that similarities between proteins may not necessarily be detected through traditional, sequence-based methods only. Deducing the relationship between sequence and structure is at the root of the 'protein-folding problem' and current research on the problem has been the focus of a number of recent reviews.

```
1–307    MAGAIASRMSFSSLKRKQPKTFTVRIVTMD
         AEMEFNCEMKWKGKDLFDLVCRTLGLRETW
         FFGLQYTIKDTVAWLKMDKKVLDHDVSKEE
         PVTFHFLAKFYPENAEEELVQEITQHLFFL
         QVKKQILDEKIYCPPEASVLLASYAVQAKY
         GDYDPSVHKRGFLAQEELLPKRVINLYQMT
         PEMWEERITAWYAEHRGRARDEAEMEYLKI
         AQDLEMYGVNYFAIRNKKGTELLLGVDALG
         LHIYDPENRLTPKISFPWNEIRNISYSDKE
         FTIKPLDKKIDVFKFNSSKLRVNKLILQLC
         IGNHDLF
```

```
mrrrkadslevqqmkaqareekarkqmerg    308–478
rlarekqmreeaertrdelerrllqmkeea
tmanealmrseetadllaekaqiteeeakl
laqkaaeaeqemqrikatairteeekrlme
qkvleaevlalkmaeeserrakeadqlkqd
lqeareaerrakqklleiatk
```

```
479–496    PTYPPMNPIPAPLPPDIP
```

```
sfnnligdslsfdfkdtdmkrlsmeiekekv    497–587
eymekskhlqeqlnelkteiealklkeret
aldilhnensdrggsskhntikkltlqsak
s
```

```
588–595    RVAFFEEL
```

Fig. 20.4. Predicted nonglobular regions for the protein product of the neurofibromatosis type 2 gene (L11353) as deduced by SEG. The nonglobular regions are shown in the left-hand column in lowercase. Numbers denote residue positions for each block.

The most robust of the structure prediction techniques is homology model building or 'threading'. This method takes, a query sequence whose structure is not known and threads it through the coordinates of a target protein whose structure has been solved, either by X-ray crystallography or NMR imaging. The sequence is moved position by position through the structure subject to some predetermined physical constraints; for example, the lengths of secondary structure elements and loop regions may either be fixed or varying within a given range. For each placement of sequence against structure, pairwise and hydrophobic interactions between nonlocal residues are determined. These thermodynamic calculations are used to determine the most energetically favourable and conformationally stable alignment of the query sequence against the target structure. Programs such as this are computationally intensive, requiring, at a minimum, a powerful UNIX workstation; they also require knowledge of specialised computer languages. While techniques such as threading are obviously very powerful, their current requirements in terms of both hardware and expertise may prove to be obstacles to most biologists. In an attempt to lower the height of the barrier, easy-to-use programs have been developed to give the average biologist a good first approximation for comparative protein modelling (numerous commercial protein structure analysis tools, such as WHAT-IF and LOOK, provide advanced capabilities, but this discussion is limited to web-based freeware).

The use of SWISS-MODEL, a program that performs automated sequence-structure comparisons, is a two-step process. The First Approach mode is used to determine whether a sequence can be modelled at all: when a sequence is submitted, SWISS-MODEL compares it to the crystallographic database

(ExPdb) and modelling is attempted only if there is a homolog in ExPdb with sufficient sequence identity to the query protein. If the first approach finds one or more appropriate entries in ExPdb, an atomic model is built and the results are returned by e-mail. Those results can be resubmitted to SWISS-MODEL using its optimise mode, which allows for alteration of the proposed structure based on other knowledge, such as biochemical information.

The second method compares structures to structures, in the same light as does the vector alignment search tool (VAST). The DALI algorithm looks for similar contact patterns between two proteins and performs an optimisation to return the best set of structure alignment solutions for those proteins. The method is flexible in that gaps may be of any length, and it allows for alternate connectivities between aligned segments, thereby facilitating identification of specific domains that are similar in two different proteins, even if the proteins as a whole are dissimilar. The DALI Web interface will perform the analysis on either two sets of coordinates already in PDB, or by using a set of coordinates in PDB format submitted by the user. Alternatively, if both proteins of interest are present in PDB, their precomputed structural neighbours can be found by accessing the FSSP database of structurally aligned protein fold families, an 'all-against-all' comparison of PDB entries.

The final method to be discussed here expands on the PHD secondary structure method discussed above. In the TOPITS method, a searchable database is created by translating the three-dimensional structure of proteins in PDB into one-dimensional 'strings' of secondary structure. Then, the secondary structure and solvent accessibility of the query sequence is determined by the PHD method, with the results of this computation also being stored as a one-dimensional string. The query and target strings are then aligned by dynamic programming, to make the structure prediction. The results are returned as a ranked list, indicating the optimal alignment of the query sequence against the target structure, along with a probability estimate (Z score) of the accuracy of the prediction. The three methods discussed here are fairly elementary, hence their speed in returning results and their ability to be adapted to a web-style interface. Yet their level of performance is impressive in that they often can detect weak structural similarities between proteins. The ultimate potential of threading techniques is proving ground for the more complex techniques alluded to above showed that while the protein-folding problem is nowhere near being solved, numerous protein folds can reliably be identified. Since different methods proved to have different strengths and it is suggested using a 'consensus approach', similar to the approach used in the secondary structure prediction examples given earlier. The timing of these developments is quite exciting, in as much as concurrence with the human genome project will give investigators a powerful handle for predicting structure-function relationships as putative gene products are identified.

Internet resources for topics presented in this chapter.

Prediction of physical properties

Compute pI/MW	http://expasy.hcuge.ch/ch2d/pi_tool.html
PeptideMass	http://expasy.hcuge.ch/sprot/peptide-mass.html
TGREASE	ftp://ftp.virginia.edu/pub/fasta/
SAPS	http://ulrec3.unil.ch/software/SAPS_form.html

Prediction of protein identity based on composition

AACompIdent	http://expasy.hcuge.ch/ch2d/aacompi.html
AACompSim	http://expasy.hcuge.ch/ch2d/aacsim.html
PROPSEARCH	http://www.embl-heidelberg.de/prs.html

(Contd...)

Prediction of secondary structure and folding classes

nnpredict	http://www.cmpharm.ucsf.edu/~nomi/nnpredict.html
PredictProtein	http://www.embl-heidelberg.de/predictprotein/
SOPMA	http://www.ibcp.fr/predict.html
SSPRED	http://www.embl-heidelberg.de/sspred/sspred_info.html

Prediction of specialised structures or features

COILS	http://ulrec3.unil.ch/software/COILS_form.html
MacStripe	http://www.wi.mit.edu/matsudaira/macstripe.html
SignalP	http://www.cbs.dtu.dk/services/SignalP/
TMAP	http://www.embl-heidelberg.de/tmap/tmap_sin.html
TMpred	http://ulrec3.unil.ch/software/TMPRED_form.html

Structure prediction

Bryant-Lawrence	ftp://ncbi.nlm.nih.gov/pub/pkb
DALI	http://www.embl-heidelberg.de/dali/dali.html
FSSP	http://www.embl-heidelberg.de/dali/fssp/fssp.html
SWISS-MODEL	http://expasy.hcuge.ch/swissmod/SWISS-MODEL.html
TOPITS	http://www.embl-heidelberg.de/predictprotein/ phd_help.html

Chapter 21

Phylogenetic Analysis

INTRODUCTION

When comparing sequence homologs from different source species, there is recognition that they are related. The questions often asked are 'how are they related'? and 'when did they diverge'? These are not new questions. Before people started making comparisons at the molecular level, they were using other types of data such as morphology and developmental processes to try to answer these questions. Phylogenetics attempts to reconstruct evolutionary history. In a phylogenetic analysis, one compares the results of evolutionary processes, be its shape and size of specific bones or patterns of DNA or protein sequences, in an attempt to determine how different groups or species may have been derived during evolution. Looking at the molecular sequences can give insight into the nature of the processes, which lead to divergence, in addition to analysing the relative degree of relatedness.

MECHANISM OF CHANGE

The mechanisms of change include:
1. Random mutation, which can be seen as genetic drift in the absence of selective pressure.
2. Sequence duplication, which may be duplication of small segments, genes or even whole genomes.
3. Recombination, which includes transposons, translocations and viral activity, to mix up sequences within an organism, to remove sequences or to introduce sequences from another organism.

There is considerable debate regarding the best approach to take when analysing sequence alignments for phylogenetic relationships. Accepted approaches include distance calculations, parsimony and maximum likelihood. New on the scene is Bayesian analysis, which is expected to gain popularity as people become familiar with it. It is good to become familiar with the different methods of analysis. It helps in understanding the arguments being made, both in terms of how things should be done and of the resulting analyses. When examining the results of molecular phylogenetic analysis, care should be taken to compare the results to other independent means of analysis and/or to other data sets.

Associated Concepts

The associated concepts in phylogenetic analysis are:
1. Phylogenetics vs. taxonomy.
2. Cladistic vs. phenetic.
3. Clustering.
4. Parsimony vs. maximum likelihood.

445

Charles Darwin was the first to recognise that the systematic hierarchy represented a rough approximation of evolutionary history. However, it was not until the 1950s that the German entomologist Willi Hennig proposed that systematics should reflect the known evolutionary history of lineages as closely as possible, an approach he called phylogenetic systematics. The followers of Hennig were referred to as 'cladists' by his opponents, because of the emphasis on recognising, only monophyletic groups, a group plus all of its descendants or clades. However, the cladists quickly adopted that term as a helpful label and nowadays, cladistic approaches to systematics are used routinely.

Phylogenetic systematics

Phylogenetic systematics is that field of biology that does deal with identifying and understanding the evolutionary relationships among the many different kinds of life on earth, both living (extant) and dead (extinct). Evolutionary theory states that similarity among individuals or species is attributable to common descent, or inheritance from a common ancestor. Thus, the relationships established by phylogenetic systematics often describe a species evolutionary history and hence, it is phylogeny, the historical relationships among lineages or organisms or their parts, such as their genes.

EVOLUTIONARY PROCESS

Following points will facilitate the discussion of evolutionary process:

Genetic Variation: Changes in a Gene Pool

Evolution is not always discrete with clearly defined boundaries that pinpoint the origin of a new species, nor is it a steady continuum. Evolution requires genetic variation, which results from changes within a gene pool, the genetic make-up of a specific population. A gene pool is the combination of all the alleles; alternative forms of a genetic locus; for all traits that population may exhibit. Changes in a gene pool can result from mutation-variation within a particular gene; or from changes in gene frequency; the proportion of an allele in a given population.

Occurrence of Genetic Variation

Every organism possesses a genome that contains all of the biological information needed to construct and maintain a living example of that organism. The biological information contained in a genome is encoded in the nucleotide sequence of its DNA or RNA molecules and is divided into discrete units called genes. The information stored in a gene is read by proteins, which attach to the genome and initiate a series of reactions called gene expression.

Every time a cell divides, it must make a complete copy of its genome, a process called DNA replication. DNA replication must be extremely accurate to avoid introducing mutations or changes in the nucleotide sequence of a short region of the genome. Inevitably, some mutations do occur, usually in one of two ways; either from errors in DNA replication or from damaging effects of chemical agents or radiation that react with DNA and change the structure of individual nucleotides. Many of these mutations result in a change that has no effect on the functioning of the genome, referred to as silent mutations. Silent mutations include virtually all changes that happen in the noncoding components of genes and gene-related sequences.

Mutations in the coding regions of genes are much more important. Here we must consider the importance of the same mutation in a somatic cell compared with a germ line cell. A somatic cell is any cell of an organism other than a reproductive cell, such as a sperm or egg cell. (A germ cell line is any line of cells that gives rise to gametes and is continuous through the generations.) Because a somatic cell does not pass on copies of its genome to the next generation, a somatic cell mutation is important only for the organism in which it occurs and has no potential evolutionary impact. In fact, most somatic mutations have no significant effect because there are many other identical cells in the same tissue.

On the other hand, mutations in germ cells can be transmitted to the next generation and will then be present in all of the cells of an individual who inherits that mutation. Even still, mutations within germ line cells may not change the phenotype of the organism in any significant way. Those mutations that do have an evolutionary effect can be divided into two categories, loss-of-function mutations and gain-of-function mutations. A loss-of-function mutation results in reduced or abolished protein function. Gain-of-function mutations, which are much less common, confer an abnormal activity on a protein.

The randomness with which mutations can occur is an important concept in biology and is a requirement of the Darwinian view of evolution, which holds that changes in the characteristics of an organism occur by chance and are not influenced by the environment in which the organism lives. Beneficial changes within an organism are then positively selected for, whereas harmful changes are negatively selected.

Drivers of Evolution: Selection, Drift and Founder Effects

We just discussed that new alleles appear in a population because of mutations that occur in the reproductive cells of an organism. This means that many genes are polymorphic, that is, two or more alleles for that gene are present in a population. Each of these alleles has its own allele or gene frequency, a measure of how common an allele is in a population. Allele frequencies vary over time because of two conditions, natural selection and random drift.

Natural selection

Natural selection is the process whereby one genotype, the hereditary constitution of an individual, leaves more offspring than another genotype because of superior life attributes, termed fitness. Natural selection acts on genetic variation by conferring a survival advantage to those individuals harbouring a particular mutation that tends to favour a changing environmental condition. These individuals then reproduce and pass on this 'new' gene, altering their gene pool. Natural selection, therefore, decreases the frequencies of alleles that reduce the fitness of an organism and increases the frequency of alleles that improve fitness. Thus, 'natural selection' is the principle by which each slight variation, if useful, is preserved.

It is important to point out that natural selection does not always represent progress, only adaptation to a changing surrounding, that is evolution attributable to natural selection is devoid of intent something does not evolve to better itself, only to adapt. Because environments are always changing, what was once an advantageous mutation can often become a liability further down the evolutionary line.

Random drift

The term random drift actually encompasses a number of distinct processes, sometimes referred to as outcomes. They include indiscriminate parent sampling, the founder effect and fluctuations in the rate of evolutionary processes such as selection, migration and mutation. Parent sampling is the process of determining which organisms of one generation will be the parents of the next generation. Parent sampling may be discriminate, that is, with regard to fitness differences or indiscriminate, without regard to fitness differences. Discriminate parent sampling is generally considered natural selection, whereas indiscriminate parent sampling is considered random drift.

SAMPLING

Suppose a population of red and brown squirrels share a habitat with a colour blind predator. Although the predator is colour blind, the brown squirrels seem to die in greater numbers than the red squirrels, suggesting that the brown squirrels just seem to be unlucky enough to come into contact with the predator more often. As a result, the frequency of brown squirrels in the next generation is reduced.

More red squirrels survive to reproduce or are sampled, but it is without regard to any differences in fitness between the two groups. The physical differences of the groups do not play a causal role in the differences in reproductive success. Now, let's say that the predator is not colour blind and can now see the red squirrels better than the brown squirrels, resulting in a better survival rate for the brown squirrels. This would be a case of discriminate parent sampling or natural selection.

FOUNDER EFFECT

Another important cause of genetic drift is the founder effect, the difference between the gene pool of a population as a whole and that of a newly isolated population of the same species. The founder effect occurs when population are started from a small number of pioneer individuals of one original population. Because of small sample size, the new population could have a much different genetic ratio than the original population. An example of the founder effect would be when a plant population results from a single seed. Thus far, we have discussed natural selection and random drift as events that occur in isolation from one another. However, in most population, the two processes will be occurring at the same time. Furthermore, there is great debate over whether, in particular instances and in general, natural selection is more prevalent than random drift.

PHYLOGENETIC TREES: PRESENTING EVOLUTIONARY RELATIONSHIPS

Systematics describes the pattern of relationships among taxa and is intended to help us understand the history of all life. But history is not something we can see it has happened once and leaves only clues as to the actual events. Scientists use these clues to build hypotheses, or models, of life's history. In phylogenetic studies, the most convenient way of visually presenting evolutionary relationships among a group of organisms is through illustrations called phylogenetic trees.

Node: represents a taxonomic unit. This can be either an existing species or an ancestor.

1. Branch: defines the relationship between the taxa in terms of descent and ancestry.
2. Branch length: represents the number of changes that have occurred in the branch.
3. Topology: the branching patterns of the tree.
4. Root: the common ancestor of all taxa.
5. Distance scale: scale that represents the number of differences between organisms or sequences.
6. Clade: a group of two or more taxa or DNA sequences that includes both their common ancestor and all of their descendants.
7. Operational taxonomic unit (OTU): taxonomic level of sampling selected by the user to be used in a study, such as individuals, populations, species, genera or bacterial strains.

A phylogenetic tree is composed of nodes, each representing a taxonomic unit (species, populations, individuals) and branches, which define the relationship between the taxonomic units in terms of descent and ancestry. Only one branch can connect any two adjacent nodes. The branching pattern of the tree is called the topology, and the branch length usually represents the number of changes that have occurred in the branch. This is called a scaled branch. Scaled trees are often calibrated to represent the passage of time. Such trees have a theoretical basis in the particular gene or genes under analysis. Branches can also be unscaled, which means that the branch length is not proportional to the number of changes that has occurred, although the actual number may be indicated numerically somewhere on the branch. Phylogenetic trees may also be either rooted or unrooted. In rooted trees, there is a particular node, called the root, representing a common ancestor, from which a unique path leads to any other node. An unrooted tree only specifies the relationship among species, without identifying a common ancestor, or evolutionary path.

Phylogenetic trees, a convenient way of representing evolutionary relationships among a group of organisms can be drawn in various ways. Branches on phylogenetic trees may be scaled representing the amount of evolutionary change, time or both, when there is a molecular clock or they may be unscaled and have no direct correspondence with either time or amount of evolutionary change. Phylogenetic trees may be rooted or unrooted. In the case of unrooted trees, branching relationships between taxa are specified by the way they are connected to each other, but the position of the common ancestor is not. For example, on an unrooted tree with five species, there are five branches (four external, one internal) on which the tree can be rooted. Rooting on each of the five branches has different implications for evolutionary relationships.

METHODS OF PHYLOGENETIC ANALYSIS

Two major groups of analyses exist to examine phylogenetic relationships: phenetic methods and cladistic methods. It is important to note that phenetics and cladistics have had an uneasy relationship over the last 40 years or so. Most of today's evolutionary biologists favour cladistics, although a strictly cladistic approach may result in counterintuitive results.

Phenetic Method of Analysis

Phenetics, also known as numerical taxonomy, involves the use of various measures of overall similarity for the ranking of species. There is no restriction on the number or type of characters (data) that can be used, although all data must be first converted to a numerical value, without any character 'weighting'. Each organism is then compared with every other for all characters measured and the number of similarities (or differences) is calculated. The organisms are then clustered in such a way that the most similar are grouped close together and the more different ones are linked more distantly. The taxonomic clusters, called phenograms, that result from such an analysis do not necessarily reflect genetic similarity or evolutionary relatedness. The lack of evolutionary significance in phenetics has meant that this system has had little impact on animal classification and as a consequence, interest in and use of phenetics has been declining in recent years.

Cladistic Method of Analysis

An alternative approach to diagramming relationships between taxa is called cladistics. The basic assumption behind cladistics is that members of a group share a common evolutionary history. Thus, they are more closely related to one another than they are to other groups of organisms. Related groups of organisms are recognised because they share a set of unique features (apomorphies) that were not present in distant ancestors but which are shared by most or all of the organisms within the group. These shared derived characteristics are called synapomorphies. Therefore, in contrast to phenetics, cladistics groupings do not depend on whether organisms share physical traits but depend on their evolutionary relationships. Indeed, in cladistic analysis two organisms may share numerous characteristics but still be considered members of different groups.

Cladistic analysis entails a number of assumptions. For example, species are assumed to arise primarily by bifurcation or separation, of the ancestral lineage; species are often considered to become extinct upon hybridisation (crossbreeding); and hybridisation is assumed to be rare or absent. In addition, cladistic groupings must possess the following characteristics: all species in a grouping must share a common ancestor and all species derived from a common ancestor must be included in the taxon. The application of these requirements results in the following terms being used to describe the different ways in which groupings can be made:

1. A monophyletic grouping is one in which all species share a common ancestor, and all species derived from that common ancestor are included. This is the only form of grouping accepted as valid by cladists.

2. A paraphyletic grouping is one in which all species share a common ancestor, but not all species derived from that common ancestor are included. A polyphyletic grouping is one in which species that do not share an immediate common ancestor are lumped together, while excluding other members that would link them.

ORIGINS OF MOLECULAR PHYLOGENETICS

Macromolecular data, meaning gene (DNA) and protein sequences, are accumulating at an increasing rate because of recent advances in molecular biology. For the evolutionary biologist, the rapid accumulation of sequence data from whole genomes has been a major advance, because the very nature of DNA allows it to be used as a 'document' of evolutionary history. Comparisons of the DNA sequences of various genes between different organisms can tell a scientist a lot about the relationships of organisms that cannot otherwise be inferred from morphology or an organism's outer form and inner structure. Because genomes evolve by the gradual accumulation of mutations, the amount of nucleotide sequence difference between a pair of genomes from different organisms should indicate how recently those two genomes shared a common ancestor. Two genomes that diverged in the recent past should have fewer differences than two genomes whose common ancestor is more ancient. Therefore, by comparing different genomes with each other, it should be possible to derive evolutionary relationships between them, the major objective of molecular phylogenetics. Molecular phylogenetics attempts to determine the rates and patterns of change occurring in DNA and proteins and to reconstruct the evolutionary history of genes and organisms. Two general approaches may be taken to obtain this information. In the first approach, scientists use DNA to study the evolution of an organism. In the second approach, different organisms are used to study the evolution of DNA. Whatever the approach, the general goal is to infer process from pattern: the processes of organismal evolution deduced from patterns of DNA variation and processes of molecular evolution inferred from the patterns of variations in the DNA itself.

Molecular Phylogenetic Analysis

Fundamental elements as we just discussed, macromolecules, especially gene and protein sequences, have surpassed morphological and other organismal characters as the most popular forms of data for phylogenetic analysis. Therefore, this next section will concentrate only on molecular data. It is important to point out that a single, all-purpose recipe does not exist for phylogenetic analysis of molecular data. Although numerous algorithms, procedures, and computer programs have been developed, their reliability and practicality are, in all cases, dependent upon the size and structure of the dataset under analysis. The merits and shortfalls of these various methods are subject to much scientific debate, because the danger of generating incorrect results is greater in computational molecular phylogenetics than many other fields of science. Occasionally, the limiting factor in such analyses is not so much the computational method used, but the users' understanding in of what the method is actually doing with the data. Therefore, the goal of this section is to demonstrate to the reader that practical analysis should be thought of both as a search for a correct model (analysis) as well as a search for the correct tree (outcome). Phylogenetic tree-building models presume particular evolutionary models. For any given set of data, these models may be violated because of various occurrences, such as the transfer of genetic material between organisms. Therefore, when interpreting a given analysis, a person should always consider the model used and entertain possible explanations for the results obtained. For example, models used in molecular phylogenetic analysis.

Methods make 'default' assumptions

The sequence is correct and originates from the specified source:
1. The sequences are homologous—all descended in some way from a shared ancestral sequence.
2. Each position in a sequence alignment is homologous with every other in that alignment.
3. Each of the multiple sequences included in a common analysis has a common phylogenetic history with the other sequences.
4. The sampling of taxa is adequate to resolve the problem under study.
5. Sequence variation among the samples is representative of the broader group.
6. The sequence variability in the sample contains phylogenetic signal adequate to resolve the problem under study.

Four Steps of Phylogenetic Analysis

A straightforward phylogenetic analysis consists of four steps:
1. Alignment-building the data model and extracting a dataset.
2. Determining the substitution model-consider sequence variation.
3. Tree building.
4. Tree evaluation.

Tree building

Key features of DNA-based phylogenetic trees: Studies of gene and protein evolution often involve the comparison of homologs, sequences that have common origins but may or may not have common activity. Sequences that share an arbitrary level of similarity determined by alignment of matching bases are homologous. These sequences are inherited from a common ancestor that possessed similar structure, although the ancestor may be difficult to determine because it has been modified through descent.

Homologs are most commonly defined as orthologs, paralogs or xenologs. Orthologs are homologs produced by speciation. They represent genes derived from a common ancestor that diverged because of divergence of the organism. Orthologs tend to have similar function.

Paralogs are homologs produced by gene duplication and represent genes derived from a common ancestral gene that duplicated within an organism and then diverged. Paralogs tend to have different functions. Xenologs are homologs resulting from the horizontal transfer of a gene between two organisms. The function of xenologs can be variable, depending on how significant the change in context was for the horizontally moving gene. In general, though, the function tends to be similar.

A typical gene-based phylogenetic tree is shown in Fig. 21.1. This tree shows the relationship between four homologous genes: A, B, C and D. The topology of this tree consists of four external nodes (A, B,

C and D), each one representing one of the four genes and two internal nodes (e and f) representing ancestral genes. The branch lengths indicate the degree of evolutionary differences between the genes. This particular tree is unrooted it is only an illustration of the relationships between genes A, B, C and D and does not signify anything about the series of evolutionary events that led to these genes. A rooted tree is often referred to as an inferred tree.

This is to emphasise that this type of illustration depicts only the series of evolutionary events that are inferred from the data under study and may not be the same as the true tree or the tree that depicts the actual series of evolutionary events that occurred.

Fig. 21.1. Gene based phylogenetic tree.

To distinguish between the pathways, the phylogenetic analysis must include at least one outgroup, a gene that is less closely related to A, B, C and D than these genes are to each other (panel below). Outgroups enable the root of the tree to be located and the correct evolutionary pathway to be identified. Let's say that the four case, an outgroup could be a gene from another primate, such as baboon, which is known to have branched away from the four species above before the common ancestor of the species. Homologous genes used in the previous tree examples come from human, chimpanzee, gorilla and orangutan. In this case, an outgroup could be a gene from another primate, such as baboon, which is known to have branched away from the four species above before the common ancestor of the species.

GENE TREES VERSUS SPECIES TREES—WHY ARE THEY DIFFERENT?

It is assumed that a gene tree, because it is based on molecular data, will be a more accurate and less ambiguous representation of the species tree that is obtainable by morphological comparisons. This may indeed be the case, but it does not mean that the gene tree is the same as the species tree. For this to be true, the internal nodes in both trees would have to be precisely equivalent, and they are not. An internal node in a gene tree indicates the divergence of an ancestral gene into two genes with different DNA sequences, usually resulting from a mutation of one sort or another.

An internal node in a species tree represents what is called a speciation event, whereby the population of the ancestral species splits into two groups that are no longer able to interbreed. These two events, mutation and speciation, do not always occur at the same time.

MOLECULAR PHYLOGENETICS TERMINOLOGY
Monophyletic

Two or more DNA sequences that are derived from a single common ancestral DNA sequence.

Clade

A group of monophyletic DNA sequences that make up all of the sequences included in the analysis that are descended from a particular common ancestral sequence.

Parsimony

An approach that decides between different tree topologies by identifying the one that involves the shortest evolutionary pathway. This is the pathway that requires the smallest number of nucleotide changes to go from the ancestral sequence, at the root of the tree, to all of the present-day sequences that have been compared.

MOLECULAR CLOCK HYPOTHESIS

Molecular clock hypothesis states that nucleotide substitutions, or amino acid substitutions in proteins are being compared, occur at a constant rate, that is, the degree of difference between two sequences can be used to assign a date to the time at which their ancestral sequence diverged. The rate of molecular change differs among groups of organisms, among genes, and even among different parts of the same gene. Furthermore, molecular clocks require calibration with fossils to determine timing of origin of clades and thus their accuracy is crucially dependent on the fossil record, or lack thereof, for the groups under study. Fossil DNA older than about 25,000–50,000 years is virtually empty of phylogenetic signal except in rare instances and therefore traditional morphological studies of extinct and extant organisms remain a crucial component of phylogenetic analysis.

IMPORTANCE OF MOLECULAR PHYLOGENETICS

The field of molecular phylogenetics has grown, both in size and in importance, since its inception in the early 1990s, attributable mostly to advances in molecular biology and more rigorous methods for phylogenetic tree building. The importance of phylogenetics has also been greatly enhanced by the successful application of tree reconstruction, as well as other phylogenetic techniques. Today, a survey of the scientific literature will show that molecular biology, genetics, evolution, development, behaviour, epidemiology, ecology, systematics, conservation biology and forensics are but a few examples of perplexing issues in the many disparate fields conceptually united by the methods and theories of molecular phylogenetics. Phylogenies are used essentially the same way in all of these fields, either by drawing inferences from the structure of the tree or from the way the character states map onto the tree. Biologists can then use these clues to build hypotheses and models of important events in history. Broadly speaking, the relationships established by phylogenetic trees often describe a species' evolutionary history and hence, its phylogeny; the historical relationships among lineages or organisms or their parts, such as their genes. Phylogenies may be thought of as a natural and meaningful way to order data, with an enormous amount of evolutionary information contained within their branches. Scientists working in these different areas can then use these phylogenies to study and elucidate the biological processes occurring at many levels of life's hierarchy.

COMMON TREE-BUILDING METHODS USED IN PHYLOGENETIC INFERENCE

Phylogenetic inference can be defined as the process of determining the estimated evolutionary history by analysis of a given data set. Increasingly, molecular data sets, such as DNA and protein sequences, are used to develop these phylogenies. The reasons for building a phylogenetic tree are as diverse as the methods used to produce the trees. The process of phylogenetic analysis can be summarised by the following steps. The first two steps are preparatory for the subsequent steps that involve tree building and evaluation of the resultant tree.

1. The first step is the alignment of either the nucleotide or the amino acid sequences for the taxa of interest. It is generally agreed upon that amino acid sequences produce a tree closest to the true tree. This is due to the higher rate of conservation of amino acid sequences and protein structure. Manual alignment editing is recommended over fully computational multiple alignments as the algorithms and programs are not yet optimal for phylogenetic alignment. Regardless of the method for alignment, the final alignment should be carefully scrutinised with any independent phylogenetic evidence and other assumptions of structure and function. Once one proceeds to tree building, the computer-generated alignment will be blind to any errors in alignment.

2. The second step will be to determine the presence of a phylogenetic signal. Most of the sequence analyses fall between two extremes: identical sequences and sequences which have become so divergent as to become randomised in relation to the phylogenetic history. The former case dictates no further analysis. The latter will result in an inferred phylogeny, though the randomness of the resulting phylogeny may not be worth the effort. Those sequence alignments that fall in between will have a mixture of conserved and random positions and will be the most useful in phylogenetic inference.

Once the alignment is complete, the next steps in phylogenetic inference are to decide the most appropriate tree-building method for a specified data set followed by choosing a strategy to find the best tree under the selected optimality criterion. Finally, the tree obtained must be scrutinised to determine the level of confidence that can be placed on the results. One of the most complex issues faced during the process of phylogenetic inference is choosing the tree-building method.

Classification of Tree-Building Methods

Tree-building methods can be classified in two ways.

The first way to classify these methods is to define them as either algorithm-based or criterion-based

Though the procedure involved in each of these methods is different, the same algorithm could potentially be used in either method. An algorithm-based method generates a tree by following a series of steps, whereas criterion-based methods define an optimality criterion for comparing alternative phylogenies to one another and deciding, which one is better. Therefore, there is a big advantage when working with criteria-based methods because scores are assigned to every examined tree and can be used to rank the resultant phylogenies in order of preference. This provides, the user with immediate knowledge about the strength of support for that tree. Strictly algorithmic methods are computationally much faster than the criteria-based methods, because they do not require evaluation of a large number of competing trees. Due to the large number of possible solutions, criteria-based methods do not produce exact results for data sets with more than 8–20 taxa.

Alternatively, tree-building methods can be classified into distance-based versus character-based methods

A distance-based method computes pairwise distances according to some measure. Then, the actual data is discarded and the fixed distances are used in the derivation of trees. Trees derived by way of a character-based method have been optimised according to the distribution of actual data patterns in relation to a specified character.

Cluster analysis and neighbour joining are examples of methods defined solely on the basis of an algorithm or of methods that are unable to separate the task of finding an optimal tree from that of evaluating a specific tree, unlike the criteria-based methods. Cluster analysis constructs trees by linking the least distant pairs of taxa, followed by successively more distant taxa or groups of taxa. Once two taxa are linked, they lose their individual identities and are subsequently referred to as a single cluster. Neighbour joining is related to this traditional cluster analysis except it removes the assumption that data are ultrameric. The tree is constructed by linking the least distant pairs of nodes as defined by a modified matrix. The modified distance matrix is constructed by adjusting the separation between each pair of nodes on the basis of the average divergence from all other nodes.

There are three common types of optimality criteria that will be briefly discussed including parsimony, likelihood and pairwise distance. Both maximum parsimony and maximum likelihood use the original data set for inference. Maximum parsimony falls under the philosophy of 'the simpler hypotheses are preferable to the complicated ones'. It works in such a way as to choose from the alternative trees, the one with the fewest character-state transformations, thus minimising homoplasy (e.g. convergence, reversal). Thus, this optimality criterion operates by selecting trees that minimise the total tree length. This method tends to yield numerous trees with the same score, which is not characteristic of other methods such as distance or maximum likelihood. Parsimony is less dependent upon assumptions about the sequence evolution than some other methods and amenable to weighting in order to accommodate any substitution bias. The drawbacks for parsimony include slowed computation with weighting and poor performance when there is substantial among-site rate heterogeneity. Though there are several modifications that can correct for heterogeneity, such as modifying the data set or reweighting positions according to their propensity to change (successive approximation), this could potentially lead to errors in a prior step if the preliminary tree contains any errors.

An area of trouble using maximum parsimony is referred to as the Felsenstein zone. This zone is created when there exists strongly unequal rates of change along different branches of a tree or even with equal rates of change in cases of long-branch attraction. Long-branch refers to a lineage that evolved so much between nodes in the phylogeny that its character states have been effectively randomised with respect to the other taxa. Once in the Felsenstein zone misleading inferences are produced. At the ends of these long branches, character states are exhibited that no longer retain genealogical information leading to a distortion in the inference. Particularly deceptive are taxa on long branches that have converged on character states present in other taxa within the analysis. This appears as a false phylogenetic signal, obscuring the true signal. There are several ways to fix this problem including weighted parsimony, the use of relative apparent synapomorphy analysis (RASA) or using maximum likelihood that incorporates models of evolutionary change.

Parsimony once took the lead as the most favoured method; however, maximum likelihood appears to be replacing parsimony, particularly as this method becomes better defined. The critical difference between these two methods is that parsimony minimises the amount of evolutionary change required for data explanation, while maximum likelihood attempts to estimate the actual amount of change according to the evolutionary model in place. Maximum likelihood works with a prior nucleotide substitution model to compute a likelihood score for each tree given the original data. Before beginning, either an evolutionary model must be specified that can account for the conversion of one sequence into another or parametres must be selected that can be estimated from the data. Then the maximum likelihood approach evaluates the probability that the selected evolutionary model will have generated the observed sequences. The trees yielding the highest likelihoods are used to infer phylogeny. The substitution model should be optimised to fit the observed data as modifying the substitution parametres modify the likelihood of the data associated with particular trees.

The greatest drawback to using maximum likelihood is the vast amount of computation time required.

Maximum likelihood is not always available for use. An alternative method that also minimises the impact of the underestimation problem present in parsimony is the pairwise distance method. It works on the idea that corrected distances to account for superimposed changes can be obtained by estimating the number of unseen events using the same models used with maximum likelihood. The corrected distances are estimates of the true evolutionary distance. The drawback for this method is the loss of data during the process.

Because many of the more complex models require an enormous amount of time to complete the computations, heuristic methods are often selected in place of the alternative search methods. A heuristic method does not guarantee finding the optimal solution, but does provide a large increase in speed. Such is the case with maximum likelihood. Likelihood has several advantages including consistency, lower variance in estimation, and its robustness to violations of its assumptions, so many attempts have been made to incorporate maximum likelihood into a heuristic method that will simultaneously optimise the substitution model and the tree for a given data set.

In applying any of these methods, there are two key ideas that have been emphasised in the literature throughout the development of phylogenetics. The importance of the starting data cannot be stressed enough. The type of data not only determines which method to choose for analysis, but also determines the validity of the results obtained from a selected method. It follows, then, that the validity of the resulting tree is dependent upon the appropriateness of the model used in tree generation. Phylogenetic inference methods are under continual evaluation and improvement upon the accuracy and speed of computation in these methods is a continual process. In several cases, it has been determined that trees obtained from the simpler methods produce as good results as those obtained by more sophisticated methods. Though this may be an accurate assessment, the more complex methods have the advantage of producing several alternatives, which allow for the different topologies to be evaluated for statistical significance. There is no agreement, yet, on which method is the best method and more than likely there never will be as the best method is dependent upon the type of data with which one begins. As long as the method has a theoretical justification, then it is more important to choose a good gene or a large number of amino acids than it is to choose a particular tree-building method.

## Chapter 22

Phylogenetic Prediction

INTRODUCTION

On one level, it is interesting to understand and study how the evolution of species has occurred. There are many different resources discussing the evolution of species. This includes the NCBI taxonomy web sites and the University of Arizona's tree of life project.

TREE OF LIFE

Evolutionary Trees

An evolutionary tree is a two-dimensional graph showing the evolutionary relationship among a set of items being compared. This set can be organisms, genes or DNA sequences. Consider for the moment that each of the units in the set are referred to as a taxon. Each taxon will be defined by a distinct unit on the tree. An evolutionary tree is composed of outer branches or leaves that represent the taxa and nodes and branches representing the relationships among the taxa. Two taxa that are derived from the same common ancestor will share a node in the graph. In general, approaches to designing evolutionary trees attempt are made to define the length of each branch to the next node according to the number of sequence level changes that occurred. One thing to be careful of in phylogenetic analysis is that this distance may not be in direct relation to evolutionary time. Analyses that prescribe to the theory of a uniform rate of mutation are known as the molecular clock hypothesis.

Rooted Trees

In a rooted tree topology, one sequence (the root) is defined to be the common ancestor of all of the other sequences. A unique path leads from the root node to any other node and the direction of the path indicates evolutionary time. The root is chosen by including a sequence from an organism that is thought to have branched off earlier than the other sequences. If the molecular clock hypothesis holds, it is also possible to predict a root. As the number of sequences increase, the number of possible rooted trees increases very rapidly. In some cases, a bifurcating binary tree is the best model to simulate evolutionary events in which case one species branches off into two separate species. Example of a rooted tree is shown in Fig. 22.1.

Star Topology (Unrooted Trees)

An unrooted tree (sometimes referred to as a star topology) shows the evolutionary relationship among sequences, without revealing the location of the oldest ancestry.

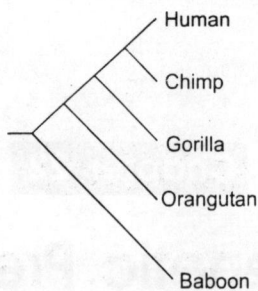

Fig. 22.1. Example of a rooted tree.

There are fewer choices for an unrooted tree than a rooted tree. Example of an unrooted tree is shown in Fig. 22.2.

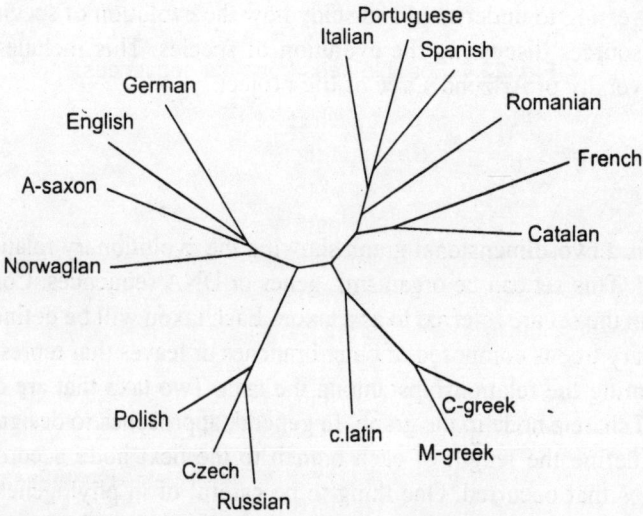

Fig. 22.2. Example of an unrooted tree.

METHODS FOR DETERMINING EVOLUTIONARY TREES

There are three methods used to calculate the tree(s) that best account for the observed variation in a set of sequences. These methods are maximum parsimony, distance and maximum likelihood.

Maximum Parsimony

Maximum parsimony methods predict the evolutionary tree that minimises the number of steps required to generate the observed variation in the sequences. In order to construct a tree using maximum parsimony, a multiple sequence alignment must first be obtained. For each aligned position, phylogenetic trees that require the smallest number of evolutionary changes to produce the observed sequence changes are identified. This continues for each position in the alignment. Those trees that produce the smallest number of changes overall for all sequence positions are identified. This is a rather time consuming algorithm that only works well if the sequences have a strong sequence similarity.

Consider the example above. There are a total of four sequences, (Fig. 22.3), which gives a possibility of three different unrooted trees as shown in Fig. 22.4. In this case some sites are informative and other sites are not. An informative site has the same sequence character in atleast two different sequences. Only the informative sites need to be considered.

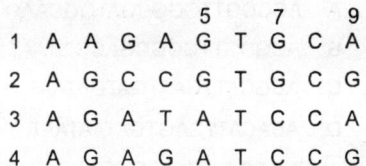

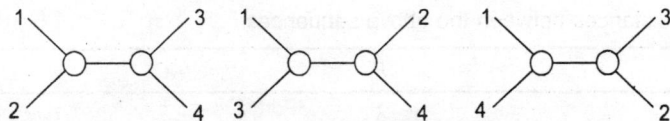

Fig. 22.3. Multiple alignment for phylogeny.

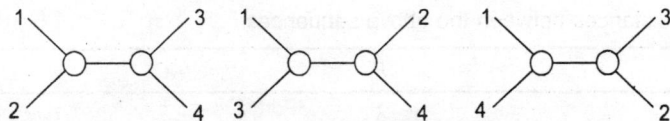

Fig. 22.4. Possible trees from four sequences.

In this case, adding the number of changes at each informative site for each tree and picking the tree requiring the least total number of changes obtain the optimal tree.

For a large number of sequences the number of trees to examine becomes so large that it might not be possible to examine all possible trees. Some programs, such as PAUP, add features that will allow the user to invoke a heuristic that will keep representative trees that best fit the data.

The informative sites in the example of alignment are position 5, 7 and 9 in Fig. 22.3.

Let's go through the possible trees and figure out the number of rearrangements for each in the informative sites.

One problem with determining evolutionary distance between sequences is that columns representing greater variation dominate the analysis. In order to overcome this problem of determining long branch lengths is to look only at transversion events, which are the most significant base changes (i.e. changes a purine to a pyrimidine or *vice versa*). This is referred to as Lake's method of invariants.

Distance Methods

The distance method for construction of phylogenetic trees looks at the number of changes between each pair in a group of sequences to produce a phylogenetic tree of the group. The goal of distance methods is to identify a tree that positions neighbours correctly and that also has branch lengths, which reproduce the original data as closely as possible.

CLUSTALW uses the neighbour-joining method as a guide to multiple sequence alignments. The PHYLIP suite of programs employs neighbour-joining methods.

Phylip http://evolution.genetics.washington. edu/phylip.html

Distance analysis programs in PHYLIP:

FITCH: estimates a phylogenetic tree assuming additivity of branch lengths using the Fitch-Margoliash method.

KITSH: same as FTCH, but under the assumption of a molecular clock.

NEIGHBOUR: estimates phylogenies using the neighbour joining (no molecular clock assumed) or unweighted pair group method with arithmetic mean (UPGMA) (molecular clock assumed).

For phylogenetic analysis, the distance score counted as either the number of mismatched positions in the alignment or the number of sequence positions that must be changed to generate the other sequence is used. The success of distance methods depends on the degree to which the distances among a set of sequences can be made additive on a predicted evolutionary tree. The alignment is shown in Fig. 22.5.

A   ACGCGTTGGGCGATGGCAAC

B   ACGCGTTGGGCGACGGTAAT

C   ACGCATTGAATGATGATAAT

D   ACACATTGAGTGATAATAAT

Fig. 22.5. The alignment.

The distances between these sequences are shown in Table 22.1.

Table 22.1. Showing distances between the above sequences.

	A	*B*	*C*	*D*
A	–	3	7	8
B	–	–	6	7
C	–	–	–	3
D	–	–	–	–

Note: Distances are nothing but the number of changes in bases/aminoacids between any two sequences under comparison.

Using this information, an unrooted tree showing the relationship between these sequences can be drawn as shown in Fig. 22.6.

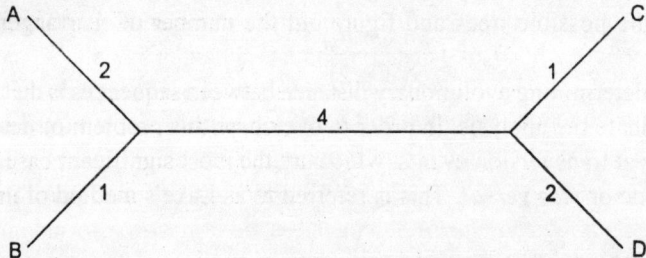

Fig. 22.6. Unrooted tree resulting from the above four sequences.

Fitch and Margoliash Method

The Fitch and Margoliash method uses a distance table. The sequences are combined in threes to define the branches of the predicted tree and to calculate the branch lengths of the tree. The Fitch and Margoliash method can be extended to three or more sequences.

The Fitch-Margoliash algorithm can be extended to three or more sequences.

Repeat the process until all lengths have been identified, in which case there is only single composite node left. Thus the steps involved in Fitch-Margoliash algorithm are summarised here pointwise.

1. Find the most closely related pairs of sequences (A, B).
2. Treat the rest of the sequences as a composite. Calculate the average distance from A to all others; and from B to all others.
3. Use these values to calculate the length of the edges a and b.
4. Treat A and B as a composite. Calculate the average distances between AB and each of the other sequences. Create a new distance table.

5. Identify next pair of related sequences and begin as with step 1.
6. Subtract extended branch lengths to calculate lengths of intermediate branches.
7. Repeat the entire process with all possible pairs of sequences.
8. Calculate predicted distances between each pair of sequences for each tree to find the best tree.

NEIGHBOUR-JOINING ALGORITHM

The neighbour-joining method is very similar to the Fitch-Margoliash method. The sequences that should be joined are chosen to give the best least-squares estimates of the branch lengths that most closely reflect the actual distances between the sequences. The neighbour-joining method begins by creating a star topology in which no neighbours are joined (Fig. 22.7).

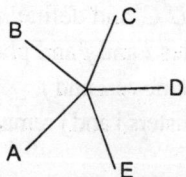

Fig. 22.7. Star topology of neighbour join method.

The tree is modified by joining pairs of sequences. The pair to be joined is chosen by calculating the sum of the branch lengths for the corresponding tree. The sum of the branch lengths is calculated as follows:

$$S_{mn} = \frac{\Sigma d_{im} + d_{in}}{2(N-2)} + \frac{d_{mn}}{2} + \frac{\Sigma d_{ij}}{N-2}$$

where, i, j represent all sequences except m and n and $i < j$.

For example, consider the tree when A and B are joined: See Fig. 22.8 below:

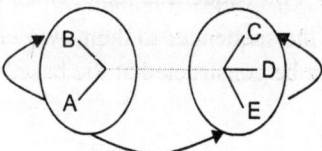

Fig. 22.8. Modified tree after joining pairs of sequences.

The pair that results in the smallest branch length is then chosen to be the pair that is joined. Based on this choice, the Fitch-Margoliash algorithm is used to compute the actual branch lengths.

After the pair has joined, a new distance table is created with the recently joined sequences now entered as a composite. The neighbour-joining algorithm chooses the next pair of sequences to join and the F-M algorithm computes the branch lengths.

The process continues until the correctly branched tree and distances have been identified.

UNWEIGHTED PAIR GROUP METHOD WITH ARITHMETIC MEAN (UPGMA)

Works by clustering the sequences, starting with more similar sequences and working towards more distant sequences. The process assembles a tree upwards, with each node being added above the others and the edge lengths being determined by the difference in the heights of the nodes.

The distance d_{ij} between two clusters C_i and C_j are number, of sequences in clusters i and j is defined to be the average distance between pairs of sequences from each cluster:

$$d_{ij} = \frac{1}{|C_i||C_j|} \sum_{pinC_i, qinC_j} d_{pq}$$

where, $|C_i|$ and $|C_j|$ are the number of sequences in clusters i and j, respectively.

The algorithm for UPGMA clustering is as follows:

1. Assign each sequence i to its own cluster C_i.
2. Define one leaf of the tree T for each sequence and place it at height 0.
3. Determine the two clusters, i and j for which d_{ij} is minimal.
4. Define a new cluster k by $C_k = C_i \cup C_j$ and define d_{kl} for all 1.
5. Define a node k with daughter nodes i and j and place it at height $d_{ij}/2$.
6. Add k to the current clusters and remove i and j.
7. Continue steps 3–6 until only two clusters i and j remain and place the root of the tree at height $d_{ij}/2$.

Example of UPGMA

Consider the case where there are five sequences represented by dots on a graph. See Fig. 22.9, the spacing between each of these is representative of the distance between them.

Fig. 22.9. Five sequences represented by dots.

The first step is to assign each of the sequences to their own cluster, which now gives a number to each of these. In addition, the tree can be constructed at the base, where each sequence is a leaf of the tree as shown in Fig. 22.10.

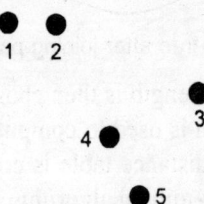

Fig. 22.10. Sharing assignment of sequences to their own cluster.

Now select the two clusters that are closest to each other. These are the sequences 1 and 2. Create a single cluster for these two sequences and create a parent node in the tree at height $d_{12}/2$ see Fig. 22.11.Continue on, selecting the two clusters that are closest: in this case, it is 4 and 5. Combine into a single cluster and update the tree, see Fig. 22.12.

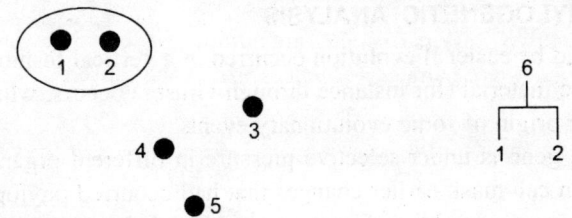

Fig. 22.11. Clumping of close clusters to create a single cluster.

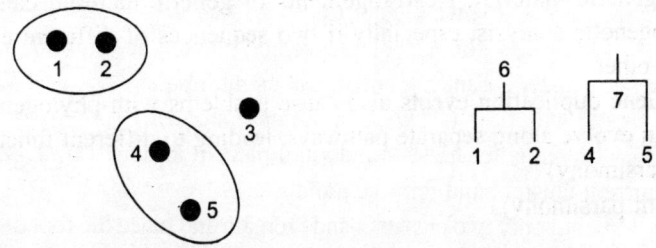

Fig. 22.12. Clustering process being extended.

The next two clusters are the one containing 4 and 5 and the one containing 3, see Fig. 22.13.

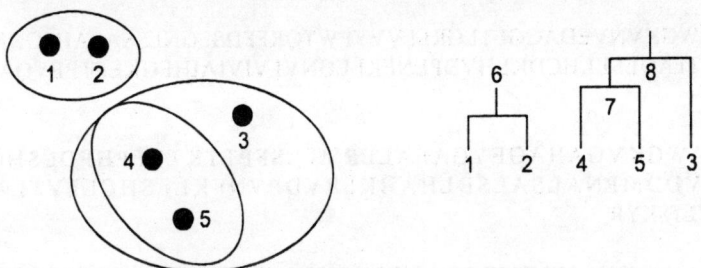

Fig. 22.13. Clustering further extended.

There are now only two clusters left, so join them to complete the tree, Fig. 22.14.

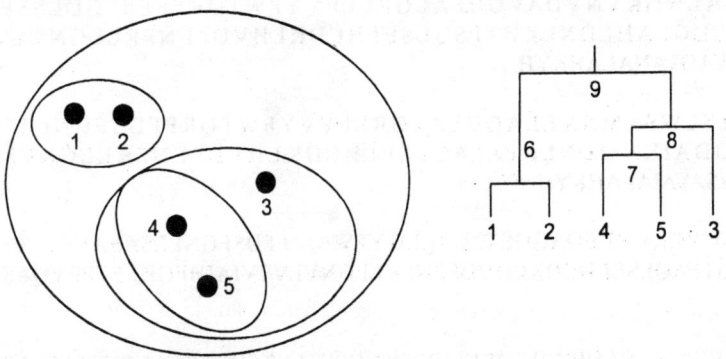

Fig. 22.14. Completion of clustering.

DIFFICULTIES WITH PHYLOGENETIC ANALYSIS

Phylogenetic analysis would be easier if evolution occurred in a vertical fashion. However, horizontal or lateral transfer of genetic material (for instance through viruses) occurs, which makes it difficult to determine the phylogenetic origin of some evolutionary events.

Selective Pressure: If a gene is under selective pressure in different organisms, it can be rapidly evolving. Such an evolution can mask earlier changes that had occurred phylogenetically. In addition, different regions of a genome are under different pressures and therefore different sites within two comparative sequences may be evolving at different rates.

Rearrangement of genetic material: Rearrangements of genetic material can also lead to false conclusions with phylogenetic analysis, especially if two sequences of different evolutionary origins are placed next to each other.

Gene duplication: Gene duplication events also cause problems with phylogenetic analysis, since the duplicated genes can evolve along separate pathways, leading to different functions.

PAUP (maximum parsimony)

MacClade (maximum parsimony)

CONSENSE

PHYLIP—(distance—neighbour joining)

CLUSTALW—distance-based tree

Consider the following list of Globin sequences:

>gamma_A
MGHFTEEDKATITSLWGKVNVEDAGGETLGRLLVVYPWTQRFFDSFGNLSSASAIMGNPKVKAHGKKVLT
SLGDAIKHLDDLKGTFAQLSELHCDKLHVDPENFKLLGNVLVIVIAIHFGKEFTPEVQASWQKMVTAVAS
ALSSRYH
>alfa
VLSPADKTNVKAAWGKVGAHAGEYGAEALERMFLSFPTTKTYFPHFDLSHGSAQVKGHGK
KVADALTNAVAHVDDMPNALSALSDLHAHKLRVDPVNFKLLSHCLLVTLAAHLPAEFTPA
VHASLDKFLASVSTVLTSKYR
>beta
VHLTPEEKSAVTALWGKVNVDEVGGEALGRLLVVYPWTQRFFESFGDLSTPDAVMGNPKV
KAHGKKVLGAFSDGLAHLDNLKGTFATLSELHCDKLHVDPENFRLLGNVLVCVLAHHFGK
EFTPPVQAAYQKVVAGVANALAHKYH
>delta
VHLTPEEKTAVNALWGKVNVDAVGGEALGRLLVVYPWTQRFFESFGDLSSPDAVMGNPKV
KAHGKKVLGAFSDGLAHLDNLKGTFSQLSELHCDKLHVDPENFRLLGNVLVCVLARNFGK
EFTPQMQAAYQKVVAGVANALAHKYH
>epsilon
VHFTAEEKAAVTSLWSKMNVEEAGGEALGRLLVVYPWTQRFFDSFGNLSSPSAILGNPKV
KAHGKKVLTSFGDAIKNMDNLKPAFAKLSELHCDKLHVDPENFKLLGNVMVIILATHFGK
EFTPEVQAAWQKLVSAVAIALAHKYH
>gamma_G
MGHFTEEDKATITSLWGKVNVEDAGGETLGRLLWYPWIQRFFDSFGNLSSASAIMGNPKVKAHGKKVLT
SLGDAIKHLDDLKGTFAQLSELHCDKLHVDPENFKLLGNVLVTVIAIHFGKEFTPEVQASWQKMVTGVAS
ALSSRYH
>myoglobin
MGLSDGEWQLVLNVWGKVEADIPGHGQEVLIRLFKGHPETLEKFDKFKHLKSEDEMKASEDLKKHGATVL
TALGGILKKKGHHEAEIKPLAQSHATKHKIPVKYLEFISECIIQVLQSKHPGDFGADAQGAMNKALELFR
KDMASNYKELGFQG
>tetal

ALSAEDRALVRALWKKLGSNVGVYTTEALERTFLAFPATKTYFSHLDLSPGSSQVRAHGQ
KVADALSLAVERLDDLPHALSALSHLHACQLRVDPASFQLLGHCLLVTLARHYPGDFSPA
LQASLDKFLSHVISALVSEYR
>zeta
SLTKTERTIIVSMWAKISTQADTIGTETLERLFLSHPQTKTYFPHFDLHPGSAQLRAHGS KVVAAVGDAVKSI
DDIGGALSKLSELHAYILRVDPVNFKLLSHCLLVTLAARFPADFTAE AHAAWDKFLSVVSSVLTEKYR

Create a phylogeny from these.

PHYLOGENETIC TREE

Methods to Build a Tree

1. Genetic distances.
2. Phylogenetic analysis programs and where to get them.
3. Our interface.
4. Common mistakes in making trees.
5. What to do when your tree looks funny.

First of all, it is important to realise that all tree-building methods assume that the alignment is correct; errors in the alignment can lead to a very misleading tree. Once the alignment is optimal, there are many different methods to create phylogenies. Roughly, the methods can be divided into distance-based and character-based methods. Character-based methods use the individual substitutions among the sequences to determine the most likely ancestral relationships, while distance-based methods first calculate the overall distance between all pairs of sequences and then calculate a tree based on those distances. Maximum parsimony (MP) and maximum likelihood (ML) are the most important character based methods. In most comparative studies, ML seems to be the method that yields the best trees.

The most important drawback of ML is that it is very computationally intensive; it is almost unusable with more than a few dozen sequences. MP is much faster than ML, but still slow compared to most distance-based methods. Both these programs calculate large numbers of trees and compare them by either the likelihood or the parsimony score. There are programs available which speed up the process considerably, such as FastDNAml but for large numbers of sequences the computational burden is still a major hurdle.

The distance-based methods are generally much faster than the character-based ones. In this group, neighbour joining (NJ) is by far the most popular method. It is very fast and generally quite good, although there are conditions under which it systematically produces a wrong tree (bias). NJ is not the only biased method: in fact, under the right conditions (mostly when evolutionary rates are different for different sites, which is frequently the case for HIV) any method is biased, i.e. systematically produces the wrong tree. The importance of the bias for the everyday tree is a matter of fierce debate.

Weighbor (short for 'weighted neighbour-joining') is a new method by Bruno, Socci and Halpern, which gives less weight to the longer distances in the distance matrix. The resulting trees are less sensitive to specific biases than NJ and MP and negative branch lengths are avoided. The method is much faster than ML and usually faster than MP, but much slower than NJ.

To some extent the choice between methods can be based on the purpose of the tree. For subtyping sequences, an NJ tree based on a matrix of genetic distances is generally good enough. It is not vital that the tree is correct in every branch, only that the sequence of interest is clustered with the right subtype. Almost any method will solve this problem correctly.

However, when more detailed information on the evolutionary relationships is important, for instance in forensic analyses or when studying rates of evolution or trying to resolve key relationships (for example, short domains and potential recombination), more realistic models of evolution and unbiased tree reconstruction methods should be used.

Genetic distances

The simplest way to calculate a distance between two sequences is to count the number of differences. This measure is often called the hamming distance. It reflects the difference between sequences, but ignores their evolutionary relationship. The most intuitive way to show how this can be misleading to think of superimposed or reversed mutations: a nucleotide in a sequence, say an A, gets mutated and becomes a G. This results in a difference of 1. Many replication rounds later the same site gets mutated again. If it becomes an A, the difference now goes down, even though the genetic distance (the number of mutational events) has gone up. If it becomes a T or a C, the differences doesn't change, but the evolutionary distance should increase, because there have now been two evolutionary events.

The oldest attempt to adjust the number of differences between two sequences for the chances of a parallel or back mutation was designed by Jukes and Cantor. They proposed the corrective formula $D = -3/4 \ln[1-(4p/3)]$, where, D = Distance, ln = Leen, P = Base frequency. First, the effect of the correction increases with the difference between the sequences and is negligible with very homologous sequences. Second, the effect of saturation can be seen beyond a certain number of differences (75 per cent), it becomes impossible to tell what the true genetic distance is.

Since this formula was first proposed in the 1980s, many different models have been proposed to accurately estimate the underlying evolutionary distance from the observed number of differences between the sequences, taking into account new knowledge about the behaviour of DNA, such as different transition/transversion rates, different base frequencies and nonuniform substitution rates between sites. Not all of these sophisticated methods are easily available (Dnadist, for example, only offers Jukes-Cantor, Kimura 2-parametre, Jin-Nei and the F84 model Phylip uses for its maximum likelihood trees; Mega also offers Tamura and Tamura-Nei and a set of Gamma distribution-based distances).

A relatively new development is the use of models that incorporate variable/evolutionary rates across sites. This is an important extension of the existing models, especially for HIV, which is well known to show dramatically different evolutionary rates (e.g. under the influence of immune escape) over the length of the genome.

Gary Olsen has a program called DNA rates, which can estimate the rates of evolution in different sites, given an initial tree. The number of categories for the rates can be specified by the user. Using the DNA rates program can quite dramatically increase the quality of the resulting trees.

Many simulations show that the importance of using a realistic substitution model for estimating the genetic distance depends very much on the divergence of the sequences. If the expected number of substitutions per site is small (below 0.2), the resulting tree will not change much when different substitution models are used. If the sequences are highly diverged, however and especially when the number of substitutions per site rises above 1, the differences become marked, the choice of the substitution model is very important.

Tree-building programs

Probably the most widely used program suite is Felsenstein's PHYLIP. It offers a large array of methods, including ML, MP and NJ. The choice of genetic distance is fairly limited and learning to use the programs requires some time investment, but their versatility makes them very popular. Most allow input of user trees, jumbling (randomising input orders) and out group designation.

MEGA is a nifty little program for DOS/Windows. It offers NJ and MP (although in a quirky implementation) and the sophisticated Tamura-Nei genetic distance estimation. MEGA is able to build trees on the basis of silent or nonsilent mutations only and has a fast bootstrapping option built in. It is available for minimal cost from the authors. Downsides are that the program is fairly unstable and has memory problems with large sets of sequences and the printing of the trees often gives problems.

PHYLOWIN is a UNIX/Linux based program with a very nice graphical user interface. It does ML, MP and NJ, allows selection of sequences (rows) and position (columns) and bootstrapping. It allows the User to define subsets of sequences and positions and save them. It is available free of charge for academic users.

FastDNAml computes fast(er) ML trees. It is not very easy to use, but is often the only option if one wants to calculate ML trees for more than 20 sequences. It uses input file or command line parametres to specify the trees. The C source code for the program and an executable for Powermac are available by ftp.

PAUP is a very versatile program that does maximum likelihood tree building in addition to parsimony and allows incorporation of variable rates per site. It is presently distributed as a beta version. The Mac version is entirely menu-driven, but the user interface is very clumsy. There are no user interfaces for the Windows and Unix versions.

HIV-WEB Treemaker Interface

This interface is just that: it interfaces between the user and the phylogenetic programs Dnadist, Neighbour and Drawtree/Drawgram from Joe Felsenstein's PHYLIP suite. The interface can only be used to make Neighbour-Joining trees, which may not be optimal for all circumstances, but usually form a good starting point for more sophisticated analysis; and as mentioned above, if the inferences made from the tree need not be very exact, for example for subtyping a small region or for a quick contamination check, this tree can suffice. Please note that the interface does not do bootstrapping.

The interface takes a sequence alignment in several formats, allows the adjustment of a few parametres (transition/transversion ratio, outgroup and the shape of the tree). It uses the F84 genetic distance estimate (i.e. the option called 'ML' in Dnadist).

Common Mistakes in Making a Tree

Presenting the output from PHYLIP's consense program as the final tree

This tree gives only a branching order. The 'branchlengths' are not true branch lengths, but rather reflect the per cent bootstrap values. For this reason, the Treefile that consense produces does not contain branch lengths and when printed, all branches in the tree have the same length.

Remedy: If you want to include bootstrap values in a tree created with PHYLIP, the simplest method is to simply paste the values into the nonbootstrapped tree with valid branchlengths. The better way is to use the tree you get from the Consense program as input for another run of the tree-building program to have the branch lengths estimated for that particular tree. This also solves the (infrequent) problem where the topology of the consensus tree doesn't exactly match the one of the original tree.

Visible alignment errors and/or unrecognised hypermutation

When one sequence protrudes far out beyond all the others and there is no inherent reason for it to be so different, further inspection is needed. Frequently the cause is an alignment error or a hypermutated sequence.

Remedy
1. Visually check the alignment of your sequences. There are many alignment editors available that make it very easy to do this.
2. Check your sequence for hypermutation. Hypermutation, a relatively common phenomenon in HIV, means a very high incidence of G - > A mutations, usually resulting in a nonviable sequence. An interface that was designed to detect hypermutation: HYPERMUT.

Unrecognised recombination

When an isolate branches off close to the root between two subtypes, especially if it has a long branch or if it is not from a particularly old isolate, there is a chance that it is a recombinant. In this case the MAL isolate, an A/D/I recombinant. Similarly, when a sequence branches off between two clusters from one patient isolate, it can be a within-patient recombinant. In this case it can be the result of a real recombination event or a PCR artifact.

Remedy

If you suspect your sequence may be a recombinant, there are a multitude of ways to look at this more closely. On this we have RIP, which produces an alignment and an easy-to-read plot that shows the similarity of your sequence to a set of reference sequences over the entire length of the sequence. If there are major changes in what the most similar sequence is over the length of your sequence, this suggests recombination. There are many more methods to detect recombination.

Assuming a molecular clock

The graphical representation of this assumption is that all branches end on one vertical line, representing the present day. This assumption is not realistic for HIV and it is very uncommon for other organisms. The most commonly used method that produces these trees is UPGMA; the Kitsch (which explicitly assumes a molecular clock) program from the PHYLIP suite also results in this type of tree.

Remedy

Use a different tree reconstruction method. Neighbour joining, maximum parsimony and maximum likelihood all produce trees that do not assume a strict molecular clock.

What to do When Your Tree Looks Funny

If none of these errors describe your situation, but you still think your tree is off, there are a few things you can do.
1. Try a different method or a different distance estimate. In rare cases (when there are many equivalent trees) even the input order of the sequence can make a difference; use the Jumble option provided in DNAML or rearrange your input file.
2. Try using a different program that uses the same tree reconstruction method and compare the results.
3. Use a different outgroup: although the outgroup does not affect the structure of the tree, it can sometimes make it easier to interpret.
4. Split your sequences in half and see if the resulting trees are different. This suggests either recombination or dramatic evolutionary rate differences. In some cases (an example is the Rev-responsive element or RRE in HIV) two adjacent regions can be under such different constraint that they evolve very differently; building a tree from a sequence that spans both regions can give confusing results.

Tree 'Reliability'

By far the most popular test for trees is the bootstrap. Contrary to what many people think, this is not a test of how accurate your tree is; it only gives information about the stability of the tree topology (the branching order) and it helps assess whether the sequence data is adequate to validate the topology. The bootstrap randomly resamples columns from your alignment, so that some positions will not be used and others will be used more than once and builds a new tree from this dataset. This is done as many times as you specify.

The bootstrap value is a count or percentage of how often each branch was present in exactly the same topology in all the resampled trees, so it gives an impression of how much the tree topology could change if, for example, you'd reconstruct it using a different gene. There are many rules of thumb about how to interpret the bootstrap. It is known to be a conservative measure, so a bootstrap of 95 per cent gives more than 95 per cent confidence in that branch. The number of 70 per cent is often cited as a cut-off for a 'reliable' branch.

SEQUENCE ALIGNMENTS AND TREE BUILDING

Alignment tools and methods for building phylogenetic trees.

Objectives

1. Gain a basic appreciation of phylogenetics:
   (a) Know the difference between phylogeny and taxonomy.
   (b) Explore phenetic and cladistic approaches.
   (c) Examine criteria of data selection and analysis.
2. Become familiar with on-line resources helpful in studying the phylogeny of organisms:
   (a) Explore and use sites, such as phylodendron web and PHYLIP servers.
   (b) Examine phylogenetic literature on-line.
3. Learn to use alignment and tree building tools and to analyse the results:
   (a) BLAST2 and ALIGN for selected pairwise alignments.
   (b) ClustalW and ClustalX for multiple sequence alignments.
   (c) Build trees using DRAWTREE and DRAWGRAM.

An excellent resource for this unit is below

If you intend to use these methods in your work or research, this following practical is highly recommended to extend beyond the basic introduction in this exercise. It contains both basic information and guided tutorials in the use of a variety of tools.

Pre-exercise

1. Review basic background on evolution, review it thoroughly before proceeding further. Dr. Jasper's site, which has excellent notes and interesting links, is also good for your cause.
   The site is mentioned below:
   http://www.zo.utexas.edu/faculty/sjasper/bio304/syl 304.html.
2. Jargon and the associated concepts, you need to know:
   (a) Phylogenetics vs. taxonomy.
   (b) Cladistic vs. phenetic.

    (c) Clustering.

    (d) Parsimony vs. maximum likelihood.

Part A

Multiple sequence alignments [MSA] and pairwise alignments:

1. You have already tried using Clustalw to do multiple sequence alignments. It is now time to dust off the cobwebs [tis the season!] and get back to it. Recall that you need to start with sequences in FASTA format or have files in Biology Workbench. For this exercise, please use the following set of accession numbers to obtain some protein sequences of glutamate synthase. These were chosen because they have similar enzymatic function and are therefore conserved, while being drawn from five kingdoms as shown in Table 22.2.

Table 22.2. Multiple sequence analysis.

A38596	Maize	Plant
CAC05496	*Arabidopsis*	Plant
AAC08261	*Porphyra*	Algae
CAA76602	*Plasmodium*	Protozoa
AAF49409	*Drosophila*	Animal
CAB92626	*Neurospora*	Fungi
CAA61505	*Saccharomyces*	Fungi
BAB05447	*Bacillus*	Bacteria
AAA58014	*E. Coli*	Bacteria
AAK94787	*Klebsiella*	Bacteria
CAB64595	*Nostoc*	Bacteria
AAG44102	*Staphylococcus*	Bacteria

These numbers can be used to obtain the protein sequences from NCBI. FASTA format is recommended for easy transfer into your log and uploading into Biology Workbench or elsewhere.

2. In your log, you need to remove the spaces on the line preceding '>gi | xxx...' for each entry. [Don't disturb the sequence lines.] This is necessary when running Clustal, because any extra spaces will terminate the alignment for all entries beyond those spaces.

3. At this point, you have two options. Choose the one you like [You can always return to try another option]:

    (a) You can use ClustalW at EBI. You need to be careful when you paste in your sequences that you remove any spaces at the beginning of lines. You may leave a blank line between sequence entries.

    http://www.ebi.ac.uk/clustalw/ or

    http://www.ebi.ac.uk/clustalw/

    Explore the site. You can read about the windows by clicking on them. [For the next steps, see 4b.] Once you have an alignment, you can save it or transfer it to another application or to Biology Workbench.

    (b) You can upload your sequences directly into Biology Workbench before aligning them. Be sure to check each sequence entry for inadvertent spaces at the beginning of lines. If you find any, remove them. Within Workbench, you can use ClustalW in either Protein Tools or Nucleotide Tools [see 4c] and then use other applications in Alignment Tools for analysis.

4. Follow the directions according to the option you selected in 3 above:

   (a) Paste your grouped FASTA sequences into the text box. For your first run, use the defaults. The alignments will take a few minutes. You may want to enter your e-mail to retrieve the report. If your run fails, the first check to see if the FASTA format and the left-hand spaces are OK. If a run seems to take too long, try 'off-hours', keeping in mind that this is a European site or try making your alignment request smaller. You can do this by selecting only 4–6 sequences.

   Alternatively, you may want to focus on just one region or domain of your sequences. In that case, you can select portions of the FASTA reports. After using the defaults, try changing some of the settings after reading about them in the support pages. For report viewing, see 5 below. *Note*: When running Clustal on a set of sequences, you may need to edit your sequences before you get reasonable alignments. It doesn't hurt to try a test run first. As you work through the following, consider what might be some of the causes of misalignments.

   (b) Select the sequences you want to compare by checking the boxes. Choose ClustalW. Initially accept the defaults. On repeated runs, try changing some of the settings [Go to the EBI site for documentation support]. Try running subgroups of sequences and try changing the order of sequences. You can change order by selecting a sequence and choosing a menu item, then return. The selected sequence is at the top of the list. You can easily scramble your list by randomly selecting and copying different sequences. You can also create edited sequences to select a region or to remove nonstandard characters. To save alignments, select 'Import alignments'. Then you can use the Alignment Tools. [See 6 below. You should skip 5.]

5. For option b only. [Option b, skip to 6 below.] Once you have the report, browse to see what you have. Click on Jalview for a graphical display. Wait for the calculations and colour assignment to be complete before trying to navigate. For your convenience, consensus notations and colours used in Jalview are assigned as follows.

Consensus line notations:

   * = identical or conserved residues in all sequences in the alignment.

   : = indicates conserved substitutions.

   . = Indicates semi-conserved substitutions.

Characteristics	*Amino acids*
red: small and hydrophobic	AVFPMILW
R groups	
blue: acidic	DE
magenta: basic	RHK
green: hydroxyl + X	STYHCNGQ
gray: other	Symbols for amino acids

Compare the results of your different runs. Which parametres did you change? What was the effect? Record for future reference. Upload some alignments into Biology Workbench.

6. At this point, everyone should have some aligned sequences in Biology Workbench. To check, select Alignment Tools after selecting the appropriate session. You should see blocks of sequences listed. If that is not true, go back and continue working on alignments and/or uploads until you do:

   (a) Use Boxshade and Textshade to easily view conserved and nonconserved regions. Note that these are similar, but not identical to Jalview. These can be saved and used as graphic inserts in reports and manuscripts. Use one of these to browse your alignments and to make comparisons between your different alignments.

(b) Make note of conserved regions.

Part B: Tree building

1. Neighbour joining [NJ] is a clustering method to group pairwise distances. It is the favoured distance calculation method because equal rates of evolution are not assumed, as in the arithmetic approach. In biology workbench's alignment tools, try the following:

    (a) Use Clustaldist to obtain a set of distance calculations.

    (b) Choose either DNAdist or Protdist, depending on whether you have nucleotide or protein alignments. Run the same alignments again to obtain a second set of distance results. How do these results differ from the first set? Which application appears to be more sensitive to differences?

    (c) Sketch a tree based on distance calculations obtained from Clustaldist. Sketch another tree based on the calculation results obtained from DNAdist or Protdist.

    (d) Use Drawtree to produce a PHYLIP unrooted tree. Compare this tree to your sketches.

2. Parsimony [also known as max pars, for maximum parsimony and as MP] is a method, which looks for the minimum number of changes, which satisfy the data. It examines sequence comparisons rather than a numerical result, as in NJ.

    Use DNAPars or ProtPars to generate a tree, which maximises parsimony. How many calculation steps were required to obtain the tree? Do different alignment runs affect the outcome of the final tree? If so, how?

3. Next try using Drawgram, a PHYLIP rooted tree tool. This allows you to build a variety of tree types from the same alignment. You can generate a phenogram, based on neighbour joining, which can then be compared to your drawtree result. You can generate a cladogram, based on parsimony, which can then be compared to both the phenogram and to the tree obtained using DNAPars or ProtPars. If you are feeling adventurous, try out some of the other tree types.

4. OK, now you are at the point where computational intensity increases considerably. To try running maximum likelihood [ML] or Bayesian analysis on your alignments, it is recommended that you download suitable software, along with any server-stored alignments of interest and run them on your PC. This is required if you want to examine protein alignments.

    For nucleotide alignments, you can use WebPHYLIP's DNAML to do maximum likelihood. This is a good site to explore for other programs within PHYLIP. Try it now or come back while you are working on the project:

    http://sdmc.krdl.org.sg: 8080/~lxzhang/phylip/

## Chapter 23

Search Engines

INTRODUCTION

As anyone who has surfed the internet has discovered, a search isn't necessarily successful and may turn up nothing or thousands of irrelevant links. Thus, the relevance of the dynamic database links created by interacting with a typical web-accessed search engine is primarily a function of the search engine's selectivity and sensitivity, the ingenuity and knowledge of the search engine user and the availability of relevant content. In addition, the amount of irrelevant content and its similarity with the desired content, together with the peculiarities of database design, limit the ease of finding the sought-after data. The exponentially increasing amounts of data accessible over the Internet, from gene sequences and clinical disease findings to related issues in other fields, is primarily accessible through search engine technologies. As such, this chapter explores the status of search engine technology, focusing on bioinformatics resources, within the context of the overall knowledge management of on-line data.

Figure 23.1 illustrates a partial view of this mesh of interrelationships, in which everything is related to everything else to some degree. The linking isn't limited to relationships between major categories such as demographics and medical history, but links exist within each sub-mesh as well. For example, within the genomic profile, there are links to nucleotide sequences, protein sequences, enzyme profiles and disease predisposition.

At issue is the fact that these links may not be explicit, or even known. In this regard, linking or associating facts from disparate fields is a metaphor for knowledge. The dynamic links or associations that are defined by a human or computer-directed search represent knowledge discovery when the user becomes aware of the links and the contexts in which they can be successfully applied.

Today, most of the potential links between data in digital form aren't readily available because the relevant data, when they exist, are in disparate databases. In addition, each database is typically based on different and incompatible database technologies and uses different languages and vocabularies to access data. These incompatibilities are especially significant when nontextual data, such as 3D images of protein structures, accessed by author-specified keywords, need to be linked with nucleotide sequences in other databases. Because each database is typically created as a stand-alone application to support one function, linking between databases is most often an afterthought.

Although static links between databases can be established programmatically, a more common approach is to create links dynamically by using search engines. In addition, even when static links are established between databases, extracting meaningful content from these linked databases invariably involves using a search engine of some sort.

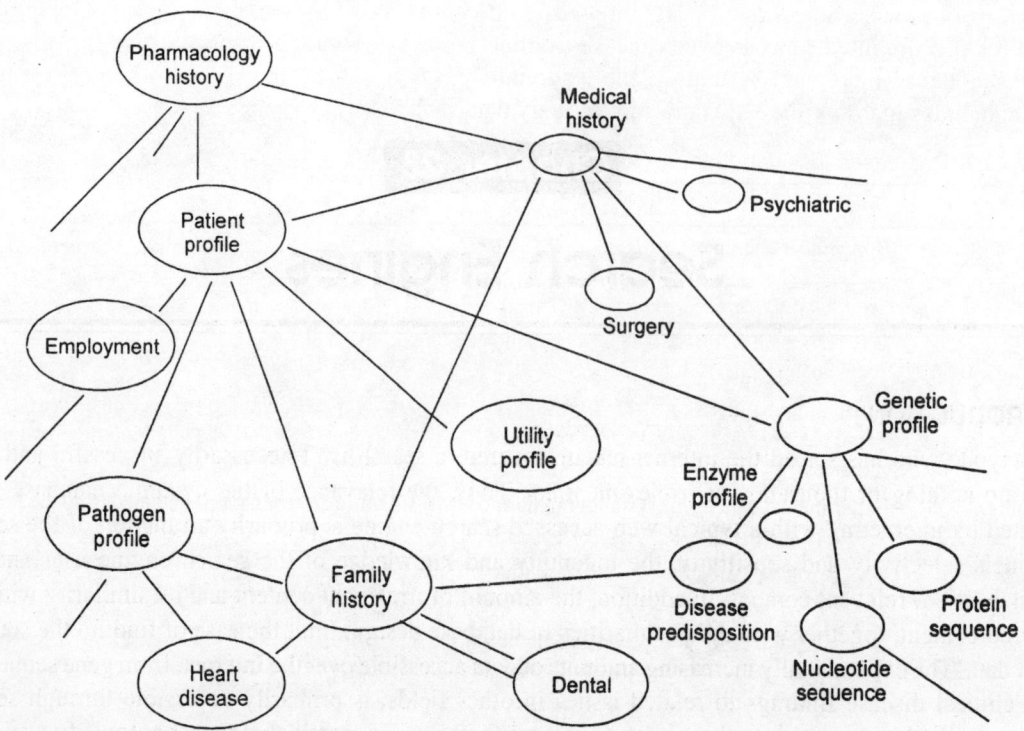

Fig. 23.1. Relationship mesh. Dynamic links created by searching medical, genomic and other databases can make use of this multi-dimensional mesh of relationships.

'The search process' section of this chapter introduces many of the challenges and concepts involved in a typical search of molecular biology databases accessible through the Internet, based on the Entrez integrated searching environment. 'Search engine technology' explores the various technologies that researchers can use to differentiate required data from the noise, from portals and intelligent agents, to natural-language processing (NLP) and other user interface tools. In particular, this section explores dynamic, search-based linking as a form of database integration. The 'searching and information theory' section explores the basic Information Theory model as it relates to online searching and defines the concepts of the sensitivity and specificity of a search and the issues of false positives and negatives in search results. 'Computational methods' explores several exact and approximate search algorithms and provides an overview of methods applicable to searching for text as well as sequence data. The 'searching, dynamic linking and knowledge management' section explores searching and the underlying process of dynamic linking from the perspective of knowledge management. The 'on the horizon' section examines the likely future of search engine technologies designed to access online resources, especially those related to the prospect of ubiquitous computing. Finally, 'endnote' explores the technical challenge of not only providing a unified image of scientific knowledge in the hard and biological sciences, but of the societal implications of achieving this capability.

SEARCH PROCESS

Pursuing a solution to a molecular biology problem with bioinformatics methods invariably involves significant backtracking, stepping and jumping around from one database to the next. In support of this typical work process, integrated information-retrieval systems have been created to provide a mesh of 'hard' or precomputed links between the key online molecular biology databases. By far, the most popular of these integrated systems is the National Centre for Biotechnology Information's Entrez, which includes many of the key molecular biology databases listed in Table 23.1.

Table 23.1. Databases included in the Entrez system.

Database	Description
PubMed	Biomedical literature
Protein	Protein sequences from the Protein information resource (PIR). SWISS-PROT, Protein research foundation (PRF) and Protein data bank (PDB) and from the translated coding regions from DNA sequences in GenBank, the European molecular biology laboratory (EMBL) and the DNA Database of Japan (DDBJ)
Nucleotide	Nucleotide sequence data from GenBank, EMBL and DDBJ, the Genome sequence data base (GSDB) and patent sequences from US patent and trademark office (USPTO) and other international patent offices
Structure	Experimental data from crystallographic and NMR structure determinations obtained from the Protein data bank (PDB)
Genome	Views of genomes, chromosomes, contiged sequence maps and integrated genetic and physical maps
PopSet	Aligned nucleotide and protein sequence data submitted as a set resulting from a population, a phylogenetic or mutation study
OMIM	Human genes and genetic disorders
Taxonomy	Names of all organisms represented NCBI's genetic database
Books	A collection of biomedical books
ProbeSet	The Gene expression omnibus (GEO) gene expression and hybridisation array
3D Domains	Protein domains from NCBI's Conserved domain database

The entrez system supports both inter- and intra-database linking. For example, not only are there links between PubMed and the Nucleotide database and between proteins and the nucleotide sequences from which the proteins were generated (Fig. 23.2), but there are BLAST-computed links between all similar sequences within the Nucleotide database. There are two versions of the entrez system—one that uses an application that runs locally on the user's workstation, called networked entrez and one that is accessible through a web browser. Networked entrez communicates directly to the NCBI's dispatcher through a client-server connection. Each version provides the same core functionality—that of providing a single interface through which all databases in the entrez suite of databases can be accessed. However, because the networked entrez can make use of local computing power, it can execute much faster than the browser-based version. In addition, it provides a more flexible user interface with multiple windows and graphical viewers for genome sequences and 3D protein structures.

The major downside of networked entrez is that data outside of the entrez system aren't available by simply clicking on hypertext links, as they are in the web version of entrez. A minor limitation of the local version is that it must be updated periodically in order to have the latest version. The most obvious benefit of a web-delivered system that runs under a browser is that updates to the interface and the underlying search engine are transparent and instantaneous. The burden of application maintenance is fully on the shoulders of the NCBI staff and their affiliates, freeing users from having to manually update local copies of a search engine or user interface.

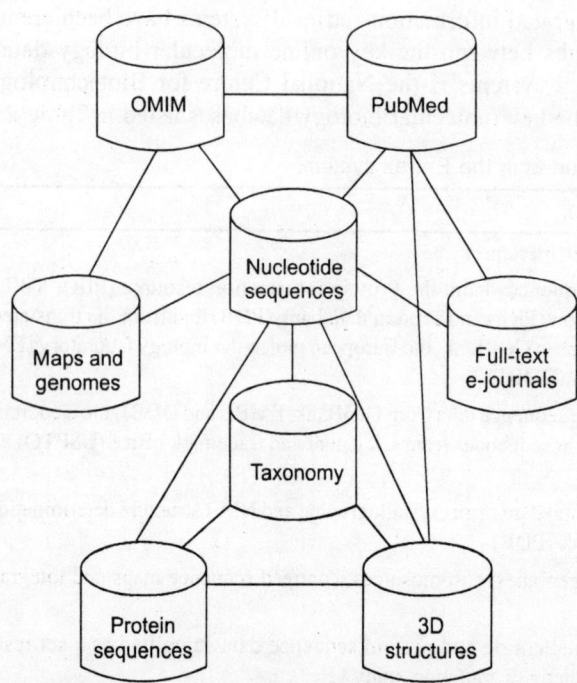

Fig. 23.2. Entrez database integration. Entrez is a link-integrated search system for accessing a growing number of linked molecular biology databases. In addition to the major databases shown here, entrez includes PopSet, ProbeSet and 3D Domains.

Trading a more flexible user interface and faster execution for lack of instant connectivity to other online resources and the need to periodically update the local application is more of a personal decision that doesn't affect the quality of data available through the entrez system. Both versions of entrez provide a common user interface, specifying subjects, ranges, Boolean operators and other search criteria. Search results may be reviewed in a variety of formats, saved to disk or to the clipboard or printed. In addition, the results can be incrementally refined if the user continually narrows the search criteria, working from the results of previous searches that are temporarily maintained in the system's memory. The discussion that follows assumes that the more popular web browser version of entrez is used. The major search features of the entrez system include a variety of tools to define and refine a database search (Fig. 23.3). These tools support selecting a database, linking, imposing limits on searches, using indexes and the search history in searches and saving results to a clipboard. In addition, the tools support searching by a variety of topics, searching within a specified range, truncating searches, using Boolean operators to narrow searches and advanced search authoring capabilities to supplement menu-driven search commands.

Search

The first step in the process of initiating a search in the entrez system is to define, through the use of a pull-down menu system, which database to search. Once a database is selected, the next step is to specify a search topic. Entrez supports searching by subject, subject phrase, author, unique identifier and where applicable, molecular weight. Search topics are defined by keying terms into a free-text query box. As in the most popular general-purpose search engines on the web, such as Google and Yahoo!, the words in a phrase are automatically treated as a Boolean AND unless they are included in double quotes. That is, the sequence of words in a nonquoted phrase is ignored. Conversely, a quoted phrase results in a much narrower search, because word order and position are additional search criteria.

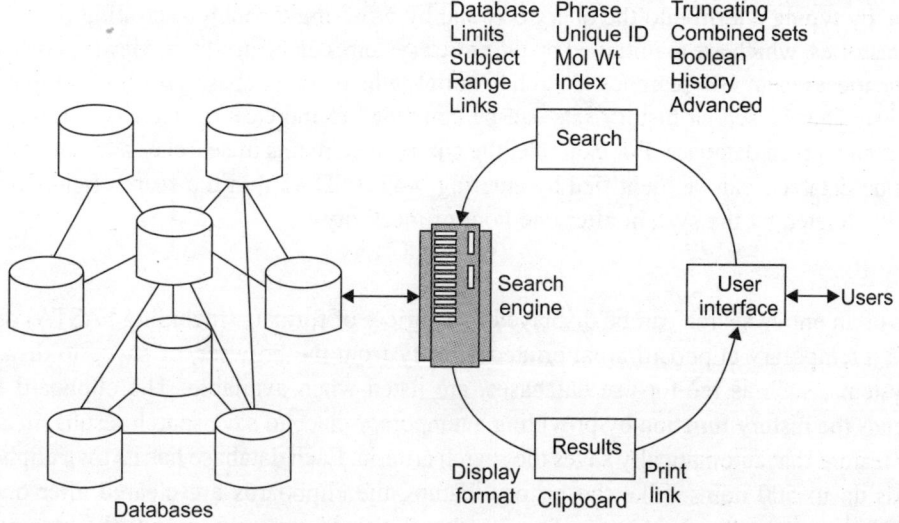

Fig. 23.3. Entrez-enabled search process. Entrez hides the underlying complexity of online molecular biology databases, facilitating the iterative process of submitting search criteria, viewing results and refining or narrowing the search until the desired results are achieved.

A search can also be specified by a unique identifier, which can be an accession number for the complete sequence record in a database or a sequence number assigned by NCBI. The format for the accession number depends on the database. For example, the format of an accession number in GenBank is one letter followed by five digits, compared to a series of six or seven digits followed by a letter for the PRF database. Entrez also supports a search based on molecular weight, including a range of weights, based on calculations of protein structures. This search capability applies only to the entrez protein database.

Regardless of the topic, searches can be narrowed and refined by the use of Boolean operators AND, OR and NOT, which are interpreted from left to right, except that expressions enclosed in parentheses are evaluated first. Boolean operators are especially helpful in performing advanced, manual searches that bypass menu-driven search choices. Complex, multi-parametre searches can be defined by keying a search directly in the Query field. In addition to operations on the search topics, the results of a search can be narrowed through the use of limits. Limits can be used to restrict a search to a particular database or database field, exclude certain types of sequences, limit the search to a particular molecule type or gene location, only the master or only the parts of segmented sets of sequences, or by date. Limits, which can be used singly or in combination with other limits, are defined through standard browser pull-down menus, a free-text query box and check boxes in the Web browser version.

For example, to perform a search in the Nucleotide database for mitochondria carriers that excludes working drafts of nucleotide sequences, the researcher first selects the Nucleotide database from the Search pull-down menu, then types 'mitochondria carrier' in the query box and then select Limits. From the Limits panel, the researcher puts a check next to the 'exclude working drafts' check box and then selects the 'Go' button. The particular limits available are a function of the database used. For example, when the Protein database is selected, exclusion check boxes are limited to 'exclude patents'.

A search can be further refined through the use of indexes, which are alphabetical lists of terms from searchable database fields. The indexes available through entrez are a function of the particular database selected. Indexes can be specified by the usual web browser tools—by selecting terms from a pull-down menu, by typing a term into the query box and by browsing through a scrolling list of terms.

Search histories, which are maintained by the entrez system, can be used to review, revise or combine results of the most recent 100 searches. Search histories, which are database-specific, are maintained as a numeric list. That is, search history sets can be combined to increase or decrease the specificity of searches within a given database. For example, the common elements of searches #45 and #56 based on the nucleotide database can be identified by entering '#45 AND #56' in the search field. Histories are automatically deleted by the system after one hour of inactivity.

Results

The results of an entrez search can be displayed in a variety of formats (including FASTA) or they can be saved to a temporary clipboard area, printed directly from the browser, or saved to disk. Links to external systems, such as fee-for-use databases, are listed when available. The clipboard feature of entrez extends the history function by providing a temporary place to save search results, in addition to the history feature that automatically saves the search criteria. Each database has its own clipboard area, which holds up to 500 items. Like the history feature, the clipboards are cleared after one hour of inactivity. However, unlike the history feature, the clipboard isn't automatic; the researcher must intentionally place results in the clipboard area for later retrieval.

SEARCH ENGINE TECHNOLOGY

Working with the entrez system illustrates several points regarding search engine technology. The first is that the state of the art in search engine integration provides only partial, high-level integration with the growing number of rapidly expanding molecular biology databases. As a result, most intra- and inter-database links are database-specific. Furthermore, the granularity or depth of integration depends on the features that front-end or portal developers have the time and resources to implement.

Even a well-designed system such as Entrez is a compromise from the perspective of user interface. One purpose of a user interface is to hide the complexity of the underlying data structures and database systems. However, entrez requires users to have some low-level knowledge of the databases included in the system. For example, different limits options are available as a function of the database selected and it's up to the user to understand the lack of uniformity in options available through the user interface. That is, it's possible for a relatively naive user to try a search that will fail because he or she assumes that what works in the search of one database will also work in any other. As a result, for optimum use of entrez or any other internet-based, link-integrated database system, users should be familiar with the underlying databases. The popular entrez system also illustrates that the links available through specialised search engines, like general-purposes systems, yield results of varying quality. A researcher will quickly discard many results. Furthermore, data contained in so-called secondary databases are calculated from data contained in primary databases. Entrez supports searches on molecular weight, for example, based on molecular weights calculated from the amino acid sequence data. As a result, errors in the primary databases propagate to secondary databases in a way that may not be obvious by examining the data in the secondary database because it's internally consistent. Furthermore, errors may not be discovered until the data are validated by a wet lab experiment months or years later. The point is that data validation isn't ensured simply because databases are integrated at some level. In contrast, the process of creating a central integrated database, such as PubMed Central (PAC), necessarily involves the validation of data during the integration process. PAC provides integration of life-science journal literature in a common format and in a single repository, providing a single, unified access portal to scientific literature instead of combination of links to disparate databases, each with their own idiosyncrasies in vocabularies and infrastructures.

Working with the entrez system demonstrates several knowledge management issues and challenges, beyond data validation. These include what to do with search results, how to update databases so that propagation of errors is controlled and traceable, how to determine who is responsible for maintenance, and how to communicate information to users on database updates and corrections. For the databases included in the Entrez system, third parties provide the maintenance. However, for private and commercial databases, these and other knowledge management activities must be assigned, monitored and assessed.

In addition to the shortcomings of link-based database integration, entrez also highlights the benefits of a high-level database search system. Without a system like entrez or a related system like the NCBI discovery space that is designed to facilitate single nucleotide polymorphism (SNP) research, users would have to alternatively login, copy and paste or otherwise transfer results from one search to the input of another. Entrez saves users time and minimises errors owing to mistakes made by transferring data from one database to another. Unfortunately, creating systems such as entrez is a major endeavour. Most search engines simply create dynamic links to content that last for the duration of the session or that at best can be saved for future reference.

Intelligent Agents

As illustrated in Table 23.2, search engine technology isn't limited to dynamically interlinking databases, but includes a range of capabilities that apply to bioinformatics work. One particularly active area of R&D is in the area of intelligent agents—search engines with advanced pattern-matching capabilities. They automatically search multiple databases using a variety of heuristics and return results preformatted according to user preferences.

Table 23.2. Search engine technologies. Many of the technologies applicable to general-purpose search engines can be applied to searching bioinformatics databases.

Search engine technology	Example
General-purpose intelligent agents (desktop)	Intelliseek, Copernic, Lexibot, WebFerret, SearchPad, WebStorm and NetAttache
General-purpose intelligent agents (internet)	Dogpile, Ixquick, MetaCrawler, QbSearch, ProFusion, SurfWax and Vivisimo
Internal (intranet) search engines	AskMe, Cadenza
General-purpose search engines	Google, Lycos, Yahoo!, Excite, AltaVista, AllTheWeb, CompletePlanet
Sequence match (desktop and internet)	FASTA, BLAST and BLAST derivatives
Utilities	Connection optimisers, browser extensions, personal firewalls, file-transfer programs, download managers
Bioinformatics portals	Entrez, SRS, BioKRIS, PubMed central, Discovery space
Interface tools	Natural Language Processing (NLP), Query by example, controlled vocabula

Although intelligent agents vary in capabilities, in general they automatically convert simple keyword searches to advanced pattern-matching searches and, in some systems, concept searches. Instead of basing a search on a literal match for a keyword, intelligent agents increase search resolution through restriction of word proximity and exclusion of user-specified associations through Boolean operators.

Intelligent agents that support concept searching perform searches based on the concept represented by the keywords entered by the user. A concept search can be as simple as executing a search on a synonym list or as complex as inferring relationships between the keywords entered in the system. For example, an agent-mediated search on 'hypertension' could perform multiple keyword searches on 'hypertension' as well as 'high blood pressure'. A more sophisticated system could infer additional search terms, such as comorbidities of hypertension-specific renal and retinal diseases resulting from high blood pressure, for example.

Concept-based searching is especially applicable in instances where the vocabulary may not be consistent. For example, in a patient's medical record, a clinician might record the patient's complaint of 'chest pain' as 'angina'. A simple keyword search, whether mediated by an agent or submitted directly to a search engine, would miss the alternate phrasing.

Advanced pattern search techniques don't necessarily involve concepts or recognisable keywords. Nucleotide sequence searches use advanced techniques to identify incomplete or approximate sequence matches. At this point in the development of molecular biology databases, higher-level concept searches are still rare. However, researchers are quickly moving to provide the capability of searching a database with a term such as 'obesity' and viewing not only the physiological and psychological components of obesity, but related protein structures and nucleotide sequences as well.

Portals

Entrez is an example of a portal—a prelinked gateway to databases selected by the portal designer. sequence retrieval service (SRS) and BioKRIS (as well as entrez) are examples of portals that provide access to link-integrated databases through a variety of special support tools. For example, SRS allows users to search multiple databases simultaneously because of a powerful and unique set of link operators that dynamically link multiple databases. Portals can make better use of intelligent agents because the search engine designer can design the heuristics to fit the databases included in the portal, as opposed to working with every database on the internet. Similarly, special operators can be defined to facilitate working with the databases encompassed by the portal.

For example, SRS uses two link operators '<' and '>' to combine two sets from different databases in the portal system, such as SWISS-PROT and PDB. The statement SWISS-PROT > PDB gives those entries in the PDB database of solved tertiary protein structures that are referenced by or linked to entries in SWISS-PROT. Conversely, the statement SWISS-PROT < PDB gives those entries in SWISS-PROT that reference or are linked to entries in PDB. As a result, the statement [swissprot-def:kinase] > PDB retrieves all kinase sequences from the SWISS-PROT protein sequence database, which are then linked to the PDB. The result is a set of all the PDB entries with atomic coordinates for all kinases for which the tertiary structure has been determined.

The SRS portal supports linking from any database to any other database in the system. If two databases are not directly connected by a link, then a series of intermediary links is created. As illustrated in Fig. 23.4, SRS attempts to find the shortest possible way for linking two databases. Ideally this is the direct link as between EMBL and SWISS-PROT. However, with a link request such as EMBL > PDB, when there are no nucleotide sequences in EMBL that are referenced by the PDB database of tertiary protein structures, then SRS automatically links the two databases through a SWISS-PROT intermediary, which relates both databases.

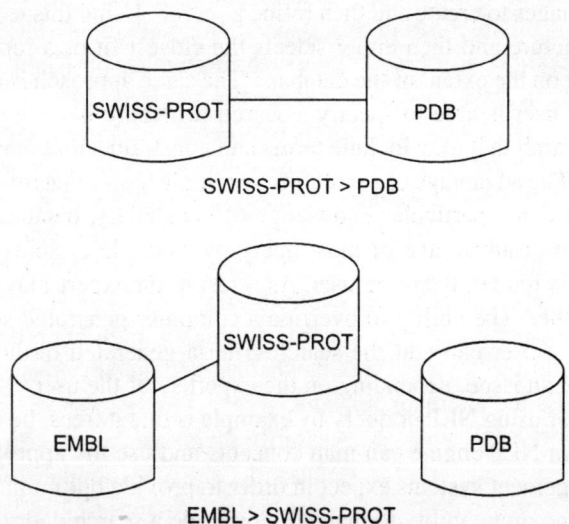

SWISS-PROT > PDB

EMBL > SWISS-PROT

Fig. 23.4. SRS Database linking. When instructed to link databases without relevant references, SRS identifies the best intermediary database to support the link. In this example, a link between EMBL and PDB is automatically facilitated by SRS-directed links through the SWISS-PROT database.

User Interface Tools

Getting information out of a database is as important as putting it in. The point of human-computer communication—the user interface—is to maximise the quality and efficiency of the interchange. The better the search engine interface, the easier it is for users to interact with the data. A major function of the user interface is to decrease the cognitive load on the researcher so that the data created by the underlying application can be quickly and easily absorbed. It also provides a mechanism for the user to painlessly communicate to the application. A variety of visualisation tools have been developed to aid researchers by presenting data so researchers can evaluate complex protein sequences, identify the location of genes on chromosomes and in general, make the otherwise unintelligible and seemingly endless strings of data intelligible.

From a data input perspective, the pull-down menus and check boxes supported by a standard Web browser, as demonstrated by the Web version of Entrez, represent standard user interface tools. Of the tools available to extend database search functionality within a Web browser environment, the most popular are free-text entry, query by example, and controlled vocabulary.

NLP is the technology that allows free-text searches of databases, whether in a Web browser or local application. A statement such as:

What is the molecular weight of the haemoglobin molecule?

Automatically generates a different statement, for example, a SELECT statement for a SQL database of the form:

SELECT molecular_wt FROM protein_database
WHERE protein = haemoglobin

In addition to NLP, there are a number of technologies that are useful in locating textual and graphic data in very large databases as well. One of them is image-based query by example, where the user selects from a library of images to create and then refine a search. Using this technology, the user selects an image of a protein structure and then either selects the closest fit or a representative of additional image libraries, depending on the extent of the database. The same approach is often used in commercial search engines, where the user is able to specify a search for 'more like these'. The system takes the exemplars and creates a search that may include terms and constraints that may not have been included in the user's initial search. The advantage of a search-by-example tool is that refining a search is relatively painless and doesn't require any particular knowledge of vocabulary, database contents or other low-level details. However, the disadvantage of most query-by-example systems is that the search query that is actually generated is hidden from the user. As a result, an expert may not be able to manually refine the search even further. The ability to override a computer-generated search, such as the utility provided in Entrez where a user can edit the search criteria generated through the use of pull-down menus, may or may not be an issue, depending on the expertise of the user.

One of the advantages of using NLP or query by example is that it frees the user from having to learn a controlled vocabulary. An NLP engine can map concepts and use the appropriate synonyms that the underlying database management systems expect in order to provide optimum search results. However, the power of an NLP engine or an ability to manually override a search query lies in the granularity of the vocabulary used to index the data originally. For example, if all genes dealing with the heart are indexed under 'cardiac', without distinguishing between normal and diseased conditions, then a researcher won't be able to narrow a search to normal heart pathology.

The optimum condition exists when the controlled vocabulary is made available to users during the search process. For example, PubMed is indexed using the medical subject heading (MeSH) vocabulary, maintained by the US national library of medicine. Knowing this, a researcher can use the online MeSH browser to identify the most appropriate search terms to use to retrieve the data of interest.

For a research group establishing an internal database, MeSH may not be the most appropriate controlled vocabulary for indexing and searching. Even within the relatively narrow domain of clinical medicine, there are several popular controlled vocabulary systems use. In addition to MeSH, there is the unified medical language system (UMLS), the read classification system (RCS), systemised nomenclature of human and veterinary medicine (SNOMED), international classification of diseases (ICD-10) and current procedural terminology (COPT). Each system has its strengths, weaknesses and primary purpose. For example, SNOMED is optimised for accessing and indexing clinical information in human and veterinary medicine databases, whereas the COPT is optimised to identify medical procedures.

The advantage of using one of these public controlled vocabularies is that the vocabulary is immediately available. Time-consuming tasks such as removing redundancies in the vocabulary, which ultimately limits scalability, have been performed by someone else—presumably experts in the field. Another advantage is that databases indexed with a public controlled vocabulary can more readily share the database with others without having to distribute the indexing vocabulary. For example, if an academic research centre wants to publish its research on SNPs and drug responses on the Internet, it can provide a simple keyword search interface to the database and simply list the appropriate search vocabulary, such as MeSH. The major disadvantage of using a public controlled vocabulary or its given representation, is that its granularity may not exactly fit the needs of the laboratory. Another limitation is that the public vocabulary may be updated periodically, forcing whoever manages the database to expend the resources necessary to reindex areas of the index affected by the updates. Failing to do so would likely lead to user frustration, because users may not have the latest version of the vocabulary, either because they aren't aware of the update or because they don't have access to an older version of the vocabulary for reference.

For internal databases where the user population can be informed about changes in indexing, there is much more flexibility in selecting or developing an indexing and search vocabulary. The most common approaches to developing an in-house controlled vocabulary range from a totally unconstrained ad-hoc system to creating a huge, potentially unwieldy combination of public vocabularies. The ad-hoc approach of creating a new vocabulary as data are generated is reasonable only if the vocabulary is relatively small and isn't expected to grow beyond 1000 or 2000 words. For larger indexing tasks requiring the breadth of a published controlled vocabulary, a reasonable approach is to modify a standard vocabulary, adding granularity in specific areas. This approach takes advantage of an extensive vocabulary that may exceed 1,00,000 terms, but comes at a cost of incompatibility with the published standard. The approach of combining standards is clearly the most challenging because of the inevitable redundancies and internal inconsistencies of the vocabularies used that must somehow be controlled. Whether or not the advantage of this approach—a vocabulary that exceeds several hundred-thousand terms and is likely to cover the spectrum of indexing needs—is worth the investment depends on the scope of the database project and the resources available. Regardless of whether a controlled vocabulary is designed from scratch or is based on a published standard, the main technological issue is providing a means of using it consistently and without error. For example, without rudimentary utilities such as text auto-completion, simply misspelling a search term can render the sought-after data inaccessible.

Utilities

Many of the generic utilities originally intended to extend the functionality of browsers can be used to facilitate searching molecular biology databases. These utilities include connection optimisers, browser add-ons, personal firewalls, file-transfer programs and download managers. Connection optimisers are designed to improve Internet connection speed and reliability. Optimisers work by allowing manual override of network communications configuration settings so that the connection throughput can be optimised for sequence data (text strings), 3D protein structures (graphics) or specific combination of data formats. Browser extensions enhance browsers with features, such as automatic form-filling, supporting searching within a document, dictionary tools that define or complete the spelling of words on-the-fly, providing visual previews of web pages before they are accessed and adding buttons of frequently accessed sites to the browser. Privacy and security utilities include personal firewalls that take up where network firewalls leave off. They block advertisements, cookies and other nuisances that can interfere with the efficient use of a browser-based search engine.

Download managers are intended to accelerate searches by opening multiple connections to one or more servers simultaneously, grabbing different parts of the file through each connection and reassembling the file on the workstation. File-transfer managers add flexibility to standard FTP clients by adding additional security through encryption and by providing users with a graphical user interface instead of a command-line prompt. Most of these utilities are available on Windows, Linux and UNIX environment platforms.

SEARCHING AND INFORMATION THEORY

Information Theory forms the basis for our understanding of modern communications networks, and provides a model for understanding the principles of search engines. Information Theory specifies the amount of meaningful information that can be communicated from the web server to the browser as a function of the signal-to-noise level and the bandwidth of the medium. The greater the strength of the desired signal compared to that of the noise—that is, the higher the signal-to-noise ratio—the greater the amount of relevant data that can be propagated from the database through the Internet to the user (Fig. 23.6). Figure 23.5 shows the application of information theory to search engine technology, where the molecular biology database constitutes the information source, a Web server is the transmitter, the Internet or other network serves as the medium, the search engine is the receiver and the user's Web browser or local application is the destination. Similarly, the relevant data in the database constitutes the message to be transmitted, irrelevant data constitutes the noise source and the message presented to the user through a Web browser consists of both relevant and irrelevant data.

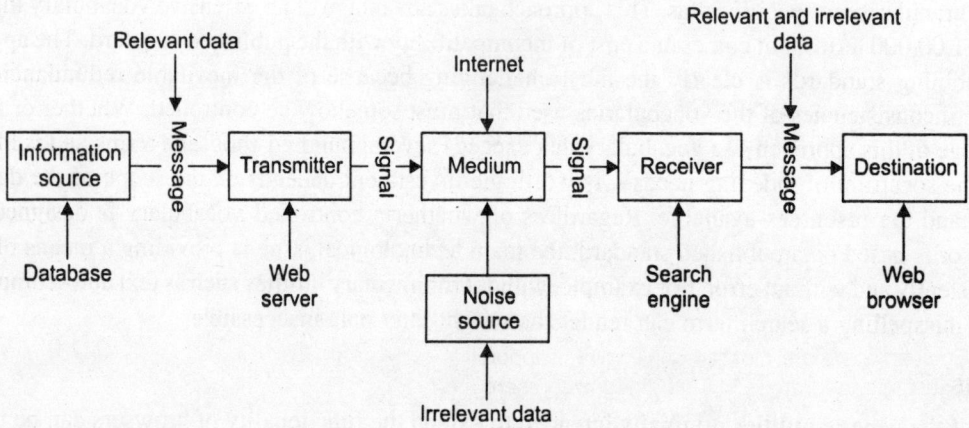

Fig. 23.5. Searching and information theory. Following information theory, both relevant and irrelevant data reach the user through the Internet as a function of the search engine (receiver) and the relative amounts of relevant and irrelevant data in the information source.

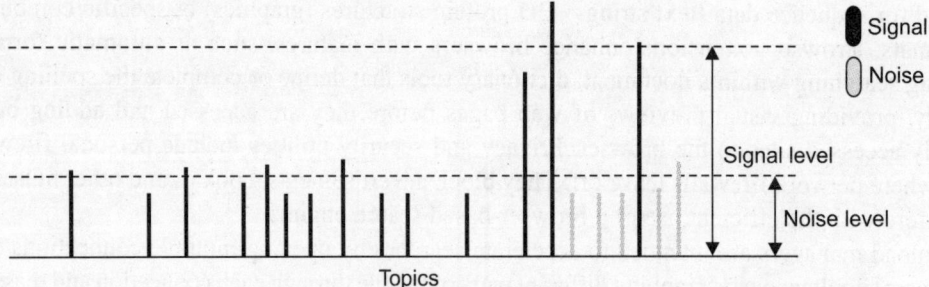

Fig. 23.6. Signal-to-Noise ratio. Line height corresponds to the amount of data available on a particular topic.

Information theory specifies the amount of meaningful information that can be communicated from the Web server to the browser as a function of the signal-to-noise level and the bandwidth of the medium. The greater the strength of the desired signal compared to that of the noise—that is, the higher the signal-to-noise ratio—the greater the amount of relevant data that can be propagated from the database through the Internet to the user (Fig. 23.6).

Searches generally fail in one of two ways: Either they retrieve too much noise with the desired data, so that the time it takes to look through results isn't worth the trouble or they retrieve the wrong data, because the search criteria were incorrect.

The best searches are sensitive enough to return all or most of the desired data and selective enough to limit undesired data or noise to the least level possible.

One way to limit the amount of noise returned by a search is to increase the selectivity of a search by using a Boolean operator, such as AND, OR or NOT. As illustrated in Fig. 23.7, the OR operator provides the least amount of selectivity. Conversely, the AND operator provides the greatest selectivity, returning data that contains all of the keywords submitted in a query. The NOT operator generally provides an intermediate amount of selectivity. The relative selectivity of the Boolean operators assumes that there is a significant signal-to-noise ratio—that there are a significant number of Web sites or nucleotide sequences that fulfill the search requirements compared to the other results that may be returned by the search.

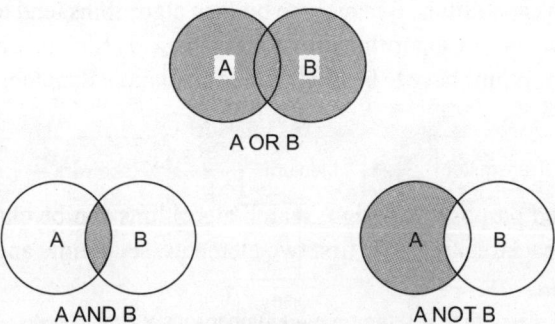

Fig. 23.7. Boolean operators. Most search engines support the Boolean AND, OR and NOT operators, illustrated graphically here. Shaded areas in each image represent the data returned by the search.

Regardless of the search technology used, the retrieval process is a trade-off between sensitivity and selectivity. A nonselective search using only general terms normally returns a large amount of irrelevant data. As shown in Fig. 23.8, a more selective search, while returning less noise or irrelevant data, may miss some of the desired data. Using an excessively selective search results in less noise at the expense of relevant data.

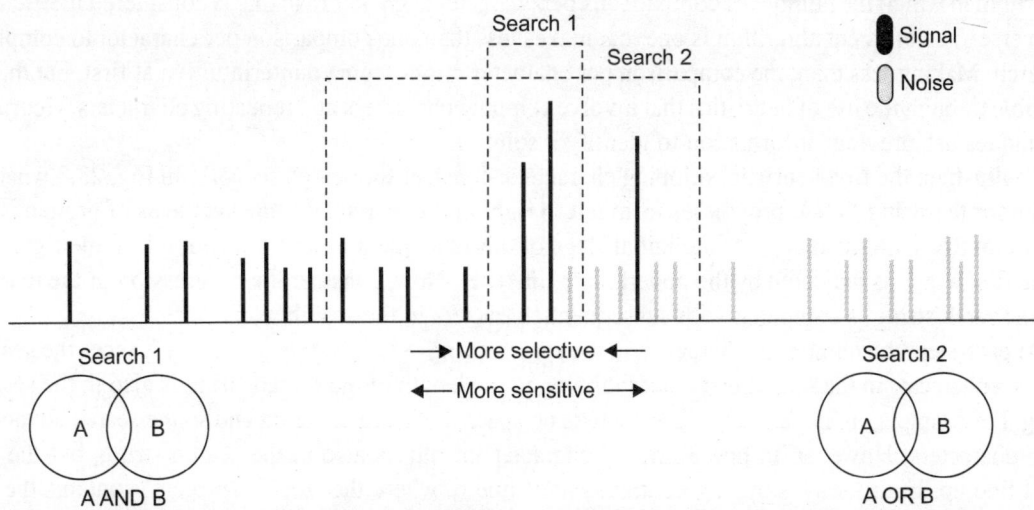

Fig. 23.8. Search sensitivity versus selectivity. Search 1 is more selective, resulting in less noise in the search results, but also misses relevant data. Search 2 is more sensitive, including more relevant data but more noise as well.

COMPUTATIONAL METHODS

A common activity in bioinformatics work is to search through a database and locate a substring—a nucleotide sequence, for example—that matches a target string. Some computational methods provide results faster, allowing a researcher to check the results of an experiment frequently, at the expense of more false positive matches. Later, more selective, albeit slower techniques can be used to verify the results of these quick screening techniques. The performance and selectivity of a search are also a function of the search string and how the data are represented in the database to be searched.

Most programming languages provide string search capabilities, but these tend to be unacceptably inefficient when performed on large data sets typical of nucleotide sequence databases, and most don't support approximate match capabilities. Because the built-in algorithms tend to use brute-force methods that don't make use of heuristics or algorithmic tricks to increase efficiency or to accelerate the search process, special-purpose algorithms have to be used with computationally intensive tasks such as sequence searching.

Search Algorithms

Regardless of their intended purpose or design, search algorithms can be characterised by setup time, running time and need for backtracking. The first two elements, setup time and running time, are related by the function:

$$\text{search time} = \text{setup time} + (\text{comparisons} \times \text{characters})$$

In this relationship, comparisons is the number of comparisons made per character in the text body to be searched and characters is the number of characters in the text body of text or sequence data that is to be searched. Setup time is the time invested prior to the actual search and includes programming to establish lookup tables and other data that can be used to simplify or accelerate the search once it's initiated.

A search algorithm is considered inefficient if, in the process of a search, the number of comparisons made is equal to or greater than the number of characters in the source text. For example, a search algorithm in which the number of comparisons per character is greater than one is considered inefficient. Conversely, an efficient algorithm is one that makes less than one comparison per character to complete a search. Making less than one comparison per character might seem counterintuitive at first, but this is possible through the use of heuristics that involve skipping characters and repeating characters. Heuristic techniques use previous information to identify a solution.

To illustrate the first heuristic, skipping characters, consider the search scenario in Fig. 23.9 where a search for the string 'RNA' progresses from left to right in the search text 'the synthesis of protein is by way of an RNA intermediary'. At the initial stage of this example, the search position is at the right end of the first word, as indicated by the underline 'e' in 'The'. Now, consider the progression of the marker as the search string is compared with subsequent characters in the search text.

At each step, the number of characters in the search string—in this case, three—advances the search unless a character in the search text corresponding to the length of the search string is also in the search string. For example, in line 2 of Fig. 23.9, there is no space in the search string and so the search advances three characters. However, in line 3, the 'n' character in 'nth' is also in the search string, but the n's don't line up. In this way, skipping continues until line 6, where the 'rot' in 'protein' contains the 'r' character in the search string. A comparison of the first characters is made, which matches and so the second characters are compared. This comparison fails and the search is again advanced. In line 7, there is again a possible match and the search string is advanced one character to verify a match, as in line 8.

However, the space at the end of 'protein' doesn't match the 'A' in 'RNA' and the search position is shifted three places to the right, as in line 10.

Search string: RNA
Search text: The synthesis of protein is by way of an RNA intermediary

1.   Th⬚ synthesis of protein is by way of an RNA intermediary
2.   The s⬚nthesis of protein is by way of an RNA intermediary
3.   The synt⬚esis of protein is by way of an RNA intermediary
4.   The synthes⬚s of protein is by way of an RNA intermediary
5.   The synthesis ⬚f protein is by way of an RNA intermediary
6.   The synthesis of ⬚rotein is by way of an RNA intermediary
7.   The synthesis of pro⬚ein is by way of an RNA intermediary
8.   The synthesis of prote⬚n is by way of an RNA intermediary
9.   The synthesis of protein⬚is by way of an RNA intermediary
10. The synthesis of protein is⬚by way of an RNA intermediary
       ⋮
18. The synthesis of protein is by way of an ⬚RNA⬚ intermediary

Fig. 23.9. Character skipping. The search, indicated by the marker box, progresses from left to right, skipping ahead up to three characters at a time until a character in the search string 'RNA' is found in the skipped-to region of the search text.

This process continues, stopping to check for matches whenever the next three characters contains an 'r', 'n' or 'a'. That is, if the algorithm is examining a character that doesn't occur in the search string at all, the algorithm moves ahead by the length of the entire search string. If a character does appear in the search string, the algorithm advances the search marker by the distance between that character and the right end of the string. By step 18, the search is complete, on a total of 44 characters (including spaces). The number of comparisons per character is approximately 0.4—an efficient search algorithm.

A second search heuristic makes use of repeating patterns in the search string, such as 'hand to hand', 'door to door' and attempts to match the first repeating word, according to the algorithm described for skipping characters. When a match is made, the search string is advanced to the point that the first occurrence of the repeated word is aligned with the first occurrence of the matching term in the main text. A comparison is now made for the second occurrence of the search term in the text. Obviously, the major gain in computational efficiency and performance is obtained by the first heuristic and the advantage of the second heuristic is dependent on the appearance of repeating words in the search pattern.

In addition to running time, another major metric for characterising search algorithms is the need for backtracking. Some search algorithms are linear, working efficiently from the beginning of the sequence to be searched to the end, whereas others move back and forth in the text to be searched during processing. For example, the skipping search algorithm moves the index ahead by the number of characters in the search string but then backs up to compare characters if a possible match exists.

Approximate Searches

Algorithms that efficiently locate exact matches have many applications in bioinformatics, including searching for data in PubMed or some other bibliographic reference database by a specific disease or author, searching a clinical database by a specific disease or patient identification number or searching any database where data are indexed by a known, controlled vocabulary. However, search algorithms that look for approximate matches are more useful in one of the most computationally challenging tasks in bioinformatics—that of searching sequence databases for homologies of particular sequences. Approximate match algorithms vary from the use of templates, to the use of a distance function and the use of how words sound when spoken.

String search algorithms based on templates use metacharacters to specify the range of permissible strings that must be matched exactly. For example, the UNIX-utility 'grep' (general regular expression parser) uses metacharacters such as '*', '\', 'g', '+' and '^' to perform a brute-force search. As such, applications such as grep don't do true approximate searches. Similarly, the Find function in the Windows operating system allows a search string such as '*research.doc' to locate Microsoft Word documents that include 'MyResearch.doc', 'DNAResearch.doc' and 'ProteinResearch.doc'. However, the search wouldn't locate documents such as 'MyResearch.doc', 'DNAResearch.doc' or 'ProteinRsch.doc', because of missing or transposed characters in the file names compared to the search string.

True approximate search algorithms allow approximate matches, permit the transposition of adjacent characters, substitution of characters and assign different weights to different types of errors. An approximate match algorithm for nucleotide sequences should be able to locate nucleotide sequences despite the presence of single nucleotide polymorphism, for example. Searching with an approximate match algorithm for a nucleotide sequence that contains the string 'AAGGTTAA' should be able to locate the sequence 'ATGGTTAA', where the second 'A' in the first string is replaced by a 'T' in the second string.

Phonetic comparison algorithms, typified by Soundex and Metaphone, are examples of true approximate search algorithms that have application in bioinformatics. For example, they can be used to search Bibliographic databases by author name when the exact spelling of the author's name may be unknown, or search a taxonomy database by phonetically spelling a species name. The Soundex approximate search algorithm addresses the problem of uncertain spelling by indexing and searching databases by an encoded string. These encoded strings are created by dropping vowels and silent consonants and assigning one of six values to the remaining consonants (Table 23.3).

Table 23.3. Soundex codes. Vowels and silent consonants are dropped from the word and the consonants are converted to a three-digit numeric codes, headed by the first character in the word. The Soundex algorithm is especially useful in performing approximate searches for names of authors, taxonomies and other text strings that can be pronounced.

Characters	Value
AEIOUHWY	Dropped
BFPV	1
CGJKQSXZ	2
DT	3
L	4
MN	5
R	6

Soundex encoding uses the first letter of the word, followed by up to three codes, depending on the length of the word. Double consonants and repetitions of the same consonant group are dropped. For example, 'protein' is converted to 'P635' and 'Pill', 'Phil' and 'Philly' are converted to 'P4'. Soundex errs on the side of sensitivity instead of specificity, in that it tends to pick up strings that are only vaguely similar to the search string. The major limitations of Soundex are that the first letter of a word must match exactly and that the string must be intended to be spoken. That is, Soundex isn't intended to work with a text string such as 'ATTAATTGGA'. Similarly, a search for a word that begins with 'ph' won't find a word that actually begins with 'f', even though the words may sound identical.

A major improvement on the Soundex approach of encoding search and index strings is the Metaphone algorithm. Like Soundex, Metaphone disposes of vowels—unless the word begins with a vowel. However, Metaphone encoding is based on diphthongs rather than consonants. For example, the Metaphone algorithm transforms 'X' to 'KS' before encoding the text string. As a result, a search using Metaphone is generally more specific than Soundex. However, the Metaphone encoding scheme doesn't overcome the limitation of being unable to encode and search for unpronounceable text strings, such as nucleotide sequence data.

When it comes to searching sequence databases for sequence homologs, the gold standard is to use a search engine based on a dynamic programming algorithm. Dynamic programming is a computationally expensive but thorough search algorithm that recursively searches through a database for a sequence that approximates the search string. Not only does a dynamic programming algorithm search a database from beginning to end, but it keeps the results of previous match attempts in memory. As a result, running a search for a sequence only a few dozen nucleotides long against a database such as the human genome database can take hours, even with a dedicated supercomputer.

Because the routine use of dynamic programming search techniques is unreasonably expensive in time and computer resources, modified versions of dynamic programming, such as the FASTA algorithm, are more practical. FASTA makes a dynamic programming approach to string search tenable by limiting the area of the sequence database that is searched. The downside to an algorithm such as FASTA is that it's possible to miss potential matches because the search isn't exhaustive.

When it comes to performing approximate searches on sequence data, by far the most popular algorithm is the Basic Local alignment search tool (BLAST), which achieves computational efficiency by using heuristics that are weighted toward local sequence alignments. The BLAST heuristic assumes that sections of protein are often conserved without gaps, so that the gaps can be ignored. As such, it's able to detect relationships among sequences that share only isolated regions of similarity. BLAST is used by virtually all of the major bioinformatics centres, including NCBI. Using BLAST over the Internet, sequence searches against the full human genome can be completed in only a few seconds, even when the system is being used by multiple users.

Because of the statistical techniques used to narrow the focus of the BLAST algorithm, it can miss potential matches in a nucleotide database. To extend the capabilities of BLAST so that it finds additional matches, NCBI developed position-specific iterated BLAST (PSI-BLAST) that extends the original BLAST algorithm using a position-specific scoring matrix that is capable of detecting subtle nucleotide sequence similarities. NCBI and other research centres have similarly created specialised versions of BLAST that are tuned to specific problems or areas. There are versions of BLAST that are optimised for human, microbial and malaria genomes, vector contamination and immunoglobins.

SEARCH ENGINES AND KNOWLEDGE MANAGEMENT

The ability to search through a molecular biology database assumes that an effective knowledge management process is in place. Using the DNA sequencing process as an example, consider the steps involved in making sequence data available to a researcher through a search engine. First, there is the lengthy process of acquiring the data from a sequence machine. This involves identifying a set of clones that span a region of the genome to be sequenced, making sets of smaller clones from mapped clones, purifying DNA from the smaller clones and finally setting up and performing the sequencing using gel electrophoresis. Then there is the verification and annotation of the sequence data. Annotation is especially critical, because it enables the sequence data to be accessed by name and linked to other databases. In this way, researchers in other labs and in other fields can access the sequence data. A newly discovered nucleotide sequence might be linked to (and linked from) a protein database, an inherited disease database and perhaps a drug interaction database, for example. Ultimately, providing name and linking hooks to the new data facilitates discovery of associations or links between different but related fields in a way that extends our knowledge. As involved as this initial stage of knowledge management can be, it's a waste of time and resources without a comprehensive knowledge management program. This includes a defined means of transforming data for other purposes, such as using the data in a tightly linked secondary database of clinical disease. It also includes archiving data so that they can be recovered in the event of failure in the primary database system and providing the infrastructure capable of tracking the location of particular data elements and of controlling access to the data.

Although every component of the knowledge management process is critical, the data that are managed are of little value unless they can be easily accessed in a timely manner. From a practical perspective, knowledge management should support the retrieval of data from an online database with a search engine while making provision for security through user authentication or other methods. As such, factors that affect usability include the quality and appropriateness of the user interface, the vocabulary used to index and retrieve data, ease of use, ease of learning and the time required for specific data to be searched for and retrieved define the value of the system.

As described earlier, using one of the integrated, database systems such as Entrez, SRS or BioKRIS can significantly reduce the time and difficulty associated with performing a successful search. Although having databases online facilitates link integration through the search process, the interface challenges begin at the time databases are first defined. The issue with creating databases of any type is that they are necessarily defined for a particular use. For example, the HomoloGene online database is optimised to manage putative homologies among the human, mouse, rat and zebra fish genomes, whereas SWISS-PROT is optimised to locate protein sequence data. Moving outside of the molecular biology arena, the online professional databases including LexisNexis, Dialog and Ingenta each provide comprehensive, efficient access to information in their domains. Similarly, PAC provides integration of life-science journal literature in a common format and in a single repository, providing a single, unified access portal to scientific literature instead of a combination of links to disparate databases, each with their own idiosyncrasies in vocabularies and infrastructures.

Information technology challenges aside, there is a limit to how far systems like entrez can be further refined, because of our incomplete understanding of how a database can and should be linked. For example, molecular biology has yet to fully explain how single genes can code tor multiple proteins or how all of the proteins in the human proteome interact with each other and the cellular environment under various conditions. That said, the future of bioinformatics lies clearly in the integration of disparate databases in molecular biology as well as with those in other fields to provide a unified view of life.

As an illustration of the degree of linking that will eventually be needed to even approximate this unified view, consider the experiences—which can be represented by links—typical of physician training in the United States. As listed in Table 23.4, the traditional premedical curriculum includes the basic sciences, including chemistry, physics and genetics. Medical school provides exposure to preclinical studies such as physiology and anatomy, followed by clinical exposure to everything from nutrition and dermatology to psychology and oncology.

Table 23.4. Typical physician training. The typical preclinical and clinical curricula, with a sampling of a possible premedical experience, illustrate the mesh of knowledge required for physicians to adequately understand and manage the disease process.

Premedical	Preclinical	Clinical
Differential equations	Anatomy	Anesthesia
Physics	Biochemistry	Dermatology
Calculus	Microbiology	Endocrinology
Chemistry	Parasitology	Geriatrics
Genetics	Pharmacology	Hematology
Molecular biology		Internal medicine
Organic chemistry		Neonatology
Strength of materials		Nutrition
Statistics		OB/GYN
Dynamics		Oncology
Computer science		Orthopedics
Art		Pediatrics
History		Plastic surgery
Languages		Psychology
Sociology		Pulmonary medicine
Psychology		Radiology
Engineering		Surgery
Management		Tropical medicine
Biology		Urology

It's possible for someone to practice medicine without learning the interconnectedness of the underlying anatomy with the biochemical basis for disease—many advances in medicine were based on accidental discoveries, as opposed to reasoning from first principles. However, for true understanding of the disease process and how to treat it, the interconnectedness of organic chemistry, biochemistry, anatomy, and physiology generally have to be mastered. Because of human memory limitations, most clinicians specialise in relatively limited areas that they can master—that is, areas in which they can develop and maintain linkages.

An orthopedic surgeon may not need to understand the intricacies of the Central Dogma in his daily practice. Similarly, real understanding of the germ theory isn't required to perform an aseptic operation, such as a hip replacement—as long as proper procedure is followed. However, when things don't go as expected—for example, if the patient requires a new hip replacement after three years instead of the usual five—it's in the patient's best interest if the surgeon can reason from first principles, using his interlinked knowledge of skeletal and muscle anatomy, engineering and clinical experience with hip prostheses to prevent a reoccurrence of premature failure. Often, as in the use of a search engine, the solution involves innovation—creating new links between existing knowledge.

Innovators rely on predefined links and create links on their own. For example, substituting a beneficial organism for a potentially hazardous one, as in replacement therapy, has been practiced for decades. Eating yogurt, for example, populates the stomach with benign acidophilus bacilli, displacing less beneficial bacteria. The same technique is being used with Streptococcus bacteria that have been modified by recombinant DNA techniques so as not to produce cavity-producing acids that attack the tooth's enamel. The idea is to displace the natural bacteria that cause tooth decay by using a mouthwash composed of benign bacteria that will displace the acid-producing variety.

Innovation in bioinformatics is occurring in the same way. Researchers are using the links provided by Entrez and other online services and supplementing them with their own to test new hypotheses, verify the findings or theories of others and otherwise advance their understanding of life.

On the Horizon

The current interest in bioinformatics is primarily focused on accelerating the expensive drug discovery process. Bioinformatics is currently viewed by the Pharma industry as a means of weeding out problem drugs more quickly and earlier in the R&D process. Although this view has yet to be validated by a viable product produced by bioinformatics methods alone, firms that rely heavily on bioinformatics techniques are projecting an R&D investment of 20 per cent on sales. This may seem prohibitively expensive, given the industry standard of 12 per cent on sales. However, the hope is that new bioinformatics methods will more accurately reject drugs that may cause serious side effects, drugs that as of now aren't discovered until millions of dollars have been invested in marketing and sales efforts.

Over the life of a drug, the initial R&D investment in bioinformatics methods could more than pay for itself if computational methods could be used to identify molecules that behave like other molecules known to cause serious side effects. Over the past 25 years, half of the dangerous side effects of drugs were recognised over 7 years after the drugs were approved. Pulling a drug from the market because of lethal side effects at this late stage is not only expensive, but these findings typically extend the FDA's approval time because of public pressure to be more vigilant.

Clearly, if bioinformatics is to solve the drug side-effect dilemma, practitioners in the field will have to work not only with gene expression and proteomic databases, but with clinical medicine databases as well. However, given the exponential growth of data in molecular biology as well as in virtually every clinical medicine domain, it's unlikely that molecular biology researchers will have sufficient knowledge or resources to manually establish and maintain links between findings in their field. Furthermore, it's even less likely that complete, up-to-date predefined links to databases in other fields can be maintained. More likely is continued work in the area of search engine technology that can create dynamic links between protein folding, DNA sequence and inherited disease databases, as well as links between these databases and those in fields as diverse as physics, biochemistry and the law.

Endnote

One potential endpoint of creating search capabilities that dynamically and completely integrate databases in medicine, law, the genome, individual IQ and education test scores and personal employment records is revealed in Aldus Huxley's 'Brave New World', in which everything is known about every citizen before their birth. In this novel, embryos are immunised *in vitro* in a central hatchery against all known infectious diseases; old age itself is a disease. Furthermore, citizens, are indoctrinated at birth to the social order, based on their made-to-order, genetic profile that determines whether they are leaders or obedient followers. Another possibility is that, like other disruptive technologies—the electric light, antibiotics, the PC and the automobile, for example—our ability to manipulate nucleotide and amino acid sequences will simply become an invisible part of the social fabric. Thanks to bioinformatics, new, more powerful drugs will be available to treat HIV and similar acquired diseases, as well as correct for genetic errors that would otherwise result in lifelong suffering for individuals and a cost burden for the healthcare system.

## Chapter 24

Submitting DNA Sequences to the Databases

INTRODUCTION

DNA sequence records from the public databases (DDBJ/EMBL/GenBank) are essential components of any computational analysis in molecular biology. Accurate and informative biological annotation of sequence records is critical in every attempt to determine the function of a disease gene by similarity to a gene that was isolated and sequenced because of its biological function. The names or functions of the encoded protein products, the name of the genetic locus and the link to the original publication of that sequence (why was it sequenced?) make a sequence record of immediate value to the scientist who retrieves it as the result of a BLAST or entrez search.

This chapter is about getting these sequences and their annotations into the public databases, with an emphasis on the nucleotide sequence databases involved in the International Nucleotide Sequence Database Collaboration: DDBJ, EMBL and GenBank. We present two different approaches for submitting sequences to the databases, one World Wide Web-based (e.g. using BankIt) and the other using Sequin, a multiplatform program that can use a network connection to great advantage but does not require one. Sequin is also an ASN.1 editing tool that takes full advantage of the NCBI data model and will become a platform for many sequence analysis tools that NCBI will incorporate in the years to come. Because of this, Sequin is the update tool of choice.

The genome sequencing era (the period during which ESTs and genomic sequences are deposited at great speed, has already affected the scientific community in many ways. For example, many scientists release their sequences before the article detailing them is in press. This practice is now the rule for large genomic centres and although some individual laboratories still wait for acceptance of publication before making their data available, others consider the release of a record as a publication in its own right.

Most of the sequence records in the early years were submitted by individual scientists studying a gene of interest. A program suitable for these submissions must allow manual annotation of arbitrary biological information. However, the databases recently have had to adapt to new classes of data and to a substantially higher rate of submission. Not long after the beginning of EST sequencing, it became clear that a separate submission protocol was going to be necessary for receiving these records, which would be coming into the databases at the rate of thousands per day, with some peak submission periods reaching 1,00,000 per week. Fortunately, these records are fairly simple and uniform in content and thus amenable to automatic processing. The bulk submission protocol is discussed later. The submission process is also part of an international activity and it is noted again that sequences submitted to anyone of the three international collaborative databases. Sequence records then are distributed worldwide by various user groups and centres, including those that reformat the records for use within their own suites of programs and databases. Thus by submitting a sequence to only one of the three database researchers can avoid any possible duplication of work for the database staff at these three locations and also avoid the possibility that redundant records will be released. Also, most journals expect that all nucleotide sequences presented in a publication and of central importance to the publication, will be referenced by an accession number provided by one of the international collaborative databases.

WHERE TO SUBMIT?

Historically, investigators would submit to a specified database, depending on the journal in which they wanted to publish. This is no longer true, although some journals still improperly indicate a preferred database. Rather, one should submit to whichever database is most convenient. This may be the database in the closest geographical area (if, for example, a telephone conversation will be required); it may be the repository one has always submitted to; or it may be simply the place one's submission is likely to receive the best attention. All three databases have knowledgeable staff who are able to help submitters throughout the process. Under normal circumstances, an accession number will be returned within a workday, and a finished record in 5–10 working days, depending on the state of things that work week and the state of the submitted sequence.

Presently, it is assumed that all submissions of sequences are done electronically: via the world wide web, by electronic mail or (at the very least) on a computer disk sent via regular postal mail. These two modes of submission replace the earlier method using the Authorin software, which is now outdated. Submissions prepared with Authorin are nonetheless still accepted and processed, but users of Authorin should be aware of its limitations and of the availability of superior alternatives.

WHAT TO SUBMIT?

All three databases want the same end result: a richly annotated, biologically and computationally sound record, one that allows other scientists to be able to reap the benefits of the work already performed by the submitting biologist and affords links to the protein, bibliographic and genomic databases. The databases are a repository of all experimentally derived sequences and so the newly determined sequence of an mRNA or of a genomic region can be submitted to a database, whose staff will assist the submitter in providing sufficient information to make the sequence useful for others. There is available a rich set of biological features and other annotations, but the important components are definitely the ones that lend themselves to analysis. These include the nucleotide and protein sequences: the CDS (coding sequence, also known as coding region), gene and mRNA features (i.e. features representing the central dogma of molecular biology); the organism from which the sequences were determined; and the bibliographic citation that links them to the information sphere and will have all the experimental details that give this sequence its *raison d'être*.

DNA/RNA

The submission process is quite simple, but care must be taken to provide information that is accurate (free of errors and vector contamination) and as biologically sound as possible, to ensure maximal usability by the scientific community. Here are a few matters to settle before starting a submission, regardless of its form.

Nature of the sequence

Is it of genomic or mRNA origin? Users of the databases like to know the nature of the physical DNA that is the origin of the molecule being sequenced. For example, although cDNA sequencing is performed on DNA (and not RNA), the type of the molecule present in the cell is mRNA. The same is true for the genomic sequencing of rRNA genes, where the sequenced molecule is almost always genomic DNA. Copying the rRNA into DNA, like direct sequencing of rRNA, although possible, is rarely done. Bear in mind also that since the sequence being submitted should be of a unique molecular type, it must not represent (for example) a mixture of genomic and mRNA molecule types that cannot actually be isolated from a living cell.

Is the sequence synthetic, but not artificial?

There is a special division in the nucleotide databases for synthetic molecules, sequences put together experimentally that do not occur naturally in the environment (e.g. protein expression vector sequences). The DNA sequence databases do not accept computer-generated sequences, such as consensus sequences, and all sequences in the databases are experimentally derived from the actual sequencing of the molecule in question. They can, however, be the compilation of a shotgun sequencing exercise.

How accurate is the sequence?

This question is poorly documented in the database literature, but the assumption that the submitted sequence is as accurate as possible usually means at least two-pass coverage (opposite orientations) on the whole submitted sequence.

Equally important is the verification of the final submitted sequence. It should be free of vector contamination (this can be verified with a BLASTN search against the vector database and possibly checked with known restriction maps, to eliminate the possibility of sequence rearrangement or to confirm correct sequence assembly.

Organism

Having the proper organism assigned to a record is of crucial importance, although in most cases this is easily done. All DNA sequence records must have an organism assigned to them. Many inferences are made from the phylogenetic position of the records present in the databases. If these are wrongly placed, an incorrect genetic code may be used for translation, with the possible consequence of an incorrectly truncated protein product sequence. Just knowing the genus and species is usually enough to permit the database staff to identify the organism and its lineage. NCBI offers an important taxonomy service and the staff taxonomists maintain the taxonomy that is used by all the nucleotide databases and by Swiss-Prot, the protein database.

Citation

As good as the annotations can be, they will never surpass a published article in fully representing large amounts of biology. It is, therefore, imperative to ensure the proper link between the research publication and the primary data it will cite. For this reason, having a citation in the submission being prepared is of great importance, even if it consists of just a temporary list of authors and a working title. Updating these citations at publication time is also important to the value of the record. (This is done routinely by the database staff and will happen more promptly if the submitter notifies the staff upon publication of the article.)

Coding Sequence(s)

A submission of nucleotide also means the inclusion of the protein sequences it encodes. This is important for two reasons:

1. Protein databases (e.g. Swiss-Prot and PIR) are almost entirely populated by protein sequences present in DNA sequence database records.
2. The inclusion of the protein sequence serves as an important, if not essential, validation step in the submission process.

Proteins include the enzyme molecules that carry out many of the biological reactions we study and their sequences are an intrinsic part of the submission process. Their importance, is also reflected in the submission process, where this information must be captured for representation in the various databases. Also important are the protein product and gene names, if these are known. There are a variety of resources (many present in the lists that conclude these chapters) that offer the correct nomenclature for a given organism's gene nomenclature.

The coding sequence features or CDS, are the links between the DNA or RNA and the protein sequences and their correct positioning is central in the validation, along with the correct translation table. The nucleotide databases now use 13 different genetic codes, which are maintained by the taxonomy and molecular biology staff at NCBI. Because protein sequences are so important, comprising one of the main pieces of molecular biology information on which biologists can compute, they receive much deserved attention from the staff at the various databases. It is usually simple to find the correct open reading frame in an mRNA and various tools are available for this (e.g. NCBI's ORF finder and also as a function within Sequin). Getting the correct CDS intervals in a genomic sequence from a higher eukaryote is a little trickier: the different exon-coding sequences must be joined and this involves a variety of approaches. (The suggest intervals function in Sequin will calculate CDS intervals if given the sequence of the protein and the proper genetic code.) What a submission includes will be validated by the database staff, but even more appropriately, by the submission tool used, as well, on the www or with Sequin. Validation checks that the start and stop codons are included in the CDS intervals, that these intervals are using legal exon/intron consensus boundaries and that the provided amino acid sequence can be translated from the designated CDS intervals using the appropriate genetic code.

Other Features

There are a variety of other features available for the feature sections of a submitted sequence record and many of these will enhance the record. The complete set of these is represented in the Feature Table documentation, which is available on the www or as PostScript files available by anonymous FTP. While many features are available, there is much inconsistent usage in the databases, mainly due to a lack of consistent guidelines and poor agreement among biologists as to what they really mean. Getting the organism, bibliography, gene, CDS and mRNA correct usually suffices and makes for a record that can be validated, is informative and allows a biologist to grasp in a few lines of text what biology is there to be captured. Nonetheless, the full renditions of the feature table documentation are available for use as appropriate, but with care taken as to the intent of the annotations.

Population, Phylogenetic and Mutational Studies

The nucleotide databases are now accepting population, phylogenetic, and mutational studies as submitted sequence sets and although this information is not adequately represented in the flatfile records, it is appearing in the various databases. This new type of submission allows, if only for a practical reason, the submission of a group of related sequences together, with entry of shared information required only once. Sequin also allows the user to include the alignment generated with a favourite alignment tool, and to submit this information with the DNA sequence. At the time of writing, NCBI was the only database accepting this information, although it is clear to all databases that the information is important for a great number of records now on hand. New ways to display this information (such as entrez) should soon make this kind of data more visible to the general scientific community.

Protein-Only Submissions

In most cases, protein sequences come with a DNA sequence. There are some exceptions—people do sequence proteins directly—and such sequences must be submitted without a corresponding DNA sequence. SWISS-PROT presently is the best venue for these submissions, which can be processed at the EBI which will accept them for submission into SWISS-PROT.

HOW TO SUBMIT ON THE WORLD WIDE WEB

The decline in the usability of Authorin led the three databases to decide to use the forms-based approach on the world wide web. This new medium lent itself well to the submission process. Each of the three repositories engineered a form for the submission of DNA sequences to its database: Sakura (cherry blossoms) at DDBJ, WebIn at EBI and BankIt at GenBank. The www is the preferred submission path for simple submissions (Fig. 24.1) or those that do not require complicated annotations or too much repetition (i.e. 30 similar sequences, as typically found in a population study, would best be done with Sequin). The www form is ideal for a research group that makes few sequence submissions and needs something simple, entailing a short learning curve, or none. The www forms will be appropriate, sufficient and more than adequate for the majority of the submissions: some 60–80 per cent of submitters make their DNA or RNA sequence submissions via the www at NCBI.

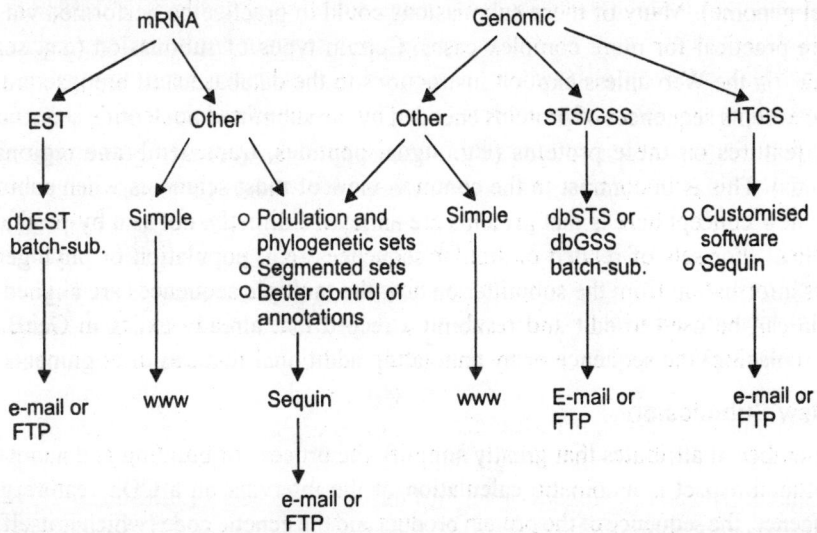

Fig. 24.1. Flowchart for deciding which protocol to follow for DNA sequence submissions to one of the DNA sequence databases. WWW is BankIt, WebIn or Sakura.

Although this part of the chapter emphasises NCBI's BankIt submission tool, submission to any one of the principal databases will ensure that a sequence is appropriately processed and will be deposited in the two others, as well.

Upon entering a BankIt submission, the user is asked about the length of the nucleotide sequence to be submitted. This is because a www browser limitation makes it impossible to enter more than 29,000 nucleotides (characters) in a window. If it is necessary to submit 40,000 base pairs (a common size for people submitting cosmid sequences), BankIt presents two windows, so that by copying and pasting 20,000 characters per window, the 29,000 characters/window limit can be accommodated.

The next BankIt form is also straightforward: it asks about the contact person (the individual to whom the database staff may address any questions), the citations (who gets the scientific credit), the organism (the top 100 organisms are on the form; all others must be typed in), the location (nuclear vs. organelle), some map information and the nucleotide sequence itself. At the end of the form, there is a BankIt button, which calls up the next form. At this point some validation is made, and if any necessary fields were not filled in, the form is presented again. If all is well, the next form asks how many features are to be added and prompts the user to indicate their type(s). If no features were added, BankIt will issue a warning and ask for confirmation that not even one CDS is to be added to the submission. The user can say no (0 new CDS) or take the opportunity to add one or more CDS. At this point structural RNA information or any other legal DDBJ/EMBL/GenBank features can be added, as well.

HOW TO SUBMIT WITH SEQUIN

Sequin is a program that is designed to assist scientists in preparing new sequence and update data for submission to DDBJ, EMBL and GenBank. It is a tool that works on most computer platforms and is suitable for a wide range of sequence lengths and complexities, including traditional (gene-sized) nucleotide sequences, segmented entries (e.g. genomic sequences of a spliced gene for which not all intronic sequences have been determined), long (genome-sized) sequences with many annotated features and sets of related sequences (i.e. population, phylogenetic or mutation studies of a particular gene, region, or viral genome). Many of these submissions could in practice be performed via the www, but Sequin is more practical for more complex cases. Certain types of submission (e.g. segmented sets) cannot be made via the Web unless explicit instructions to the database staff are inserted.

Sequin also accepts sequences of proteins encoded by the submitted nucleotide sequences and allows annotation of features on these proteins (e.g. signal peptides, transmembrane regions, or cysteine disulphide bonds). This is in contrast to the common view of most scientists when submitting a DNA sequence. The new concept here is that proteins are annotated directly, not as a by-product of the DNA that encodes them. For sets of related or similar sequences (e.g. population or phylogenetic studies), Sequin accepts information from the submitter on how the multiple sequences are aligned to each other. Finally, Sequin can be used to edit and resubmit a record that already exists in GenBank, either by extending (or replacing) the sequence or by annotating additional features or alignments (see below).

Entering a New Submission

Sequin has a number of attributes that greatly simplify the process of building and annotating a record. The most profound aspect is automatic calculation of the intervals on a CDS feature given only the nucleotide sequence, the sequence of the protein product and the genetic code (which is itself automatically obtained from the organism name). This 'Suggest Intervals' process takes consensus splice sites into account in its calculations. Traditionally these intervals were entered manually, a time-consuming and error-prone process, especially on a genomic sequence with many exons, in cases of alternative splicing or on segmented sequences.

Another important attribute is the ability to enter relevant annotation in a simple format in the Definition line of the sequence datafile. Sequin recognises and extracts this information when reading the sequences, then puts it in the proper places in the record. For nucleotide sequences, it is possible to enter the organism's scientific name, the strain or clone name and several other source modifiers. For protein sequences, the gene and protein names can be entered. (If this information is not present in the sequence definition line, Sequin will prompt the user for it before proceeding. But annotations of the Definition line can be very convenient, since the information stays with the sequence and can't be forgotten or mixed up later.) In addition to building the proper CDS feature, Sequin will automatically make gene and protein features with this information.

Since the majority of submissions contain a single nucleotide sequence and one or more coding region features (and their associated protein sequences), the functionality just outlined can frequently result in a finished record, ready to submit without any further annotation. And with gene and protein names properly recorded, the record becomes informative to other scientists, who may retrieve it as a BLAST similarity result or from an Entrez search.

Validation

To ensure the quality of data being submitted, Sequin has a built-in validator that searches out, for example, missing organism information, incorrect coding region lengths (compared to the submitted protein sequence), internal stop codons in coding regions, mismatched amino acids or nonconsensus splice sites. Double-clicking on an item in the error report launches an editor on the 'offending' feature.

The validator also checks for inconsistent use of 'partial' indications, especially among coding regions, the protein product and the protein feature on the product (Unless told otherwise, the CDS editor will automatically synchronise these separate partial indicators, facilitating the correction of this kind of inconsistency).

Viewing the Sequence Record

Sequin provides a number of different views of a sequence record. The traditional flatfile can be presented in FASTA, GenBank or EMBL format (these can be exported to files on the user's computer, which can then be entered into other sequence analysis packages). A graphical view shows feature intervals on a sequence. This is particularly useful for viewing alternatively spliced coding regions (the graphical view's style can be customised and these views can also be copied to the personal computer's clipboard, for pasting into a word processor or drawing program that will be used in preparing a manuscript for publication). There is a more detailed view that shows the features on the actual sequence. For records containing alignments (e.g. alignments between related sequences entered by a user or the results of a PowerBLAST search), one can request either a graphical overview showing insertions, deletions and mismatches, or a detailed view showing the alignment of sequence letters.

The above-mentioned viewers are active. Clicking on a feature, a sequence or the graphical representation of an alignment between sequences will highlight that object. Double-clicking will launch the appropriate editor. Multiple viewers can be used on the same record, permitting different formats to be seen simultaneously. For example, it is quite convenient to have the graphical view and the GenBank (or EMBL) flatfile view present at the same time, especially on larger records containing more than one CDS. The graphical view can be compared to a scientist's lab notebook drawings, providing a quick reality check on the overall accuracy of the feature annotation.

Advanced Annotation and Editing Functions

The sequence editor built into Sequin automatically adjusts feature intervals as the sequence is edited. This is particularly important if one is adding a 5′ sequence to a record submitted earlier. Prior to Sequin, this entailed manually correcting the intervals on all biological features on the sequence or more likely, redoing the entire submission from scratch. The sequence editor is used much like a text editor, with new sequence being pasted in or typed in at the position of a cursor.

A major class of submissions involves multiple related sequences (i.e. phylogenetic, population or mutation studies). These records are most informative if the user submits information on how the sequences align to each other. This alignment can be entered with the sequence data (e.g. in PHYLIP, NEXUS or FASTA+GAP format) or calculated by Sequin after the sequences have been read.

For these records, Sequin allows annotation of one sequence, whereupon features from that sequence can be propagated to all other sequences. (In the case of a CDS feature, the feature intervals can be calculated automatically by reading in the sequence of its protein product, rather than having to enter them by typing.) To do this, feature propagation is chosen (from the alignment editor). Selected features are then copied onto the remaining sequences, with feature intervals adjusted using the alignment information. The result is the same that would have been achieved if features had been manually annotated on each sequence, but with feature propagation the entire process can be completed in minutes rather than hours.

Feature propagation and the sequence editor combine to provide simple and automatic methods for updating an existing sequence. The update sequence functions allow the user to enter an overlapping sequence or a replacement sequence. Sequin makes an alignment, merges the sequences if necessary, propagates features onto the new sequence in their new positions and uses these to replace the old sequence and features.

Sequin as an Analysis Workbench

Sequin also provides a number of sequence analysis functions. For example, one function will reverse complement the sequence and the intervals of its features. New functions can easily be added. These functions appear in a window called the NCBI DeskTop, which directly displays the internal structure of the records currently loaded in memory. This window can be understood as a Venn diagram, with descriptors on a set (such as a population study) applying to all sequences in that set. With the DeskTop, the user can read the results of a PowerBLAST analysis, then drag and drop this information onto a sequence record, thus adding the alignment data to the record. The modifications are immediately displayed on any active viewers. Note, however, that not all annotations are visible in all viewers. The flatfile view does have its limitations; for example, it does not indicate that alignments are present.

The NCBI data model supports sets of sequences and Sequin allows complete navigation around these sets, for purposes of display or annotation. For example, Nuc-prot sets contain a nucleotide sequence and its protein products. The nucleotide sequence can itself be segmented. In this case, a Seg set contains the segmented sequence and a Parts set, which in turn contains the raw sequence data for the individual segments. And the Population, Phylogenetic and Mutation sets can contain multiple related sequences or Nuc-prot sets. The NCBI DeskTop is the quickest way of examining the internal structure of a record at a glance.

Consequences of Data Model

Sequin is an ASN.1 editor. The NCBI data model, written in the ASN.1 data description language, is designed to keep associated information together in descriptors or features. Features are typically biological concepts (e.g. genes, coding regions, RNAs, proteins) that always have a location (of one or more intervals) on a sequence. Descriptors were introduced to carry information that can apply to multiple sequences, eliminating the need to enter multiple copies of the same information.

For example, the BioSource descriptor contains an organism's scientific name, preferred common name, taxonomic lineage and GenBank division, as well as modifiers (e.g. strain, clone, chromosome, map location) specific to a given entry. Collecting this information in one place in the data specification makes it easier for the user to enter or edit this information. And placing a single BioSource descriptor on a Nuc-prot set satisfies the validator's desire (and the databases' policy) to have biological source information applying to each sequence, including the proteins.

Double-clicking on a paragraph in the GenBank flatfile view or on a feature in a graphical view, launches an editor that can edit all pertinent information on that item. In some cases, particularly BioSource or Publications, the items may be descriptors or features and discerning which is which from looking at the flatfile may be difficult. (It is easy to tell what is a descriptor and what is a feature in the NCBI DeskTop. And only features and sequences are shown in the Summary, Graphic, Alignment and Sequence views.)

The data model results in conventions that may not be obvious to the casual user (looking at the GenBank or EMBL flatfile views) but can, in fact, simplify entry of biological information. For example, a publication, which appears in the header section of the GenBank flatfile, can contain a remark subsection. Text explaining the biological conclusions of the reference, as these pertain to the sequence record, can be entered here. The text always remains with the reference in the report. In contrast, putting explanatory information in a large comment section and referring to publications by number (e.g. '[5]') is a risky practice because the numbering may change (e.g. due to addition of new publications), making the numbers out of synch with the publications.

Similarly, citations on features (e.g. justifying ribosomal slippage in a coding region) internally reference the publication, not a publication number, even though in the flatfile a number is displayed. This is another convention that allows the publication numbering to change without 'breaking' the integrity of the citations. And it means that there is only one full copy of the citation, which makes updating any information on the publication easier.

Nevertheless, literature references on sequence records should be used sparingly. A sequence record is not meant to be a review of the subject. Using links and neighbours in Entrez (and in Sequin with a network connection) is a much more reliable method of collecting relevant information and of making original discoveries using the sequence databases.

For the simplest case, that of a single nucleotide sequence with one or more protein products, Sequin allows the user to work without needing to be aware of the data model's structural hierarchy. The CDS feature editor can be used to enter the protein sequence (or translate it from an entered location) and to enter or edit the protein feature (which supplies the protein name) on that sequence. The user can access the (single) protein feature without having to 'navigate' to the protein sequence. And the CDS editor can also create a separate gene feature with the gene name.

Navigation is necessary, as is at least a cursory understanding of the data model, if extensive annotation on protein product sequences is contemplated. Many proteins have cysteine disulphide bonds, binding sites, active sites, glycosylation sites, signal peptides or transmembrane regions. Annotating these can make a record more informative to biologists who come across it as the result of a BLAST or entrez search. Setting the Target control to a given sequence changes the viewer to show a graphical view or text report on that sequence. Any features or descriptors created with the Annotation submenus will be packaged on the currently targeted sequence.

Although Sequin does provide full navigation among all sequences within a structured record, building the original structure from the raw sequence data is a job best left to Sequin's 'create new submission' functions. Sequin asks up front for information (e.g. organism and source modifiers, gene and protein names) and knows how to correctly package everything into the appropriate place. This was, in fact, one of the main design goals of Sequin. Manual annotation requires a more detailed understanding of the data model and expertise with the more esoteric functions of Sequin.

A finished submission can be saved to disk (File -> Prepare Submission) and e-mailed to one of the databases. It is also a good practice to save frequently throughout the Sequin session, to make sure nothing is inadvertently lost.

Submitting a Single Sequence

The simplest submission contains a single contiguous nucleotide sequence and one or more protein product sequences. These records typically come from the traditional gene-based biological research and such submissions can in most cases be done on the web or with Sequin. Sequin offers the advantages of numerous validations as well as independence from the vagaries of network access.

Sequin begins with a window that allows the user to start a new submission or load a file containing a saved record. After the initial submission has been built, the record can be saved to a file and edited later, before finally being sent to the database.

Using Sequin as a Workbench

An exploded view of a complex record, illustrating some of what would be seen with the DeskTop, is shown in Fig. 24.2. In this example, a phylogenetic study contains five components, each of which is a Nuc-prot set. There are two descriptors (Create-date and Publication) on the Phy set and these apply to all components. The first Nuc-prot set is 'blown up' to show more details: it contains nucleotide and protein bioseqs and a BioSource descriptor applying to both. (The other components of a phylogenetic set would have BioSources for different organisms.)

Both bioseqs are of type 'raw', meaning that the actual sequence data is encoded in the bioseq. ('Segmented' bioseqs contain sequence identifiers that refer to the actual raw segments. This is how the Entrez Genomes division is built.) The nucleotide bioseq has a MolInfo descriptor, which says that the molecule sequenced was genomic [as opposed to mRNA (cDNA), or tRNA or rRNA]. The protein bioseq's MolInfo states that it is a peptide and that it is an author-supplied conceptual translation (as opposed to having been directly sequenced by Edman degradation or other methods).

Features in a DeskTop view show a text label and information on the feature's location and optional product. For example, the CDS feature location points to intervals on the nucleotide bioseq. Its product points to the entire protein bioseq. The text label ('alcohol dehydrogenase') is in fact taken from the Protein feature on the protein bioseq. This can easily be verified by editing the protein name in the Protein feature. (The GenBank flatfile view does the same kind of mapping, with a CDS taking the Protein feature's name for its /product qualifier and the protein bioseq's sequence data for its /translation qualifier.) Those who want to become familiar with the NCBI data model will find that viewing records of different kinds with the NCBI DeskTop is a good way to see bioseq sets, to discover the levels at which various descriptors are packaged, and to learn how the set hierarchy works. This understanding is not necessary for the casual user submitting a simple sequence, but for the advanced user it can immediately take the mystery out of the data.

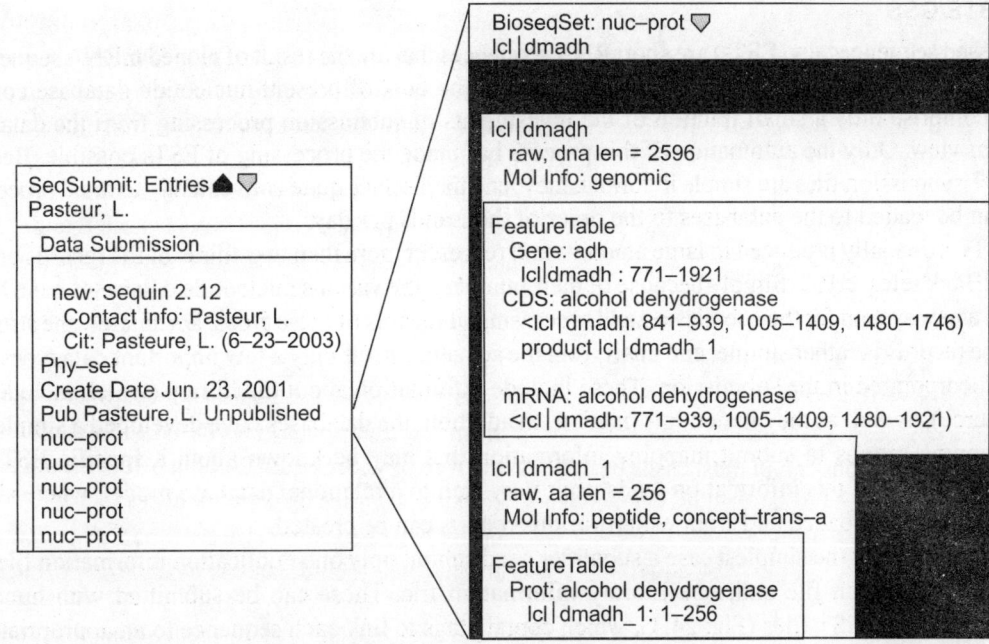

Fig. 24.2. DeskTop views of a Phylogenetic set. In this composite figure, a Phylogenetic set contains several Nuc-prot sets and applies the same publication to all components. One of the Nuc-prots is expanded in further detail. It contains a BioSource for *Drosophila melanogaster*, a nucleotide sequence with Gene, mRNA and CDS features and a protein sequence with a Protein feature that provides the name of the product.

Sequin with a Network Connection

When configured for a network connection, Sequin includes the functionality of PowerBLAST, Network Entrez Cn3D and the ability to do MEDLINE/PubMed lookups as well as Taxonomy lookups. Choose PowerBLAST from the Search menu and a dialog box appears, offering the choice of running BLASTN or BLASTX with a nucleotide query; in addition, one can choose to search the nr database or several subset databases, including est and vector. The results are automatically added to the sequence record and will appear in Summary, Graphic, Alignment and Sequence views.

Double-clicking on an alignment in one of these views will retrieve the corresponding sequence record from the Entrez network service. At the bottom of the window of the resulting viewer will be neighbour and link controls. So a user who sequences a disease gene and runs PowerBLAST within Sequin can immediately view the database 'hit' and in one step will be able to retrieve the MEDLINE article that discusses its biology. Or sequence neighbours of that record can be retrieved, then passed (with the Refine button) into the Entrez query window, where, for example, the results can be refined by selecting for or against any taxonomic category.

To configure for network usage, choose Net Configure from the Misc menu. The 'outgoing connections only' checkbox is used if the network has a firewall. In general, unless there is a temporary problem with the network, the 'Test connection during configuration' checkboxes should be set.

At the time of writing, numerous enhancements were being added to Sequin. The best way to stay abreast of new developments (e.g. new versions of Sequin; bug fixes) is to visit the Sequin Web page and register as a Sequin user. The Sequin home page also contains information about the latest enhancements and complete documentation and FAQ listings.

EST/STS/GSS

Expressed sequence tags (ESTs) are short RNA sequences that are the result of cloned mRNA sequencing survey projects. Although these sequences represent the bulk of present nucleotide database content, ESTs comprise only a small fraction of the investments of submission processing from the databases point of view. Only the automation of this process has made the processing of ESTs possible. Because the EST submission files are simple in format, they lend themselves quite conveniently to rapid processing and can be loaded to the databases to the order of thousands per day.

ESTs are usually produced in large amounts and represent more than two-thirds of the records present in GenBank release 102. Simply because of their numbers, the various nucleotide databases have had to design a new system for the submission and processing of records of these types. Fortunately the structure of these records is rather simple, and apart from the sequence itself only a few important data types need to be incorporated in the submission. These include information about the library (which includes the BioSource), as well as the citation information. In addition, the databases have developed a simple way for mapping groups to submit mapping information that may be known about a specific EST. The simple structure of this information lends itself very well to a relational database model, where simple data items can be loaded and from which various reports can be created.

For example, in the simplest case a submitter need submit only one Publication information file, one Contact information file and, one Library information file. These can be submitted with hundreds (or thousands) of EST files (Fig. 24.3), which contain tags to link each sequence to an appropriate file of the other type. The files are normally built by customised programs, ensuring that the information is constant between the various records. The files are then submitted by e-mail (if the numbers are in the hundreds) or by FTP (if the numbers are in the thousands).

This submission model was so successful that it was cloned for the sequence tagged sites (STS) and genome survey sequences (GSS) database submissions process. Here again the same simple file format is used with a few variants. The finer details of how to submit these records are also included in their respective Web pages.

GENOME CENTRES

Centres that specialise in sequencing large segments of DNA (hundreds of thousands to millions of base pairs per year) have their own information-handling systems. Not only have they designed their own database systems, but their programmers maintain software and databases that keep track of the various sequencing projects and will organise this information to allow assemblies to be tracked, performances followed and problems spotted at an early stage. The genome centres format their results in a variety of ways, often including the www pages, making the information they produce available directly to the community as a whole or to their customers. If these genome centres want their sequences available in the public databases, they communicate with one of the databases to ensure that correct data exchange can take place. All three database centres (DDBJ, EBI and NCBI) have extensive experience in working with the various genome centres to ensure timely and effortless (insofar as is possible) exchange of information. This includes the setting up of automatic exchange of data, the creation of special FTP accounts so that data can exchanged in a most accurate and convenient way, and the generation of tools to ensure data exchange in the most useful format. At NCBI, for example, FTP accounts have been set up for all genome sequencing centres that submit to the organisation, and a variety of tools for accelerating the submission of high-throughput genome sequences (HTGS) have been created.

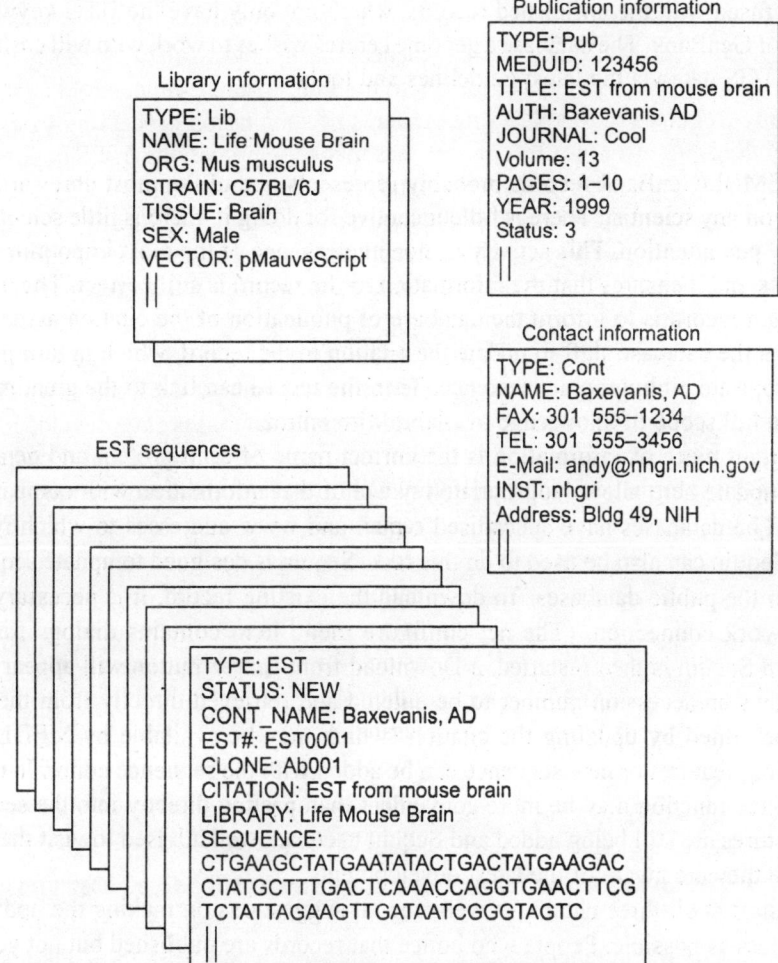

Fig. 24.3. The EST submission. Submitting ESTs (or STS and GSS records) requires the generation of simple files from which the database staff will build the GenBank and dbEST records. Single contact information, publication information, and one or more library information files will be joined with the many-sequence files that will result in as many complete EST records. All these files start with a TYPE line and end with ll on the last line.

These HTGS records are found in two different divisions of GenBank, depending on their status of completion. Unfinished records (phase 1 or 2) are in the HTG division of GenBank and finished records (phase 3) are in the taxonomic division to which they belong. Throughout their existence, HTGS records keep the same DDBJ/EMBL/GenBank accession number. One of the tools devised by NCBI to build these records is fa2htgs, a command line program that can easily be incorporated in scripts and allows the user to generate HTGS submissions from FASTA files and a Sequin template. As for all other NCBI products, this program is available for most computer platforms.

High-throughput genome sequencing also implies a change in the way the sequences are used. This is why sequences generated by these centres are marked with an HTG keyword, making it possible for users of the data to selectively use it in their analyses or to simply be aware of its origin. Data so tagged should not be confused with the unfinished records, which not only have the HTG keyword but are in the HTG division of GenBank. The database a genome centres wishes to work with will ensure appropriate handling of the HTGS data via the latest guidelines and tools.

UPDATES

Updating DDBJ/EMBL/GenBank records probably represents one of the most unrewarding tasks that could be imposed on any scientist. There is little incentive for doing it, there is little scientific credit and it appears that few pay attention. This activity is, nonetheless, one of the most important steps after the submission process and it ensures that the information in the record is still correct. The most important aspect of updating a record is to inform the database of publication of the citation associated with the record. This allows the database staff to update the citation in the record, which in turn permits it to be linked to the appropriate bibliographic reference. Then the record can link to the great mass of related references and the full scope of knowledge available with entrez.

Another important piece of information is the correct name of each protein and gene present in a record; again, an update here allows appropriate linkage of that information with comparable material in the databases. The databases have specialised e-mail and www addresses to which record updates can be sent, and Sequin can also be used to do this task. Sequin is designed to update sequence records that are already in the public databases. To download the existing record, it is necessary to configure Sequin for a network connection. (The net configure menu item contains dialogs for making this connection.) When Sequin is then restarted, a Download from Entrez button will appear in the startup window. This allows an accession number to be entered and retrieved directly from the ID database. The record can be edited by updating the citation (which may be available by MEDLINE/PubMed lookup) or by adding features or new sequence can be added with the sequence editor. In the latter case, the Update Sequence function may be more convenient than pasting directly into the sequence editor. New updating features are still being added and Sequin users are well advised to visit the Sequin www page to make sure they are aware of the latest developments.

The database staff at all three databases welcome all suggestions on making the update process as efficient and painless as possible. People who notice that records are published but not yet released are strongly encouraged to notify the databases as well. If errors are detected, these should also be forwarded to the updates addresses; the owner of the record is notified accordingly (by the database staff) and a correction usually results. This chain of events is to be distinguished from third-party annotations, which are presently not accepted by the databases. The record belongs to the submitter(s); the database staff offers some curatorial, formatting guideline suggestions, but substantive changes come only from a listed submitter.

Thus, the act of depositing records into a database and seeing these made public has always been an exercise of pride on the part of submitters, a segment of the scientific activity from their laboratory which they present to the scientific community. It is also a step that has been imposed by publishers as part of the publication process. In this process submitters always hope to provide information in the most complete and useful fashion, allowing maximum use of their data by the scientific community.

Very few users are aware of the complete array of intricacies present in the databases, but they do know the biology they want to represent. It has become the task of the databases to provide tools that will facilitate this process. The database staff also provides expertise with their indexers (some databases also call them curators or annotators), who have extensive training in biology and are very familiar with the databases, ensuring that nothing is lost in the submission process. The submission exercise itself has not always been easy and was not even encouraged at the beginning of the sequencing era, simply because databases did not know how to handle this information. Now, however, the databases strongly encourage the submission of sequence data and of all appropriate updates. Many tools are available to facilitate this task and together the databases support Sequin as the tool to use for new submissions, in addition to their respective www submissions tools. Submitting data to the databases has now become an enjoyable task and scientists no longer have good excuses for neglecting it.

Glossary

Ab initio	:	Describing an analysis method carried out from first principle.
Accession number	:	A unique number or code (identifier) given to mark the entry of a sequence (protein or nucleic acid) or pattern (regular expression, finger-print, profile) to a primary or secondary database.
Adenine	:	A purine base found in DNA and RNA.
Affine gap penalty	:	A gap penalty score that is a linear function of gap length, consisting of a gap opening penalty and a gap extension penalty multiplied by the length of the gap.
Algorithm	:	Any sequence of actions (e.g. computational steps) that perform a particular task.
Alignment	:	Arrangement of two or more nucleotides or protein sequences to maximise the number of matching monomers.
Alignment score	:	An algorithmically computed score based on the number of matches, substitutions, insertions and deletions (gaps) within an alignment. Alignment scores are in log odds units, often bit units (log to the base 2).
Alphabet	:	The total number of symbols in a sequence—4 for DNA sequences and 20 for protein sequences.
Amino acid	:	The fundamental building block of proteins. There are 20 naturally occurring amino acids in animals and around 100 more found only in plants.
Analogs	:	In phylogenetics, nonhomologous proteins that have similar folding architectures, or similar functional sites, which are believed to have arisen through convergent evolution.
Annotation	:	A combination of comments, notations, references and citations, either in free format or utilising a controlled vocabulary that together describes all the experimental and inferred information about a gene or protein.
Applet	:	Small software applications loaded from a server via HTML pages.
Archive	:	A collection of files.
ASCII	:	The American Standard Code of Information Interchange. ASCII specifies 128 characters that are mapped to the values 0–127.
Assembly	:	The process of aligning overlapping sequence fragments into a contig or series of contigs.
Attachment	:	A file that is sent appended to an e-mail.
Base	:	Distinct chemical structures found in → nucleic acids and part of → nucleotides. The bases of nucleotides form the signature letters allowing sequence information to be stored in → DNA and → RNA strands.

509

Basepair (bp)	:	Any possible pairing between bases in opposing strands of DNA or RNA. Adenine pairs with thymine in DNA or with uracil in RNA; and guanine pairs with cytosine.
Bioinformatics	:	Computational analysis of biological information such as → nucleic acid and → protein sequences and protein structures.
Bit units	:	A bit denotes the amount of information required to distinguish between two equally likely possibilities (from information theory). The number of bits of information, N, required to convey a message that has N possibilities is $\log_2 M = N$ bits.
Bit	:	A binary digit.
BLAST	:	A program for sequence database similarity searching.
Block	:	An ungapped, aligned motif consisting of sequence segments that are clustered to reduce multiple contributions from groups of highly similar or identical sequences.
BLOSUM matrix	:	It is a matrix derived using local multiple alignment of more distantly related sequences. It is used to assess similarity of sequences when performing alignments.
Branch length	:	In sequence analysis, the number of sequence changes along a particular branch of a phylogenetic tree.
Browser	:	A computer program (commonly known as a web client) that permits information retrieval from the internet and the www.
cDNA (complementary DNA)	:	A DNA strand copied from mRNA using reverse transcriptase.
cDNA library	:	A gene library composed of cDNA inserts synthesised from mRNA using reverse transcriptase.
Cell culture	:	Artificially (*in vitro*) maintained cell population in growth medium containing specifically isolated cell types which grow indefinitely; used to express → recombinant DNA or → proteins for physiological studies simulating experiments that would have been done in living organisms.
Cell	:	Basic, self-sustaining unit of living organisms. Composed of cell → membrane as outer boundary surrounding the → cytoplasm and internal → organelles that carry out specialised functions (see → mitochondrion).
Central dogma	:	A fundamental principle of molecular biology, first expounded by Francis Crick in 1958, essentially stating that the transfer of information from nucleic acid to nucleic acid or from nucleic acid to protein is possible, while transfer from protein to nucleic acid or from protein to protein is impossible.
Chaperone	:	A protein that assists the correct noncovalent assembly of folding proteins *in vivo*; chaperones do not themselves form part of the structures they help to assemble.
Characters and character states	:	In phylogenetics, characters are homologous features in different organisms. The exact condition of that feature in a particular individual is the character state. For example, the character 'hair colour' might have the character states 'gold', 'red' and 'yellow'. In molecular biology, the character states can be one of the four nucleotides (A, C, T, G) or one of the 20 amino acids. Some authors define 'character' to mean the character state as defined here.

Chromosome	:	Structurally independent unit of a → genome (see also karyotype).
Cladogram	:	A dendrogram in which each node has two branches, representing evolutionary history as speciation by bifurcation of the evolutionary lineage.
Client	:	A computer, or the software running on a computer, that interacts with another computer at a remote site (server). Note the difference between client and user.
Clone	:	A copied fragment of DNA, maintained in circular form, identical to the template from which it is derived: also a population of genetically identical cells derived from a single ancestor.
Cloning vector	:	A DNA molecule originating from a virus, a plasmid or the cell of a higher organism into which another DNA fragment can be integrated without compromising the vector's capacity for self-replication.
Cloning	:	The process of generating identical copies of a DNA fragment (that may encode a complete gene) from a single template DNA or producing identical copies of cells from single ancestor.
Cluster analysis	:	A method for grouping together a set of objects those are most similar from a larger group of related objects. The relationships are based on some criterion of similarity or difference.
Cluster	:	The grouping of similar objects in a multidimensional space.
Coding sequence (CDS)	:	A region of DNA or RNA whose sequence determines the sequence of amino acids in a protein.
Codon	:	A sequence of three adjacent nucleotides that designates a specific amino acid or start/stop site for transcription.
Command language	:	The language used for giving instructions to a computer operating system.
Command line	:	The basic level at which a computer prompts the user for input.
Communication protocol	:	An agreed set of rules for structuring communication between programs (allowing, for example, data exchange between nodes on the internet).
Comparative genomics	:	A comparison of gene numbers, gene locations and biological functions of genes in the genomes of diverse organisms, one objective being to identify groups of genes that play a unique biological role in a particular organism.
Comparative modelling	:	The process of predicting protein structure based on related sequence of known structure.
Composite database	:	A database that amalgamates a number of primary sources, using a set of defined criteria that determine the priority of inclusion of the different sources and the level of redundancy retained.
Conceptual translation	:	The computational process of interpreting the sequence of nucleotides in mRNA via the genetic code to a sequence of amino acid which may or may not code for protein.
Conformation	:	The precise three-dimensional arrangement of atoms and bonds in a molecule describing its geometry and hence its molecular function.
Consensus sequence	:	A pseudo-sequence that summarises the residue information contained in a multiple alignment.

Conserved sequence	:	A sequence of bases in a DNA molecule (or an amino acid sequence in a protein) that has remained essentially unchanged during evolution.
Contig	:	Contiguous → DNA sequence obtained from individually sequenced DNA fragments that contain overlapping sequences at their ends.
Contig	:	Sequences of clones, representing overlapping regions of a gene presented as an assembly or multiple alignment.
CORBA	:	The Common Object Request Broker Architecture (CORBA) is an open industry standard for working with distributed objects, developed by the Object Management Group. CORBA allows the interconnection of objects and applications regardless of computer language, machine architecture, or geographic location of the computers.
Cytoplasm	:	Content of cell in which most metabolic processes occur.
Cytosine	:	A pyrimidine base found in DNA and RNA.
Database	:	A collection of data records either in a single file or as multiple files.
Dendrogram	:	A branching graph used to represent phylogenetic relationships.
Descriptor	:	Information about a sequence or set of sequences whose scope depends on its placement in a record. A descriptor is placed on a set of sequences to reduce the need to save multiple redundant copies of information.
Discriminator	:	A mathematical abstraction of a conserved motif or set of motifs (e.g. a regular expression pattern, a profile or a fingerprint), used to search either an individual query sequence or a full database for the occurrence of that same or similar motif(s).
DNA (deoxyribonucleic acid)	:	The molecule that encodes genetic information. DNA is a double-stranded molecule held together by weak bonds between basepairs of nucleotides. The four nucleotides in DNA contain the bases: adenine (A), guanine (G), cytosine (C) and thymine (T). In nature, basepairs form only between A and T and between G and C; thus the base sequence of each single strand can be deduced from that of its partner.
DNA sequence	:	The linear sequence of base pairs, whether in a fragment of DNA, a gene, a chromosome or an entire genome.
DNAse (deoxyribonuclease)	:	One of a series of enzymes that can digest DNA.
Domain name	:	Refers to one of the levels of organisation of the internet; used to both classify and identify host machines. Top-level domain names indicate the type of site or the country in which the host is located.
Domain	:	A compact, local, semi-independent folding unit, presumed to have arisen via gene fusion and gene duplication events. Domains need not be formed from contiguous regions of an amino acid sequence: They may be discrete entities joined only by a flexible linking region of the chain; they may have extensive interfaces, sharing many close contacts: and they may exchange chains with domain neighbours. The combination of domains within a protein determines its overall structure and function.
Dot matrix	:	Dot matrix diagram provides a graphical method for comparing two sequences.
Download	:	Transferring files from a computer network to a local computer.
Download	:	To transfer a file from a remote host to a local machine via FTP.

Drug	:	An agent that affects a biological process.
Dumb	:	A dumb terminal is a desktop display device that is not capable of local processing, this being entirely carried out by the central computer. Such terminals, do not support windowing applications.
Dynamic programming	:	A method for the comparison and alignment of strings or sequences in a way that allows the computationally efficient incorporation of gaps.
Edman degradation	:	A method used in sequencing polypeptides, whereby amino acid residues are removed sequentially from N-terminus by reaction with phenyl-isothiocyanate, to form phenylthiocarbamyl-peptide (PTC-peptide). This is cleaved in anhydrous acid, releasing a thiazolinone intermediate and the remainder of the peptide.
E-mail	:	Electronic mail. Refers to messages that can be composed on the computer and transmitted via the internet to a remote location within seconds [Ant: snail mail, postal mail].
Enzyme	:	A protein that acts as a catalyst, speeding the rate at which a biochemical reaction proceeds but not altering the direction or nature of the reaction.
EST	:	Expressed sequence tag. ESTs are usually short (300–500 bp) single reads from mRNA (cDNA) which are usually produced in large numbers. They represent a snap shot of what is expressed in a given tissue and/or at a given developmental stage. They represent tags (some coding, others not) of expression for a given cDNA library. These records usually are very poor in annotation and have only library and BioSource information. They are represented in a variety of databases, notably DDBJ/EMBL/GenBank, dbEST and Unigene.
Eukaryote	:	Group of organisms that contain organelles within their → cytoplasm, specifically a nucleus containing all → chromosomal material.
Evolution	:	(Biological evolution) the perpetual change of the genetic composition of living organisms.
Exon	:	Gene sequence on chromosome that belongs to the coding sequence; exon sequences are interrupted by → introns.
Expressed sequence tag (EST)	:	A partial sequence of a clone, randomly selected from a cDNA library and used to identify genes expressed in a particular tissue.
Expression profile	:	The characteristic range of genes expressed at different stages of a cell's development and functioning.
Expression vector	:	A cloning vector that is engineered to allow the expression of protein from a cDNA.
False-negative	:	A true match that incorrectly fails to be recognised by a discriminator.
False-positive	:	A false match incorrectly recognised by a discriminator.
FAQ	:	A computer file of frequently asked questions. Exactly what it sounds like: A compiled list of questions and answers intended for new users of a computer-based resource, such as a mailing list or a newsgroup.
Feature	:	Annotation on a specific location on a given sequence.
Feature	:	Annotation on a specific location on a given sequence.
File transfer protocol (FTP)	:	A method of transferring files to remote computers.

File	:	A discrete collection of bytes that can be manipulated as a single-entity.
Fingerprint	:	A group of ungapped motifs excised from a sequence alignment and used to build a characteristic signature of family membership by means of interactive searching of a primary (or composite) database.
Firewall	:	Refers to the separation of a company or organisation's internal network from the public part, if any, of the same network. Intended to prevent unauthorised access to private computer systems.
Flat-file	:	A human-reliable data-file in a convenient form for interchange of database information. Flat-files may be created as output from relational databases, in a format suitable for loading into other databases.
Fold	:	The basic tertiary structure of a protein, including the secondary structure elements, their sequential connections and relative spatial positions.
Folding problem	:	The problem of determining how a protein folds into its final 3D form given only the information encoded in its primary structure.
Frameshift	:	An alteration in the reading sense of DNA resulting from an inserted or deleted base, such that the reading frame for all subsequent codons is shifted with respect to the number of changes made (e.g. if a sequence should read UCU-CAA-AGG-UUA and a single U is added to the beginning, the new sequence would read UUC-UCA-AAG-GUU, etc.). Frameshift may arise through random mutations or via errors in reading sequencing output.
FTP	:	File transfer protocol. The method by which files are transferred between hosts.
Gopher	:	A document delivery system allowing the retrieval and display of text-based files.
Functional genomics	:	Assessment of the function of genes identified by genome comparisons. The function of a newly identified gene is tested by introducing mutations into the gene and then examining the resultant mutant organism for an altered phenotype.
Gap penalty	:	A penalty subtracted from a sequence similarity score to account for gaps in a sequence alignment.
Gap	:	A part of a sequence alignment where one sequence contains no aligned monomer.
Gene duplication	:	A genetic alteration in which a segment of DNA is repeated. Duplications may appear anywhere, but where the duplicated segment is adjacent to the original one, this is termed as tandem duplication.
Gene expression	:	The process by which a gene's coded information is converted into the structures present and operating in the cell. Expressed genes include those that are transcribed in mRNA and then translated into protein and those that are transcribed into RNA but not translated into protein (e.g. transfer and ribosomal RNAs).
Gene families	:	Groups of closely related genes that encode similar protein products.
Gene pool	:	Collection of all genes or coding sequences within a population of an organism.
Gene product	:	The protein resulting from the expression of a gene. In some cases, the gene product may be an RNA molecule that is never translated.
Gene	:	The fundamental physical and functional unit of heredity. A gene is an ordered sequence of nucleotides located in a particular position on a particular

chromosome that encodes a specific functional product (i.e. a protein or RNA molecule).

Genetic algorithm : A kind of search algorithm that was inspired by the principles of evolution. A population of initial solutions is encoded and the algorithm searches through these by applying a predefined fitness measurement to each solution, selecting those with the highest fitness for reproduction.

Genetic code : The rules that relate the four DNA or RNA bases to the 20 amino acids. There are 64 possible three-base (triplet) sequences, which are known as codons. A single triplet uniquely defines one amino acid, but an amino acid may be coded by as many as six codons. The code is thus said to be degenerate.

Genetic map : The relative positions of known genes or markers.

Genome : All the genetic material in the chromosomes of a particular organism; its size is generally given as its total number of basepairs.

Genotype : Hereditary unit of the → genome (usually a → gene or group of genes).

Global alignment : Attempts to match as many characters as possible, from end to end, in a set of more than two sequences.

GSS : Genome survey sequences. This DDBJ/EMBL/GenBank division is similar in nature to the EST division, except that its sequences are genomic in origin, rather than cDNA (mRNA). The GSS division contains (but will not be limited to) the following types of data: random 'single-pass read' genome survey sequences; single-pass reads from cosmid/BAC/YAC ends (these could be chromosome specific,but need not be); exon-trapped genomic sequences; Alu PCR sequences.

Guanine : One of the nitrogenous purine bases found in DNA and RNA.

GUI : Graphical user interface. Refers to software front ends that rely on pictures and icons to direct the interaction of users with the application.

Heuristic algorithm : An economical strategy for deriving a solution to a problem for which an exact solution is computationally impractical or intractable. Consequently, a heuristic approach is not guaranteed to find the optimal or 'true' solution.

Hidden Markov Model (MMM) : A probabilistic model consisting of a number of interconnecting states. Like profiles, HMMs encode full domain alignments. They are essentially linear chains of match, delete or insert states; a match state denotes a conserved column in an alignment; an insert state allows insertions relative to match states; and delete states allow match positions to be skipped.

High throughput screening : The technique of using automated assays to search through large numbers of compounds for desired activity.

Home page : The HTML document that acts as the first contact point between a browser and a server.

Homologous : In phylogenetics, describing particular features in different individuals that are genetically descended from the same feature in a common ancestor. In molecular biology, often 'homologous' simply means similar, regardless of genetic relationship.

Homology : Being related by the evolutionary process of divergence from a common ancestor. Homology is not a synonym for similarity.

Homoplasy	:	Similarity that has evolved independently and is not indicative of common phylogenetic origin.
Host	:	Any computer on the internet that can be addressed directly through a unique IP address.
HTGS (HTG)	:	High-throughput genome sequences (HTG is the HTGS division in DDBJ/EMBL/ GenBank). Various genome sequencing centres worldwide have begun the large-scale sequencing of human and other higher eukaryotic genomes. The databases have deemed it beneficial to put the unfinished sequences that are the result of such sequencing efforts in a separate division. These unfinished records, in most cases, are potable for important numbers of gaps in the nucleotides, low accuracy and no annotations on the record. These sequences do not achieve the high standard expected in the standard DDBJ/EMBL/GenBank records.
HTML	:	Hypertext markup language. The standard, text-based language used to specify the format of World Wide Web documents. HTML files are translated and rendered through the use of Web browsers.
Hybridisation	:	The process of joining two complementary strands of DNA or one each of DNA and RNA to form double-stranded molecule.
Hydropathy profile	:	A graph in which hydropathy values are calculated within a sliding window and plotted for each residue in a protein sequence. Such graphs show characteristic peaks and troughs, corresponding to the most hydrophobic and hydrophilic regions of the sequence respectively.
Hydropathy	:	Having the property of hydrophobicity, a low affinity for water.
Hyperlink	:	A graphic or text within a World Wide Web document that can be selected by means of a mouse. Clicking on a hyperlink transports the user to another part of the same Web page or to another Web page, regardless of location.
Hypermedia	:	Formatted web documents containing a variety of information types, including text, image, movie and audio.
Hypertext transport protocol (HTTP)	:	The communication protocol used by web servers.
Hypertext	:	Text that contains embedded links (hyperlinks) to other documents.
Hypertext	:	Within a Web page, text that is differentiated by colour or by underlining and functions as a hyperlink.
Idiotype	:	The numbers and size of chromosomes in a cell of an organism.
In silico	:	The use of computers to stimulate, process or analyse biological experiment.
Indel	:	Acronym for 'INsertion or DELetion'. Applied to length-variable regions of a multiple alignment when it is not specified whether sequence length differences have been created by insertions or deletions.
Information theory	:	A branch of mathematics that measures information in terms of bits, the minimal amount of structural complexity needed to encode a given piece of information.
Insertion	:	Part of a sequence alignment where one sequence appears to have extra monomers compared with another sequence.
Internet inter-ORB protocol (IIOP)	:	The communication protocol used by object-request brokers to communicate over the internet.

Internet	:	A system of linked computer networks used for the transmission of files and messages between hosts.
Intranet	:	A computer network internal to a company or organisation. Intranets are often not connected to the internet or are protected by a firewall.
Intron	:	Chromosomal DNA sequences interrupting the coding sequence of genes (called → exons).
Introns	:	The sequence of DNA bases that interrupts the protein-coding sequence of a gene; these sequences are transcribed into RNA but are edited out of the message before it is translated into protein.
IP address	:	The unique, numeric address of a computer host on the internet.
IP	:	Internet protocol.
Iterative	:	A sequence of operations in a procedure that is performed repeatedly.
Java script	:	A scripting language designed for web-based applications.
Java	:	A programming language developed by Sun Microsystems that allows small programs (applets) to be run on any computer. Java applets are typically invoked when a user clicks on a hyperlink on a web page.
Karyotype	:	The number and size of chromosomes in a cell of an organism presented diagrammatically.
Kilobase (kb)	:	Unit of length for DNA fragments equal to 1000 nucleotides.
k-tuple	:	Identical short stretches of sequences, also called words.
LAN	:	Local area network. A network that connects computers in a small, defined area, such as the offices in a single wing or a group of buildings.
Lead compound	:	A substance that has many of the characteristics of an ideal drug and which interacts with a specific target.
Library	:	An unordered collection of clones (i.e. cloned DNA from a particular organism), generated from genomic DNA or cDNA.
Ligand	:	Any small molecule that binds to a protein or receptor.
Local alignment	:	Attempts to align regions of sequences with the highest density of matches in two short sequences.
Log odds score	:	The logarithm of an odds score.
Machine code	:	The binary code interpreted by a computer's processor.
Maximum likelihood	:	The most likely outcome (tree or alignment), given a probabilistic model of evolutionary change in DNA sequences.
Maximum parsimony	:	The minimum number of evolutionary steps required to generate the observed variation in a set of sequences, as found by comparison of the number of steps in all possible phylogenetic trees.
Megabase (mb)	:	Unit of length for DNA fragments equal to 1 million nucleotides.
Membrane	:	Semi-permeable cell envelope made of phospholipids and membrane proteins; while phospholipids provide stability of membranes, proteins provide transport and signalling processes across this otherwise impermeable structure.

Metabolism	:	Chemical reactions in → cells for the degradation and biosynthesis of molecules. Chemical energy is extracted from nutrients and used to synthesise macromolecules, promote transport, signalling and growth.
Microarray	:	A miniature device, also known as a chip (microchip, biochip), containing hundreds or thousands of different molecules immobilised in a regular pattern.
Mirror	:	Identical web sites, hosted on different computers such that the data might be acquired more quickly by users in specific countries.
Mitochondrion	:	Organelle in → eukaryotic organisms responsible for oxygen-dependent energy → metabolism.
Molecular clock	:	The hypothesis that nucleotide or amino acid substitutions occur at more or less fixed rate over evolutionary time, like the slow ticking of a clock. It has been proposed that given a calibration date and a constant molecular clock, the amount of sequence divergence can be used to calculate the time that has elapsed since two molecules diverged.
Monte carlo	:	A method that samples possible solutions to a complex problem as a way to estimate a more general solution.
Mosaic	:	A mosaic protein is a modular protein that, rather than including multiple tandem repeats of the same module, is composed of a number of different modules, each conferring different aspects of the parent protein's overall functionality.
Motif	:	A consecutive string of amino acids in a protein sequence whose general character is repeated or conserved, in all sequences in a multiple alignment at a particular position. Motifs are of interest because they may correspond to structural or functional elements within the sequence they characterise.
mRNA	:	(messenger RNA) Complementary RNA copy of DNA formed from a single stranded DNA template during transcription that migrates from the nucleus to the cytoplasm.
Mutation studies	:	In Sequin, a set of sequences for the same gene in the same species, perhaps the same individual, in which several different induced mutations are isolated and sequenced.
Mutation	:	Any change in DNA sequence.
Mutation	:	Change in the → base or → nucleotide sequence in a gene or → chromosomal structure.
Nanometre nanotechnology	:	One nanometre is one billionth of a metre; nanotechnology pertains to molecular devices with dimensions in the nanometre range.
Needleman-Wunsch algorithm	:	Uses dynamic programming to find global alignments between sequences.
Neighbour-joining method	:	Clusters together alike pairs within a group of related objects to create a tree whose branches reflect the degrees of difference among the objects (genes with similar sequences).
Neural network	:	From artificial intelligence algorithms, techniques that involve a set of many simple units that hold symbolic data, which are with numeric weights. Units operate only on their symbolic data and on the inputs that they receive through their connections.

Neuron	:	Nerve cell in the brain responsible for electrical and chemical signal transmission.
Normalised library	:	cDNA library generated such that all the genes in the library are represented at the same frequency.
Northern blotting	:	A technique to identify RNA molecules by hybridisation.
Nucleotide	:	A molecule consisting of a nitrogenous base (A, G, T and C in DNA; A, G, U or C in RNA); a phosphate moiety and a sugar group (deoxyribose in DNA and ribose in RNA). Thousands of nucleotide are linked to form a DNA or RNA molecule.
Nucleotides	:	Building blocks of → DNA and → RNA; composed of → base, ribose (sugar) and phosphate groups.
Object-oriented database	:	A database in which data are stored as abstract objects, with abstract relationships between them. The data representations are potentially very varied, including, for example, character string, digitised images, tables, etc. An object may subsume many other objects and the database allows retrieval of the objects as a whole. The flexibility of data representation and the ability to group objects together, renders object-oriented databases potentially very powerful systems.
Odds score	:	The ratio of the likelihoods of two events or outcomes. In sequence alignments and scoring matrices, the odds score for matching two sequence characters is the ratio of the frequency with which the characters are aligned in related sequences divided by the frequency with which those same two characters align by chance alone, given the frequency of occurrence of each in the sequences. Odd scores for a set of individually aligned positions are obtained by multiplying the odd scores for each position. Odd scores are often converted to logarithms to create log odd scores that can be added to obtain the log odd score of a sequence alignment.
Ontology	:	Relationship between objects, especially in artificial intelligence systems.
Open reading frame (ORF)	:	A series of DNA codons, including a 5' initiation codon and a termination codon that encodes a putative or known gene.
Operating system	:	A program or suite of programs, that controls the entire operation of the computer, handling input/output operations, interrupts user requests, etc. (e.g. UNIX, VMS, Window NT, etc.).
Operon	:	A unit of transcription consisting of one or more structural genes, an operator and a promoter.
Optimal alignment	:	The highest-scoring alignment found by an algorithm capable of producing multiple solutions. This is the best possible alignment that can be found, given any parametre supplied by the user to the sequence alignment program.
Organelle	:	Small → membrane-encapsulated particle in the cytoplasm of → eukaryotes.
Ortholog	:	A homologous sequence that is derived from a common ancestor found in individuals of different species.
Orthologs	:	Homologous proteins that perform the same function in different species.
Orthologs/orthologous	:	Homologous sequences are said to be orthologous when they are direct descendants of a sequence in the common ancestor (i.e. without having under gone a gene duplication event). See also homologous and paralogs.
Packet	:	A self-contained message or component of a message, comprising address, control.

Pairwise alignment	:	An alignment performed between two sequences.
PAM matrix	:	PAM (per cent accepted mutation) and BLOSUM (blocks substitution matrix) are matrices that define scores for each of the 210 possible amino acid substitutions. The scores are based on empirical substitution frequencies observed in alignments of database sequences and in general reflect similar physicochemical properties (e.g. a substitution of leucine for isoleucine, two amino acids of similar hydrophobicity and size, will score higher than a substitution of leucine for glutamate).
Paralogs/paralogous	:	Homologous sequences in two organisms A and B that are descendants of two different copies of a sequence that was created by a duplication event in the genome of the common ancestor. See also homologous and orthologs.
Parametric sequence alignment	:	An algorithm that finds a range of possible alignments based on varying the parametres of the scoring system for matches, mismatches and gap penalties.
Pattern	:	Molecular biological patterns usually occur at the level of the characters making up the gene or protein sequence.
PCR, polymerase chain reaction	:	An enzyme-mediated DNA amplification mechanism which allows sequence-specific selection of the DNA to be amplified.
Penalties	:	Scores or weights, used by programs in the computation of sequence alignments; such scores are normally supplied as parametres to the programs and thus may be modified by the user.
Peptide	:	A short stretch of amino acids each covalently coupled by a peptide bond between two nucleotide or amino acid sequences.
Per cent similarity	:	An alignment score used for amino acid sequences in which a substitution matrix is used to rank the substitution scores of different amino acids.
Phantom INDELs	:	Spurious insertions or deletions that arise when physical irregularities in a sequencing gel cause the reading software either to call a base too soon or to miss a base altogether.
Pharmainformatics	:	The branch of information science that deals with handling biological and chemical data in the pharmaceutical industry.
Phylogenetic analysis	:	Study of the evolutionary relationships between a species and its predecessors (e.g. using phylogenetic trees).
Phylogenetic studies	:	In Sequin, a set of sequences for the same gene in individuals of different species. The presumption is that the individuals cannot interbreed. Sequin does not allow a single organism name, but expects the organism to be encoded in the Definition line. It does, however, present a control for setting the proper genetic code.
Phylogenetic tree	:	A graphical representation of the putative evolutionary relationships between groups of organisms, e.g. as calculated from multiple protein or nucleic acid sequence alignments.
Platform	:	Properly, the operating system running software on a computer (e.g. Unix or Windows95). More often used to refer to the type of computer, such as a Macintosh or PC-compatible.
Polymerase-chain Reaction (PCR)	:	A method for amplifying a DNA base sequence using a heat-stable polymerase and two primers, one complementary to the (+) strand, at one end of the sequence to be amplified and the other complementary to the (–) strand at the other end.

Polymorphism	:	Sequence differences among individuals found on specific → chromosome locations within a population.
Population studies	:	In Sequin, a set of sequences for the same gene in individuals of a single species. The presumption is that the individuals can interbreed. Sequin allows entry of a single organism name, though some distinguishing source information, such as strain, clone, or isolate, must be entered for each sequence if the program is to function properly.
Position-specific scoring matrix	:	Represents the variation found in the columns of an alignment of a set of related sequences. Each subsequent matrix column corresponds to the next column in the alignment and each row corresponds to a particular sequence character.
Post-translational modification	:	An enzyme-catalysed alteration to a protein made after its translation from mRNA (e.g. glycosylation, phosphorylation, myristoylation, methylation).
Primary database	:	A database that stores biomolecular sequences (protein or nucleic acid) and associated annotation information (organism, species, function, mutations, linked to particular diseases, functional/structural patterns, bibliographic, etc.).
Primary structure	:	The linear sequence of amino acids in a protein molecule.
Primer	:	A short polynucleotide chain to which new deoxyribonucleotides can be added by DNA polymerase.
Probe	:	A DNA or protein sequence used as a query in a database search.
Profile	:	A position-specific scoring table that encapsulates the sequence information within complete alignments. Profiles define which residues are allowed at given positions; which positions are conserved and which degenerate; and which positions or regions, can tolerate insertions. In addition to data implicit in the alignment, the scoring system may include evolutionary weights and results from structural studies. Variable penalties are specified to weight against insertions and deletions occurring in secondary structure elements.
Prokaryote	:	An organism lacking a membrane-bound, structurally discrete nucleus and other subcellular compartments. Bacteria are prokaryotes.
Promoter	:	A site on DNA to which RNA polymerase will bind and initiate transcription.
Protein	:	A molecule composed of one or more chains of amino acids in a specific order; the order is determined by the base sequence of nucleotides in the gene coding for the protein. Proteins are required for the structure, function and regulation of cells, tissues and organs, each protein having a specific role (e.g. hormones, enzymes and antibodies).
Proteome	:	The entire complement of proteins produced by a particular genome, including variants of the same basic protein generated by post-translational modifications, etc.
QSAR	:	QSAR is a mathematical function used to relate the structural features of a molecule to its biological function.
Quaternary structure	:	The arrangement of separate protein chains in a protein molecule with more than one subunit.
Query sequence	:	A DNA, RNA or protein sequence used to search a sequence database in order to identify close or remote family members of known function.

Receptor	:	Protein that serves as binding site for signalling molecules such as growth factors, hormones or neurotransmitters.
Recombinant DNA	:	Genetically modified or structurally altered → nucleic acid sequence (usually a → gene) within a → vector or host DNA.
Regular expression	:	A single consensus expression derived from a conserved region of a sequence alignment, and used as a characteristic signature of family membership. Synonymous terms: rule, pattern.
Regulator regions or sequences	:	A DNA base sequence that controls gene expression.
Relational database	:	A database that uses a relational data model, in which data are stored in two-dimensional tables. The tables embody different aspects or properties of the data, but contain overlapping information.
R-factor	:	In X-ray chrystallography, this parametre is used to express the extent of agreement between theoretical calculations and the measured data; the lower the R-factor, the better the fit (R means either residual or reliability).
RNA (ribonucleic acid)	:	A molecule chemically similar to DNA that plays a central role in protein synthesis. The structure of RNA is similar to that of DNA but it is inherently less stable. There are several classes of RNA molecule, including messenger RNA (mRNA), transfer RNA (tRNA), ribosomal RNA (rRNA) and other small RNAs, each serving a different purpose.
Rooted tree	:	A phylogenetic tree in which the least common ancestor of all the species in the tree is present as an ancestral outgroup.
Rule	:	A short regular expression (typically 4–6 residues in length) used to identify genome (nonfamily specific) patterns in protein sequences. Rules tend to be used to encode particular functional sites: e.g. sugar attachment sites, phosphorylation, hydroxylation, sulphation sites, etc. However, their small size means that the patterns do not provide good discrimination and can only give a guide as to whether a certain functional site might exist in a sequence.
Secondary database	:	A database that contains information derived from primary sequence data, typically in the form of regular expressions (patterns), fingerprints, blocks, profiles or Hidden Markov Models. These abstractions represent distillations of the most conserved
Secondary structure	:	Regions of local regularity within a protein fold (e.g. α-helices, β-turns, β-strands).
Sequence alignment	:	A linear comparison of amino (or nucleic) acid sequences in which insertions are made in order to bring equivalent positions in adjacent sequences into the correct register. Alignments are the basis of sequence-analysis methods and are used to pinpoint the occurrence of conserved motifs.
Sequence tagged site (STS)	:	Short (200–500 basepairs) DNA sequence that has a single occurrence in the human genome and whose location and base sequence are known. Detectable by polymerase chain reaction (PCR), STSs are useful for localising and orienting the mapping and sequence data reported from many different laboratories and serve as landmarks on the developing physical map of the human genome. Expressed sequence tags (ESTs) are STSs derived from cDNA.

Sequencing	:	Determination of the order of nucleotides (base sequences) in a DNA or RNA molecule or the order of amino acids in a protein.
Server	:	A computer that processes requests issued from remote locations by client machines.
Shotgun method	:	Cloning of DNA fragments randomly generated from a genome.
Silent mutation	:	A nucleotide substitution that does not result in an amino acid substitution in the translation product, because of the redundancy of the genetic code.
Site	:	An individual column of residues in an amino acid or nucleotide alignment. The residues at a site are presumed to be homologous.
Six frame translation	:	Translation of a stretch of DNA taking into account three forward translation and three reverse translations, arising from the three possible reading frames of an uncharacterised stretch of DNA.
Smith-waterman algorithm	:	Uses dynamic programming to find local alignments between sequences. The key feature is that all negative scores calculated in the dynamic programming matrix are changed to zero in order to avoid extending poorly scoring alignments and to assist in identifying local alignments starting and stopping anywhere with the matrix.
SNP	:	(Single nucleotide polymorphism) A change in DNA sequence at a single residue.
Spam	:	Postings to newsgroups or mail broadcast to a large number of e-mail accounts that usually are irrelevant or not of interest to the recipients. Analogous to postal junk mail.
Splice variants	:	Proteins of different length that arise through translation of mRNAs that have not included all available exons in the template DNA.
SRS	:	(Sequence retrieval system) A data retrieval tool.
Structure prediction	:	Algorithms that predict the secondary, tertiary and even quaternary structure of proteins from their sequences.
STS	:	Sequenced tagged site. STSs are operationally unique sequences that identify the combinations of primer pairs used in PCR assays that generate mapping reagents, each of which maps to a single position within the genome. Variations on this definition are also present in this division. This division of GenBank is intended to facilitate cross-comparison of STSs with sequences in other divisions for the purpose of correlating map positions of anonymous sequences with known genes.
Subunit	:	A distinct polypeptide chain within a protein that may be separated from other chains (whether identical or different) without breaking covalent bonds.
Super-secondary structure	:	The arrangement of α-helices and/or β-strands in a protein sequence into discrete folded structures (e.g. β-barrels, β α β units, Greek keys, etc.).
Target	:	A molecule that is critical to a disease that may be targeted with a potential therapeutic agent.
Telnet	:	An internet protocol or application that allows users to connect to computers at remote locations and use these computers as if they were physically operating the remote hardware.

Tertiary database	:	A database derived from information housed in secondary (pattern) databases (e.g. the BLOCKS and eMOTIF databases, which draw on data stored within PROSITE and PRINTS). The value of such resources is in providing a different scoring perspective on the same underlying data, allowing the possibility to diagnose relationships that might be missed using the original implementation.
Tertiary structure	:	The overall fold of a protein sequence, formed by the packing of its secondary and/or super-secondary structure elements.
Threading	:	In protein structure prediction, the aligning of the sequence of a protein of unknown structure with a known 3D structure to determine whether the amino acid sequence is spatially and chemically compatible with that structure.
Transcript	:	The single stranded mRNA chain that is assembled from a gene template.
Transcription	:	The synthesis of an RNA copy from a sequence of DNA (a gene); the first step in gene expression.
Translation	:	The process in which the genetic code carried by mRNA directs the synthesis of
Transmembrane domain	:	A region of a protein sequence that traverses a membrane; for α-helical structures, this requires a span of 20–25 residues.
Transmission control protocol/internet Protocol (TCP/IP)	:	The rules that govern data transmission between two computers over the internet.
True-negative	:	A false match that correctly fails to be recognised by a discriminator.
True-positive	:	A true match correctly recognised by a discriminator.
Uniform resource locator (URL)	:	The address of a source of information. The URL comprises four parts—the protocol, the host name, the directory path and the file name.
Upstream	:	Further back in the sequence of a DNA molecule, with respect to the direction in
URL	:	Uniform resource locator. Used Web browsers, URLs specify both the type of site being accessed (FTP, Gopher or Web) and the address of the Web site.
User	:	The person using client-server or other type of software.
Vector DNA	:	Small piece of → DNA containing regulatory and coding sequences of interest; vector → DNA functions to insert and amplify a gene into a target → genome.
Western blot	:	Technique in which specific antibodies are used to identify their antigens from a mixture of proteins.
Widow	:	Amino acid residues isolated from neighbouring residues by spurious gaps, usually the result of over-zealous gap insertion by automatic alignment programs.
World wide web (www)	:	The information system or network on the internet that uses HTTP as the primary communication medium.
World wide web	:	A document delivery system capable of handling nontext-based media of various types.
X-ray crystallography	:	A technique to determine the three-dimensional structure of a protein.

Appendices

SYMBOLS

2D-PAGE	:	Two-dimensional polyacrylamide gel electrophoresis
AC	:	Approximate correlation
ACeDB	:	A *C. elegans* DataBase
ADIT	:	AutoDep input tool
AE	:	Annotated exon
AN	:	Actual negative
AP	:	Actual positive
AQL	:	ACeDB query language
BDGP	:	Berkeley *Drosophila* Genome project
BIND	:	Biomolecular interaction network database
BIOS	:	Basic input-output system
BRET	:	Bioluminescent resonance energy transfer
CASP	:	Critical assessment of structure prediction
CD	:	Circular dichroism
CD	:	Candidate drug
CDE	:	Common desktop environment
cDNA	:	copy DNA
CDS	:	Coding sequence
CGI	:	Common gateway interface
CIP	:	Cahn–Inglod–Prelog
CORBA	:	Common object request brokering architecture
DBMS	:	Database management system
DDBJ	:	DNA databank of Japan
DEC	:	Digital equipment corporation
DIP	:	Database of interacting proteins
DNS	:	Domain name server
EBI	:	European bioinformatics institute
EMBL	:	European molecular biology laboratory
ENU	:	Ethylnitrosourea
EP	:	Expression profiler
ES cells	:	Embryonic stem cells
ESI	:	Electrospray ionisation
EST	:	Expressed sequence tag
ExPASy	:	Export protein analysis system (Switzerland)
FE	:	False exon
FN	:	False negative

FP	:	False positive
FRET	:	Fluorescent resonance energy transfer
FTP	:	File transfer protocol
GASP	:	Gene annotation assessment project
GEO	:	Gene expression omnibus
GFP	:	Green fluorescent protein
GGTC	:	German gene trap consortium
GNOME	:	GNU network object model environment
GOLD	:	Genomes online database
GOR	:	Garnier–Osguthorpe–Robson
GRAIL	:	Gene recognition and assembly Internet link
GSS	:	Genome survey sequence
GST	:	Glutathione S-transferase
GUI	:	Graphical user interface
HIV	:	Human immunodeficiency virus
HMM	:	Hidden Morkov model
HSP	:	High-scoring segment pair
HTG	:	High-throughput genomic sequence
HTML	:	Hypertext markup language
HTS	:	High-throughput screening
http	:	Hypertext transfer protocol
IP	:	Internet protocol
ISP	:	Internet service provider
KDE	:	K desktop environment
KEGG	:	Kyoto encyclopedia of genes and genomes
LCA	:	Last common ancestor
LOG	:	Laplacian of Gaussian
m/e or m/z	:	mass/charge ratio
MAD	:	Multiwavelength anomalous diffraction
MAGE	:	Microarray and gene expression
MAGE-ML	:	Microarray gene expression markup language
MAGE-OM	:	Microarray gene expression object model
MALDI	:	Matrix-assisted laser desorption/ionisation
ME	:	Missing exon
MGED	:	Microarray gene expression database
MIAME	:	Minimum information about a microarray experiment
MIME	:	Multiple Internet Mail Extensions
MIR	:	Multiple isomorphous replacement
MMDB	:	Molecular modeling database
mRNA	:	messenger RNA
MS	:	Mass spectrometry
MSD	:	Macromolecular structure database
MS-DOS	:	Microsoft Disk Operating System
MSF	:	Multiple sequence format

NBRF	:	National biomedical research foundation
NCBI	:	National centre for biotechnology information
NDB	:	Nucleic acid data bank
NJ	:	Neighbour joining
NMR	:	Nuclear magnetic resonance
NNSSP	:	Nearest neighbour secondary structure prediction
NOE	:	Nuclear overhauser effect
OMIM	:	OnLine Mendelian Inheritance in Man
ORF	:	Open reading frame
PAGE	:	Polyacrylamide gel electrophoresis
PAM	:	Accepted point mutations
PAUP	:	Phylogenetic analysis using parsimony
PCNA	:	Proliferating cell nuclear antigen
PCR	:	Polymerase chain reaction
PDB	:	Protein data bank
PE	:	Prediction exon
PERL	:	Practical extraction and reporting language
PH	:	Pleckstrin homology
PHYLIP	:	Phylogenetic inference package
pI	:	Isoelectric point
PIR	:	Protein information resource
PN	:	Prediction negative
PP	:	Predicted positive
RCSB	:	Research collaboratory for structural bioinformatics
RMSD	:	Root mean square deviation
rRNA	:	Ribosomal RNA
RT	:	Reverse transcription
SAGE	:	Serial analysis of gene expression
SDS	:	Sodium dodecyl sulphate
SELDI	:	Surface-enhance laser desorption/ionisation
SH2, SH3	:	Src – homology domain
SMART	:	Simple modular architecture research tool
SMILES	:	Simplified molecular input line entry specification
SNP	:	Single nucleotide polymorphism
SOM	:	Self-organising map
SPR	:	Surface plasmon resonance
SQL	:	Symbolic query language
SRS	:	Sequence retrieval system
SSE	:	Secondary structure element
STS	:	Sequence tagged site
T_C	:	Tanimoto coefficient
TCP	:	Transmission control protocol
TE	:	True exon
TN	:	True negative

TP	:	True positive
TrEMBL	:	Translated EMBL
tRNA	:	Transfer RNA
UML	:	Unified modelling language
UPGMA	:	Unweighted pair group method using arithmetic mean
UPGMC	:	Unweighted pair group method using centroid value
URL	:	Uniform resource locator
WE	:	Wrong exon
WPGMA	:	Weighted pair group method using arithmetic mean
WPGMC	:	Weighted pair group method using centroid value
WST	:	Watershed transformation
WWW	:	World wide web
XML	:	eXtensible markup language
Y2H	:	Yeast two-hybrid

APPENDIX II

Important World Wide Web

Name of site	Web address
Activity	URL:http://www.mgs.bionet.nsc.ru/systems/Activity/
Aligned	URL:http://sgi.sscc.ru/srs5/
Arabidopsis thalliang	http://lenti.med.umn.edu/arabidopsis/arab/arab_top_page.html
	http://cbil.humgen.upenn.edu/-atgc/ATGCUP.html
	http://www.arabidopsis.com/bb/b950928z.html
	http://nasc.nott.Ac.uk/JIC-contigs/
Bombyx mor	http://www.ab.a.u-tokyo.ac.jp/sericulture/shimada.html
Caenorhabditis	http://www.sanger.ac.uk/Projects/C_elegans/
	http://moulon.inra.fr/acedb/acedb.html
	http://www.ddbj.nig.ac.jp/htmls/c-elegans/html/CE_INDEX.html
Candido albicans	http://glamdring.ucsd.edu/others/dsmith/dictydb.html
Chicken	http://www.ri.bbsrc.ac.uk/chickmap/chickgbase/manager.html
COG: Clusters of orthologous groups	http://www.ncbi.nlm.nih.gov/COG/
Cow	http://locus.jouy.inra.fr/cgi-bin/bovmap/lintro2.pl
Database of genetics of disease	http://www.ncbi.nlm.nih.gov/omin/
	http://www.geneclinics.org/profiles/all.html
Database on electronic access to the scientific literature	http://www.nature.com/nature/debates/e-access/
dBEST (EST sequences)	http://www.ncbi.nih.gov/dbEST/linex.html
Dictyostelium discoideum	http://glamdring.ucsd.edu/others/dsmith/dictyab.html
Dog	http://mendel.berkeley.edu.dog.html
Drosophila melanogaster	http://flybase.bio.indiana.edu/
ESRG-TRRD	http://www.bionet.nsc.ru/trrd/
Ethical, legal, social issues	http://www.nhgri.nih.gov/ELSI/
Gene map99	http://www.ncbi.nlm.nih.gov/genemap99/
Gene express	http://www.mgs.bionet.nsc.ru/
General NCBI	info@ncbi.nlm.nih.gov
GeNet	www.csa.ru/Inst/gorb_dep/inbios/genet/genet.htm
Genethon (SSLP maps)	http://www.genethon.fr/
Geneome statistics	http://bioinformatics.weizmann.ac.il/mb/statistics.html
GR-TRRD	http://www.icg.bionet.nsc.ru/trrd/34/gluc.htm
Hidden Markov models	http://cse.ucsc.edu/research/compbio/sam.html
	http://cse.ucsc.edu/research/compbio/HMM-apps/HMM-applications.html
	http://hmmer.wustl.edu/

(Contd...)

Name of site	Web address
HOBACGEN: Homologous bacterial genes database	http://pbil.univ-lyon1.fr/database/hobacgen.html
Homology Modeling	
SWISS-MODEL (automatic homology modeling)	http://www.expasy.ch/swissmod/SWISS-MODEL.html
HOVERGEN: Homologous vertebrate genes database	http://pbil.univ-lyon1.fr/databases/hovergen.html
HOX-PRO DB	http://www.iephb.ru/~spirov/hox_pro/hox-pro00.html
	http://www.mssm.edu/molbio/hoxpro/new/hox-pro00.html
Human genetic disease	http://www.ncbi.nlm.nih.gov/Omim/
	http://www.geneclinics.org/profiles/all.html
Human genome project information	http://www.ornl.gov/hgmis/project/info.html
HG-TRRD	http://www.bionet.nsc.ru/trrd/
Images of chromosomes, maps, loci	http://www.ncbi.nlm.nih.gov/genome/guide/
Interactive access to DNA and protein sequences (human)	http://www.ensembl.org/
Interactive dotplottin	http://www.isrec.isb-sib.ch/java/dotlet/exonintron.html
List of completed genomes	http://www.ncbi.nlm.nih.gov/PMGifs/Genomes/allorg.html
	http://www.ebi.ac.uk/genomes/mot/index.html
	http://pir.georgetown.edu/pirwww/search/genome.html
Lists of databases	http://www.infobiogen.fr/services/dbcat/
	http://www.ebi.ac.uk/biocat/
LM system genes obtained through the SRS	http://www.mgs.bionet.nsc.ru/
Mekada fish	http://nioll.bio.nagoya.u.ac.jp:8000/
Membrane protein explorer (S. White)	http://blanco.biomol.uci.edu/mpex/
MODBASE, a database of comparative models of proteins from complete genomes	http://guitar.rockefeller.edu/modbase/
Mosquito	http://klab.agsci.colostate.edu/
Mouse	http://www.genome.wi.mit.edu/cgi-bin/mouse
	http://www.genethon.fr/
	http://www.informatics.jax.org/

(Contd...)

Name of site	Web address
Organism-specific databases	http://www.unl.edu/stc-95/ResTools/biotools/biotools10.html
	http://www-fp.mcs.anl.gov/~gaasterland/genomes.html
	http://www.hgmp.mrc.ac.uk/GenomeWeb/genome-db.html
	http://www.bioinformatik.de/cgi-bin/browse/Catalog/Databases/Genome_Projects/
Overview of human genome structure	http://hgrep.ims.u-tokyo.ac.jp
Pfam: protein families database	http://www.sanger.ac.uk/Software/Pfam/
PHDhtm (B. Rost)	http://dodo.bioc.columbia.edu/predictprotein
Phylogenetic trees	http://evolution.genetics.washington.edu/phylip/software.html
Pig	http://www.ri.bbsrc.as.uk/pigmap/pigbase/pigbase.html
Plasmodium falciparum	http://ben.vub.ac.be/malaria/mad.html
	http://www.wehi.edu.au/biology/malaria/who.html
	http://parasite.arf.efl.edu/malaria.html
Protein and nucleic acid structures	Home page of protein data bank
	http://www.rcsb.org
	Home page of EBI macromolecular structure database
	http://msd.ebi.ac.uk/
	Home page of BioMagResBank
	http://www.bmrb.wisc.edu/
	Searching the protein data bank
	Home page of SCOP (Structual classification of protiens)
	http://scop.mrc-lmb.cam.ac.uk/scop/
	List of browsers
	http://pdb-browsers.ebi.ac.uk/browser_it.shtml
	OCA
	http://oca.ebi.ac.uk/oca-bin/ocamain
	Database of protein quanternary structure
	http://pqs.ebi.ac.uk/
Pufferfish	http://fugu.hgmp.mrc.ac.uk
Radiation hybrid database	http://www.ebi.ac.uk/RHdb
Rat	http://ratmap.gen.gu.se/
Reports of structure quality	http://www.cmbi.kun.nl/gv/pdbreport
Regulatory sequences in the eukaryotic genome	http://www.mgs.bionet.nsc.ru/Systems/GeneExpress/
Saccharomyces cerevisiae	http://genome-www.standford.edu/Saccharomyces/
	http://www.mips.biochem.mpg.de/
	http://www.sanger.ac.uk/Projects/

(Contd...)

Name of site	Web address
Samples has a EMBL-like format, is under the SRS5	URL http://sgi.sscc.ru/srs5/
Schizosaccharomyces pombe	http://www.mips.biochem.mpg.de/
SegNet: the expression pattern field incorporates the images of expression pattern of segmentation genes in the fruit fly	http://www.csa.ru/%20Inst/gorb_dep/inbios/genet/krueppel.html
D. melanogaster	
Sheep	http://dirk.invermay.cri.nz/
Single-nucleotide polymorphisms	http://snp.cshl.org/
Site relevant to the	CEPH (YAC mapping)
Human genome project	http://www.cephb.fr/bio/ceph-genethon-map.html
Specific protein families	Protein kinases http://www.sdsc.edu/kinases/ HIV proteases http://www-fbsc.ncifcrf.gov/HIVdb/
Icosahedral viruses	http://mmtsb.scripps.edu/viper/main.html
Immunology IGMT	http://imgt.cines.fr
KABAT	http://immuno.bme.nwu.edu/
MHCPEP	http://wehih.wehi.edu.au/mhcpep/
Collections of links of databases on specific protein families	http://www2.ebi.ac.uk/msd/Links/family.shtml
TAED: The adaptive evolution database	http://www.sbc.su.se/~liberless/TAED.html
Taxonomy sites	Species 2000-a comprehensive index of all known plants, animals, fungi and micro-organisms http://www.sp2000.org
Tools for analysis	http://www.ebi.ac.uk/Tools/index.html
Transmembrane helix prediction	TMHMM (A. Krogh and E. Sonnammer) – based on a Hidden Markov Model http://www.cbs.dtu.dk/krogh/TMHMM/
Tree of life—phylogeny and biodiversity	http://phylogeny.arizona.edu/tree
TRRD is installed under the SRS	http://sgi.sscc.ru/
Whitehead institute (physical mapping)	http://www.genome.mit.edu/
Zebrafish	http://zfish.uoregon.edu/

APPENDIX III

A Collection of Useful Bioinformatic Tools and Molecular Tables

The Genetic Code

		2nd Position				
		U	C	A	G	
1st position	U	UUU Phe	UCU Ser	UAU Tyr	UGU Cys	U
		UUC Phe	UCC Ser	UAC Tyr	UGC Cys	C
		UUA Leu	UCA Ser	UAA Stop	UGA Stop	A
		UUG Leu	UCG Ser	UAG Stop	UGG Trp	G
	C	CUU Leu	CCU Pro	CAU His	CGU Arg	U
		CUC Leu	CCC Pro	CAC His	CGC Arg	C
		CUA Leu	CCA Pro	CAA Gin	CGA Arg	A
		CUG Leu	CCG Pro	CAG Gin	CGG Arg	G
	A	AUU Ile	ACU Thr	AAU Asn	AGU Ser	U
		AUC Ile	ACC Thr	AAC Asn	AGC Ser	C
		AUA Ile	ACA Thr	AAA Lys	AGA Arg	A
		AUG Met	ACG Thr	AAG Lys	AGG Arg	G
	G	GUU Val	GCU Ala	GAU Asp	GGU Gly	U
		GUC Val	GCC Ala	GAC Asp	GGC Gly	C
		GUA Val	GCA Ala	GAA Glu	GGA Gly	A
		GUGVal	GCG Ala	GAG Glu	GGG Gly	G

The codons are read as triplets in the 5' → 3' direction, i.e. left to right. Termination codons are in bold.

IUPAC Nucleotide Codes

Code	Members	Nucleotide
A	A	Adenine
C	C	Cytosine
G	G	Guanine
T	T	Thymine (DNA)
U	U	Uracil (RNA)
Y	C or T(U)	pYrimidine
R	A or G	puRine
M	A or C	aMino

(Contd...)

Code	Members	Nucleotide
K	G or T(U)	Keto
S	G or C	Strong interaction (3H bonds)
W	A or T(U)	Weak interaction (2H bonds)
H	A or C or T(U)	not-G
B	G or T(U) or C	not-A
V	G or C or A	not-T
D	G or A or T(U)	not-C
N	G, A, C or T(U)	aNy base

IUPAC Amino Acid Codes

3-Letter code	1-Letter code	Amino acid
Ala	A	Alanine
Arg	R	Arginine
Asn	N	Asparagine
Asp	D	Aspartic acid
Cys	C	Cysteine
Gln	Q	Glutamine
Glu	E	Glutamic acid
Gly	G	Glycine
His	H	Histidine
Ile	I	Isoleucine
Leu	L	Leucine
Lys	K	Lysine
Met	M	Methionine
Phe	F	Phenylalanine
Pro	P	Proline
Ser	S	Serine
Thr	T	Threonine
Trp	W	Tryptophan
Tyr	Y	Tyrosine
Val	V	Valine
Asx	B	Aspartic acid or Asparagine
Glx	Z	Glutamic acid or Glutamine
Xaa	X	Any amino acid

Converting Base Size of a Nucleic Acid → Mass of Nucleic Acid

Number of bases	Mass of nucleic acid
1 kb ds DNA (Na$^+$)	6.6×10^5 Da
1 kb ss DNA (Na$^+$)	3.3×10^5 Da
1 kb ss RNA (Na$^+$)	3.4×10^5 Da
1.52 kb ds DNA	1MDa ds DNA (Na$^+$)
Average MW of a dsDNA	660 Da
Average MW of a ssDNA	330 Da
Average NW of an RNA	340 Da

Converting Base Size of a Nucleic Acid → Maximum Moles of Protein

DNA	Molecular Weight (Da)	Amino Acids	1 µg	1 nmol
270 bp	10,000	90	100 pmol or 6×10^{13} molecules	10 µg
1.35 Kbp	50,000	450	20 pmol or 1.2×10^{13} molecules	50 µg
2.7 Kbp	1,00,000	900	10 pmol or 6×10^{12} molecules	100 µg
4.05 Kbp	1,50,000	1350	6.7 pmol or 4×10^{12} molecules	150 µg

Average MW of an amino acid = 110 (Da).

3 bp are required to encode 1 amino acid.

Sizes of Common Nucleic Acids

Nucleic acid	Number of nucleotides	Molecular weight
lambda DNA	48502 (dsDNA)	3.2×10^7
pBR322 DNA	4361 (dsDNA)	2.8×10^6
28S rRNA	4800	1.6×10^6
23S rRNA (E. coli)	2900	1.0×10^6
18S rRNA	1900	6.5×10^5
16S rRNA (E. coli)	1500	5.1×10^5
5S rRNA (E. coli)	120	4.1×10^4
tRNA (E. coli)	75	2.5×10^4

Mass of Nucleic Acid ↔ Moles of Nucleic Acid

Mass	Moles
1 µg/ml of nucleic acid	3.0 µM phosphate
1 µg of a 1 kb DNA fragment	1.5 pmol; 3.0 pmol ends
0.66 µg of a 1 kb DNA fragment	1 pmol

Sizes of Various Genomes

Organism	Approximate size (million bases)
Human	3000.0
M. Musculus (mouse)	3000.0
Drosophila (fruit fly)	135.6
Arabidopsis (plant)	100.0
C. elegans (round worm)	97.0
S. cerevisiae (yeast)	12.1
E. coli (bacteria)	4.7
H. influenzae (bacteria)	1.8

Genomic Equivalents of Species

Organism	Source of DNA	pg/haploid[a] Genome	Average[b]	µg quantity for Genome equivalence	Number of Genomes × 10^6
Human	diploid	3.50	3.16	10.0	2.86
Mouse	diploid	3.00	3.21	8.57	2.86
Rat	diploid	3.00	3.68	8.57	2.86
Bovine	haploid	3.24	3.24	9.26	2.86
Annelid	haploid	1.45	1.45	4.14	2.86
Drosophila	diploid	0.17	0.18	0.486	2.86
Yeast	haploid	0.016	0.0245	0.0457	2.86

[a] pg/haploid genome was calculated as a function of the tissue source. Genomic equivalence was calculated given that 10 µg of human genomic DNA contains 2.86×10^6 genome copies.

[b] Average of all values given in each tissue for that species.

APPENDIX IV

Simple UNIX Commands

The following tables contain a brief list of simple but useful UNIX commands. (Most commands have options. To see what options are available, use the *man* command to open the manual pages for the command, e.g. type *man Is* to open the manual for the *Is* command.) These commands can be used to move around the file system, examine files and copy, delete or rename files. They can also be used to do housekeeping on a user's account and to communicate with other users on the local system or on remote systems.

Directory Operations

Command	Action
pwd	Present working directory (show directory name)
cd	Change directory: *cd/path/name*
cd	Change to your home directory: *cd*
mkdir	Make (create) new directory: *mkdir Name*
rmdir	remove directory (if empty): *rmdir Name*
quota	Check disk space quota: *quota -v*

File Operations

Command	Action
Is	List files
cp	Copy files: *cp/path/name newname*
rm	Remove (i.e. delete) files: *rm name*
mv	Move or rename files: *mv name newname*
more	Page file contents (spacebar to continue): *more name*
cat	Scroll file contents: *cat name*
less	Better pager than more? (q to quit): *less name*
vi	Visual text editor (:wq to save and quit): *vi name*
pico	Pico text editor (*Ctrl-X* to quit): *pico name*
chmod	Change mode of file permissions: *chmod xxx name*

Manual Pages

Command	Action
man	Open the man pages for a command: *man command*

Communications

Command	Action
write	Write messages to another user's screen
talk	Talk split-screen with another user: *talk username*
mail	UNIX e-mail command
pine	Send or read e-mail with pine mail system
telnet	Connect to another computer via the network
ftp	File transfer over the network
lynx	Text-based Web browser

System Operations

Command	Action
df	Show free disk space
du	Show disk usage
ps	List your processes
kill	Kill a process: kill ###
passwd	Change your password
date	Show date and time
w	Who is doing what on the system
who	Who is connected to the system
ping	Ping another computer (is it alive?)
finger	Get information on users
exit	Exit or logout, from the system

X Windows

Command	Action
clock &	Display a clock (&: run in background)
cmdtool &	Command tool window
filemgr &	File manager
mailtool &	E-mail program
perfmetre &	System performance metre
seqlab &	SeqLab interface for GCG
setenv DISPLAY	For setting the DISPLAY environment variable
shelltool &	Shell tool window
textedit &	Text editor
xterm &	X terminal window

References

Attwood, T.K., Parry-Smith and D.J., *Introduction to Bioinformatics*, Addison Wesley Longman, Harlow, Essex.

Brazma, A., Jonassen and T. Schneider, *Approaches to Automatic Discovery of Patterns in Biosequences*, Butterworth, London.

Bryan Bergeron, *Bioinformatics Computing*, Pearson Education, Singapore.

Dayhoff, M.O., Schwartz, R.M., *Database Searching*, Academic Press, London.

Durbin, R. Eddy., *Computational and Biological Sequences*, Academic Press, London.

Freund, R. Kri, L., *Theory of Computing Systems*, John Wiley and Sons, New York.

Gorodkin, J., Heyer, *Structure Comparison and Computational Analysis*, Applied Science Publishers, London.

Henikoff, S. and Benner, S.A., *Basic Principles of Computing in Bioinformatics*, Academic Press, London.

Johnson, C., *Analog Computer Techniques*, Tata McGraw Hill, New York.

K.A. De Jong, *Evolutionary Computation*, Chapman and Hall, London.

Kanehisa, M., *Linking Databases and Organism*, Pergamon Press, Oxford, London.

Kari, L. and Paun, G., *Bioinformatics and Computation*, Chilton Book Co., USA.

Mount, D.W., *Bioinformatics Sequence and Genome Analysis*, Cold Spring Horbor Press, UK.

Munn, R.F., *Fundamentals of Database Searching*, John Wiley & Sons, New York.

Painter, D.E., *Finding the Genes in Genomic DNA*, Reston Publishing Co., Reston, Virginia.

Pevzner, P.A., *Computational Molecular Biology*, Chapman and Hall, New York.

Ricci, F., *Computer Programming and Simulation*, Johny Wiley and Sons, New York.

Richard Dybowshi and Stephen Roberts, *Probabilistic Modelling in Bioinformatics and Medical Informatics*, Springer-Verlog, London.

Richard M. Twyman, *Bioinformatics*, Bio Scientific Publishers, Oxford.

Richardson, D. and Coffee, L., *Threading a Database Protein Cores*, University Press, Cambridge.

Schrowebel, J., *DNA Sequencing*, Pergamon Press, New York.

Smith, T.F. and Waterman, M.S., *Identification of Common Molecular Substances*, Prentice Hall, London.

Snell, I.D. and Snell, C.T., *Protein Evolution*, D. Van Nostrand, New York.

Stephen Misener and Stephen A. Krawetz, *Bioinformatics Methods and Protocols*, Human Press Inc., New Jersey.

Wilbur, W.J. and Lipman, D.J., *Statistics and Datavisualisation in Bioinformatics*, Heinemann, London.

Index

Reader's Notes

Reader's Notes